HYPERTENSION AND HORMONE MECHANISMS

CONTEMPORARY ENDOCRINOLOGY

R. M. Carey, SERIES EDITOR

HYPERTENSION AND HORMONE MECHANISMS

Edited by

ROBERT M. CAREY, MD, MACP

David A. Harrison III Distinguished Professor of Medicine,
Division of Endocrinology and Metabolism, Department of Medicine,
University of Virginia School of Medicine, Charlottesville, VA

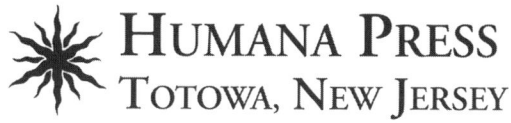
HUMANA PRESS
TOTOWA, NEW JERSEY

This publication is printed on acid-free paper. ∞

ANSI Z39.48-1984 (American National Standards Institute) Permanence of Paper for Printed Library Materials.

Cover design by Karen Schulz

Production Editor: Amy Thau

For additional copies, pricing for bulk purchases, and/or information about other Humana titles,contact Humana at the above address or at any of the following numbers: Tel: 973-256-1699; Fax: 973-256-8341; E-mail: orders@ humanapr.com or visit our website at http://humanapress.com

Printed in the United States of America. 10 9 8 7 6 5 4 3 2 1
eISBN 13: 978-1-59259-987-5

Library of Congress Cataloging-in-Publication Data
Hypertension and hormone mechanisms / edited by Robert M. Carey.
        p. ; cm. -- (Contemporary endocrinology)
        Includes bibliographical references and index.
        ISBN 978-1-58829-408-1 (alk. paper)
1. Hypertension--Endocrine aspects. 2. Hypertension--Pathophysiology. 3. Hormones--Therapeutic use. I. Carey, Robert M. II. Series: Contemporary endocrinology (Totowa, N.J.: Unnumbered)
[DNLM: 1. Hypertension--physiopathology. 2. Hypertension--therapy. 3. Autacoids--therapeutic use. 4. Hormones--therapeutic use. WG 340 H998 2007]
RC685.H8H7692 2007
616.1'32--dc22
2007005797

PREFACE

Hypertension, a major risk factor for cardiovascular disease and stroke, is present in approximately one-quarter of the adult population of Western societies. Seven percent of deaths worldwide are attributed to hypertension, and the rate of end-stage renal disease due to hypertension has doubled since 1982. In the United States, 77% of persons with hypertension go untreated and 31% of these individuals are unaware of their high blood pressure. The substantial public health problem of hypertension, compounded by the recognition of health hazards of "high normal" blood pressure, has raised a call for better understanding of the pathophysiological mechanisms underlying primary hypertension.

Hormones and autocoids are substances of major critical importance to the pathophysiology of hypertension. Remarkable advances during the past 25 yr, and particularly in the last decade, have identified several hormonal mechanisms in the regulation of blood pressure. Among the hormonal systems playing a major role in blood pressure and hypertension are the renin–angiotensin system, the sympathetic nervous system, the renal dopaminergic system, insulin and other metabolic factors, endothelium-dependent factors, natriuretic peptides, sex steroids, and the lipoxygenase system. This book represents a systematic treatment of each of these hormonal systems in the pathogenesis of primary (essential) hypertension.

The renin–angiotensin system is undoubtedly the best-studied hormonal system in the regulation of blood pressure. However, in spite of the voluminous literature on this subject, an understanding of this complex system is far from complete. During the past decade, truly remarkable advances have been made in the identification of new components of the renin–angiotensin system. The renin–angiotensin system is increasingly being regarded as a tissue rather than a circulating hormonal system. The intrarenal renin–angiotensin system, discussed by Drs. Minolfa Prieto-Carrasquero, Hiroyuki Kobori and L. Gabriel Navar, is the best-developed of these cell-to-cell (paracrine/ autocrine) systems. The cardiac and vascular renin–angiotensin systems, becoming widely appreciated as localized independent tissue systems, are covered by Drs. Rajesh Kumar, Kenneth M. Baker and Jing Pan. Angiotensin (1–7), a new peptide of the renin–angiotensin system and its newly discovered biosynthetic pathway, angiotensin converting enzyme-2 (ACE-2), are discussed by the pioneers of this area, Drs. Carlos M. Ferrario, David B. Averill, K. Bridget Brosnihan, Mark C. Chappell, Debra I. Diz, Patricia E. Gallagher, Liomar A. A. Neves, and E. Ann Tallant. Two relatively new angiotensin receptors, AT_2 and AT_4, are discussed by Drs. Robert M. Carey and Helmy M. Siragy (AT_2) and Drs. T. A. Jenkins, F. A. O. Mendelsohn, A. L. Albiston and S. Y. Chai (AT_4). The emerging role of the renin–angiotensin system in inflammation is covered by Drs. Rhian M. Touyz and Ernesto L. Schiffrin, and the role of aldosterone in vascular damage is discussed by Drs. Hylton V. Joffe, Gordon H. Williams, and Gail K. Adler.

The sympathetic nervous system has long been regarded as critical in blood pressure regulation. In this book, Drs. David Robertson, Andre Diedrich, and Italo Biaggione discuss the recent and compelling evidence for neurogenic human hypertension, and

Drs. Donald J. DiPette and Scott C. Supowit introduce the new role of calcitonin gene-related peptide in hypertension. Drs. Pedro A. Jose, Robert M. Carey, and Robin A. Felder cover important emerging area of renal proximal tubule dopamine and D_1 receptors and their regulation induced by Gprotein kinase-4 (GRK-4). Mutations of GRK-4 in humans are associated with salt-sensitivity and hypertension in several populations.

During the recent years, the importance of diabetes and obesity in hypertension has become evident. Dr. James R. Sowers discusses the insulin resistance (metabolic) syndrome, Dr. Brent M. Egan covers fatty acid metabolism, and Drs. Gregory M. Singer, John F. Setaro and Henry R. Black elaborate on goal-oriented hypertension management in diabetic and nondiabetic patients.

The 1998 Nobel Prize in medicine was awarded to Drs. Furchgott, Ignarro, and Murad for their discovery of nitric oxide and cyclic guanosine monophosphate as an endogenous vasodilator pathway. Their work highlighted the importance of the endothelium in hypertension. In a section devoted to endothelial factors, Drs. David L. Mattson and Alan W. Cowley discuss nitric oxide, Dr. Ernesto L. Schiffrin covers endothelin, and Drs. Julie and Lee Chao cover the kallikrein–kinin system in hypertension.

Recent advances in natriuretic peptides in hypertension are covered by Dr. Kailash N. Pandey. The role of sex steroids is discussed by Drs. Suzanne Oparil and Andrew P. Miller. The lipoxygenase system is elaborated by Drs. Naftali Stern and Michael Tuck.

The focus of *Hypertension and Hormone Mechanisms* is on new developments in hormones/autocoids related to hypertension. Each of the chapters is written by the world's experts in their fields. My hope is that the discussions in this book will open new doors to the understanding that will help propel us closer to knowing the etiology and pathogenesis of primary (essential) hypertension. I further hope that this book will stimulate active research in the fundamental mechanisms of hypertension so that new therapies and even prevention can be realized in the not-too-distant future.

Robert M. Carey, MD, MACP

Contents

Contributors

GAIL K. ADLER, PhD • *Division of Endocrinology, Diabetes, and Hypertension, Brigham and Women's Hospital, Harvard Medical School, Boston, MA*

A. L. ALBISTON, PhD • *Howard Florey Institute of Experimental Physiology and Medicine, University of Melbourne, Parkville, Victoria, Australia*

DAVID A. AVERIL, PhD • *Hypertension and Vascular Disease Center, Wake Forest University School of Medicine, Winston-Salem, NC*

KENNETH M. BAKER, MD • *Division of Molecular Cardiology, The Cardiovascular Research Institute, Texas A&M Health Science Center, College of Medicine; Scott & White Hospital; and Central Texas Veterans Health Care System, Temple, TX*

ITALO BIAGGIONI, MD • *Division of Clinical Pharmacology, Department of Medicine, Autonomic Dysfunction Center, Vanderbilt University Medical Center, Nashville, TN*

HENRY R. BLACK, MD • *Department of Preventive Medicine, Rush Medical College, Rush University Medical Center, Chicago, IL*

K. BRIDGET BROSNIHAN, PhD • *Hypertension and Vascular Disease Center, Wake Forest University School of Medicine, Winston-Salem, NC*

ROBERT M. CAREY, MD, MACP • *David A. Harrison III Distinguished Professor of Medicine, Division of Endocrinology and Metabolism, Department of Medicine, University of Virginia School of Medicine, Charlottesville, VA*

S. Y. CHAI, BSc, PhD • *Howard Florey Institute of Experimental Physiology and Medicine, University of Melbourne, Parkville, Victoria, Australia*

JULIE CHAO, PhD • *Department of Biochemistry and Molecular Biology, Medical University of South Carolina, Charleston, SC*

LEE CHAO, PhD • *Department of Biochemistry and Molecular Biology, Medical University of South Carolina, Charleston, SC*

MARK C. CHAPPEL, PhD • *Hypertension and Vascular Disease Center, Wake Forest University School of Medicine, Winston-Salem, NC*

ALLEN W. COWLEY, JR., PhD • *Department of Physiology, Medical College of Wisconsin, Milwaukee, WI*

ANDRE DIEDRICH, MD • *Division of Clinical Pharmacology, Department of Medicine, Autonomic Dysfunction Center, Vanderbilt University Medical Center, Nashville, TN*

DONALD J. DIPETTE, MD • *Department of Internal Medicine, The Texas A&M Health Science Center, College of Medicine, Scott & White Hospital, Temple, TX*

DEBRA I. DIZ, PhD • *Hypertension and Vascular Disease Center, Wake Forest University School of Medicine, Winston-Salem, NC*

BRENT M. EGAN, MD • *Department of General Internal Medicine and Hypertension, Medical University of South Carolina, Charleston, SC*

ROBIN A. FELDER, PhD • *Department of Pathology, Medical Automation Research Center, University of Virginia Health System, Charlottesville, VA*

CARLOS M. FERRARIO, MD • *Hypertension and Vascular Disease Center, Wake Forest University School of Medicine, Winston-Salem, NC*

PATRICIA GALLAGHER, PhD • *Hypertension and Vascular Disease Center, Wake Forest University School of Medicine, Winston-Salem, NC*

T. A. JENKINS, BSc • *Howard Florey Institute of Experimental Physiology and Medicine, University of Melbourne, Parkville, Victoria, Australia*

HYLTON W. JOFFE, MD • *Division of Endocrinology, Diabetes, and Hypertension, Brigham and Women's Hospital, Harvard Medical School, Boston, MA*

PEDRO A. JOSE, MD, PhD • *Department of Pediatrics, Georgetown University Medical Center, Washington, DC*

HIROYUKI KOBURI, MD, PhD • *Departments of Physiology and Medicine, Molecular Core in Hypertension and Renal COE, Tulane University Health Sciences Center, New Orleans, LA*

RAJESH KUMAR, PhD • *Division of Molecular Cardiology, The Cardiovascular Research Institute, Texas A&M Health Science Center, College of Medicine; Scott & White Hospital; and Central Texas Veterans Health Care System, Temple, TX*

DAVID L. MATTSON, PhD • *Department of Physiology, Medical College of Wisconsin, Milwaukee, WI*

F. A. O. MENDELSOHN, MD, BS, PhD, FRACP • *Howard Florey Institute of Experimental Physiology and Medicine, University of Melbourne, Parkville, Victoria, Australia*

ANDREW P. MILLER, MD • *Division of Cardiovascular Disease, Vascular Biology and Hypertension Program, University of Alabama at Birmingham, Birmingham, AL*

L. GABRIEL NAVAR, PhD • *Department of Physiology, Tulane University Health Sciences Center, New Orleans, LA*

LIOMAR NEVES, PhD • *Hypertension and Vascular Disease Center, Wake Forest University School of Medicine, Winston-Salem, NC*

SUZANNE OPARIL, MD • *Division of Cardiovascular Disease, Vascular Biology and Hypertension Program, University of Alabama at Birmingham, Birmingham, AL*

JING PAN, MD, PhD • *Division of Molecular Cardiology, The Cardiovascular Research Institute, Texas A&M Health Science Center, College of Medicine; Scott & White Hospital; and Central Texas Veterans Health Care System, Temple, TX*

KAILASH N. PANDEY, PhD • *Department of Physiology, Tulane University Health Sciences Center and School of Medicine, New Orleans, LA*

MINOLFA C. PRIETO-CARRASQUERO, MD, PhD • *Section of Diabetes, Hypertension, and Metabolism, Department of Medicine, University of Arizona, Tucson, AZ*

DAVID ROBERTSON, MD • *Elton Yates Professor of Medicine, Pharmacology and Neurology, Vanderbilt University, Nashville, TN*

ERNESTO L. SCHIFFRIN, MD, PhD, FRCPC • *Department of Medicine, Sir Mortimer B. Davis Jewish General Hospital, McGill University, Montreal Quebec, Canada*

JOHN F. SETARO, MD, FACC • *Section of Cardiovascular Medicine, Department of Internal Medicine, Cardiovascular Disease Prevention Center, Yale University School of Medicine, New Haven, CT*

GREGORY SINGER, MD • *Section of Cardiovascular Medicine, Yale University School of Medicine, New Haven, CT*

HELMY M. SIRAGY, MD • *Department of Medicine and Endocrinology, University of Virginia Health System, Charlottesville, VA*

JAMES R. SOWERS, MD • *Diabetes Center, Departments of Medicine and Physiology, University of Arizona, Tucson, AZ*

NAFTALI STERN, MD • *Institute of Endocrinology, Metabolism and Hypertension, Tel Aviv Sourasky Medical Center, Tel Aviv, Israel*

SCOTT C. SUPOWIT, PhD • *Texas A&M University Medical Research Building, Temple, TX*

E. ANN TALLANT, PhD • *Hypertension and Vascular Disease Center, Wake Forest University School of Medicine, Winston-Salem, NC*

RHIAN M. TOUYZ, MD, PhD • *Kidney Research Center, University of Ottowa/Ottowa Health Research Institute, Ottowa, Ontario, Canada*

MICHAEL L. TUCK, MD • *Department of Medicine, David Geffen School of Medicine, University of California at Los Angeles, Los Angeles, CA*

GORDON H. WILLIAMS, MD • *Division of Endocrinology, Diabetes, and Hypertension, Brigham and Women's Hospital, Harvard Medical School, Boston, MA*

List of Color Plates

The images listed below appear in the color insert:

I

NEW DEVELOPMENTS
IN THE RENIN–ANGIOTENSIN SYSTEM

1

The Intrarenal Renin–Angiotensin System

Minolfa C. Prieto-Carrasquero,
Hiroyuki Kobori, and L. Gabriel Navar

CONTENTS

1. INTRODUCTION

We enter a new phase in our understanding of the intrarenal renin–angiotensin system (RAS) in which its intriguing complexities are appreciated. Indeed, it is apparent that the RAS with its multiple components operates in autocrine and intracrine manners as well as an endocrine system. The new developments have raised our awareness of distinct regulatory mechanisms for the intratubular and intracellular as well as the interstitial RAS in the kidney. In this chapter, we will briefly review the current understanding of the intrarenal RAS and discuss how its inappropriate activation alters the capability of the kidney to maintain an adequate sodium and fluid balance at normal arterial pressures, thus setting the stage for the development of hypertension.

2. RENIN–ANGIOTENSIN SYSTEM AND REGULATION OF ARTERIAL BLOOD PRESSURE

RAS plays a pivotal role in the regulation of renal sodium and water excretion, and thus in maintaining body sodium and fluid balance *(1,2)*. It has generally been held

From: *Contemporary Endocrinology: Hypertension and Hormone Mechanisms*
Edited by: R. M. Carey © Humana Press Inc., Totowa, NJ

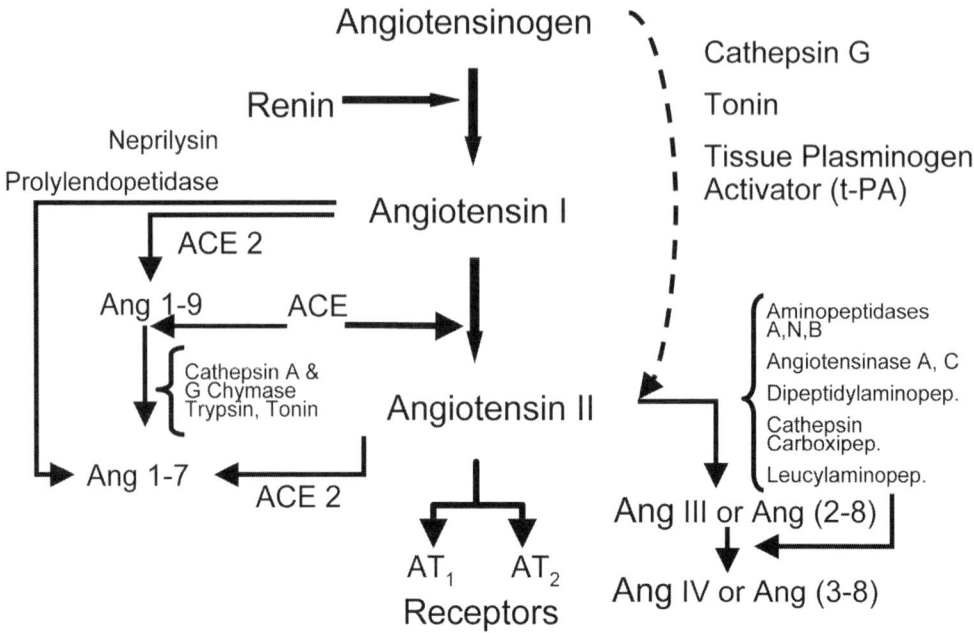

Fig. 1. Known and postulated enzymatic pathways responsible for formation and metabolism of angiotensin peptides.

that renin produced by the kidney cleaves liver-derived angiotensinogen (AGT) to form angiotensin (Ang) I in circulating blood. Subsequently, Ang I is converted into Ang II, the main effector peptide of the RAS, by angiotensin-converting enzyme (ACE) located at the luminal side of the endothelium in many tissues. Ang II exerts its effects via stimulation of Ang II receptors, of which at least two types have been described, AT_1 and AT_2. Several studies have drawn attention to other enzymatic pathways that form Ang I and Ang II as well as other Ang peptides, which may also have significant biological actions such as tonin, cathepsin G or tissue plasminogen activator, that may form Ang II directly from AGT. There are also alternative pathways for Ang I conversion in the various tissues, such as chymase in cardiac tissue *(3,4)* and in the clipped kidney of the 2-kidney-1-clip (2K1C) Goldblatt hypertension model in dogs, which appears to have a marked upregulation of chymase activity *(5)*. Chymase upregulation has also been reported in human subjects with diabetic nephropathy *(6)*. Indeed, chymase seems to play a greater role in vascular Ang II generation under conditions associated with vascular injury and inflammation *(7)*. Endopeptidases such as neprilysin and prolyl endopeptidase may bypass Ang II and convert Ang I directly to Ang 1–7 *(8)*. Further, metabolism of Ang II to Ang III (2–8) and Ang IV (3–8) is catalyzed by the amino-peptidases A, N, and B and dipeptidylaminopeptidase II *(9)*. Ang I conversion to Ang II via chymase, kallikrein, trypsin as well as tonin, and cathespin G provide non-renin, non-ACE pathways for Ang I and Ang II formation *(8,10)* (Fig. 1). Finally, the recently described enzyme, termed ACE2, is capable of cleaving a single amino acid from Ang I to form Ang 1–9 and from Ang II to form Ang 1–7 *(8,11,12)*. Ang 1–7 exerts significant vasodilator and natriuretic actions that may partially counteract the effects of Ang II *(8,13)*. Thus, actions of ACE2 could have a substantial impact on the balance of Ang peptides found in the kidney by diverting the RAS cascade from Ang II to Ang 1–7.

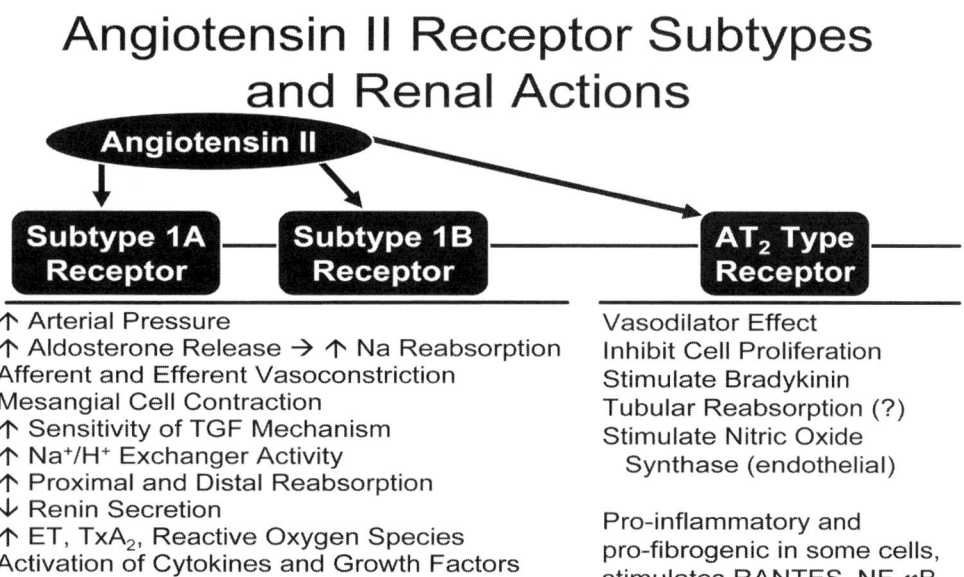

Fig. 2. Intrarenal and intratubular processing of the renin–angiotensin system. All components of the renin–angiotensin system are present in the kidney providing multiple pathways for enhanced intrarenal formation. PT, proximal tubule; DT, distal tubule; CD, collecting duct; AGT, angiotensinogen; JGA, juxtaglomerular apparatus; AA, afferent arteriole; EA, efferent arteriole; ACE, angiotensin-converting enzyme.

The systemic RAS maintains arterial pressure by controlling extracellular fluid volume and through the vasoactive actions of Ang II and related peptides on vascular smooth muscle cells. Ang II enhances myocardial contractility, stimulates aldosterone release, stimulates release of catecholamines from the adrenal medulla and sympathetic nerve endings, increases sympathetic nervous system activity, stimulates thirst and salt appetite, and influences epithelial salt and water reabsorption in the intestine and kidney $(1,14)$. Ang II directly activates postganglionic sympathetic neurons by activating voltage-gated Ca^{2+} channels and increasing intracellular Ca^{2+} (15). Ang II also has long-term effects on growth and remodeling, development, vascular hypertrophy, and erythropoiesis. In pathological situations, Ang II exerts significant long-term proliferative effects leading to tissue injury because of the activation of cytokines $(16,17)$ as well as the alteration of the immune system. Indeed, it has been found that in Ang II-induced hypertension there is an increase in the number of α-interferon-secreting T-cells that is prevented by a treatment with an AT_1 receptor blocker (18), which may explain some of the beneficial effects of AT_1 blockers as modulators of immunological responses (Fig. 2).

3. INTRARENAL RAS COMPONENTS AND LOCALLY FORMED ANGIOTENSIN PEPTIDES

RAS has been portrayed as an endocrine, paracrine, autocrine, and intracrine system $(19–21)$ and thus it has been difficult to delineate the quantitative contributions of systemically delivered vs locally formed Ang peptides to the levels existing in any given tissue. Emerging evidence indicates that local formation is of major significance in the regulation of the Ang peptide levels in many organs and tissues $(22,23)$. Various studies have demonstrated the importance of tissue RAS in the brain, heart, adrenal glands, vasculature, as well as in the kidney *(1,24)*. Although every organ in the body has the elements of the RAS, the kidney is unique in having every component of the RAS with compartmentalization in the tubular and interstitial networks as well as intracellular accumulation. In addition, the kidneys, as well as the adrenal glands, have tissue concentrations of Ang II much greater than can be explained by the concentrations delivered by the arterial blood flow *(25–28)*. There is substantial evidence that the major fraction of Ang II present in renal tissues is generated locally from the AGT delivered to the kidney and from the AGT locally produced by proximal tubule cells. Ang I delivered to the kidney can also be converted to Ang II *(29,30)*. Renin secreted by the juxtaglomerular apparatus (JGA) cells and delivered to the renal interstitium and vascular compartment also provides a pathway for the local generation of Ang I. ACE is abundant in the rat kidney and has been located in the proximal and distal tubules, the collecting ducts and renal endothelial cells *(31–33)*. Therefore, all of the components necessary to generate intrarenal Ang II are present along the nephron.

3.1. Renin

Although in the strictest sense renin is not a hormone, it can be considered as such because of its role in determining Ang I generation and because it is subject to tight control. Hence, the plasma renin concentration or activity is often used as a measure of the overall activity of the RAS. In most species, renin synthesized by JGA cells is the primary source of both circulating and intrarenal renin levels. However, some strains of mice also produce substantial amounts of renin in the submandibular and submaxillary glands as expression of the duplicated renin gene, *Ren-2 (34,35)*.

The secreted active form of renin contains 339–343 amino acid residues after proteolytic removal of the 43-amino acid residue at the N-terminus (prorenin). Although circulating active renin is derived exclusively from the kidney, the kidneys and other tissues also secrete prorenin into the circulation and its concentration may exceed that of renin *(36)*. Besides serving as the precursor for active renin, it has been suggested that circulating prorenin is taken up by some tissues through which it may contribute to the local synthesis of angiotensin peptides *(37)*. In the heart under normal conditions, renin is not produced and its transcript is undetectable or extremely low *(38,39)*. Nevertheless, transgenic rats expressing the *Ren-2* renin gene exhibit high circulating prorenin levels in absence of the cardiac transgene owing to prorenin internalization into cardiomyocytes with the generation of angiotensins *(40)*. These effects suggest that the uptake of circulating prorenin but not active renin may play an important role in cardiac hypertrophy.

Although there have been suggestions that renin itself or perhaps prorenin may directly elicit cellular effects, independent of the generation of Ang II, the only well-established role of renin is to act on AGT, a protein with a non-glycosylated weight of 52 kDa and synthesized primarily by the liver to form the decapeptide Ang I. Recent evidence indicates the existence of a renin receptor that may also initiate intracellular signaling to activate ERK1/ERK2 *(41)*. In the heart and kidney, the recently described renin receptor *(41–44)* binds renin and prorenin leading to an increase in the catalytic efficiency of Ang I formation from AGT.

It should be recognized that JGA cells are not the only intrarenal structures in which renin has been localized. Kidneys from rats that are treated chronically with ACE inhibitors also exhibit renin immunoreactivity on the afferent arteriole extending well beyond the JGA loci up toward the interlobular artery, suggesting that ACE inhibition induces a recruitment of cells that in the basal state were not expressing the renin gene *(45)*. Positive renin immunoreaction has also been observed in cells of glomeruli and of proximal and distal nephron segments *(46–49)*. In addition, renin mRNA and protein expression have been also reported in proximal and distal nephron segments *(47,49–53)*. Using immunoblotting, Rohrwasser et al. *(53)* found that renin was secreted by microdissected arcades of connecting tubule cells indicating that renin is probably secreted into the distal tubular fluid, leading to Ang I formation within the distal nephron lumen.

3.2. Angiotensin-Converting Enzyme

Ang I is rapidly converted into the major effector of this system, Ang II, by ACE, which is located on endothelial cells in many vascular beds and on membranes of various other cells including brush border membranes of proximal tubules *(54,55)*. The localization of ACE within the kidney in various species has been well characterized. However, there are some important differences between humans and commonly used experimental animals *(56)*. Indeed, Metzger et al. *(56)* reported that kidneys from normal human subjects predominantly expressed ACE in the brush border of proximal tubular segments, and very little ACE expression was observed on vascular endothelial cells. ACE was not detectable in the vasculature of the glomerular tuft, or even in the basolateral membranes of epithelial cells. In contrast, there was intense labeling on the endothelial cells of almost all the renal microvasculature of rats. However, kidneys from human subjects with non-neoplastic diseases manifested increased expression on vascular endothelial cells *(56)*. Data indicating much lower endothelial expression in renal vascular endothelial cells in humans help explain the much lower Ang I to Ang II conversion rates that have been reported for human kidneys as compared to other species *(57,58)*. Danser et al. *(57)* reported that less than 10% of arterially delivered Ang I is converted to Ang II, which is much lower than reported for dogs *(59)*. The reduced ACE on renal vascular endothelial cells in humans implies that the influence of intrarenal Ang II formed from circulating precursors may have less significance than in experimental animals.

The recently described ACE2, which acts on Ang II to form Ang 1–7, is a membrane-associated and secreted enzyme expressed predominantly on endothelium, but highly restricted to heart, kidneys, and testis in humans *(11)*. It has been suggested that Ang 1–7 acts on its own receptor, postulated to be the orphan Mas receptor *(60,61)*. Recent studies demonstrated that genetic deletion of the G protein-coupled receptor encoded by the Mas protooncogene abolished the binding of Ang 1–7 to mouse renal cells *(61)*. Ang 1–7 is thought to serve as an endogenous antagonist of the Ang II-induced actions mediated via AT_1 receptors *(62)*. Thus, ACE2 could have substantial impact on the balance of Ang peptides found in the kidney by diverting the RAS cascade from Ang II to Ang 1–7. This helps explain the elevated Ang II levels in the ACE2 knockout mice *(61)*. Collectrin, a novel homolog of ACE2, has been identified in mouse, rat and humans *(63,64)*. Both ACE2 and collectrin have tissue-restricted expression in the kidney. Collectrin is localized on the luminal surface and in the cytoplasm of collecting duct cells and its mRNA is expressed in renal collecting ducts cells *(64)*, whereas ACE2 is present throughout the endothelium and in proximal tubular epithelial cells. Collectrin is upregulated in the hypertrophic phase of the ablated kidney in 5/6 nephrectomized rat model *(65)*. In contrast to ACE and ACE2, collectrin does not contain dipeptidyl carboxy-peptidase domains, and thus it may play a role in the hypertrophic phase through other pathways. Other peptides with reported biological activity formed as part of the Ang cascade include Ang 2–8 and Ang 3–8 as a consequence of action by aminopeptidases and other degradating enzymes *(66)*. Although there is an increasing interest in the potential roles of these other Ang peptides, the majority of the evidence continues to support the established premise that most of the vascular and transport actions attributed to the RAS that lead to vascular constriction, enhanced sodium transport and hypertension are because of the actions of Ang II and also Ang III or Ang 2–8 acting primarily on AT_1 receptors *(67–69)*. Nevertheless, Ang 1–7, Ang IV and Ang II-mediated activation of AT_2 receptors may exert significant counteracting or protective actions partially buffering the AT_1-mediated effects under certain circumstances *(8,70–73)*.

3.3. Angiotensinogen

Although most of the circulating AGT is produced and secreted by the liver, it is also produced by the kidneys. Intrarenal AGT mRNA and protein have been localized to prox-imal tubule cells indicating that the intratubular Ang II could be derived from locally formed and secreted AGT *(27,74–76)*. Furthermore, AGT is regulated by an amplification mechanism such that AGT mRNA and protein are enhanced by Ang II *(77)*. This effect helps to maintain or even increase further the production of Ang II in Ang II-dependent hypertension *(74,75)*. The AGT produced in proximal tubule cells appears to be secreted directly into the tubular lumen in addition to producing its metabolites intracellularly and secreting them into the tubule lumen *(27,51,53,78,79)*. Ding et al. *(80)* demonstrated in mice harboring the gene for human AGT fused to the kidney androgen–protein promoter that human AGT was localized primarily to proximal tubule cells. They found abundant human AGT in the urine but only slight traces in the systemic circulation. This finding suggests that most of the AGT formed in proximal tubule cells is destined for secretion into the lumen. Rohrwasser et al. *(53)* demonstrated luminal localization of AGT in proximal tubular cells in vivo and showed, in monolayer proximal tubule cell cultures, that most of the AGT was detected near the apical membrane. They also reported that AGT was detected at low nanomolar concentrations in urine from mice and human volunteers.

Proximal tubule AGT concentrations in anesthetized rats have been reported in the range of 300 nM, which greatly exceed the free Ang I and Ang II tubular fluid concen-trations *(81)*. Because of its molecular size, it seems unlikely that much of the plasma AGT filters across the glomerular membrane further supporting the concept that proximal tubule cells secrete AGT directly into the tubule *(53,76,80,82)*. Kobori et al. *(83)* infused human AGT into hypertensive rats in order to determine whether AGT from the circu-lation could be detected in the urine. The human AGT was not detectable suggesting that most of the AGT in the urine is of renal origin *(83)*. Formation of Ang I and II in the tubular lumen subsequent to AGT secretion may be possible because some renin is filtered and/or secreted from JGA cells. The identification of renin in distal nephron segments also indicates a possible pathway for Ang I generation from proximally delivered AGT. Intact AGT in urine reflects its presence throughout the nephron and, to the extent that renin and ACE are available along the nephron, substrate availability supports continued Ang I generation and Ang II conversion in distal segments *(22,51,53,80)*.

Once Ang I is formed, conversion readily occurs because there are abundant amounts of ACE associated with the proximal tubule brush border. Casarini et al. *(32)* found that ACE activity is present in tubular fluid throughout the nephron except in the late distal tubule, being higher at the initial portion of the proximal tubule but then decreasing to the distal nephron and increasing again in the urine. This evidence suggests proximal ACE secretion, degradation, and/or reabsorption associated with secretion in the collecting duct. Therefore, intratubular Ang II formation may occur not only in the proximal tubule but also beyond the connecting tubule. Thus, renal tissue ACE activity is critical to maintain the steady-state Ang II levels in the kidney. Indeed, Modrall et al. *(84)* demonstrated that tissue-ACE (*tis*ACE–/–) knockout mice exhibit 80% lower intrarenal Ang II levels compared to wild-type mice *(84)*. In addition to the marked reduction of intrarenal Ang II levels, this *tis*ACE–/– mouse model showed significant depletion of its immediate precursor Ang I in renal tissue, which supports the concept that Ang II exerts a positive feedback loop on proximal AGT *(74,75,77)*. However, at present there are no data indicating how much of the Ang peptides are formed intracellularly and secreted and how much are formed in the tubule lumen from secreted substrate.

4. INTRARENAL ANGIOTENSIN II RECEPTORS

Most of the actions of Ang II on renal function are the consequence of activation of Ang II receptors, which are widely distributed in various regions and cell types of the kidney (Fig. 2). Two major categories of Ang II receptors, AT_1 (subtype AT_{1a} and AT_{1b}) and AT_2 have been described, pharmacologically characterized, and cloned *(85–90)*. However, most of the Ang II hypertensinogenic actions are generally attributed to the AT_1 receptor *(91–93)*.

AT_1 receptor transcript has been localized to proximal tubules, thick ascending limb of the loop of Henle, glomeruli, arterial vasculature, vasa recta, arcuate arteries, and juxtaglomerular cells *(94,96)*. In rodents, there are two AT_1 receptor subtypes, with the AT_{1a} being the predominant subtype in all nephron segments, whereas the AT_{1b} is more abundant than AT_{1a} only in the glomerulus *(97,98)*. The AT_{1a} receptor subtype has been found in ureteric bud derivatives as early as the embryonic day E11.5 *(99)*. In mature kidneys, AT_{1a} receptors have been localized to the luminal and basolateral membranes of several segments of the nephron, as well as on the renal microvasculature in both cortex and medulla, smooth muscle cells of afferent and efferent arterioles, epithelial cells of the thick ascending limb of Henle, proximal tubular apical and basolateral membranes, mesangial cells, distal tubules, collecting ducts, and macula densa cells *(100–106)*. This evidence is consistent with the localization of the transcript for the AT_1 receptor subtypes in all of the renal tubular and vascular segments *(106)*. Nevertheless, renal microvascular functional studies obtained from transgenic mice lacking the AT_{1a} receptor gene have shown that the afferent arteriole has both AT_{1a} and AT_{1b} receptors, whereas the efferent arteriole only expresses AT_{1a} receptors *(107)*.

The regulation of intrarenal Ang II receptors in hypertensive conditions is complex because vascular and tubular receptors respond differently during high Ang II states *(2)*. In general, high Ang II levels associated with a low salt diet decrease glomerular AT_1 receptor expression but increase tubular AT_1 receptor levels *(108)*. Studies in 2K1C Goldblatt hypertensive rats demonstrated that glomerular AT_1 receptors were decreased within 2 wk after clipping, but vascular receptors were not decreased until

16 wk *(109)*. However, glomerular AT_1 receptor density was not increased in the 1K1C model although vascular AT_1 receptor density was increased *(110)*. In the Ang II-infused rat model of hypertension, total kidney AT_1 mRNA levels and receptor protein were not significantly altered by 2 wk Ang II infusion sufficient to cause marked hypertension *(111)*. However, Wang et al. *(112)* reported that AT_{1a} receptor protein was reduced in both ischemic and contralateral kidneys of 2K1C Goldblatt and 2-kidney-1-wrap hypertensive models, and in kidneys of Ang II-infused rats. AT_2 receptors were downregulated only in ischemic kidneys. In the transgenic rat TGR(*mRen*2) harboring the mouse renin gene, Zhuo et al. *(113)* found increased AT_1 receptor binding in vascular smooth muscle of afferent and efferent arterioles, JGA, glomerular mesangial cells, proximal tubular cells, and renomedullary interstitial cells. It was suggested that upregulation of AT_1 receptors in multiple renal cells may contribute to the pathogenesis of hypertension in these rats. Harrison-Bernard et al. *(114)* extended the analysis in Ang II-infused rats with in vitro autoradiography and showed differential responses with significant decreases in glomeruli and inner stripe but not in proximal tubules. Furthermore, ACE binding was significantly increased in proximal tubules of Ang II-infused rats. Thus, vascular and glomerular AT_1 receptors are downregulated, but the proximal tubular receptors are either upregulated or not significantly altered in Ang II-dependent hypertension.

The AT_2 receptor is highly expressed in human and rodent kidney mesenchyme during fetal life and decreases dramatically after birth *(115)*. AT_2 receptors have been localized to the glomerular epithelial cells, proximal tubules, collecting ducts, and parts of the renal vasculature of the adult rat *(106,112)*. Although the role of AT_2 receptors in regulating renal function remains uncertain, it has been suggested that AT_2 activation counteracts AT_1 receptor effects by stimulating the formation of bradykinin and nitric oxide leading to increases in interstitial fluid concentration of cyclic guanosine monophosphate (cGMP) *(116–118)*. AT_2 receptor activation appears to influence proximal tubule sodium reabsorption either by a cell membrane receptor-mediated mechanism or via an interstitial nitric oxide–cGMP pathway *(119)*. Ang II infusion into AT_2 knockout mice leads to exaggerated hypertension and reductions in renal function, probably because of the decreased renal interstitial fluid levels of bradykinin and cGMP available, which counteract the direct effect of Ang II *(120)*.

5. INTRARENAL LEVELS OF ANGIOTENSIN II

5.1. Interstitial and Tubular Angiotensin II

Intrarenal Ang II is not distributed in a homogenous fashion but is compartmentalized in both regional and segmental manners *(121)*. Earlier studies indicated that medullary Ang II-levels are higher than the cortical levels in normal rats and increase further in Ang II infused hypertensive rats *(81)*. The combination of high Ang II levels in the medulla coupled with the high density of Ang II receptors suggest that Ang II exerts a major role in regulating hemodynamics and tubular function in the medulla *(2,114)*. The higher Ang II levels in the medulla suggest that there may be specialized Ang II forming pathways or accumulation mechanisms in medullary tissues that are subject to local regulation. However, Ingert et al. *(26,122)* failed to confirm that medullary Ang II contents are higher than cortical Ang II contents. These authors found that Ang I and Ang II

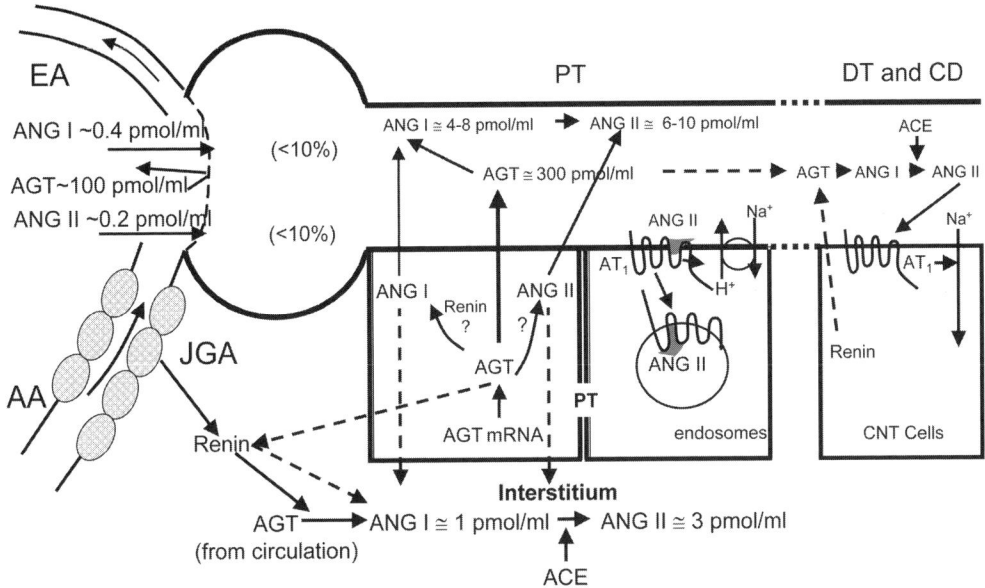

Fig. 3. Major renal actions exerted by Ang receptor subtypes.

levels in cortex and medulla are equivalent and respond in a similar manner to alterations in dietary salt intake.

Within the cortex, there is a distribution of Ang II in the interstitial fluid, tubular fluid and the intracellular compartments. The interstitial as well as the intratubular compartments contribute to the disproportionately high total Ang II (Fig. 3) levels. Studies using microdialysis probes implanted in the renal cortex demonstrated that Ang II concentrations in interstitial fluid are much higher than the plasma concentrations with recent results suggesting values in the range of 3–5 pmol/mL *(117,123–125)*. Interestingly, Nishiyama et al. *(124,125)* demonstrated that ACE inhibitors administered either directly into the renal artery or via the microdialysis probe were not able to substantially suppress the renal interstitial fluid Ang II levels. These studies suggest that much of the Ang II in the renal interstitial compartment is formed through non-ACE-dependent pathways or by ACE that is not easily accessed by the exogenously administered ACE inhibitors. Increases in renal interstitial fluid Ang II levels have been reported for two models of hypertension. Siragy et al. *(117)* found that renal interstitial Ang II is increased in the wrapped kidney of rats with Grollman hypertension. Nishiyama et al. *(126)* reported that renal interstitial fluid Ang II concentrations are also increased in rats infused with Ang II for 2 wk. Because the renal interstitial values are much higher than can be explained on the basis of equilibration with the plasma concentrations, the data suggest local regulation of Ang II formation in the renal interstitial compartment and an enhancement of interstitial Ang II production in Ang II-dependent hypertension.

As shown in Fig. 3, micropuncture studies have shown that proximal tubule fluid concentrations of Ang I and Ang II are also much greater than the plasma concentrations *(27)*. The finding that tubular fluid samples collected from perfused segments had Ang II concentrations similar to those measured in nonperfused tubules indicates that the proximal tubule secretes Ang II or a precursor into the proximal tubule fluid *(127)*.

In addition to AGT, proximal tubule cells also have renin mRNA that is stimulated by a low sodium diet, which may thus act on AGT to generate Ang I *(47)*. Evidence for the presence of distal nephron renin mRNA and protein *(49,51,53)* also provides a pathway for Ang I generation from proximally delivered AGT. Furthermore, distal nephron renin regulation by Ang II differs from that in JGA cells because chronic Ang II infusion in rats enhances renin protein in principal cells but suppresses renin in JGA cells *(49)*. Ang II stimulatory effects on collecting duct renin could help explain the marked impairment of sodium excretion and suppression of the pressure–natriuresis relationship observed in Ang II-infused hypertensive rats *(128)*. Because renal AGT mRNA and protein levels are upregulated by increases in circulating Ang II levels *(129,130)*, we postulate that renin in connecting tubule and collecting duct cells may be secreted into the tubular fluid and it acts on proximally delivered AGT to form Ang I in the luminal fluid. In turn, the presence of ACE in the distal nephron would lead to maintained renal Ang II-generating capacity that occurs in Ang II-dependent hypertension leading to high intrarenal Ang II levels and the maintenance of high blood pressure.

Measurements of proximal tubular fluid Ang II concentrations in anesthetized rats have not revealed significant differences among control rats and in several hypertensive models *(131–133)*. Considering that kidneys of the hypertensive rats have marked depletion of JGA renin and are exposed to elevated arterial pressures, the maintenance of high proximal tubular Ang II concentrations reflects an inappropriate maintenance of intrarenal Ang II formation levels. Nevertheless, the results so far have not demonstrated further elevations in proximal tubule Ang II concentrations above the levels found in normal anesthetized rats. In normal rats, volume expansion failed to suppress proximal tubule Ang II concentrations, but increased levels were documented following reductions in renal perfusion pressure *(134)*.

The Ang II concentrations in tubular fluid from the other segments of the nephron remain unknown. Several studies support an important role for Ang II in regulating reabsorptive function in distal nephron and collecting duct segments, as well as in proximal tubule segments, which activate the Ang II receptors on the luminal borders *(27,135)*. Recently, a direct action of Ang II on the luminal amiloride-sensitive sodium channel (ENaC) was reported *(136)*. These data indicate that when luminal distal nephron Ang II concentrations are augmented, they could contribute directly to the regulation of distal tubule and collecting duct sodium reabsorption.

5.2. Intracellular Angiotensin II

As indicated earlier, some of the Ang II that binds to receptors is internalized via AT_1 receptor-mediated endocytosis *(26,137,138)*. Zhuo et al. *(139)* reported direct evidence for accumulation of Ang II in intermicrovillar clefts and endosomes of Ang II-infused hypertensive rats. It was also shown that AT_1 receptor blockade with candesartan prevented the ensodomal accumulation even though plasma Ang II increased further, demonstrating the importance of AT_1 receptor-mediated uptake. The presence of Ang II in renal endosomes indicates that some of the internalized Ang II remains intact and contributes to the total Ang II content measured in tissue homogenates *(25,127,138–141)*. As shown for proximal tubule cells, endocytosis of the Ang II–AT_1 receptor complex seems to be required for the full expression of functional responses coupled to the activation of signal transduction pathways *(142,143)*. In Ang II-dependent hypertension, a higher fraction of the total kidney Ang II is internalized into intracellular endosomes (light endosomes as well as intramicrovillar clefts) via an AT_1 receptor-mediated process *(139)*. The demonstration that AT_1 receptor blockade prevents the augmentation of intrarenal Ang II that occurs during chronic infusions of Ang II suggests AT_1 receptor-mediated accumulation of Ang II into an intracellular compartment, and that some of the internalized Ang II is protected from degradation *(26,139)*. Van Kats *(138)* infused labeled Ang II and showed six- to sevenfold increase in intrarenal Ang II, which was prevented by an AT_1 receptor antagonist.

There are several possible functions of the internalized Ang II. Ang II could be recycled and secreted in order to exert further actions by binding to Ang II receptors on the cell membranes. Ang II may also act on cytosolic receptors to stimulate IP3 as has been described for vascular smooth muscle cells *(144)*. A particularly intriguing hypothesis is that Ang II migrates to the nucleus to exert genomic effects *(141)*. Nuclear binding sites for Ang II in renal cells have been reported by Licea-Vargas et al. *(145)*. The nuclear receptors were primarily of the AT_1 subtype because they were displaced by losartan as well as by saralasin. Nuclear Ang II receptor density was not altered in Ang II-infused hypertension. Chen et al. *(141)* transfected Chinese hamster ovary cells with an AT_{1a} receptor fused with green fluorescent protein (GFP), which allowed the visualization of trafficking of the internalized ligand–receptor complex. Ang II increased colocalization of GFP fluorescence with nuclear markers suggesting the migration of the receptor complex to the nucleus *(141)*. Because Ang II exerts a positive stimulation on AGT mRNA and protein production, it is possible that the intracellular Ang II may have genomic actions to regulate AGT or renin mRNA expression in proximal tubule cells *(127)*.

6. AUGMENTATION OF INTRARENAL AGT AND ANG II IN HYPERTENSION

Although increased internalization of Ang II contributes to the increased intrarenal Ang II in the Ang II-infused model of hypertension, the overall Ang II levels are also due to additional Ang II formation as a consequence of enhanced AGT production. In vivo and in vitro studies have shown that Ang II stimulates intrarenal AGT mRNA localized in proximal tubule cells *(75,77,146)*. Several recent studies have focused on long-term changes in the intrarenal AGT formation in Ang II-dependent hypertension. Kobori et al. *(74,75,83,129,147)* evaluated the effects of Ang II infusions on intrarenal AGT and Ang II levels and the relationship between urinary excretion of AGT and kidney Ang II levels in hypertensive models. They reported that Ang II-infused rats had increases in renal AGT mRNA *(75)* and protein *(74)*, and an enhancement of urinary excretion rate of AGT *(147)*. Chronic Ang II infusions to normal rats significantly increased the urinary excretion rate of AGT in a time- and dose-dependent manner *(83)*. This augmentation process may be responsible for sustained or enhanced generation of AGT leading to continued intrarenal production of Ang II under conditions of elevated circulating concentrations. The intrarenally produced Ang II would be additive with the internalized Ang II by the AT_1 receptors leading to the overall increased intrarenal Ang II contents.

Kobori et al. *(83,147)* demonstrated that urinary excretion rate of AGT was closely correlated with systolic blood pressure and kidney Ang II content, but not with plasma Ang II concentration. This increase was not just because of the increased proteinuria or the development of hypertension because urinary protein excretion in volume-dependent hypertensive rats was significantly increased more than in Ang II-dependent hypertensive rats; however, urinary AGT excretion was significantly lower in volume-dependent hypertensive rats than in Ang II-dependent hypertensive rats (83). The finding of intact AGT in urine suggests its presence throughout the nephron and, to the extent that renin and ACE are available along the nephron, there may be continued Ang I generation and Ang II conversion in segments beyond the proximal tubule (22,53,80). As previously mentioned, renin has been demonstrated on the luminal side of connecting tubule cells in the kidneys of mice and humans suggesting that renin may be secreted into the distal tubular fluid (53). Collectively, these data support the concept depicted in Fig. 3 that, in angiotensin-dependent hypertension, there is an increased AGT secretion by the proximal tubule cells, leading to spillover of intact AGT into distal nephron segments. Because there is available renin and ACE or other enzymes that can subserve similar functions, there should be enhanced distal tubular formation of Ang II and increased Ang II-dependent stimulation of distal sodium reabsorption rate (136). This may help explain the markedly enhanced sodium reabsorption and suppression of pressure natriuresis that has been shown in Ang II-infused rats (128). A recent study by Komlosi et al. (30) showed that Ang I added to the luminal surface of collecting ducts was converted to Ang II and activated ENaC thus providing direct evidence of Ang I to Ang II conversion in distal nephron segments.

Although the Dahl-salt sensitive (DS) hypertensive rat is generally considered to be characterized by a low activity of circulating RAS, Ang I-converting enzyme inhibitors and AT_1 receptor antagonists reduce renal dysfunction in DS hypertensive rats fed a high-salt (HS) diet (148–151). These findings suggest that the intrarenal RAS may be inappropriately activated and contributes to the development of hypertension in this animal model. Kobori et al. (129) examined the relationship between urinary excretion of AGT and kidney AGT levels in DS rats. Kidney AGT levels were significantly increased in DS rats fed a HS diet compared to DS fed a low-salt (LS) diet, or Dahl-salt resistant rats on either high- or low-salt diets. Urinary excretion of AGT was paradoxically increased in DS rats fed a HS diet demonstrating an inappropriate response to increases in salt intake. Thus, the hypertension that results when DS rats are fed a HS diet may be because of inappropriate and paradoxical increases in intrarenal AGT levels. This may be resulting from the increased oxidative stress in response to the HS diet-stimulating AGT expression.

Collectively, the experiments evaluating the regulation of urinary AGT excretion rates have indicated that there is a quantitative relationship among urinary AGT, intrarenal AGT, and Ang II production. When intrarenal AGT formation rate is increased, some of the increased AGT secreted into the tubular fluid spills over into the distal tubule and eventually into the urine. Renin from collecting tubule cells would then act on AGT to form Ang I. Ang I can be converted to Ang II by the ACE present in the tubular fluid of collecting ducts to allow activation of luminal AT_1 receptors and stimulation of sodium transport (136). Further enhancement of this Ang II-mediated effects would also develop as a consequence of ENaC upregulation (152). Accordingly, urinary AGT excretion rates reflect the distal nephron spillover of AGT and provide an index of the magnitude of the enhanced intrarenal AGT production in angiotensin-dependent hypertension and thus, may provide a useful test in human hypertensive subjects to identify Ang II-dependent hypertension.

7. CONCLUDING REMARKS

There continues to be a great deal of interest in the mechanisms regulating the intrarenal RAS and related peptides as well as the many intrarenal actions exerted by Ang II. It is becoming apparent that intrarenal Ang II can be regulated independently from the circulating Ang II. Although the possible counteracting effects of Ang 1–7 and AT_2 receptors cannot be disregarded, the powerful actions of intrarenal Ang II acting via the stimulation of AT_1 receptors on the vascular, glomerular, and tubular structures provide a synchronous cascade of effects contributing to the ability of the kidney to retain over 99% of the filtered sodium. From a functional perspective, the additive effects of Ang II working on distal nephron transport function coupled with the associated actions of elevated aldosterone levels markedly increase the sodium-retaining capability of the kidney. When activated in a physiologically appropriate setting, these actions can be life saving. When inappropriately sustained, however, these effects contribute to the development and maintenance of hypertension. Furthermore, the sustained increases in intrarenal Ang II in a setting of hypertension can lead to progressive renal injury, proliferation, and fibrosis associated with the activation of several major cytokines and growth factors *(17,153–155)*.

ACKNOWLEDGMENTS

The authors' studies cited in this work have been supported by grants from NHLBI, NCRR, Health Excellence Fund of the Louisiana Board of Regents, and the American Heart Association. We acknowledge with appreciation the assistance of Debbie Olavarrieta for preparation of the manuscript and figures.

REFERENCES

1. Mitchell, K. D. and Navar, L. G. (1995) Intrarenal actions of angiotensin II in the pathogenesis of experimental hypertension. In: *Hypertension: Pathophysiology, Diagnosis, and Management* (Laragh, J. H. and Brenner, B. M., eds.), 2nd ed., Raven, New York, pp. 1437–1450.
2. Navar, L. G., Harrison-Bernard, L. M., Imig, J. D., and Mitchell, K. D. (2000) Renal actions of angiotensin II at AT_1 receptor blockers. In: *Angiotensin II Receptor Antagonists* (Epstein, M. and Brunner, H. R., eds.), Hanley & Belfus, Philadelphia, pp. 189–214.
3. Urata, H., Nishimura, H., and Ganten, D. (1996) Chymase-dependent angiotensin II forming system in humans. *Am. J. Hypertens.* **9,** 277–284.
4. Chen, L. Y., Li, P., He, Q., et al. (2002) Transgenic study of the function of chymase in heart remodeling. *J. Hypertens.* **20,** 2047–2055.
5. Tokuyama, H., Hayashi, K., Matsuda, H., et al. (2002) Differential regulation of elevated renal angiotensin II in chronic renal ischemia. *Hypertension* **40,** 34–40.
6. Huang, X. R., Chen, W. Y., Truong, L. D., and Lan, H. Y. (2003) Chymase is upregulated in diabetic nephropathy: implications for an alternative pathway of angiotensin II-mediated diabetic renal and vascular disease. *J. Am. Soc. Nephrol.* **14,** 1738–1747.
7. Miyazaki, M. and Takai, S. (2001) Local angiotensin II-generating system in vascular tissues: the roles of chymase. *Hypertens. Res.* **24,** 189–193.
8. Chappell, M. C., Tallant, E. A., Diz, D. I., and Ferrario, C. M. (2000) The renin–angiotensin system and cardiovascular homeostasis. In: *Drugs, Enzymes and Receptors of the Renin–Angiotensin System: Celebrating a Century of Discovery* (Husain, A. and Graham, R. M., eds.), Harwood Academic, Amsterdam, pp. 3–22.
9. Ardaillou, R. and Chansel, D. (1997) Synthesis and effects of active fragments of angiotensin II. *Kidney Int.* **52,** 1458–1468.

10. Fukamizu, A. (2000) Genomic expression systems on hierarchy and network leading to hypertension: long on history, short on facts. *Hypertens. Res.* **23**, 545–552.
11. Donoghue, M., Hsieh, F., Baronas, E., et al. (2000) A novel angiotensin-converting enzyme-related carboxypeptidase (ACE2) converts angiotensin I to angiotensin 1–9. *Circ. Res.* **87**, E1–E9.
12. Crackower, M. A., Sarao, R., Oudit, G. Y., et al. (2002) Angiotensin-converting enzyme 2 is an essential regulator of heart function. *Nature* **417**, 822–828.
13. Ferrario, C. M. (2003) Contribution of angiotensin-(1–7) to cardiovascular physiology and pathology. *Curr. Hypertens. Rep.* **5**, 129–134.
14. Corvol, P., Jeunemaitre, X., Charru, A., Kotelevtsev, Y., and Soubrier, F. (1995) Role of the renin-angiotensin system in blood pressure regulation and in human hypertension: new insights from molecular genetics. *Recent Prog. Hormone Res.* **50**, 287–308.
15. Ma, X., Chapleau, M. W., Whiteis, C. A., Abboud, F. M., and Bielefeldt, K. (2001) Angiotensin selectively activates a subpopulation of postganglionic sympathetic neurons in mice. *Circ. Res.* **88**, 787–793.
16. Wolf, G. and Ziyadeh, F. (1997) The role of angiotensin II in diabetic nephropathy: emphasis on non-hemodynamic mechanisms. *Am. J. Kidney Dis.* **29**, 153–163.
17. Wolf, G. (2002) *The Renin–Angiotensin System and Progression of Renal Diseases*, Vol. 135., Karger, Hamburg, pp. 1–268.
18. Shao, J., Nangaku, M., Miyata, T., et al. (2003) Imbalance of T-cell subsets in angiotensin II-infused hypertensive rats with kidney injury. *Hypertension* **42**, 31–38.
19. Navar, L. G., Inscho, E. W., Majid, S. A., et al. (1996) Paracrine regulation of the renal microcirculation. *Physiol. Rev.* **76**, 425–536.
20. Carretero, O. A. and Scicli, A. G. (1991) Local hormonal factors (intracrine, autocrine, and paracrine) in hypertension. *Hypertension* **18(Suppl I)**, I58–I69.
21. Re, R. N. (2003) The intracrine hypothesis and intracellular peptide hormone action. *Bioessays* **25**, 401–409.
22. Davisson, R. L., Ding, Y., Stec, D. E., Catterall, J. F., and Sigmund, C. D. (1999) Novel mechanism of hypertension revealed by cell-specific targeting of human angiotensinogen in transgenic mice. *Physiol. Genom.* **1**, 3–9.
23. Baltatu, O., Silva, J. A. Jr., Ganten, D., and Bader, M. (2000) The brain renin–angiotensin system modulates angiotensin II-induced hypertension and cardiac hypertrophy. *Hypertension* **35**, 409–412.
24. Campbell, D. J., Kladis, A., Skinner, S. L., and Whitworth, J. A. (1991) Characterization of angiotensin peptides in plasma of anephric man. *J. Hypertens.* **9**, 265–274.
25. Imig, J. D., Navar, G. L., Zou, L. X., et al. (1999) Renal endosomes contain angiotensin peptides, converting enzyme, and AT_{1A} receptors. *Am. J. Physiol. Renal. Physiol.* **277**, F303–F311.
26. Ingert, C., Grima, M., Coquard, C., Barthelmebs, M., and Imbs, J. L. (2002) Contribution of angiotensin II internalization to intrarenal angiotensin II levels in rats. *Am. J. Physiol. Renal. Physiol.* **283**, F1003–F1010.
27. Navar, L. G., Harrison-Bernard, L. M., Wang, C.-T., Cervenka, L., and Mitchell, K. D. (1999) Concentrations and actions of intraluminal angiotensin II. *J. Am. Soc. Nephrol.* **10**, S189–S195.
28. van Kats, J. P., Schalekamp, M. A., Verdouw, P. D., Duncker, D. J., and Danser, A. H. (2001) Intrarenal angiotensin II: interstitial and cellular levels and site of production. *Kidney Int.* **60**, 2311–2317.
29. Helin, K., Tikkanen, I., Hohenthal, U., and Fyhrquist, F. (1994) Inhibition of either angiotensin-converting enzyme or neutral endopeptidase induces both enzymes. *Eur. J. Pharmacol.* **264**, 135–141.
30. Komlosi, P., Fuson, A. L., Fintha, A., et al. (2003) Angiotensin I conversion to angiotensin II stimulates cortical collecting duct sodium transport. *Hypertension* **42**, 195–199.
31. Cardini, J. F., Santos, R. A., Martins, A. S., Machado, R. P., and Alzamora, F. (1988) Site of entry of kininase II into renal tubular fluid. *Hypertension* **11**, I66–I68.
32. Casarini, D. E., Boim, M. A., Stella, R. C. R., Krieger-Azzolini, M. H., Krieger, J. E., and Schor, N. (1997) Angiotensin I-converting enzyme activity in tubular fluid along the rat nephron. *Am. J. Physiol. Renal. Physiol.* **272**, F405–F409.
33. Casarini, D. E., Carmona, A. K., Plavnik, F. L., Zanella, M. T., Juliano, L., and Ribeiro, A. B. (1995) Calcium channel blockers as inhibitors of angiotensin I-converting enzyme. *Hypertension* **26**, 1145–1148.
34. Field, L. J., McGowan, R. A., Dickinson, D. P., and Gross, K. W. (1984) Tissue and gene specificity of mouse renin expression. *Hypertension* **6**, 597–603.
35. Catanzaro, D. F., Mullins, J. J., and Morris, B. J. (1983) The biosynthetic pathway of renin in mouse submandibular gland. *J. Biol. Chem.* **258**, 7364–7368.

36. Sealey, J. E. and Laragh, J. H. (1975) "Prorenin" in human plasma? *Circ. Res.* **36,** 10–16.

37. Prescott, G., Silversides, D. W., and Reudelhuber, T. L. (2002) Tissue activity of circulating prorenin. *Am. J. Hypertens.* **15,** 280–285.

38. Ekker, M., Tronik, D., and Rougeon, F. (1989) Extra-renal transcription of the renin genes in multiple tissues of mice and rats. *Proc. Natl. Acad. Sci. USA* **86,** 5155–5158.

39. Iwai, N. and Inagami, T. (1992) Quantitative analysis of renin gene expression in extrarenal tissues by polymerase chain reaction method. *J. Hypertens.* **10,** 717–724.

40. Peters, J., Farrenkopf, R., Clausmeyer, S., et al. (2002) Functional significance of prorenin internalization in the rat heart. *Circ. Res.* **90,** 1135–1141.

41. Nguyen, G., Delarue, F., Burckle, C., Bouzhir, L., Giller, T., and Sraer, J. D. (2002) Pivotal role of the renin/prorenin receptor in angiotensin II production and cellular responses to renin. *J. Clin. Investig.* **109,** 1417–1427.

42. Nguyen, G., Delarue, F., Berrou, J., Rondeau, E., and Sraer, J. D. (1996) Specific receptor binding of renin on human mesangial cells in culture increases plasminogen activator inhibitor-1 antigen. *Kidney Int.* **50,** 1897–1903.

43. Sealey, J. E., Catanzaro, D. F., Lavin, T. N., et al. (1996) Specific prorenin/renin binding (ProBP). Identification and characterization of a novel membrane site. *Am. J. Hypertens.* **9,** 491–502.

44. Danser, A. H. J. and Saris, J. J. (2002) Prorenin uptake in the heart: a prerequisite for local angiotensin generation? *J. Mol. Cell. Cardiol.* **34,** 1463–1472.

45. Gomez, R. A., Lynch, K. R., Chevalier, R. L., et al. (1988) Renin and angiotensinogen gene expression and intrarenal renin distribution during ACE inhibition. *Am. J. Physiol. Renal. Physiol.* **254,** F900–F906.

46. Taugner, R., Mannek, E., Nobiling, R., et al. (1984) Coexistence of renin and angiotensin II in epitheloid cell secretory granules of rat kidney. *Histochemistry* **81,** 39–45.

47. Tank, J. E., Henrich, W. L., and Moe, O. W. (1997) Regulation of glomerular and proximal tubule renin mRNA by chronic changes in dietary NaCl. *Am. J. Physiol. Renal. Physiol.* **273,** F892–F898.

48. Moe, O. W., Ujiie, K., Star, R. A., et al. (1993) Renin expression in renal proximal tubule. *J. Clin. Investig.* **91,** 774–779.

49. Prieto-Carrasquero, M. C., Harrison-Bernard, L. M., Kobori, H., et al. (2004) Enhancement of collecting duct renin in angiotensin II-dependent hypertensive rats. *Hypertension* **44,** 223–229.

50. Henrich, W. L., McAllister, E. A., Eskue, A., Miller, T., and Moe, O. W. (1996) Renin regulation in cultured proximal tubular cells. *Hypertension* **27,** 1337–1340.

51. Lantelme, P., Rohrwasser, A., Gociman, B., et al. (2002) Effects of dietary sodium and genetic background on angiotensinogen and renin in mouse. *Hypertension* **39,** 1007–1014.

52. Gilbert, R. E., Wu, L. L., Kelly, D. J., et al. (1999) Pathological expression of renin and angiotensin II in the renal tubule after subtotal nephrectomy. Implications for the pathogenesis of tubulointerstitial fibrosis. *Am. J. Pathol.* **155,** 429–440.

53. Rohrwasser, A., Morgan, T., Dillon, H. F., et al. (1999) Elements of a paracrine tubular renin–angiotensin system along the entire nephron. *Hypertension* **34,** 1265–1274.

54. Schulz, W. W., Hagler, H. K., Buja, L. M., and Erdos, E. G. (1988) Ultrastructural localization of angiotensin I-converting enzyme (EC 3.4.15.1) and neutral metalloendopeptidase (EC 3.4.24.11) in the proximal tubule of the human kidney. *Lab. Investig.* **59,** 789–797.

55. Erdos, E. G. (1990) Angiotensin I converting enzyme and the changes in our concepts through the years. *Hypertension* **16,** 363–370.

56. Metzger, R., Bohle, R. M., Pauls, K., et al. (1999) Angiotensin-converting enzyme in non-neoplastic kidney diseases. *Kidney Int.* **56,** 1442–1454.

57. Danser, A. H., Admiraal, P. J. J., Derkx, F. H., and Schalekamp, M. A. (1988) Angiotensin I-to-II conversion in the human renal vascular bed. *J. Hypertens.* **16,** 2051–2056.

58. Admiraal, P. J. J., Derkx, F. H. M., Danser, A. H. J., Pieterman, H., and Schalekamp, M. A. D. H. (1990) Intrarenal de novo production of angiotensin I in subjects with renal artery stenosis. *Hypertension* **16,** 555–563.

59. Rosivall, L., Rinder, D. F., Champion, J., Khosla, M. C., Navar, L. G., and Oparil, S. (1983) Intrarenal angiotensin I conversion at normal and reduced renal blood flow in the dog. *Am. J. Physiol.* **245,** F408–F415.

60. Roks, A. J. and Henning, R. H. (2003) Angiotensin peptides: ready to re(de)fine the angiotensin system? *J. Hypertens.* **21,** 1269–1271.

61. Santos, R. A., Simoes e Silva, A. C., Maric, C., et al. (2003) Angiotensin-(1–7) is an endogenous ligand for the G protein-coupled receptor Mas. *Proc. Natl. Acad. Sci. USA* **100**, 8258–8263.

62. Stegbauer, J., Vonend, O., Oberhauser, V., and Rump, L. C. (2003) Effects of angiotensin-(1–7) and other bioactive components of the renin–angiotensin system on vascular resistance and noradrenaline release in rat kidney. *J. Hypertens.* **21**, 1391–1399.

63. Tipnis, S. R., Hooper, N. M., Hyde, R., Karran, E., Christie, G., and Turner, A. J. (2000) A human homolog of angiotensin-converting enzyme. Cloning and functional expression as a captopril-insensitive carboxypeptidase. *J. Biol. Chem.* **275**, 33,238–33,243.

64. Zhang, H., Wada, J., Hida, K., et al. (2001) Collectrin, a collecting duct-specific transmembrane glycoprotein, is a novel homolog of ACE2 and is developmentally regulated in embryonic kidneys. *J. Biol. Chem.* **276**, 17,132–17,139.

65. Zhang, H., Wada, J., Kanwar, Y. S., et al. (1999) Screening for genes up-regulated in 5/6 nephrectomized mouse kidney. *Kidney Int.* **56**, 549–558.

66. Goodfriend, T. L. (1993) Angiotensinases. In: *Renin-Angiotensin System* (Robertson, J. I. S. and Nichols, M. G., eds.), Gower Med Pub, London, pp. 1–5.

67. Tharaux, P.-L., Chatziantoniou, C., Fakhouri, F., and Dussaule, J.-C. (2000) Angiotensin II activates collagen I gene through a mechanism involving the MAP/ER kinase pathway. *Hypertension* **36**, 330–336.

68. Opie, L. H. and Sack, M. N. (2001) Enhanced angiotensin II activity in heart failure—reevaluation of the counterregulatory hypothesis of receptor subtypes. *Circ. Res.* **88**, 654–658.

69. Touyz, R. M. and Schiffrin, E. L. (2000) Signal transduction mechanisms mediating the physiological and pathophysiological actions of angiotensin II in vascular smooth muscle cells. *Pharmacol. Rev.* **52**, 639–672.

70. Ferrario, C. M., Averill, D. B., Brosnihan, K. B., et al. (2002) Vasopeptidase inhibition and Ang-(1–7) in the spontaneously hypertensive rat. *Kidney Int.* **62**, 1349–1357.

71. Unger, T. and Sandmann, S. (2000) Angiotensin receptor blocker selectivity at the AT_1- and AT_2-receptors: conceptual and clinical effects. *JRAAS* **1**, 6–9.

72. Carey, R. M., Wang, Z. Q., and Siragy, H. M. (2000) Role of the angiotensin type 2 receptor in the regulation of blood pressure and renal function. *Hypertension* **35**, 155–163.

73. Carey, R. M. and Siragy, H. M. (2003) The intrarenal renin–angiotensin system and diabetic nephropathy. *Trends Endocrinol. Metab.* **14**, 274–281.

74. Kobori, H., Harrison-Bernard, L. M., and Navar, L. G. (2001) Enhancement of angiotensinogen expression in angiotensin II-dependent hypertension. *Hypertension* **37**, 1329–1335.

75. Kobori, H., Harrison-Bernard, L. M., and Navar, L. G. (2001) Expression of angiotensinogen mRNA and protein in angiotensin II-dependent hypertension. *J. Am. Soc. Nephrol.* **12**, 431–439.

76. Darby, I. A. and Sernia, C. (1995) In situ hybridization and immunohistochemistry of renal angiotensinogen in neonatal and adult rat kidneys. *Cell Tissue Res.* **281**, 197–206.

77. Ingelfinger, J. R., Jung, F., Diamant, D., et al. (1999) Rat proximal tubule cell line transformed with origin-defective SV40 DNA: autocrine ANG II feedback. *Am. J. Physiol. Renal. Physiol.* **276**, F218–F227.

78. Lalouel, J.-M., Rohrwasser, A., Terreros, D., Morgan, T., and Ward, K. (2001) Angiotensinogen in essential hypertension: from genetics to nephrology. *J. Am. Soc. Nephrol.* **12**, 606–615.

79. Loghman-Adham, M., Rohrwasser, A., Helin, C., et al. (1997) A conditionally immortalized cell line from murine proximal tubule. *Kidney Int.* **52**, 229–239.

80. Ding, Y., Davisson, R. L., Hardy, D. O., et al. (1997) The kidney androgen-regulated protein promoter confers renal proximal tubule cell-specific and highly androgen-responsive expression on the human angiotensinogen gene in transgenic mice. *J. Biol. Chem.* **272**, 28,142–28,148.

81. Navar, L. G., Imig, J. D., Zou, L., and Wang, C.-T. (1997) Intrarenal production of angiotensin II. *Sem. Nephrol.* **17**, 412–422.

82. Jeunemaitre, X., Ménard, J., Clauser, E., and Corvol, P. (2000) Angiotensinogen: molecular biology and genetics. In: *Hypertension: Pathophysiology, Diagnosis, and Management* (Laragh, J. H. and Brenner, B. M., eds.), Vol. 1, 2nd ed., Raven, New York, pp. 1653–1665.

83. Kobori, H., Nishiyama, A., Harrison-Bernard, L. M., and Navar, L. G. (2003) Urinary angiotensinogen as an indicator of intrarenal angiotensin status in hypertension. *Hypertension* **41**, 42–49.

84. Modrall, J. G., Sadjadi, J., Brosnihan, K. B., et al. (2004) Depletion of tissue angiotensin-converting enzyme differentially influences the intrarenal and urinary expression of angiotensin peptides. *Hypertension* **43**, 849–853.

85. Iwai, N. and Inagami, T. (1992) Identification of two subtypes in rat type I angiotensin II receptor. *FEBS Lett.* **298,** 257–260.
86. Sasamura, H., Hein, L., Krieger, J. E., Pratt, R. E., Kobilka, B. K., and Dzau, V. J. (1992) Cloning, characterization, and expression of two angiotensin receptor (AT-1) isoforms from the mouse genome. *Biochem. Biophys. Res. Commun.* **185,** 253–259.
87. Iwai, N., Yamano, Y., Chaki, S., et al. (1991) Rat angiotensin II receptor: cDNA sequence and regulation of the gene expression. *Biochem. Biophys. Res. Commun.* **177,** 299–304.
88. Murphy, T. J., Alexander, R. W., Griendling, K. K., Runge, M. S., and Bernstein, K. E. (1991) Isolation of a cDNA encoding the vascular type-1 angiotensin II receptor. *Nature (Lond)* **351,** 233–236.
89. Nakajima, M., Mukoyama, M., Pratt, R. E., Horiuchi, M., and Dzau, V. J. (1993) Cloning of cDNA and analysis of the gene for mouse angiotensin II type 2 receptor. *Biochem. Biophys. Res. Commun.* **197,** 393–399.
90. Tsuzuki, S., Ichiki, T., Nakakubo, H., Kitami, Y., Guo, D. F., and Shirai, H. (1994) Molecular cloning and expression of the gene encoding human angiotensin II type 2 receptor. *Biochem. Biophys. Res. Commun.* **200,** 1449–1454.
91. Ito, M., Oliverio, M. I., Mannon, P. J., et al. (1995) Regulation of blood pressure by the type 1A angiotensin II receptor gene. *Proc. Natl. Acad. Sci. USA* **92,** 3521–3525.
92. Cervenka, L., Mitchell, K. D., Oliverio, M. I., Coffman, T. M., and Navar, L. G. (1999) Renal function in the AT_{1A} receptor knockout mouse during normal and volume-expanded conditions. *Kidney Int.* **56,** 1855–1862.
93. Oliverio, M. I., Best, C. F., Smithies, O., and Coffman, T. M. (2000) Regulation of sodium balance and blood pressure by the AT(1A) receptor for angiotensin II. *Hypertension* **35,** 550–554.
94. Meister, B., Lippoldt, A., Bunnemann, B., Inagami, T., Ganten, D., and Fuxe, K. (1993) Cellular expression of angiotensin type-1 receptor mRNA in the kidney. *Kidney Int.* **44,** 331–336.
95. Tufro-McReddie, A., Harrison, J. K., Everett, A. D., and Gomez, R. A. (1993) Ontogeny of type 1 angiotensin II receptor gene expression in the rat. *J. Clin. Investig.* **91,** 530–537.
96. Gasc, J.-M., Monnot, C., Clauser, E., and Corvol, P. (1993) Co-expression of type 1 angiotensin II receptor (AT_1R) and renin mRNAs in juxtaglomerular cells of the rat kidney. *Endocrinology* **132,** 2723–2725.
97. Bouby, N., Hus-Citharel, A., Marchetti, J., Bankir, L., Corvol, P., and Llorens-Cortes, C. (1997) Expression of type 1 angiotensin II receptor subtypes and angiotensin II-induced calcium mobilization along the rat nephron. *J. Am. Soc. Nephrol.* **8,** 1658–1667.
98. Ruan, X. P., Wagner, C., Chatziantoniou, C., Kurtz, A., and Arendshorst, W. J. (1997) Regulation of angiotensin II receptor AT_1 subtypes in renal afferent arterioles during chronic changes in sodium diet. *J. Clin. Investig.* **99,** 1072–1081.
99. Prieto, M., Dipp, S., Meleg-Smith, S., and El Dahr, S. S. (2001) Ureteric bud derivatives express angiotensinogen and AT1 receptors. *Physiol. Genom.* **6,** 29–37.
100. Douglas, J. G. (1987) Angiotensin receptor subtypes of the kidney cortex. *Am. J. Physiol. Renal. Physiol.* **253,** F1–F7.
101. Mendelsohn, F. A. O., Dunbar, M., Allen, A., et al. (1986) Angiotensin II receptors in the kidney. *Fed. Proc.* **45,** 1420–1425.
102. Burns, K. D., Inagami, T., and Harris, R. C. (1993) Cloning of a rabbit kidney cortex AT_1 angiotensin II receptor that is present in proximal tubule epithelium. *Am. J. Physiol. Renal. Physiol.* **264,** F645–F654.
103. Paxton, W. G., Runge, M., Horaist, C., Cohen, C., Alexander, R. W., and Bernstein, K. E. (1993) Immunohistochemical localization of rat angiotensin II AT_1 receptor. *Am. J. Physiol. Renal. Physiol.* **264,** F989–F995.
104. Zhuo, J., Alcorn, D., McCausland, J., and Mendelsohn, F. A. O. (1994) Localization and regulation of angiotensin II receptors in renomedullary interstitial cells. *Kidney Int.* **46,** 1483–1485.
105. Harrison-Bernard, L. M., Navar, L. G., Ho, M. M., Vinson, G. P., and El-Dahr, S. S. (1997) Immunohistochemical localization of ANG II AT_1 receptor in adult rat kidney using a monoclonal antibody. *Am. J. Physiol. Renal. Physiol.* **273,** F170–F177.
106. Miyata, N., Park, F., Li, X. F., and Cowley, A. W. Jr. (1999) Distribution of angiotensin AT_1 and AT_2 receptor subtypes in the rat kidney. *Am. J. Physiol.* **277,** F437–F446.
107. Harrison-Bernard, L. M., Cook, A. K., Oliverio, M. I., and Coffman, T. M. (2003) Renal segmental microvascular responses to ANG II in AT1A receptor null mice. *Am. J. Physiol. Renal. Physiol.* **284,** F538–F545.

108. Cheng, H. F., Becker, B. N., Burns, K. D., and Harris, R. C. Angiotensin II upregulates type-1 angiotensin II receptors in renal proximal tubule. *J. Clin. Investig.* **95,** 2012–2019.

109. Amiri, F. and Garcia, R. (1997) Renal angiotensin II receptor regulation in two-kidney, one clip hypertensive rats. Effect of ACE inhibition. *Hypertension* **30,** 337–344.

110. Amiri, F., Haddad, G., and Garcia, R. (1999) Renal angiotensin II receptor regulation and renin–angiotensin system inhibition in one-kidney, one clip hypertensive rats. *J. Hypertens.* **17,** 279–286.

111. Harrison-Bernard, L. M., El-Dahr, S. S., O'Leary, D. F., and Navar, L. G. (1999) Regulation of angiotensin II type 1 receptor mRNA and protein in angiotensin II-induced hypertension. *Hypertension* **33,** 340–346.

112. Wang, Z.-Q., Millatt, L. J., Heiderstadt, N. T., Siragy, H. M., Johns, R. A., and Carey, R. M. (1999) Differential regulation of renal angiotensin subtype AT_{1A} and AT_2 receptor protein in rats with angiotensin-dependent hypertension. *Hypertension* **33,** 96–101.

113. Zhuo, J., Ohishi, M., and Mendelsohn, F. A. O. (1999) Roles of AT_1 and AT_2 receptors in the hypertensive *Ren-2* gene transgenic rat kidney. *Hypertension* **33,** 347–353.

114. Harrison-Bernard, L. M., Zhuo, J., Kobori, H., Ohishi, M., and Navar, L. G. (2001) Intrarenal AT1 receptor and ACE binding in angiotensin II-induced hypertensive rats. *Am. J. Physiol. Renal. Physiol.* **281,** F19–F25.

115. Norwood, V. F., Garmey, M., Wolford, J., Carey, R. M., and Gomez, R. A. (2000) Novel expression and regulation of the renin–angiotensin system in metanephric organ culture. *Am. J. Physiol. Regul. Integr. Comp. Physiol.* **279,** R522–R530.

116. Siragy, H. M., Jaffa, A. A., and Margolius, H. S. (1997) Bradykinin B_2 receptor modulates renal prostaglandin E_2 and nitric oxide. *Hypertension* **29,** 757–762.

117. Siragy, H. M. and Carey, R. M. (1999) Protective role of the angiotensin AT_2 receptor in a renal wrap hypertension model. *Hypertension* **33,** 1237–1242.

118. de Gasparo, M. and Siragy, H. M. (1999) The AT_2 receptor: fact, fancy and fantasy. *Regul. Pept.* **81,** 11–24.

119. Jin, X. H., Siragy, H. M., and Carey, R. M. (2001) Renal interstitial cGMP mediates natriuresis by direct tubule mechanism. *Hypertension* **38,** 309–316.

120. Siragy, H. M., Inagami, T., Ichiki, T., and Carey, R. M. (1999) Sustained hypersensitivity to angiotensin II and its mechanism in mice lacking the subtype-2 (AT_2) angiotensin receptor. *Proc. Natl. Acad. Sci. USA* **96,** 6506–6510.

121. Navar, L. G., Harrison-Bernard, L. M., and Imig, J. D. (1998) Compartmentalization of intrarenal angiotensin II. In: *Renin–Angiotensin* (Ulfendahl, H. R. and Aurell, M., eds.), Portland, London, pp. 193–208.

122. Ingert, C., Grima, M., Coquard, C., Barthelmebs, M., and Imbs, J. L. (2002) Effects of dietary salt changes on renal renin–angiotensin system in rats. *Am. J. Physiol. Renal. Physiol.* **283,** F995–F1002.

123. Siragy, H. M., Howell, N. L., Ragsdale, N. V., and Carey, R. M. (1995) Renal interstitial fluid angiotensin: modulation by anesthesia, epinephrine, sodium depletion and renin inhibition. *Hypertension* **25,** 1021–1024.

124. Nishiyama, A., Seth, D. M., and Navar, L. G. (2002) Renal interstitial fluid concentrations of angiotensins I and II in anesthetized rats. *Hypertension* **39,** 129–134.

125. Nishiyama, A., Seth, D. M., and Navar, L. G. (2002) Renal interstitial fluid angiotensin I and angiotensin II concentrations during local angiotensin-converting enzyme inhibition. *J. Am. Soc. Nephrol.* **13,** 2207–2212.

126. Nishiyama, A., Seth, D. E., and Navar, L. G. (2001) Renal interstitial concentrations of angiotensin I and angiotensin II in angiotensin II-infused hypertensive rats. *J. Am. Soc. Nephrol.* **12,** 574A.

127. Navar, L. G., Harrison-Bernard, L. M., Nishiyama, A., and Kobori, H. (2002) Regulation of intrarenal angiotensin II in hypertension. *Hypertension* **39,** 316–322.

128. Wang, C.-T., Chin, S. Y., and Navar, L. G. (2000) Impairment of pressure-natriuresis and renal autoregulation in ANG II-infused hypertensive rats. *Am. J. Physiol. Renal. Physiol.* **279,** F319–F325.

129. Kobori, H., Nishiyama, A., Abe, Y., and Navar, L. G. (2003) Enhancement of intrarenal angiotensinogen in Dahl salt-sensitive rats on high salt diet. *Hypertension* **41,** 592–597.

130. Kobori, H., Prieto-Carrasquero, M. C., Ozawa, Y., and Navar, L. G. (2004) AT1 receptor mediated augmentation of intrarenal angiotensinogen in angiotensin II-dependent hypertension. *Hypertension* **43,** 1126–1132.

131. Cervenka, L., Wang, C.-T., Mitchell, K. D., and Navar, L. G. (1999) Proximal tubular angiotensin II levels and renal functional responses to AT_1 receptor blockade in nonclipped kidneys of Goldblatt hypertensive rats. *Hypertension* **33,** 102–107.

132. Mitchell, K. D., Jacinto, S. M., and Mullins, J. J. (1997) Proximal tubular fluid, kidney, and plasma levels of angiotensin II in hypertensive ren-2 transgenic rats. *Am. J. Physiol. Renal. Physiol.* **273,** F246–F253.

133. Wang, C.-T., Navar, L. G., and Mitchell, K. D. (2003) Proximal tubular fluid angiotensin II levels in angiotensin II-induced hypertensive rats. *J. Hypertens.* **21,** 353–360.

134. Boer, W. H., Braam, B., Fransen, R., Boer, P., and Koomans, H. A. (1997) Effects of reduced renal perfusion pressure and acute volume expansion on proximal tubule and whole kidney angiotensin II content in the rat. *Kidney Int.* **51,** 44–49.

135. Wang, T. and Giebisch, G. (1996) Effects of angiotensin II on electrolyte transport in the early and late distal tubule in rat kidney. *Am. J. Physiol. Renal. Physiol.* **271,** F143–F149.

136. Peti-Peterdi, J., Warnock, D. G., and Bell, P. D. (2002) Angiotensin II directly stimulates ENaC activity in the cortical collecting duct via AT(1) receptors. *J. Am. Soc. Nephrol.* **13,** 1131–1135.

137. Zou, L., Imig, J. D., Hymel, A., and Navar, L. G. (1998) Renal uptake of circulating angiotensin II in Val^5-angiotensin II infused rats is mediated by AT_1 receptor. *Am. J. Hypertens.* **11,** 570–578.

138. van Kats, J. P., de Lannoy, L. M., Danser, A. H. J., van Meegen, J. R., Verdouw, P. D., and Schalekamp, M. A. D. H. (1997) Angiotensin II type 1 (AT_1) receptor-mediated accumulation of angiotensin II in tissues and its intracellular half-life in vivo. *Hypertension* **30,** 42–49.

139. Zhuo, J. L., Imig, J. D., Hammond, T. G., Orengo, S., Benes, E., and Navar, L. G. (2002) Ang II accumulation in rat renal endosomes during Ang II-induced hypertension: role of AT(1) receptor. *Hypertension* **39,** 116–121.

140. Hein, L., Meinel, L., Pratt, R. E., Dzau, V. J., and Kobilka, B. K. (1997) Intracellular trafficking of angiotensin II and its AT_1 and AT_2 receptors: evidence for selective sorting of receptor and ligand. *Mol. Endocrinol.* **11,** 1266–1277.

141. Chen, R., Mukhin, Y. V., Garnovskaya, M. N., et al. (2000) A functional angiotensin II receptor–GFP fusion protein: evidence for agonist-dependent nuclear translocation. *Am. J. Physiol. Renal. Physiol.* **279,** F440–F448.

142. Linas, S. L. (1997) Role of receptor mediated endocytosis in proximal tubule epithelial function. *Kidney Int.* **52(Suppl 61),** S18–S21.

143. Becker, B. N., Cheng, H.-F., and Harris, R. C. (1997) Apical ANG II-stimulated PLA_2 activity and Na^+ flux: a potential role for Ca^{2+}-independent PLA_2. *Am. J. Physiol. Renal. Physiol.* **273,** F554–F562.

144. Haller, H., Lindschau, C., Erdmann, B., Quass, P., and Luft, F. C. (1996) Effects of intracellular angiotensin II in vascular smooth muscle cells. *Circ. Res.* **79,** 765–772.

145. Licea, H., Walters, M. R., and Navar, L. G. (2002) Renal nuclear angiotensin II receptors in normal and hypertensive rats. *Acta Physiol. Hung.* **89,** 427–438.

146. Schunkert, H., Ingelfinger, J. R., Jacob, H., Jackson, B., Bouyounes, B., and Dzau, V. J. (1992) Reciprocal feedback regulation of kidney angiotensinogen and renin mRNA expressions by angiotensin II. *Am. J. Physiol. Endocrinol. Metab.* **263,** E863–E869.

147. Kobori, H., Harrison-Bernard, L. M., and Navar, L. G. (2002) Urinary excretion of angiotensinogen reflects intrarenal angiotensinogen production. *Kidney Int.* **61,** 579–585.

148. Kodama, K., Adachi, H., and Sonoda, J. (1997) Beneficial effects of long-term enalapril treatment and low-salt intake on survival rate of Dahl salt-sensitive rats with established hypertension. *J. Pharmacol. Exp. Ther.* **283,** 625–629.

149. Otsuka, F., Yamauchi, T., Kataoka, H., Mimura, Y., Ogura, T., and Makino, H. (1998) Effects of chronic inhibition of ACE and AT_1 receptors on glomerular injury in Dahl salt-sensitive rats. *Am. J. Physiol. Regul. Integr. Comp. Physiol.* **274,** R1797–R1806.

150. Hayakawa, H., Coffee, K., and Raij, L. (1997) Endothelial dysfunction and cardiorenal injury in experimental salt-sensitive hypertension: effects of antihypertensive therapy. *Circ. Res.* **96,** 2407–2413.

151. Nishikimi, T., Mori, Y., Kobayashi, N., et al. (2002) Renoprotective effect of chronic adrenomedullin infusion in Dahl salt- sensitive rats. *Hypertension* **39,** 1077–1082.

152. Beutler, K. T., Masilamani, S., Turban, S., et al. (2003) Long-term regulation of ENaC expression in kidney by angiotensin II. *Hypertension* **41,** 1143–1150.

153. Ma, L.-J., Nakamura, S., Whitsitt, J. S., Marcantoni, C., Davidson, J. M., and Fogo, A. B. (2000) Regression of sclerosis in aging by an angiotensin inhibition-induced decrease in PAI-1. *Kidney Int.* **58,** 2425–2436.

154. Nakamura, S., Nakamura, I., Ma, L., Vaughan, D. E., and Fogo, A. B. (2000) Plasminogen activator inhibitor-1 expression is regulated by the angiotensin type 1 receptor in vivo. *Kidney Int.* **58,** 251–259.

155. Taal, M. W., Chertow, G. M., Rennke, H. G., et al. (2001) Mechanisms underlying renoprotection during renin–angiotensin system blockade. *Am. J. Physiol. Renal. Physiol.* **280,** F343–F355.

2

Cardiac and Vascular Renin–Angiotensin Systems

Rajesh Kumar, Kenneth M. Baker, and Jing Pan

CONTENTS

INTRODUCTION
NOVEL COMPONENTS OF THE RAS
THE CARDIAC RAS
THE VASCULAR RAS
ANG II-MEDIATED SIGNALING PATHWAYS
AT$_1$-MEDIATED INTRACELLULAR SIGNALING
AT$_1$-MEDIATED TYROSINE PHOSPHORYLATION
NON-RECEPTOR TYROSINE KINASE ACTIVATION
RECEPTOR TYROSINE KINASES
MITOGEN-ACTIVATED PROTEIN KINASES
SMALL G PROTEINS
GENERATION OF REACTIVE OXYGEN SPECIES
SUMMARY AND CONCLUSIONS
REFERENCES

1. INTRODUCTION

Angiotensin II (Ang II), a peptide hormone, is the primary product of the renin–angiotensin system (RAS). The main effects of Ang II are related to the control of cardiovascular, renal and adrenal functions, as related to fluid and electrolyte balance, and arterial pressure. In addition, the octapeptide Ang II also affects cell growth, apoptosis, fibrosis, inflammation, and coagulation. The classical RAS involves the biosynthesis of the enzyme renin in the juxtaglomerular cells of the kidney. Active renin cleaves angiotensinogen (Ao), which is synthesized in the liver to form the deca-peptide angiotensin I (Ang I). Angiotensin I is acted upon by angiotensin-converting enzyme (ACE), a primarily membrane bound glycoprotein, which hydrolyzes the Ang I into the biologically active Ang II. The majority of the actions of Ang II are attributed to the interaction of the peptide with the Ang II, type 1 plasma membrane (AT$_1$) receptor.

From: *Contemporary Endocrinology: Hypertension and Hormone Mechanisms*
Edited by: R. M. Carey © Humana Press Inc., Totowa, NJ

The AT_1 is a seven-transmembrane spanning, heterotrimeric G protein-coupled receptor (GPCR) that activates multiple signal transduction pathways. An AT_2 receptor, which in large part couples to effector pathways that antagonize the AT_1 effects, is also present in the cardiovascular tissue. The AT_2 receptor function will be discussed in more detail in Chapter 5. In addition to the classical, circulating RAS, locally derived RASs have been described in many studies on organs and tissues, including the heart and vasculature. Clinical, animal, and cell culture studies support the concept that these local RASs can act in an autocrine, paracrine, and/or intracrine manner. In this chapter, we describe the data that support the existence of a local RAS in the heart and vasculature and detail the signaling pathways by which locally generated Ang II may effect the responses described earlier.

Approximately 25 yr ago the first data were presented that a local RAS may be functional in the kidney (1). These initial observations have now been extended to many organs and tissues. There are substantial data that suggest a biologically/physiologically and pathologically relevant intracardiac RAS in the heart. To separate the circulating RAS from a local RAS, a number of criteria need to be met. The mRNAs for the components of the system (renin, Ao, and ACE) necessary for the biosynthesis of Ang II should be present in the tissue (1). However, a caveat is that if Ao is present, alternative conversion pathways may exist in the biosynthesis of Ang II. For example, chymase is an abundant enzyme in cardiac tissue (including human heart) that can convert Ang I to Ang II. Human blood vessels can also generate Ang II by a chymase-dependent pathway. Chymase-dependent Ang II formation also affects vascular proliferation in grafted veins (2). In the heart, renin mRNA is present, though in minuscule amounts. Because circulating renin and prorenin are efficiently taken up by the heart, this may be the likely source of cardiac renin. Additionally, several studies suggest that the endothelium mediates vascular Ang II formation via the cellular uptake of renin (1). Secondly, a biologically active product (Ang II) needs to be synthesized in the tissue. Importantly, the receptors (AT_1) or recognition sites for the peptide need to be present, so that local responses can be mediated. The local system should be regulated within the tissue in a manner that is independent of the circulating RAS. Finally, the product should produce a physiological or pathophysiological response that can be separated from the circulating system (1). One of the most difficult aspects of performing research in this area has been the conclusive in vivo demonstration of separate regulation and actions for the circulating and local RASs.

There is a substantial evidence to support the role of Ang II as a modulator involved in the process of cardiac remodeling that occurs in association with pressure overload or myocardial ischemia. There are many studies that demonstrate the efficacy of ACE inhibitors and AT_1 receptor antagonists in blocking cardiac hypertrophy and extracellular matrix deposition. Additionally, recent multicenter clinical trials suggest that these agents reduce morbidity and mortality associated with heart failure, as well as among the survivors of myocardial infarction, beyond that predicted by blood pressure reduction alone. That the antihypertensive actions of ACE inhibitors correlate better with the inhibition of tissue ACE than plasma ACE and that hypertensive patients with normal or low levels of systemic RAS activity can be effectively treated with inhibitors of the RAS, strongly supports the concept of a tissue RAS (3). A number of transgenic animal studies support the functional significance of a cardiac RAS. Targeted cardiac myocyte overexpression of Ao, resulted in increases in cardiac Ang II concentration and both left and right ventricular hypertrophy, unaccompanied by any increase in arterial pressure or circulating levels of Ang II. In other experiments in which the AT_1 expression was targeted to the cardiac ventricles in transgenic rats, there was an increase in the hypertrophic response to pressure or volume overload. Thus, there was a synergism between mechanical load and AT_1 activation in inducing cardiac hypertrophy. AT_{1A} knockout mice showed diminished left ventricular remodeling and improved survival after myocardial infarction. However, in a different AT_{1A} knockout study, pressure overload-induced hypertrophy was not prevented, suggesting that compensatory mechanisms were activated following AT_{1A} gene deletion in early embryogenesis. Transgenic mice that express Ao in the liver and brain, but not in the heart, exhibited less cardiac hypertrophy, and perivascular and interstitial fibrosis *(4)*. Recent studies that used adenoviral and plasmid vectors, which were constructed to express Ang II intracellularly, demonstrated hypertrophic growth in primary cultures of cardiomyocytes and significant cardiac hypertrophy in adult mice (without an increase in blood pressure or in circulating Ang II concentrations), respectively *(5)*. These latter observations were not blocked by AT_1 antagonists, suggesting an intracellular recognition site, independent of the plasma membrane AT_1 and are consistent with an intracrine mechanism of action *(4)*. Overall, there are many in vitro (isolated cells) and in vivo (whole animal) studies, coupled with experimental observations in humans, suggest that functionally relevant tissue and organ (local) RASs exist. The remainder of this chapter details the functional aspects and the signal transduction pathways, important in mediating the cellular effects of the cardiac and vascular RASs.

2. NOVEL COMPONENTS OF THE RAS

Recently, additional components of the RAS and their biological functions have been identified. A second isoform of renin, called renin 1A, lacking the secretory signal peptide has been identified and transcripts were detected in brain, adrenal, and heart *(6)*. Kidneys express only the full-length transcript of renin. In addition to enzymatically cleaving Ao into Ang I, renin was shown to bind the mannose-6-phosphate receptor, but without functional effects. A renin receptor has now been cloned from mesangial cells *(1)*. Binding of renin or prorenin to this receptor activates mitogen-activated protein (MAP) kinase signaling and increases the catalytic efficiency of Ao to Ang I conversion. The receptor mRNA is expressed highly in heart, brain, placenta, and to lower levels in kidney and liver. A new homolog of ACE, angiotensin-converting enzyme 2 (ACE2) has been discovered *(7)*. ACE2 has significant sequence homology to ACE; however, it differs in enzymatic activity. In contrast to ACE, ACE2 cleaves Ang I to Ang (1–9) and Ang II to Ang (1–7), effectively inhibiting the formation of Ang II. In addition to Ang II, additional biological active peptide fragments of Ao have been demonstrated. Ang (1–7) is a heptapeptide that is formed, either from Ang I or Ang II, by the action of several peptidases, such as neutral-endopeptidase, prolyl-endopeptidase, prolyl-carboxypeptidase, and by ACE2. Ang (1–7) has opposite actions to Ang II, exhibiting vasodilatory and antiproliferative effects. The cardiovascular effects of ACE inhibitors are attributed to changes in Ang II and bradykinin levels. According to a recent evidence, ACE is also involved in outside-in signaling in endothelial cells, and "ACE signaling" may be an important cellular mechanism contributing to the beneficial effects of ACE inhibitors *(8)*. ACE inhibitors increased the activity of ACE-associated Jun N-terminal kinase (JNK) and elicited the accumulation of phosphorylated c-Jun in the nucleus *(8)*. Ang (3–8), known as angiotensin IV (Ang IV), is another biologically active metabolite formed from Ang II by aminopeptidases A and N. Ang IV has an important role in the memory enhancing and hypertensive effects of Ang II in animal models.

3. THE CARDIAC RAS

3.1. Synthesis and Regulation

The concept of a local cardiac RAS is generally accepted, with the demonstration of RAS components and differential regulation by physiological and pharmacological perturbations. Cardiac RAS activity is under the control of tissue-specific regulatory influences and differs from that of the systemic RAS. For example, an increase in left ventricular mass produced by abdominal aortic constriction can be prevented by an ACE inhibitor, with no change in the afterload *(9)*. There is an evidence that most of the cardiac Ang II is synthesized at the site and is not taken up from the circulation. A quantitative study using radiolabeled Ao infusion has shown that more than 90% of cardiac Ang I and 75% of cardiac Ang II are synthesized at cardiac sites *(10)*. The components for Ang II biosynthesis are present in both cardiac myocytes and fibro-blasts. The interstitial concentration of Ang II in the heart is about 100-fold more than that of plasma, though the myocardial concentration of renin and Ao is only 1–4% that of plasma *(1)*. There is a debate about which and in what amount RAS components are synthesized locally or are taken up from the plasma. Much of the controversy surrounds the source of renin in the heart. Active uptake from the plasma, by endothelial cells, cardiomyocytes and fibroblasts, in addition to de novo synthesis, has been proposed. Two uptake mechanisms have been described, one that is mediated by the mannose-6-phosphate receptor and another that is not. The former mainly represents a clearance mechanism of circulating glycosylated prorenin by heart cells; whereas the latter mechanism takes up non-glycosylated prorenin and results in an intracellular generation of angiotensin peptides *(11)*. Emerging evidence suggests that under specific circum-stances renin is synthesized in cardiovascular tissues. Renin mRNA has been detected in cardiac atria, ventricles, and primary cultures of neonatal and adult rat ventricular myocytes *(12,13)*. Increased levels of renin mRNA have been reported in patients sustaining a myocardial infarction and in the ventricles of animals with experimental models of infarction *(14)*. Renin mRNA and protein have been detected in canine cardiac myocytes, levels of which are upregulated by ventricular-pacing-induced cardiac failure *(15)*. A second renin transcript, lacking the coding region for the secre-tory signal peptide and named Exon 1A renin, has been detected in brain, adrenal, and heart *(6)*. Interestingly, Exon 1A renin is the only transcript of the renin expressed in heart. The latter observation may help to explain the discrepancy in the literature regarding renin expression in the heart. The methods applied in studies with negative results, might not have detected this newly identified transcript. This potentially intracellular renin coding mRNA is upregulated in the left ventricle following myocardial infarction. Thus, the possibility of two cardiac RASs has been suggested, one is the intracardiac RAS, and another intracellular RAS driven by Exon 1A renin *(11)*. The local production of Ao and ACE is less controversial. Ao mRNA and protein have been detected in the hearts of human, dog, and rat, as well as in rat cardiac myocytes and fibroblasts in primary cell culture *(13)*. Upregulation of the Ao gene in an experimental model of pressure overload has been reported *(16)*. ACE has been detected in human and rat heart, with higher amounts in atria compared to the ventricles. Endothelial cells and fibroblasts appear to be the major cell types of the heart that express ACE. ACE has also been detected in primary cultures of adult and neonatal cardiac myocytes *(12,17)*. There also exist other enzymes such as cathepsins, chymase, and ACE2 that can substitute for renin and ACE in the processing of Ao in the heart. Cathepsin D has been shown to cleave Ao into Ang II, and chymase can convert Ang I to Ang II. Chymase is highly specific for Ang I and does not degrade bradykinin and vasoactive intestinal peptide. In myocardial extracts from humans and dogs, chymase accounts for about 90% of Ang II forming activity, although the role in intact heart is unknown *(13)*. Thus, it remains unclear in which situation renin- or ACE-independent Ang II synthesis occurs. ACE2 affects Ang II levels by converting Ang I into Ang (1–9) and Ang II into Ang (1–7). ACE2 expression is significantly increased in failing human heart *(18)*. ACE2 knockout mice have left ventricular dysfunction and wall thinning, along with increased Ang II levels. ACE and ACE2 double-knockout completely prevents cardiac abnormalities and the increase in Ang II production *(7)*. On the other hand, transgenic mice with increased cardiac ACE2 expression show a high incidence of sudden death owing to ventricular tachycardia and ventricular fibrillation, as a result of gap junction remodeling *(19)*. Local generation of Ang (1–7) in the myocardium of dogs *(20)* and elevation of Ang (1–7) in cardiac myocytes during development of heart failure, subsequent to coronary artery ligation, has been reported *(21)*. In addition, intravenous infusion of Ang (1–7) attenuates the development of heart failure after myocardial infarction, suggesting a role for this peptide in cardiac remodeling *(22)*.

The activity of the cardiac RAS is influenced by several pathophysiological conditions. Volume overload is associated with the increased expression of renin and ACE, whereas pressure overload increases the expression of Ao and AT_1 *(13)*. Mechanical stretch of cardiac myocytes increases Ang II release from the cells. Ao gene expression is increased in the heart by cardiotrophin-1, glucocorticoids, estrogen, and thyroid hormone *(13,23)*. Ang II stimulates the production of atrial natriuretic peptide, which in turn regulates renin and Ao mRNA levels *(13)*. Ang II has a differential effect on renin and Ao expression in cardiac myocytes and fibroblasts, positively regulating the former, whereas negatively regulating the latter. Cardiac fibroblasts also secrete a factor that upregulates Ao gene expression by cardiac myocytes *(4)*. Together, these observations suggest that the cardiac RAS represents a self-sustaining paracrine–autocrine loop, involving both cardiac myocytes and fibroblasts *(4)* (Fig. 1).

3.2. Intracrine Cardiac RAS

In addition to autocrine–paracrine functions of a cardiac RAS, there is a substantial evidence for intracellular (intracrine) actions of Ang II in heart *(24)*. Our recent studies have shown that intracellular expression of Ang II in cultured cardiac myocytes, and in mice hearts using a specific promoter, results in hypertrophic cell growth and in biventricular hypertrophy, respectively *(5)*. This is accompanied by an increase in gene expression, but without any change in blood pressure. Ang II non-peptide

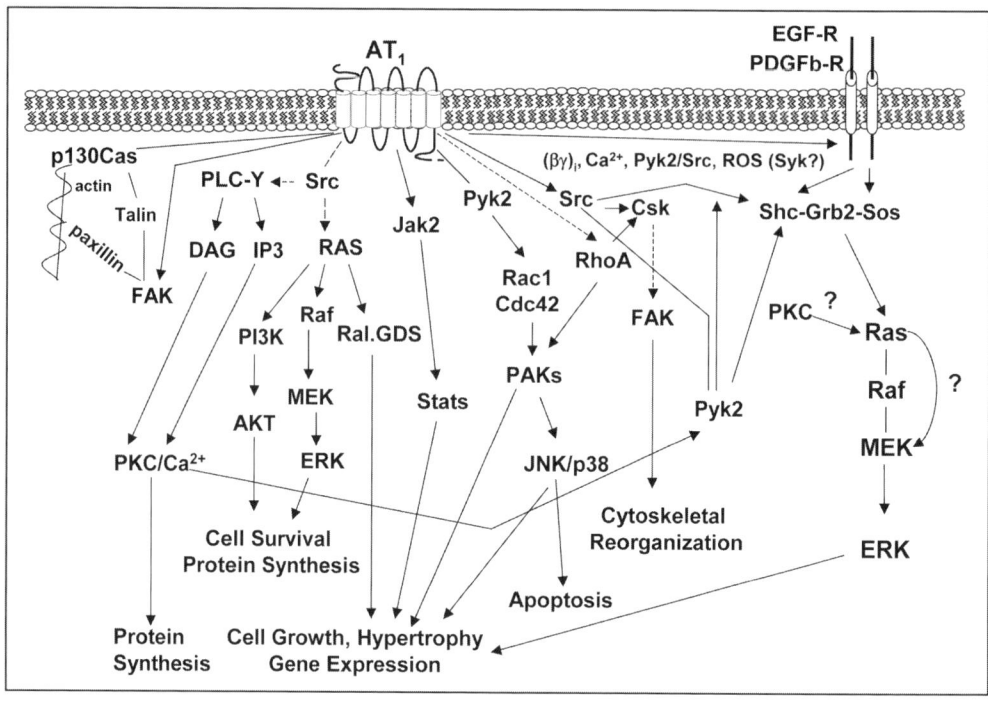

Fig. 1. Cardiac and vascular renin–angiotensin system. The components of the RAS are present in both vascular and the cardiac tissues. A significant amount of Ang II production occurs at local sites, from the precursors of local and circulatory origin. Based on the origin and site of action of Ang II, the biological effects can be categorized as endocrine, autocrine/paracrine, and intracrine.

receptor antagonists do not block the intracellular effects of Ang II in cardiac tissue. The physiological significance of intracellular effects of Ang II has not been established. An intracrine RAS might provide an essential part of a self-sustaining cardiac RAS loop.

4. THE VASCULAR RAS

4.1. Synthesis and Regulation

Local production of Ang I and Ang II in vascular smooth muscle, endothelial, and endocardial cells has been widely recognized. Angiotensinogen gene expression in the vasculature was reported in the 1980s (25,26). Angiotensinogen expression was observed in the medial smooth muscle layer, as well as in periaortic adipose tissue. Dietary sodium and vascular injury regulated the expression of angiotensinogen in the smooth muscle layer (26,27). Insulin-like growth factor (IGF)-1, as well as insulin, stimulates Ao production and vascular smooth muscle cell (VSMC) growth. In contrast, both low and high levels of insulin suppress Ao and renin expression in cultured endothelial cells; however, high doses of insulin stimulate ACE activity. These observations suggest that insulin regulates VSMC growth and endothelial function via bifunctional modulation of vascular angiotensin generation (28). ACE is constitutively expressed in endothelial cells, but can also be detected at low levels in VSMC. In rats, the ACE activity can be induced in VSMC, in vivo, by experimental hypertension or vascular injury and by corticosteroid treatment. ACE is upregulated in the human atherosclerotic plaque and more particularly at the shoulder of the plaque, the most vulnerable site for rupture. ACE-independent generation of Ang II by chymase, the latter being produced by mast cells in atherosclerotic lesions, also seems to be significant. The synthesis of renin in blood vessels is still a matter of debate. It is possible that renin expression is very low or undetectable under normal physiological conditions and increased in certain pathological situations. A transgenic mouse model, in which human renin promoter directed tissue-specific and regulated expression of a β-galactosidase reporter gene mimicking endogenous renin, has shown β-galactosidase staining in kidney afferent arterioles and in larger arteries (renal arteries, aorta to iliac arteries) outside the kidney *(29)*. In larger vessels, β-galactosidase expression is observed in discrete areas, separated by regions of non-expressing cells. Renin mRNA and protein have been detected in the spiral arteries of human uterus. Renin message and protein are increased in vascular cells following carotid artery injury in the rat, suggesting that locally synthesized renin has a role in the medial thickening that follows. Renin mRNA concentration is markedly increased in 24 h after balloon injury, and renin is transiently expressed in medial VSMC, as demonstrated by an immunohistochemical analysis *(30)*. AT_1 receptor is also expressed in the vessel wall, with the highest receptor density being found on VSMC. A significant increase in the receptor density is observed in hypercholesterolemic-induced atherosclerosis and in balloon injury *(31)*.

4.2. Functions of the Vascular RAS

Vascular diseases are triggered by a variety of factors such as growth factors, extracellular matrix proteins, cytokines, or chemokines. Ang II exerts multiple actions on vascular structure and function, including regulation of vasomotor tone, cell growth/apoptosis, fibrinolytic imbalance and inflammation, all key components of atherosclerotic progression, and of adverse coronary outcomes. Enhanced shear stress produced by increased vascular load, in concert with elevated levels of Ang II, causes vessel wall remodeling, leading to the initiation, maintenance, and destabilization of atherosclerotic lesions *(32)*. Increased production of plasminogen activator inhibitor type-1 and enhanced oxidative stress are other mechanisms by which Ang II promotes atherosclerosis. Ang II increases lipid loading into foam cells and expression of redox-sensitive gene products, such as vascular cell adhesion molecule-1 and monocyte chemoattractant protein-1. These proteins recruit macrophages and other inflammatory cells in vascular injury and in vasculopathy related to diabetes, re-stenosis, and atherosclerosis *(30)*. Ang II induces intimal proliferation and fibrosis via increased production of a number of growth factors, such as transforming growth factor (TGF)-β, platelet-derived growth factor (PDGF), basic fibroblast growth factor, parathyroid hormone-related protein, and connective tissue growth factor. Consistent with these findings, inhibitors of the RAS prevent intimal proliferation. Over-activation of the RAS promotes endothelial dysfunction by Ang II-induced oxidative stress and the release of endothelin-1, a potent vasoconstrictor *(31)*. Ang II also stimulates the production of several extracellular matrix (ECM) components, including fibronectin, collagen, laminin, and tenascin. These changes in ECM may facilitate an environment that allows cells to proliferate, grow, and migrate. Clinical and experimental data demonstrate improvement in endothelial dysfunction

and reduction in vascular inflammation, cellular proliferation, and fibrosis in atherosclerotic lesions in response to RAS blockade *(33)*.

4.3. Benefits of Vascular RAS Blockade

The beneficial effects of blockade of the RAS on experimental vascular diseases in
animal models have been demonstrated. Spontaneously hypertensive rats (SHR) show
elevated levels of aortic TGF-β1, fibronectin, and collagen type IV mRNA, compared
to Wistar–Kyoto (WKY) rats; which are significantly reduced by an ACE inhibitor or
an AT_1 receptor antagonist. Similar suppression of these mRNAs is observed with an
AT_1 blocker or ACE inhibitor, in stroke-prone SHR. These effects on gene expression
correlate with the suppression of medial hypertrophy of the aorta and the mesenteric
artery of SHR and stroke-prone SHR, respectively *(30)*. Arterial injury produced by
balloon angioplasty activates the RAS, leading to progressive neointimal thickening and
narrowing of the vascular lumen. Accumulating evidence suggests that the inhibition of
the vascular RAS results in suppression of injury-induced neointima formation. In the
porcine coronary artery balloon-injury model, an ACE inhibitor significantly inhibited
neointima formation after balloon injury that was accompanied by a significant improvement from endothelial dysfunction *(34)*. Treatment with an AT_1 blocker significantly
inhibited neointima formation caused by polyethylene cuff placement around the
femoral artery of mice *(35)*. Combined treatment with an AT_1 blocker and an ACE
inhibitor had an additive inhibitory effect on balloon-injury-elicited neointima formation
in the carotid artery of rat *(36)*. In hypercholesterolemic animals, abnormal endothelial
function and reactive oxygen species (ROS) production associated with increased AT_1
receptors are normalized by treatment with an AT_1 antagonist *(31)*.

5. ANG II-MEDIATED SIGNALING PATHWAYS

The multiple actions of Ang II are mediated via specific, highly complex intracellular
signaling pathways, which are stimulated following initial binding of the peptide to its
specific receptors. In mammalian cells, Ang II mediates effects via at least two high-
affinity plasma membrane receptors, AT_1 and AT_2. Both receptor subtypes have been
cloned and pharmacologically characterized *(37,38)*. Two other Ang II receptors have
been described, namely AT_3 and AT_4. The AT_3 receptor is peptide-specific, recognizing
mainly Ang II. This receptor does not bind nonpeptide ligands such as losartan (selective
AT_1 receptor antagonist) or PD123319 (selective AT_2 receptor antagonist), and has only
been observed in cell lines. The AT_4 receptor, which is present in heart, lung, kidney,
brain, and liver, binds Ang IV *(39)*, but not losartan or PD123319. We will focus on the
signaling pathways mediated by AT_1 and AT_2.

5.1. AT_1 Receptor

The gene for the AT_1 was first cloned in 1991 *(37)*, and consists of 359 amino acids
with a molecular mass of 41 kDa. Two AT_1 receptor subtypes have been described in
rodents, AT_{1a} and AT_{1b}, with greater than 94% amino acid sequence homology *(40)*, and
which have similar pharmacological properties and tissue distribution patterns. AT_{1a} and
AT_{1b} genes in rats are mapped to chromosomes 17 and 2 *(41)*, respectively; whereas, the
human AT_1 gene is mapped to chromosome 3 *(42)*. AT_1 receptors are primarily found

in the brain, adrenals, heart, vasculature, and kidney, and serve to regulate blood pressure and fluid and electrolyte balance. In the heart, the highest density of AT_1 is found in the conducting system (43). Punctate AT_1 binding is found in the epicardium surrounding the atria, with low binding seen throughout the atrial and ventricular myocardium (44). Moreover, AT_1 in the vasculature, including the aorta, pulmonary and mesenteric arteries, are present in high levels on VSMC, with low levels in the adventitia (45). Virtually all of the known biological actions of Ang II are mediated by AT_1, including the elevation of blood pressure, vasoconstriction, increase in cardiac contractility, release of aldosterone and vasopressin, renal tubular sodium reabsorption, stimulation of sympathetic transmission, and cellular growth (46). In addition, a recent in vitro and in vivo evidence supports the notion that Ang II, mediated by AT_1, may participate directly in the pathogenesis of various cardiovascular diseases (47–49). Thus, the molecular and cellular actions of Ang II in cardiovascular diseases are almost exclusively mediated by AT_1.

AT_1 belongs to the seven transmembrane class of GPCRs. Four cysteine residues are located in the extracellular domain, which represent the sites of disulfide bridge formation and are critical tertiary structure determinants. The transmembrane domain and the extracellular loop play an important role in Ang II binding (50). The Ang II binding site with AT_1 is different from the binding site for AT_1 antagonists, which interact only with the transmembrane domain of the receptor (51). Like most G protein-coupled receptors, AT_1 is also subject to internalization when stimulated by Ang II, a process dependent on specific residues on the cytoplasmic tail (52). AT_1 receptors interact with various heterotrimeric G proteins, including Gq/11, Gi/o, $G\alpha12$, and $G\alpha13$. The different G protein isoforms couple to distinct signaling cascades.

5.2. AT_2 Receptor

The second major isoform of the Ang II receptor, AT_2, has been cloned in a variety of species, including human (53), rat (54), and mouse (38). AT_2 is also a seven-transmembrane glycoprotein, encoded by a 363-amino-acid protein with a molecular mass of 41 kDa, and shares only 34% sequence identity with AT_1 (55). The AT_2 receptor gene is localized as a single copy on the X chromosome. Unlike AT_1, there is no evidence for subtypes of AT_2. AT_2 is normally expressed at high levels in developing fetal tissues, and decreases rapidly after birth (56). In the adult, AT_2 expression is detectable in the pancreas, heart, kidney, adrenals, myometrium, ovary, brain and vasculature. AT_2 is re-expressed in adults after vascular and cardiac injury and during wound healing and renal obstruction (57–60). Thus, AT_2 receptors appear to be involved in the control of cell proliferation, cell differentiation and development, angiogenesis, wound healing, tissue regeneration, and even apoptosis, namely, biological processes that counteract the trophic responses mediated through AT_1 (61,62).

In the heart, AT_2 inhibits growth and remodeling, induces vasodilation, and is up-regulated in pathological states (63). Conflicting data on antigrowth effects have emerged from the studies of mice lacking AT_2 (64). However, recent studies have helped to clarify the role of AT_2 in cardiac remodeling following myocardial infarction (65) and in cardiac hypertrophy and fibrosis because of Ang II infusion in mice overexpressing AT_2 selectively in the myocardium. After myocardial infarction, AT_2 overexpression resulted in preservation of left ventricular global and regional function, indicating a beneficial role of AT_2 in volume-overload states, including post-myocardial infarction remodeling

(65,66). In blood vessels, in addition to vasodilatory actions, AT_2 exerts antiproliferative and apoptotic effects in VSMC and decreases neointima formation in response to an injury by counteracting Ang II actions at the AT_1 receptor *(67)*. Part of the actions of AT_2 in blood vessels may be to downregulate the expression of AT_1 and TGF-β receptors via the bradykinin–nitric oxide (NO) pathway.

Signaling pathways through which AT_2 mediates cardiovascular actions have recently been explained. Four major cascades are involved that include: (1) activation of protein phosphatases and protein dephosphorylation, (2) regulation of the NO–cGMP system, (3) stimulation of phospholipase A_2 (PLA_2) and release of arachidonic acid (AA), and (4) sphingolipid-derived ceramide *(61,62,68,69)*. In contrast to the extensive data on the molecular and cellular functions and pathophysiological significance of AT_1, the role of AT_2 in cardiovascular diseases remains to be defined.

6. AT_1-MEDIATED INTRACELLULAR SIGNALING

There are five classical signal transduction mechanisms for AT_1, as follows: activation of PLA_2, phospholipase C (PLC), phospholipase D (PLD) and L-type Ca^{2+} channels and inhibition of adenylyl cyclase (Fig. 2). AT_1 couples to $G_{q/11}$ protein, and induces the activation of PLC-β, which results in generation of two secondary messengers, inositol (1,4,5) trisphosphate (IP_3) and diacylglycerol (DAG). IP_3 stimulates the release of Ca^{2+} from intracellular stores, and DAG activates protein kinase C (PKC), both of which are involved in cardiac hypertrophy, heart failure, and vasoconstriction *(70–73)*. Activation of PLA_2 and PLD stimulates the release of AA, the precursor molecule for the generation of prostaglandins, and is involved in the Ang II-induced growth of VSMC and cardiac hypertrophy *(74)*. Ang II-mediated stimulation of AT_1 coupled with $G_{i/o}$ protein can also inhibit adenylyl cyclase in several target tissues, thereby attenuating the production of the second messenger cAMP *(75)*. cAMP is a vasodilator and when production is decreased by AT_1 activation, vasoconstriction ensues. Moreover, AT_1 is also involved in the opening of Ca^{2+} channels and influx of extracellular Ca^{2+} into cells *(76,77)*, and the activation of L-channels is mediated by AT_1 coupled with $G_{12/13}$ proteins *(78)*.

7. AT_1-MEDIATED TYROSINE PHOSPHORYLATION

A recent development in the field of Ang II signaling is the demonstration that AT_1 activation is associated with increased protein tyrosine phosphorylation. These processes are characteristically associated with growth factors and cytokines. Accordingly, it is becoming increasingly evident that in addition to its potent vasoconstrictor properties, Ang II has mitogenic- and inflammatory-like characteristics. Ang II stimulates phosphorylation of many non-receptor tyrosine kinases including PLCγ, Src family kinases, Janus kinase (JAK), focal adhesion kinase (FAK), Ca^{2+}-dependent tyrosine kinases (e.g., proline-rich tyrosine kinase, Pyk2), p130Cas, and phosphatidylinositol 3-kinase (PI3K). In addition, Ang II influences the activity of receptor tyrosine kinases (RTK), such as epidermal growth factor receptor (EGFR), PDGF receptor (PDGFR), and IGF receptor (IGFR) (Fig. 3). Ang II mediated stimulation of cellular proliferation and growth has been demonstrated in cardiac myocytes and VSMC. These growth-like effects are associated with increased tyrosine phosphorylation and activation of MAP kinase and related pathways, which result in increased expression of early response genes, such as c-*fos*,

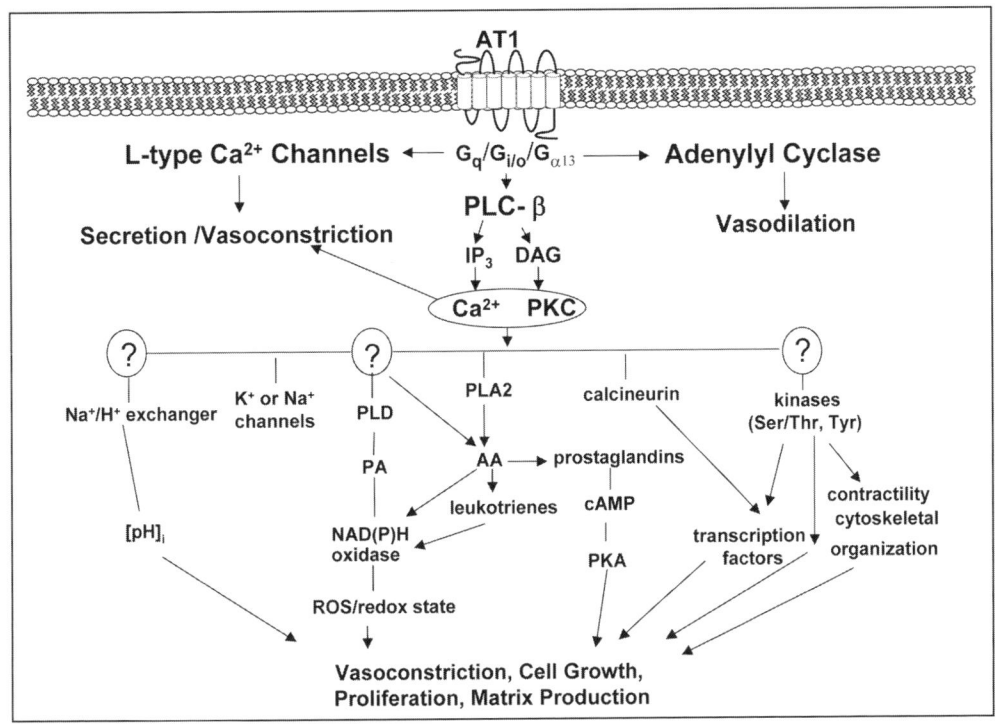

Fig. 2. Classical signal transduction mechanisms mediated by AT_1. Binding of Ang II to AT_1 leads to G protein-coupled activation of PLC, resulting in phosphatidylinositol hydrolysis, formation of IP_3, and DAG accumulation. IP_3 mobilizes Ca^{2+} from sarcoplasmic reticular stores, and DAG activates PKC.

c-*jun* and c-*myc*, which control cellular proliferation and growth *(79)*. Such actions have been linked to cardiovascular diseases, including hypertension, cardiac hypertrophy, heart failure, and atherosclerosis. The role of tyrosine kinases in Ang II-mediated signaling has been extensively reviewed *(74,79–81)* and only recent developments are discussed here.

8. NON-RECEPTOR TYROSINE KINASE ACTIVATION

8.1. Src Family Kinases

To date at least 14 Src kinase family members have been identified, of which the 60-kDa c-Src is ubiquitously expressed. All Src family members share common functional domains, including an N-terminal myristoylation sequence for membrane targeting, SH2 and SH3 domains for protein binding, a kinase domain and a C-terminal noncatalytic domain *(82)*. c-Src is abundantly expressed in cardiomyocytes and VSMC and is rapidly activated by Ang II *(83)*. Src has an important role in Ang II-induced phosphorylation of PLC-γ and IP_3 formation. Src, intracellular Ca^{2+} and PKC regulate Ang II-induced phosphorylation of p130Cas, a signaling molecule involved in integrin-mediated cell adhesion. Src has also been associated with Ang II-induced activation of Pyk2 and extracellular signal-regulated kinases (ERKs), as well as the activation of other downstream proteins including FAK, paxillin, JAK2, signal transducer and activator of transcription (STAT)-1, caveolin, and the adapter protein, Shc *(84)*. Activation of c-Src is required for cytoskeletal reorganization, focal adhesion formation, and cell migration

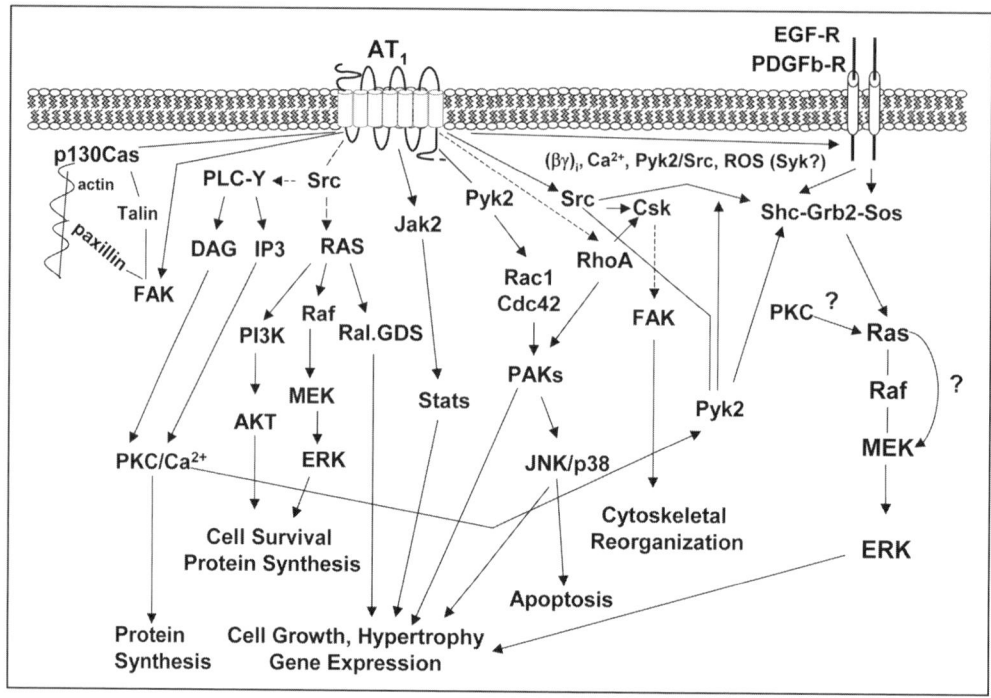

Fig. 3. Novel signal transduction mechanisms mediated by AT_1. Ang II phosphorylates multiple tyrosine kinases, such as JAK, FAK, Pyk2, p130Cas, and PI3K. Activated tyrosine kinases phosphorylate many downstream targets including the MAP kinase cascade. Src associates with the adapter protein complex, Shc–GRB2–Sos, that induces guanine nucleotide exchange on the small G protein Ras-GDP/GTP. Activated Ras-GTP interacts with Raf, resulting in phosphorylation of MEK, which in turn, phosphorylates MAP kinases, including ERK1/2, JNK/SAPK, and p38. Rho is also activated through AT_1 receptors. In addition, Ang II influences activity of receptor tyrosine kinases (RTK), such as EGFR, and PDGFR. The transactivated EGFR serves as a scaffold for downstream adapters, leading to activation of MAP kinases.

and growth. Increased activation of c-Src by Ang II may be an important mediator of cardiac hypertrophy and altered VSMC function in hypertension.

8.2. JAK-STAT Activation

Similar to cytokine receptors and RTKs, AT_1 activates the JAK/STAT signaling pathway. There are four JAK proteins in mammalian cells: JAK1, JAK2, JAK3, and TYK2 (85). JAKs bind specifically to intracellular domains of cytokine receptor signaling chains and catalyze ligand-induced phosphorylation of themselves and of intracellular tyrosine residues on the receptor, creating tyrosine-phosphorylated docking sites for STATs. Tyrosine phosphorylation of STATs leads to STAT homo- and hetero-dimerization. STAT dimers are rapidly transported from the cytoplasm to the nucleus, where they activate gene transcription. AT_1 activates JAK2 and Tyk2 in the cardiovascular system (86). AT_1 receptor-induced activation of JAKs leads to phosphorylation of the STAT proteins p91/84 (STAT1a/β), p113 (STAT2), and p92 (STAT3). The JAK–STAT signaling pathway activates early growth response genes, providing a mechanism whereby Ang II may influence vascular and cardiac growth, remodeling, and repair (87,88). The STATs have an important role in Ao gene expression in cardiac myocytes. Ang II-induced

Ao gene upregulation, by STAT3 and STAT6 activation, may constitute part of an autocrine, positive-feedback loop that contributes to cardiac hypertrophy in vivo *(86)*.

8.3. FAK and Pyk2 Activation

FAK is a cytoplasmic protein tyrosine kinase localized to regions called focal adhesions. Many stimuli can induce tyrosine phosphorylation and activation of FAK, including integrins and growth factors. The major site of autophosphorylation, tyrosine 397, is a docking site for the SH2 domains of Src family proteins. The other sites of phosphorylation are phosphorylated by Src kinases *(89)*. As a consequence of association with c-Src, FAK undergoes further tyrosine phosphorylation, which results in FAK binding to Grb2, Sos, and Ras. This in turn leads to ERK1/2 activation. Ang II-induced activation of FAK causes its translocation to sites of focal adhesion with the extracellular matrix and phosphorylation of paxillin and talin, which may be involved in the regulation of cell morphology and movement *(90)*. AT_1-induced FAK activation also has an important role in Ang II-mediated hypertrophic responses in cardiomyocytes and VSMC *(91)*. The link between the AT_1 receptor and FAK is unknown, but the Rho family of GTPases may be important.

Another FAK family member, Pyk2, also known as cell adhesion kinase-β, related adhesion focal tyrosine kinase and calcium-dependent tyrosine kinase (the rat homolog of Pyk2), is activated by AT_1 and is dependent on increased intracellular Ca^{2+} and PKC *(90,92)*. Because Pyk2 is a candidate to regulate c-Src and to link G protein-coupled vasoconstrictor receptors with protein tyrosine kinase-mediated contractile, migratory and growth responses, it may be a potential point of convergence between Ca^{2+}-dependent signaling pathways and protein tyrosine kinase pathways in cardiovascular cells.

8.4. p130Cas

p130Cas is an Ang II-activated tyrosine kinase that plays a role in cytoskeletal rearrangement. This protein serves as an adapter molecule since it contains proline-rich domains, an SH3 domain, and binding motifs for the SH2 domains of Crk and Src. p130Cas is important for integrin-mediated cell adhesion, by the recruitment of cytoskeletal signaling molecules such as FAK, paxillin and tensin to the focal adhesions *(93)*. The phosphorylation of p130Cas is dependent on Ca^{2+}, c-Src, and PKC, and requires an intact cytoskeletal network. Other studies reported that Ang II-induced activation of p130Cas is Ca^{2+} and PKC independent *(94)*. Although the exact functional significance of Ang II-induced activation of p130Cas is unclear, it might regulate α-actin expression, cellular proliferation, migration, and cell adhesion. p130Cas also has a critical role in cardiovascular development and actin filament assembly.

8.5. PI3K

PI3K-dependent signaling is involved in the control of cell growth, proliferation, survival, and cytoskeletal remodeling, and has recently been shown to have an important role in the regulation of cardiomyocyte and VSMC growth *(95,96)*. Recent findings suggest an involvement of PI3K in the pathogenesis of numerous diseases, including cancer, heart failure and autoimmune/inflammatory disorders. PI3K is a heterodimeric enzyme composed of a p85 adapter and a p110 catalytic subunit *(97)*. PI3K, characteristically associated with tyrosine kinase receptors, is also activated by AT_1. PI3Kα, which is activated by a tyrosine kinase receptor, appears to have a critical role for the induction of physiological cardiac growth; but, not pathological growth, and appears essential for maintaining contractile function in response to pathological stimuli (98). In contrast, PI3Kγ, which is activated by GPCR, appears to negatively control cardiac contractility through different signaling mechanisms (99). Akt/PKB has been identified as an important PI3K downstream target in Ang II-activated cardiomyocytes and VSMC (100). It regulates protein synthesis by activating p70 S6-kinase and modulates Ang II-mediated Ca^{2+} responses, by stimulating Ca^{2+} channel currents. Akt/PKB has also been implicated in promoting cell survival, by influencing Bcl-2 and c-Myc expression and inhibiting caspases. Although the exact role of PI3K in Ang II signaling has not been established, it is possible that this complex pathway controls the balance between mitogenesis and apoptosis.

9. RECEPTOR TYROSINE KINASES

Increasing evidence suggests that there is a cross-talk between GPCR and RTK. GPCR utilize signaling pathways downstream of RTK to exert cellular effects. AT_1 activation-mediated mitogenic responses may be regulated by activation of RTK. Ang II can activate RTK, even though it does not directly bind to RTK (101). This process of transactivation has been demonstrated for EGFR, PDGFR, and IGFR (101). Ca^{2+}, Pyk2, Src, and redox-sensitive processes are involved in Ang II-induced transactivation of RTKs. AT_1-induced EGFR transactivation is important for some of the trophic effects of Ang II. Studies have demonstrated that the EGFR activation is involved in Ang II-induced vascular contraction, cell growth, cardiac hypertrophy, and hypertension (102).

10. MITOGEN-ACTIVATED PROTEIN KINASES

MAP kinases, including ERKs, JNKs, and p38s, have a central role in cellular responses through various stress stimuli, such as cell proliferation, apoptosis, migration, or gene expression (103). Ang II induces phosphorylation of Ras, Raf, and Shc, which leads to the activation of MEK kinases and MEKs, resulting in tyrosine and threonine phosphorylation of ERK1/2, JNK2, and p38 (104). Ang II-induced activation of ERK1/2 is associated with the increased expression of the early response genes c-fos, c-myc and c-jun, DNA/protein synthesis, cell growth and differentiation, and cytoskeletal organization in cardiovascular cells (105). In addition to ERKs, Ang II activates JNKs, which regulate cardiomyocytes and VSMC growth (106,107). Ang II induces the activation of JNK via p21-activated kinase (PAK), which is dependent on intracellular Ca^{2+} mobilization and PKC activation (108). Ang II-activated ERK1/2 and JNK have opposite growth effects in VSMC, with ERK1/2 being growth promoting and JNK inhibitory. Ang II also induces the phosphorylation of p38, which has an important role in inflammatory responses, apoptosis, and regulation of cell growth (109). The p38 pathway has been implicated in various pathological conditions, such as cardiac ischemia, ischemia/reperfusion injury, cardiac hypertrophy, progression of atherosclerosis, and vascular remodeling in hypertension (109,110).

11. SMALL G PROTEINS

The small G protein superfamily consists of five subfamilies (Ras, Rho, ADP ribosylation factors, Rab, and Ran) that act as molecular switches to regulate cellular responses *(111)*. Of these, the Rho subfamily (RhoA, Rac1, and Cdc42) has been associated with Ang II signaling. Upon stimulation, Rho GTPases are activated by exchanging bound GDP for GTP. Rho kinase is one of the major downstream targets of RhoA. It has been demonstrated that Rho-kinase-mediated signaling is involved in AT_1-stimulated cardiovascular cell growth, remodeling, atherosclerosis and vascular contraction *(112)*. Ang II also activates Rac1, another small G protein, which participates in cytoskeletal organization, cell growth, inflammation, and regulation of NAD(P)H oxidase *(111)*. Ang II-activated Rac1 is an upstream regulator of PAK and JNK. Rac1 also has a role in Ang II-induced gene transcription and regulation of NAD(P)H oxidase, and the activation of JAK/STAT *(113)*.

12. GENERATION OF REACTIVE OXYGEN SPECIES

Ang II has been shown to activate the vascular NAD(P)H oxidase(s) resulting in the production of ROS, namely superoxide (O_2^-) and hydrogen peroxide (H_2O_2). ROS act as intercellular and intracellular second messengers that may have a physiological role in vascular tone and cell growth, and a pathophysiological role in inflammation, ischemia reperfusion, hypertension and atherosclerosis *(114,115)*. It has been suggested that NAD(P)H oxidase may be the most important source of ROS in vasculature and myocytes. This enzyme transfers electrons from NADH or NADPH to molecular oxygen, producing O_2^-. Generation of reactive oxygen species is regulated by various cytokines and growth factors, including Ang II, which increases O_2^- and H_2O_2 production in cardiac, VSMC, endothelial, adventitial, and mesangial cells *(116)*. ROS produced following Ang II-mediated stimulation of NAD(P)H oxidases, signal through pathways such as MAP kinases, tyrosine kinases and transcription factors, and lead to events such as inflammation, hypertrophy, remodeling, and angiogenesis *(115)*.

13. SUMMARY AND CONCLUSIONS

The RAS is a hormonal cascade that regulates cardiovascular, renal, and adrenal function, as it relates to fluid and electrolyte homeostasis and arterial pressure. The RAS has been further delineated as a local, self-contained, paracrine, autocrine, and intracrine system. The tissue RASs are likely important in normal physiological responses, as well as in the pathophysiology of disease states such as hypertension, cardiac hypertrophy, congestive heart failure, and post myocardial infarction remodeling. Although major progress has been made in our understanding of the physiology and pathophysiology of the circulating RAS, it will be important to more completely elucidate the role of tissue RASs in normal physiology and in the pathophysiology of cardiovascular diseases.

REFERENCES

1. Carey, R. M. and Siragy, H. M. (2003) Newly recognized components of the renin–angiotensin system: potential roles in cardiovascular and renal regulation. *Endocr. Rev.* **24**, 261–271.
2. Schiffrin, E. L. (2002) Vascular and cardiac benefits of angiotensin receptor blockers. *Am. J. Med.* **113**, 409–418.
3. Lavoie, J. L. and Sigmund, C. D. (2003) Minireview: overview of the renin–angiotensin system—an endocrine and paracrine system. *Endocrinology* **144**, 2179–2183.
4. Booz, G. and Baker, K. (2004) Intracellular signaling and the cardiac renin angiotensin system. In: *Renin Angiotensin System and the Heart* (De Mello, W., ed.), Wiley, Chichester, pp. 1–12.

5. Baker, K. M., Chernin, M. I., Schreiber, T., et al. (2004) Evidence of a novel intracrine mechanism in angiotensin II-induced cardiac hypertrophy. *Regul. Pept.* **120,** 5–13.
6. Clausmeyer, S., Reinecke, A., Farrenkopf, R., Unger, T., and Peters, J. (2000) Tissue-specific expression of a rat renin transcript lacking the coding sequence for the prefragment and its stimulation by myocardial infarction. *Endocrinology* **141,** 2963–2970.
7. Crackower, M. A., Sarao, R., Oudit, G. Y., et al. (2002) Angiotensin-converting enzyme 2 is an essential regulator of heart function. *Nature* **417,** 822–828.
8. Kohlstedt, K., Brandes, R. P., Muller-Esterl, W., Busse, R., and Fleming, I. (2004) Angiotensin-converting enzyme is involved in outside-in signaling in endothelial cells. *Circ. Res.* **94,** 60–67.
9. Bruckschlegel, G., Holmer, S. R., Jandeleit, K., et al. (1995) Blockade of the renin–angiotensin system in cardiac pressure-overload hypertrophy in rats. *Hypertension* **25,** 250–259.
10. van Kats, J. P., Danser, A. H., van Meegen, J. R., Sassen, L. M., Verdouw, P. D., and Schalekamp, M. A. (1998) Angiotensin production by the heart: a quantitative study in pigs with the use of radiolabeled angiotensin infusions. *Circulation* **98,** 73–81.
11. Peters, J. and Clausmeyer, S. (2002) Intracellular sorting of renin: cell type specific differences and their consequences. *J. Mol. Cell Cardiol.* **34,** 1561–1568.
12. Zhang, X., Dostal, D. E., Reiss, K., et al. (1995) Identification and activation of autocrine renin– angiotensin system in adult ventricular myocytes. *Am. J. Physiol.* **269,** H1791–H1802.
13. Dostal, D. E. and Baker, K. M. (1999) The cardiac renin–angiotensin system: conceptual, or a regulator of cardiac function? *Circ. Res.* **85,** 643–650.
14. Sun, Y., Zhang, J., Zhang, J. Q., and Weber, K. T. (2001) Renin expression at sites of repair in the infarcted rat heart. *J. Mol. Cell. Cardiol.* **33,** 995–1003.
15. Barlucchi, L., Leri, A., Dostal, D. E., et al. (2001) Canine ventricular myocytes possess a renin– angiotensin system that is upregulated with heart failure. *Circ. Res.* **88,** 298–304.
16. Baker, K. M., Chernin, M. I., Wixson, S. K., and Aceto, J. F. (1990) Renin–angiotensin system involvement in pressure-overload cardiac hypertrophy in rats. *Am. J. Physiol.* **259,** H324–H332.
17. Dostal, D. E., Rothblum, K. N., Conrad, K. M., Cooper, G. R., and Baker, K. M. (1992) Detection of angiotensin I and II in cultured rat cardiac myocytes and fibroblasts. *Am. J. Physiol.* **263,** C851–C863.
18. Zisman, L. S., Keller, R. S., Weaver, B., et al. (2003) Increased angiotensin-(1–7)-forming activity in failing human heart ventricles: evidence for upregulation of the angiotensin-converting enzyme homologue ACE2. *Circulation* **108,** 1707–1712.
19. Donoghue, M., Wakimoto, H., Maguire, C. T., et al. (2003) Heart block, ventricular tachycardia, and sudden death in ACE2 transgenic mice with downregulated connexins. *J. Mol. Cell. Cardiol.* **35,** 1043–1053.
20. Wei, C. C., Ferrario, C. M., Brosnihan, K. B., et al. (2002) Angiotensin peptides modulate bradykinin levels in the interstitium of the dog heart in vivo. *J. Pharmacol. Exp. Ther.* **300,** 324–329.
21. Averill, D. B., Ishiyama, Y., Chappell, M. C., and Ferrario, C. M. (2003) Cardiac angiotensin-(1–7) in ischemic cardiomyopathy. *Circulation* **108,** 2141–2146.
22. Loot, A. E., Roks, A. J., Henning, R. H., et al. (2002) Angiotensin-(1–7) attenuates the development of heart failure after myocardial infarction in rats. *Circulation* **105,** 1548–1550.
23. Fukuzawa, J., Booz, G. W., Hunt, R. A., et al. (2000) Cardiotrophin-1 increases angiotensinogen mRNA in rat cardiac myocytes through STAT3: an autocrine loop for hypertrophy. *Hypertension* **35,** 1191–1196.
24. De Mello, W. (2004) The heart: a target for the renin angiotensin system. Evidence of an intracrine system. In: *Renin Angiotensin System and the Heart* (De Mello, W., ed.), Wiley, Chichester, pp. 101–118.
25. Cassis, L. A., Lynch, K. R., and Peach, M. J. (1988) Localization of angiotensinogen messenger RNA in rat aorta. *Circ. Res.* **62,** 1259–1262.
26. Naftilan, A. J., Zuo, W. M., Inglefinger, J., Ryan, T. J. Jr., Pratt, R. E., and Dzau, V. J. (1991) Localization and differential regulation of angiotensinogen mRNA expression in the vessel wall. *J. Clin. Investig.* **87,** 1300–1311.
27. Rakugi, H., Jacob, H. J., Krieger, J. E., Ingelfinger, J. R., and Pratt, R. E. (1993) Vascular injury induces angiotensinogen gene expression in the media and neointima. *Circulation* **87,** 283–290.
28. Kamide, K., Rakugi, H., Nagai, M., et al. (2004) Insulin-mediated regulation of the endothelial renin–angiotensin system and vascular cell growth. *J. Hypertens.* **22,** 121–127.

29. Fuchs, S., Germain, S., Philippe, J., Corvol, P., and Pinet, F. (2002) Expression of renin in large arteries outside the kidney revealed by human renin promoter/LacZ transgenic mouse. *Am. J. Pathol.* **161,** 717–725.

30. Collidge, T. A., Lammie, G. A., Fleming, S., and Mullins, J. J. (2004) The role of the renin–angiotensin system in malignant vascular injury affecting the systemic and cerebral circulations. *Prog. Biophys. Mol. Biol.* **84,** 301–319.

31. Schmidt-Ott, K. M., Kagiyama, S., and Phillips, M. I. (2000) The multiple actions of angiotensin II in atherosclerosis. *Regul. Pept.* **93,** 65–77.

32. Grote, K., Drexler, H., and Schieffer, B. (2004) Renin–angiotensin system and atherosclerosis. *Nephrol. Dial. Transplant.* **19,** 770–773.

33. Yousufuddin, M. and Yamani, M. H. (2004) The renin–angiotensin hypothesis for the pathogenesis of cardiac allograft vasculopathy. *Int. J. Cardiol.* **95,** 123–127.

34. Matsumoto, K., Morishita, R., Moriguchi, A., et al. (2001) Inhibition of neointima by angiotensin-converting enzyme inhibitor in porcine coronary artery balloon-injury model. *Hypertension* **37,** 270–274.

35. Liu, H.-W., Iwai, M., Takeda-Matsubara, Y., et al. (2002) Effect of estrogen and AT1 receptor blocker on neointima formation. *Hypertension* **40,** 451–457.

36. Yagi, S., Morita, T., and Katayama, S. (2004) Combined treatment with an AT1 receptor blocker and angiotensin converting enzyme inhibitor has an additive effect on inhibiting neointima formation via improvement of nitric oxide production and suppression of oxidative stress. *Hypertens. Res.* **27,** 129–135.

37. Murphy, T. J., Alexander, R. W., Griendling, K. K., Runge, M. S., and Bernstein, K. E. (1991) Isolation of a cDNA encoding the vascular type-1 angiotensin II receptor. *Nature* **351,** 233–236.

38. Nakajima, M., Mukoyama, M., Pratt, R. E., Horiuchi, M., and Dzau, V. J. (1993) Cloning of cDNA and analysis of the gene for mouse angiotensin II type 2 receptor. *Biochem. Biophys. Res. Commun.* **197,** 393–399.

39. Harding, J. W., Wright, J. W., Swanson, G. N., Hanesworth, J. M., and Krebs, L. T. (1994) AT_4 receptors: specificity and distribution. *Kidney Int.* **46,** 1510–1512.

40. Iwai, N. and Inagami, T. (1992) Identification of two subtypes in the rat type I angiotensin II receptor. *FEBS Lett.* **298,** 257–260.

41. Lewis, J. L., Serikawa, T., and Warnock, D. G. (1993) Chromosomal localization of angiotensin II type 1 receptor isoforms in the rat. *Biochem. Biophys. Res. Commun.* **194,** 677–682.

42. Guo, D. F., Furuta, H., Mizukoshi, M., and Inagami, T. (1994) The genomic organization of human angiotensin II type 1 receptor. *Biochem. Biophys. Res. Commun.* **200,** 313–319.

43. Saavedra, J. M., Viswanathan, M., and Shigematsu, K. (1993) Localization of angiotensin AT_1 receptors in the rat heart conduction system. *Eur. J. Pharmacol.* **235,** 301–303.

44. Sechi, L. A., Griffin, C. A., Grady, E. F., Kalinyak, J. E., and Schambelan, M. (1992) Characterization of angiotensin II receptor subtypes in rat heart. *Circ. Res.* **71,** 1482–1489.

45. Allen, A. M., Zhuo, J., and Mendelsohn, F. A. (2000) Localization and function of angiotensin AT_1 receptors. *Am. J. Hypertens.* **13,** 31S–38S.

46. Timmermans, P. B., Wong, P. C., Chiu, A. T., et al. (1993) Angiotensin II receptors and angiotensin II receptor antagonists. *Pharmacol. Rev.* **45,** 205–251.

47. Berk, B. C., Vekshtein, V., Gordon, H. M., and Tsuda, T. (1989) Angiotensin II-stimulated protein synthesis in cultured vascular smooth muscle cells. *Hypertension* **13,** 305–314.

48. Ryan, M. J., Didion, S. P., Mathur, S., Faraci, F. M., and Sigmund, C. D. (2004) Angiotensin II-induced vascular dysfunction is mediated by the AT_{1A} receptor in mice. *Hypertension* **43,** 1074–1079.

49. Lijnen, P. and Petrov, V. (1999) Renin–angiotensin system, hypertrophy and gene expression in cardiac myocytes. *J. Mol. Cell. Cardiol.* **31,** 949–970.

50. Hunyady, L., Balla, T., and Catt, K. J. (1996) The ligand binding site of the angiotensin AT_1 receptor. *Trends Pharmacol. Sci.* **17,** 135–140.

51. Groblewski, T., Maigret, B., Nouet, S., et al. (1995) Amino acids of the third transmembrane domain of the AT_{1A} angiotensin II receptor are involved in the differential recognition of peptide and nonpeptide ligands. *Biochem. Biophys. Res. Commun.* **209,** 153–160.

52. Thekkumkara, T. J., Thomas, W. G., Motel, T. J., and Baker, K. M. (1998) Functional role for the angiotensin II receptor (AT_{1A}) 3′-untranslated region in determining cellular responses to agonist: evidence for recognition by RNA binding proteins. *Biochem. J.* **329,** 255–264.

53. Koike, G., Horiuchi, M., Yamada, T., Szpirer, C., Jacob, H. J., and Dzau, V. J. (1994) Human type 2 angiotensin II receptor gene: cloned, mapped to the X chromosome, and its mRNA is expressed in the human lung. *Biochem. Biophys. Res. Commun.* **203,** 1842–1850.

54. Koike, G., Winer, E. S., Horiuchi, M., et al. (1995) Cloning, characterization, and genetic mapping of the rat type 2 angiotensin II receptor gene. *Hypertension* **26,** 998–1002.

55. Mukoyama, M., Nakajima, M., Horiuchi, M., Sasamura, H., Pratt, R. E., and Dzau, V. J. (1993) Expression cloning of type 2 angiotensin II receptor reveals a unique class of seven-transmembrane receptors. *J. Biol. Chem.* **268,** 24,539–24,542.

56. Nahmias, C. and Strosberg, A. D. (1995) The angiotensin AT_2 receptor: searching for signal-transduction pathways and physiological function. *Trends Pharmacol. Sci.* **16,** 223–225.

57. Tsutsumi, Y., Matsubara, H., Ohkubo, N., et al. (1998) Angiotensin II type 2 receptor is upregulated in human heart with interstitial fibrosis, and cardiac fibroblasts are the major cell type for its expression. *Circ. Res.* **83,** 1035–1046.

58. Kimura, B., Sumners, C., and Phillips, M. I. (1992) Changes in skin angiotensin II receptors in rats during wound healing. *Biochem. Biophys. Res. Commun.* **187,** 1083–1090.

59. Nio, Y., Matsubara, H., Murasawa, S., Kanasaki, M., and Inada, M. (1995) Regulation of gene transcription of angiotensin II receptor subtypes in myocardial infarction. *J. Clin. Investig.* **95,** 46–54.

60. Nakajima, M., Hutchinson, H. G., Fujinaga, M., et al. (1995) The angiotensin II type 2 (AT_2) receptor antagonizes the growth effects of the AT_1 receptor: gain-of-function study using gene transfer. *Proc. Natl Acad. Sci. USA* **92,** 10,663–10,667.

61. de Gasparo, M., Catt, K. J., Inagami, T., Wright, J. W., and Unger, T. (2000) International Union of Pharmacology. XXIII. The angiotensin II receptors. *Pharmacol. Rev.* **52,** 415–472.

62. Berk, B. C. (2003) Angiotensin type 2 receptor (AT_2R): a challenging twin. *Sci. STKE.* **181,** PE16.

63. Schneider, M. D. and Lorell, B. H. (2001) AT(2), judgment day: which angiotensin receptor is the culprit in cardiac hypertrophy? *Circulation* **104,** 247–248.

64. Ichihara, S., Senbonmatsu, T., Price, E. Jr., Ichiki, T., Gaffney, F. A., and Inagami, T. (2001) Angiotensin II type 2 receptor is essential for left ventricular hypertrophy and cardiac fibrosis in chronic angiotensin II-induced hypertension. *Circulation* **104,** 346–351.

65. Yang, Z., Bove, C. M., French, B. A., et al. (2002) Angiotensin II type 2 receptor overexpression preserves left ventricular function after myocardial infarction. *Circulation* **106,** 106–111.

66. Oishi, Y., Ozono, R., Yano, Y., et al. (2003) Cardioprotective role of AT_2 receptor in postinfarction left ventricular remodeling. *Hypertension* **41,** 814–818.

67. Suzuki, J., Iwai, M., Nakagami, H., et al. (2002) Role of angiotensin II-regulated apoptosis through distinct AT_1 and AT_2 receptors in neointimal formation. *Circulation* **106,** 847–853.

68. Zhang, J. and Pratt, R. E. (1996) The AT_2 receptor selectively associates with Gialpha2 and Gialpha3 in the rat fetus. *J. Biol. Chem.* **271,** 15,026–15,033.

69. Blume, A., Kaschina, E., and Unger, T. (2001) Angiotensin II type 2 receptors: signalling and patho-physiological role. *Curr. Opin. Nephrol. Hypertens.* **10,** 239–246.

70. Griendling, K. K., Ushio-Fukai, M., Lassegue, B., and Alexander, R. W. (1997) Angiotensin II signaling in vascular smooth muscle. New concepts. *Hypertension* **29,** 366–373.

71. Capponi, A. M. (1996) Distribution and signal transduction of angiotensin II AT_1 and AT_2 receptors. *Blood Press. Suppl.* **2,** 41–46.

72. Ruan, X. and Arendshorst, W. J. (1996) Role of protein kinase C in angiotensin II-induced renal vasoconstriction in genetically hypertensive rats. *Am. J. Physiol.* **270,** F945–F952.

73. Booz, G. W., Dostal, D. E., Singer, H. A., and Baker, K. M. (1994) Involvement of protein kinase C and Ca^{2+} in angiotensin II-induced mitogenesis of cardiac fibroblasts. *Am. J. Physiol.* **267,** C1308–C1318.

74. Touyz, R. M. and Berry, C. (2002) Recent advances in angiotensin II signaling. *Braz. J. Med. Biol. Res.* **35,** 1001–1015.

75. Anand-Srivastava, M. B. (1983) Angiotensin II receptors negatively coupled to adenylate cyclase in rat aorta. *Biochem. Biophys. Res. Commun.* **117,** 420–428.

76. Kem, D. C., Johnson, E. I., Capponi, A. M., et al. (1991) Effect of angiotensin II on cytosolic free calcium in neonatal rat cardiomyocytes. *Am. J. Physiol.* **261,** C77–C85.

77. Iversen, B. M. and Arendshorst, W. J. (1999) AT_1 calcium signaling in renal vascular smooth muscle cells. *J. Am. Soc. Nephrol. Suppl.* **10(11),** S84–S89.

78. Macrez, N., Morel, J. L., Kalkbrenner, F., Viard, P., Schultz, G., and Mironneau, J. (1997) A βγ dimer derived from G13 transduces the angiotensin AT_1 receptor signal to stimulation of Ca^{2+} channels in rat portal vein myocytes. *J. Biol. Chem.* **272,** 23,180–23,185.

79. Kim, S. and Iwao, H. (2000) Molecular and cellular mechanisms of angiotensin II-mediated cardio-vascular and renal diseases. *Pharmacol. Rev.* **52,** 11–34.

80. Yin, G., Yan, C., and Berk, B. C. (2003) Angiotensin II signaling pathways mediated by tyrosine kinases. *Int. J. Biochem. Cell. Biol.* **35,** 780–783.

81. Haendeler, J. and Berk, B. C. (2000) Angiotensin II mediated signal transduction. Important role of tyrosine kinases. *Regul. Pept.* **95,** 1–7.

82. Tatosyan, A. G. and Mizenina, O. A. (2000) Kinases of the Src family: structure and functions. *Biochemistry (Mosc)* **65,** 49–58.

83. Thomas, S. M. and Brugge, J. S. (1997) Cellular functions regulated by Src family kinases. *Annu. Rev. Cell. Dev. Biol.* **13,** 513–609.

84. Erpel, T. and Courtneidge, S. A. (1995) Src family protein tyrosine kinases and cellular signal transduction pathways. *Curr. Opin. Cell. Biol.* **7,** 176–182.

85. Aaronson, D. S. and Horvath, C. M. (2002) A road map for those who don't know JAK-STAT. *Science* **296,** 1653–1655.

86. Booz, G. W., Day, J. N., and Baker, K. M. (2002) Interplay between the cardiac renin angiotensin system and JAK-STAT signaling: role in cardiac hypertrophy, ischemia/reperfusion dysfunction, and heart failure. *J. Mol. Cell. Cardiol.* **34,** 1443–1453.

87. Bolli, R., Dawn, B., and Xuan, Y. T. (2003) Role of the JAK-STAT pathway in protection against myocardial ischemia/reperfusion injury. *Trends Cardiovasc. Med.* **13,** 72–79.

88. Mascareno, E. and Siddiqui, M. A. (2000) The role of Jak/STAT signaling in heart tissue renin–angiotensin system. *Mol. Cell. Biochem.* **212,** 171–175.

89. Parsons, J. T. (2003) Focal adhesion kinase: the first ten years. *J. Cell. Sci.* **116,** 1409–1416.

90. Guan, J. L. (1997) Role of focal adhesion kinase in integrin signaling. *Int. J. Biochem. Cell. Biol.* **29,** 1085–1096.

91. Schnee, J. M. and Hsueh, W. A. (2000) Angiotensin II, adhesion, and cardiac fibrosis. *Cardiovasc. Res.* **46,** 264–268.

92. Sabri, A., Govindarajan, G., Griffin, T. M., Byron, K. L., Samarel, A. M., and Lucchesi, P. A. (1998) Calcium- and protein kinase C-dependent activation of the tyrosine kinase PYK2 by angiotensin II in vascular smooth muscle. *Circ. Res.* **83,** 841–851.

93. O'Neill, G. M., Fashena, S. J., and Golemis, E. A. (2000) Integrin signalling: a new Cas(t) of characters enters the stage. *Trends Cell Biol.* **10,** 111–119.

94. Takahashi, T., Kawahara, Y., Taniguchi, T., and Yokoyama, M. (1998) Tyrosine phosphorylation and association of p130Cas and c-Crk II by ANG II in vascular smooth muscle cells. *Am. J. Physiol.* **274,** H1059–H1065.

95. Prasad, S. V., Perrino, C., and Rockman, H. A. (2002) Role of phosphoinositide 3-kinase in cardiac function and heart failure. *Trends Cardiovasc. Med.* **13,** 206–212.

96. Saward, L. and Zahradka, P. (1997) Angiotensin II activates phosphatidylinositol 3-kinase in vascular smooth muscle cells. *Circ. Res.* **81,** 249–257.

97. Cantley, L. C. (2002) The phosphoinositide 3-kinase pathway. *Science* **296,** 1655–1657.

98. McMullen, J. R., Shioi, T., Zhang, L., et al. (2003) Phosphoinositide 3-kinase (p110alpha) plays a critical role for the induction of physiological, but not pathological, cardiac hypertrophy. *Proc. Natl Acad. Sci. USA* **100,** 12,355–12,360.

99. Alloatti, G., Montrucchio, G., Lembo, G., and Hirsch, E. (2004) Phosphoinositide 3-kinase gamma: kinase-dependent and -independent activities in cardiovascular function and disease. *Biochem. Soc. Trans.* **32,** 383–386.

100. Chen, Q. M., Tu, V. C., Purdon, S., Wood, J., and Dilley, T. (2001) Molecular mechanisms of cardiac hypertrophy induced by toxicants. *Cardiovasc. Toxicol.* **1,** 267–283.

101. Saito, Y. and Berk, B. C. (2001) Transactivation: a novel signaling pathway from angiotensin II to tyrosine kinase receptors. *J. Mol. Cell. Cardiol.* **33,** 3–7.

102. Shah, B. H. and Catt, K. J. (2003) A central role of EGF receptor transactivation in angiotensin II-induced cardiac hypertrophy. *Trends Pharmacol. Sci.* **24,** 239–244.

103. Strniskova, M., Barancik, M., and Ravingerova, T. (2002) Mitogen-activated protein kinases and their role in regulation of cellular processes. *Gen. Physiol. Biophys.* **21,** 231–255.

104. Kim, S. and Iwao, H. (1999) Activation of mitogen-activated protein kinases in cardiovascular hypertrophy and remodeling. *Jpn. J. Pharmacol.* **80,** 97–102.

105. Ravingerova, T., Barancik, M., and Strniskova, M. (2003) Mitogen-activated protein kinases: a new therapeutic target in cardiac pathology. *Mol. Cell. Biochem.* **247,** 127–138.

106. Kim, S. and Iwao, H. (2003) Stress and vascular responses: mitogen-activated protein kinases and activator protein-1 as promising therapeutic targets of vascular remodeling. *J. Pharmacol. Sci.* **91,** 177–181.
107. Wang, Y., Su, B., Sah, V. P., Brown, J. H., Han, J., and Chien, K. R. (1998) Cardiac hypertrophy induced by mitogen-activated protein kinase kinase 7, a specific activator for c-Jun NH2-terminal kinase in ventricular muscle cells. *J. Biol. Chem.* **273,** 5423–5426.
108. Schmitz, U., Ishida, T., Ishida, M., et al. (1998) Angiotensin II stimulates p21-activated kinase in vascular smooth muscle cells: role in activation of JNK. *Circ. Res.* **82,** 1272–1278.
109. Behr, T. M., Berova, M., Doe, C. P., et al. (2003) p38 mitogen-activated protein kinase inhibitors for the treatment of chronic cardiovascular disease. *Curr. Opin. Investig. Drugs* **4,** 1059–1064.
110. Liang, Q. and Molkentin, J. D. (2003) Redefining the roles of p38 and JNK signaling in cardiac hypertrophy: dichotomy between cultured myocytes and animal models. *J. Mol. Cell. Cardiol.* **35,** 1385–1394.
111. Laufs, U. and Liao, J. K. (2000) Targeting Rho in cardiovascular disease. *Circ. Res.* **87,** 526–528.
112. Yamakawa, T., Tanaka, S., Numaguchi, K., et al. (2000) Involvement of Rho-kinase in angiotensin II-induced hypertrophy of rat vascular smooth muscle cells. *Hypertension* **35,** 313–318.
113. Pelletier, S., Duhamel, F., Coulombe, P., Popoff, M. R., and Meloche, S. (2003) Rho family GTPases are required for activation of Jak/STAT signaling by G protein-coupled receptors. *Mol. Cell. Biol.* **23,** 1316–1333.
114. Hanna, I. R., Taniyama, Y., Szocs, K., Rocic, P., and Griendling, K. K. (2002) NAD(P)H oxidase-derived reactive oxygen species as mediators of angiotensin II signaling. *Antioxid. Redox. Signal* **4,** 899–914.
115. Cai, H., Griendling, K. K., and Harrison, D. G. (2003) The vascular NAD(P)H oxidases as therapeutic targets in cardiovascular diseases. *Trends Pharmacol. Sci.* **24,** 471–478.
116. Griendling, K. K., Sorescu, D., and Ushio-Fukai, M. (2000) NAD(P)H oxidase: role in cardiovascular biology and disease. *Circ. Res.* **86,** 494–501.

3

Regulation of Cardiovascular Control Mechanisms by Angiotensin-(1–7) and Angiotensin-Converting Enzyme 2

Carlos M. Ferrario, David B. Averill,
K. Bridget Brosnihan, Mark C. Chappell,
Debra I. Diz, Patricia E. Gallagher,
Liomar Neves, and E. Ann Tallant

CONTENTS

1. INTRODUCTION

Among the molecular forms of angiotensin peptides generated by the action of renin on angiotensinogen (Aogen), both angiotensin II (Ang II) and the amino terminal heptapeptide angiotensin-(1–7) [Ang-(1–7)] are critically involved in the long-term control of tissue perfusion, cell–cell communication, development, and growth. Whereas an impressive body of literature continues to uncover pleiotropic effects of Ang II in the regulation of cell function, research on Ang-(1–7) has a shorter history as it was only 16 yr ago that a biological function for this heptapeptide was first demonstrated in the isolated rat neuro-hypophysial explant preparation *(1)*. On the contrary, the synthesis of angiotonin/hypertensin (now Ang II) was first obtained in 1957 *(2)*, three decades ahead of the discovery of Ang-(1–7) biological properties.

As Ang-(1–7) research continues to provide important and new information on the complexity of actions of the renin–angiotensin system (RAS) in homeostasis, it should be noted that one of the fundamental lessons learned from this discovery is that it

From: *Contemporary Endocrinology: Hypertension and Hormone Mechanisms*
Edited by: R. M. Carey © Humana Press Inc., Totowa, NJ

showed the existence of a feedback control mechanism whereby within the RAS a product, Ang-(1–7), regulates in an opposite manner the actions of the other product (Ang II) originating from a common substrate (angiotensin I) *(3,4)*. The current status of our knowledge about the physiological actions of Ang-(1–7), its formation and degradation, and its role in cardiovascular disease are discussed in this chapter.

2. ANG-(1–7)-FORMING AND -DEGRADING ENZYMES

The major bioactive components of the RAS are produced from the conversion of angiotensinogen to the decapeptide angiotensin I (Ang I) in both the circulation and tissues. At these sites, the reaction of Ang I with angiotensin-converting enzyme (ACE) forms Ang II, whereas Ang-(1–7) is generated from Ang I by the action of endopeptidases. Generation of the two peptides possessing different carboxy termini and contrasting biological actions diverges through enzymic reactions from which ACE functioning as a di-peptidyl carboxypeptidase cleaves the Phe^8–His^9 bond of Ang I to generate the octapeptide Ang II [Ang-(1–8)], whereas neutral endopeptidase 24.11 (neprilysin), 24.15 (thimet oligopeptidase), and 24.26 (prolyl-endopeptidase) cleave a tripeptide (Phe^8–His^9–Leu^{10}) from Ang I to produce Ang-(1–7) (Fig. 1). Both ACE and the endopeptidases have a wide tissue distribution, but our studies suggest that the conversion of Ang I to Ang-(1–7) by the various peptidases may be determined by the relative abundance of the enzyme in the tissue or in the circulation. In accord with this interpretation, we showed that neprilysin forms Ang-(1–7) from Ang I in the circulation, prolyl-endopeptidase 24.26 may be more active in brain tissue *(5)* and in vascular endothelium *(6)* whereas thimet oligopeptidase 24.15 is an Ang-(1–7)-forming enzyme in vascular smooth muscle *(7)*. The diversity of the Ang-(1–7)-forming enzymes reinforces our proposal that Ang-(1–7) may be a true *paracrine* or even *intracrine* hormone because its formation from Ang I could be determined in part by the relative abundance of the specific enzyme in either the circulation or the tissue compartment in which the Ang I substrate can react with the enzyme. The idea that tissue localization of the enzyme and its relative abundance are important is suggested by the demonstration that in renal tissue neprilysin degrades Ang-(1–7) into Ang-(1–4) *(8,9)*.

Additional studies of the catabolic pathways for Ang-(1–7) degradation showed that ACE hydrolyzes the heptapeptide into Ang-(1–5) *(10)*, a finding that signifies the contribution of the vasodilator and antiproliferative actions of Ang-(1–7) in explaining the mode of action of ACE inhibitors *(11–14)*.

Angiotensin-converting enzyme 2 (ACE2) is a newly identified enzyme of the RAS that catalyzes the conversion of Ang I to Ang-(1–9) and, more importantly, converts Ang II into Ang-(1–7) *(15–19)* (Fig. 1). ACE2 exhibits a high catalytic efficiency for the latter reaction—almost 500-fold greater than that for the conversion of Ang I to Ang-(1–9). From an array of over 120 peptides, only dynorphin A and apelin 13 were hydrolyzed by ACE2 with comparable kinetics to the conversion of Ang II to Ang-(1–7) *(18)*.

ACE2 was originally characterized as a homolog of ACE, sharing about 42% nucleotide sequence homology *(19,20)*. Although both enzymes are type I glycoproteins, there are notable differences. The somatic form of ACE has two catalytic sites; on the other hand, both the testicular form of ACE and ACE2 have only one. ACE2 is a carboxymonopeptidase with a preference for hydrolysis between a proline and the

Renin-Angiotensin Cascade

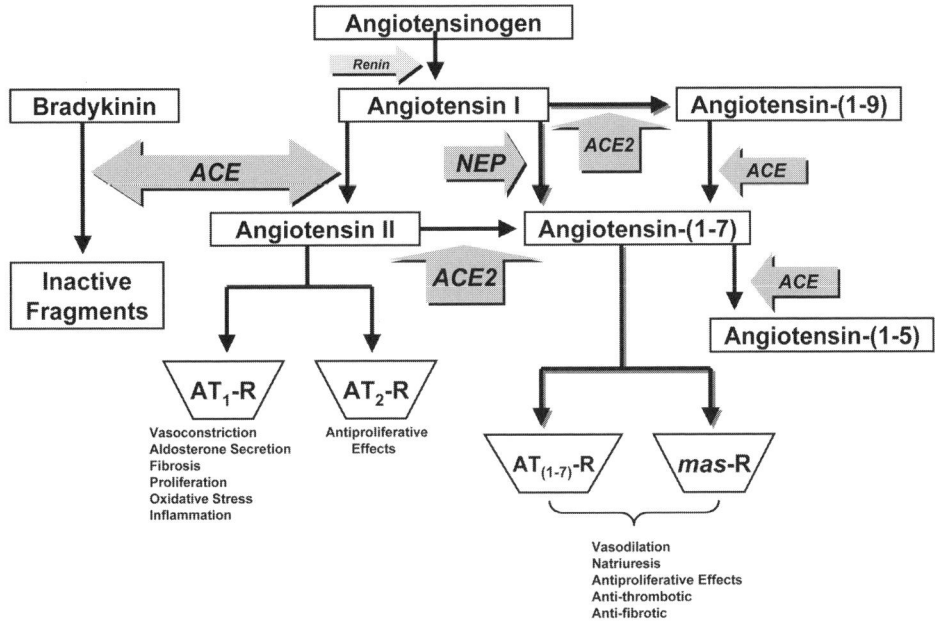

Fig. 1. Schematic representation of the biochemical cascade for angiotensin peptide formation and metabolism.

carboxy-terminal hydrophobic or basic residues, whereas ACE cleaves two amino acids from its substrate. The ACE2 sequence is similar to those of the testis-specific or germinal form of ACE (tACE) and the Drosophila homolog of ACE (AnCE; sequence identities of 43% and 35%, and similarities of 61% and 55%, respectively) *(21)*. Conformational differences between the somatic form of ACE and germinal ACE account for the demonstration that ACE2 activity is not blocked by ACE inhibitors *(15,19)*. The potential importance of ACE2, not only in the regulation of cardiac function and blood pressure but also in other disease states, has been realized with the discovery that ACE2 also serves as the cellular entry point for the severe acute respiratory syndrome (SARS) virus *(21–24)*. Prabakaran et al. *(21)* built a homology model of the ACE2 structure with a root-mean-square deviation less than 0.5 Å from the aligned crystal structures of tACE and AnCE. According to the authors a prominent feature of the model is a deep channel on the top of the molecule that contains the catalytic site *(21)*. Negatively charged ridges surrounding the channel may provide a possible binding site for the positively charged receptor-binding domain (RBD) of the *S*-glycoprotein, which they recently identified *(25)*. Several distinct patches of hydrophobic residues at the ACE2 surface were noted at close proximity to the charged ridges that could contribute to binding. These results may help explain the structure and function of ACE2.

3. LOCALIZATION OF ANG-(1–7) IN TISSUES

We have employed immunocytochemistry to identify the tissues expressing Ang-(1–7) focusing primarily on the heart, kidney, brain, vascular system, and the utero-placenta

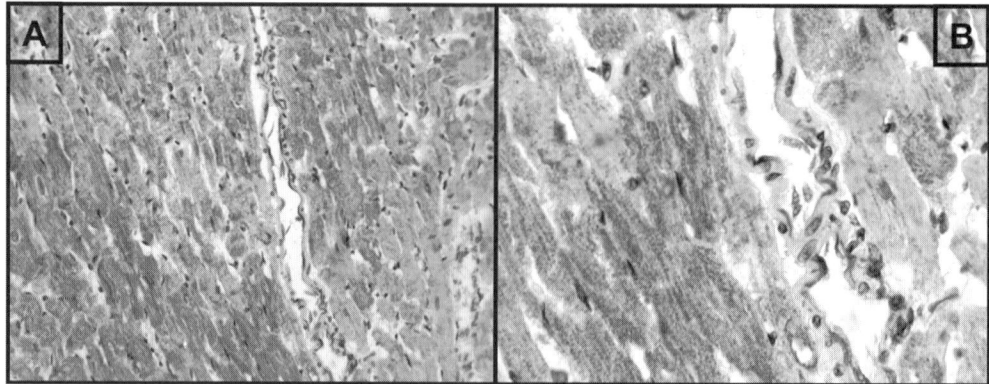

Fig. 2. Expression of Ang-(1–7)-like cardiac immunoreactivity in the rat. Ang-(1–7) staining was restricted to ventricular myocytes whereas it appeared as a granular reaction product throughout the cytoplasm (Panel **A**). The absence of Ang-(1–7) staining in endothelial and vascular smooth muscle cells of coronary vessels is best illustrated in the higher power magnification of Panel **B**. (*See* color version of this figure on color plates.)

complex. Early studies have demonstrated the Ang-(1–7) immunoreactivity in the cell bodies and in the axons of magnocellular neurons of the paraventricular nucleus (PVN) and supra-optic nucleus (SON) of the hypothalamus as well as in the neurons of the nucleus circularis *(26)*. In fact, Ang-(1–7) immunoreactivity in neurons of the PVN and SON was co-localized with vasopressin-like immunoreactivity whereas Ang-(1–7) was not co-localized in paraventricular neurons immunoreactive for oxytocin *(26,27)*. The same pattern of Ang-(1–7) immunoreactivity, seen in Sprague–Dawley rats, was also observed in the brains of (mRen2)27 transgenic rats *(28)* in which a subpopulation of nitric oxide synthase-containing neurons also contained Ang-(1–7)-like immunoreactivity. Collectively, the co-localization of Ang-(1–7) and vasopressin immunoreactivity in neurons of the magnocellular division of the PVN and the SON are congruent with functional studies demonstrating a role of Ang-(1–7) in the regulation of hydro-mineral balance involving neurons of the hypothalami-neurohypophysial pathway. In addition, the co-localization of Ang-(1–7) immunoreactivity in nitric oxide synthase-containing neurons of the PVN is especially interesting because a number of studies now show that the angiotensin peptides may modulate the disposition of reactive oxygen species in the PVN of animals with heart failure *(29)*.

Our interest in the role of Ang-(1–7) in cardiovascular regulation during heart failure led to the investigation of expression of Ang-(1–7) in the heart *(30)*. Ang-(1–7) immuno-reactivity in Lewis rats was restricted to myocytes of both the right and left ventricles. Fig. 2 shows that Ang-(1–7) staining in myocytes had a granular appearance throughout the cytoplasm. In contrast, there was a distinct absence of staining for the peptide in vascular smooth muscle as well as in interstitial cells of the heart. When Ang-(1–7) was examined in the hearts of rats subjected to ligation of the left main coronary artery, we observed a significant increase in Ang-(1–7) staining in ventricular myocytes that had undergone hypertrophic remodeling. In the region of ischemic damage there was a marked absence of Ang-(1–7) staining in fibroblasts and connective tissue. The increase in Ang-(1–7) staining in rats with congestive heart failure was positively correlated with an increase in left ventricular end-diastolic pressure and negatively correlated with

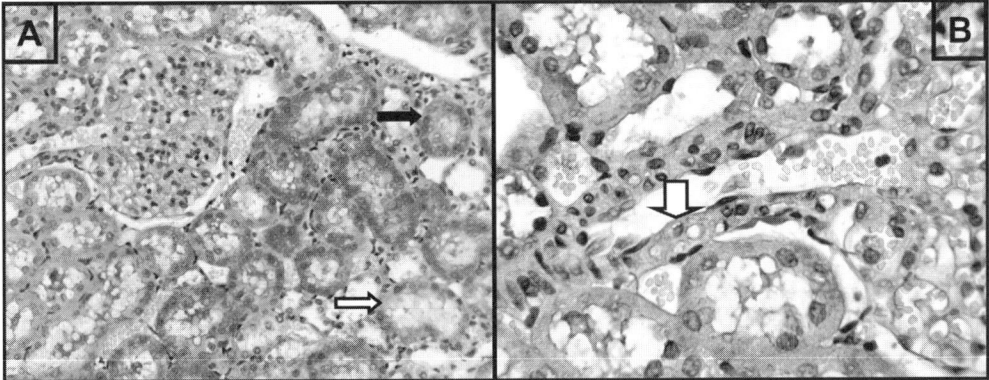

Fig. 3. Characteristics of Ang-(1–7)-like immunoreactivity in rat kidney. The most intense staining for Ang-(1–7) was in the thick-walled epithelial cells of the proximal-convoluted tubule (filled arrow in Panel **A**). A less intense staining for the peptide was observed in the thin-walled epithelial cells of collecting ducts (open arrow of Panel A). At both low (Panel A) and high (Panel **B**) power magnifications, there is essentially no staining for Ang-(1–7) in the glomerulus. Panel B also illustrates modest staining in the afferent arteriole (arrowhead in Panel B). (*See* color version of this figure on color plates.)

decreased cardiac contractility. These findings along with the report that Ang-(1–7) infusion in coronary ligated rats attenuated the development of heart failure *(31)* suggest that this peptide may play an important role in cardiac performance in cardiomyopathy.

Consistent with studies showing important actions of Ang-(1–7) in the regulation of renal function, characteristic features of Ang-(1–7) staining in the kidney are (1) varied intensity of staining in renal tubules with the degree of staining being more intense in proximal convoluted tubules and a lesser degree of staining in the thinner epithelial cells of the collecting ducts, (2) distinct absence of Ang-(1–7) immunoreactivity in the glomerulus, and (3) light staining in renal vessels (Fig. 3). Fig. 3B shows a granular reaction product for Ang-(1–7) staining in the juxtaglomerular cells of the afferent arteriole *(32)*. It is interesting that blood vessels (arterioles) of the kidney exhibit Ang-(1–7) staining whereas this was not the observation for blood vessels in the heart or in other organs.

4. PHYSIOLOGICAL ACTIONS

4.1. Effects on the Vasculature

Vasodilation produced by Ang-(1–7) was first described in 1993 by Benter et al. *(33)* in rats that were made areflexic by spinal cord destruction. The vasodilator properties of the peptide were confirmed in isolated canine *(34,35)* and porcine *(36)* coronary artery vessels, rabbit pial arterioles *(37)*, the rat mesenteric circulation *(38)*, the spontaneously hypertensive rats (SHR) *(39)*, [mRen2]27 hypertensive transgenic rats *(40)*, two-kidney one-clip hypertensive dogs *(41)*, and in the human forearm circulation *(42)*. As reviewed elsewhere *(43,44)*, the vasodilator response is mediated by release of vascular endothelium nitric oxide (NO), prostacyclin, and a receptor-mediated potentiation of bradykinin. The biological action of Ang-(1–7) satisfies the concept that the peptide acts to oppose the vasoconstrictor and hypertensive effects of Ang II by raising the activity of intrinsic vasodilator autocoids.

4.2. Effects on the Brain

Ang-(1–7) is present in hypothalamus, amygdala, and medulla oblongata at concentrations equivalent to or greater than those of Ang II *(45)* and evidence of a functional role for Ang-(1–7) exists in brain regions known to respond to other components of the RAS. Ang-(1–7) excites neurons in the PVN and in the nucleus of the solitary tract, dorsal motor nucleus of the vagus, and rostral and caudal ventrolateral medulla. The population of cells excited by Ang-(1–7) and Ang II shows some overlap, but the majority of cells respond to one or the other peptide. In addition to direct cellular actions, Ang-(1–7) releases other neurotransmitters including monoamines, substance P, vasopressin, glutamate, prostaglandins, and NO as reviewed recently *(43)*. Like Ang II, the Ang-(1–7)-mediated release of vasopressin may involve tachykinin peptides *(46–48)*. In contrast, intracerebroventricular injections of Ang-(1–7) do not increase blood pressure or promote drinking, which are thought to be mediated by Ang II acting on monoaminergic pathways *(49,50)*. An opposing action of Ang-(1–7) on central mechanisms regulating blood pressure is demonstrated by the finding that cerebroventricular injections of antibodies to Ang-(1–7) produce opposite effects to those of Ang II *(47)*. Evidence from studies using *c-fos* reveals that Ang-(1–7) activates pathways in the organum vasculosum of the lamina terminalis and median preoptic nucleus, whereas Ang II activates these pathways as well as those involving the PVN and subfornical organ *(51,52)*. Pathways in the medulla oblongata appear separate for the two peptides as well, since sino-aortic denervation potentiated the responses to Ang-(1–7) but not those to Ang II in the nucleus of the solitary tract *(53)*.

Important indicators of a role for the endogenous peptide in cardiovascular regulation come from studies using the Ang-(1–7) antagonist D-Ala[7]–Ang-(1–7) *(44)*. Blockade of endogenous Ang-(1–7) within the solitary tract nucleus augments baroreceptor reflex control of heart rate, providing an independent and opposite effect from those of Ang II *(54,55)*. A loss of tonic input by Ang-(1–7) may accompany the age-related decrease in reflex gain *(56)*. In ASrAogen animals deficient of glial angiotensinogen, a role for endogenous Ang-(1–7) to facilitate baroreflex sensitivity persists, whereas the attenuating effect of Ang II is lost *(57)*. These data suggest different sources of the two peptides consistent with their divergent functional effects. In the rostral and caudal ventrolateral medulla, Ang-(1–7) exerts excitatory actions mimicking those of Ang II *(54,55)*, although clear differences exist in terms of regulation of the responses to the two peptides *(58–60)*.

In brain, receptor subtypes exhibiting varying degrees of selectivity for either the AT_1 or AT_2 antagonists and D-Ala[7]–Ang-(1–7) appear to mediate the actions of Ang-(1–7) *(43,61,62)*. The pharmacology of the receptor involved may be dependent on the specific transmitter studied, but blockade by D-Ala[7]–Ang-(1–7) is a common feature as reviewed in detail by Ferrario et al. *(43)*. As an explanation for the fact that either D-Ala[7]–Ang-(1–7), AT_1 or AT_2 receptor antagonists, or some combination of the three antagonists is effective in blocking actions of Ang-(1–7) in brain, there is evidence that distinct subpopulations of classical AT_1 sites in the nucleus tractus solitarius (nTS) and dorsal motor nucleus of the vagus (dmnX) exist showing differential sensitivity/selectivity to Ang-(1–7) and the AT_2 antagonist *(43)*. Moreover, AT_1 receptor antagonists (either losartan or candesartan) and D-Ala[7]–Ang-(1–7) block the actions of the peptide in the nTS *(63)* and ventrolateral medulla *(64)*. It is now recognized that the *mas* gene codes for a receptor responsible for vascular and renal effects of Ang-(1–7) *(65)*. Mice deficient in the *mas* receptor show impairments in the baroreceptor reflex and alterations in responses to Ang II *(64,66)*, providing additional evidence of a role for endogenous Ang-(1–7) in these functions.

4.3. Effects on the Heart

There are few studies about the direct actions of Ang-(1–7) on heart function, although the peptide is highly expressed in rat myocardium *(30)* and can be detected in larger concentrations in the cardiac interstitium or the coronary sinus blood after acute coronary artery ligation *(67–69)*. In the isolated perfused heart of a rat, Ang-(1–7) appears to act as an anti-arrhythmogenic factor during reperfusion injury *(70,71)*, although a study from the same group showed that Ang-(1–7) increased reperfusion arrhythmias *(72)*. Functional data in whole animals suggest that Ang-(1–7) may have cardioprotective functions because an 8 wk infusion of Ang-(1–7) in Sprague–Dawley rats, started 2-wk postmyocardial infarction, attenuated heart failure progression together with restoration of vascular endothelial function *(31)*. That the heart may be an important site for Ang-(1–7) actions is highlighted by the demonstration that ACE activity in plasma and atrial tissue is inhibited by Ang-(1–7) *(73)* whereas the peptide enhances tritiated norepinephrine release from isolated atrial tissue at doses comparable to those for Ang II *(74)*.

The studies by us *(69,75)* and others on the relation between Ang-(1–7) function and cardiac ACE2 expression are shedding light on an intracardiac role for Ang-(1–7) as counterbalancing the hypertrophic and inotropic actions of Ang-(1–7) following myocardial injury. Ang-(1–7) was formed in the intact human myocardial circulation in patients with postcardiac transplantation and its levels were decreased when Ang II formation was suppressed by enalaprilat *(76)*. The evolution of myocardial infarction in the rat 28 d after coronary artery ligation was accompanied by large increases in plasma Ang-(1–7) concentrations; further plasma Ang-(1–7) augmentation accompanied by reversal of cardiac remodeling because of continuous blockade of Ang II receptors with either losartan or olmesartan was accompanied by a threefold increase in cardiac ACE2 mRNA *(75)*. In addition, emerging data suggest that Ang-(1–7) may oppose the atherogenic actions of Ang II through inhibition of smooth muscle proliferation and blockade of inflammatory cytokines. This interpretation is supported by the finding that the chronic effects of losartan in the prevention of fatty streak formation and monocyte activation in monkeys was associated with large increases in plasma Ang-(1–7) concentrations *(77–81)*.

4.4. Effects on the Kidney

Although Ang-(1–7) is processed from either Ang I or Ang II in the circulation and in many tissues, it is important to emphasize that the processing pathways for Ang-(1–7) in the circulation and kidney are distinct. The endopeptidase neprilysin is the primary enzyme forming Ang-(1–7) from Ang I or Ang-(1–9) in the circulation *(43,82)*. Although levels of neprilysin are low to undetectable, the enzyme is appropriately localized to the exocellular surface of endothelial and smooth muscle cells to contribute to the formation of Ang-(1–7). In the kidney, Ang-(1–7) is the primary product formed in preparations of isolated proximal tubules and exists in urine at significantly higher levels than Ang II *(8)*. Neprilysin may contribute to both the formation as well as the degradation of the peptide. Neprilysin cleaves Ang I to Ang-(1–7), but continues to metabolize Ang-(1–7) at the Tyr^5–Ile^6 bond to form Ang-(1–4) and Ang-(5–7) *(8,9)*. Indeed, neprilysin inhibitors increase the urinary levels of Ang-(1–7) in both human and rat *(83,84)*. Moreover, the combined ACE/neprilysin inhibitor omapatrilat augmented renal and urinary levels of Ang-(1–7), but produced a blunted Ang-(1–7) response in plasma in comparison to ACE inhibition alone *(32,84)*. Omapatrilat was also associated with increased expression of ACE2 and Ang-(1–7) in the proximal tubule *(85)*. These data suggest that upregulation of ACE2 may contribute to the renal protective effects of ACE or combined vaso-peptidase inhibitors through increased conversion of Ang II to Ang-(1–7), as well as the reduced metabolism of Ang-(1–7). Indeed, ACE2 (–/–) mice exhibit enhanced intrarenal levels of Ang II and pronounced glomerulosclerosis *(83)*.

We found that Ang-(1–7) and ACE2 are present within the proximal tubular regions of the mouse and the rat kidney *(86,87)*. These data clearly support the concept of a complete RAS within the proximal tubule including expression of renin, ACE, angiotensinogen, the AT_1 and AT_2 receptors *(88,89)*. The presence of Ang II and Ang-(1–7) in kidney supports the concept of important and divergent actions for the two peptides. For Ang II, renal actions include potent vasoconstriction, retention of sodium and water, as well as a stimulus for inflammation, and oxidative stress. In contrast, Ang-(1–7) stimulates diuresis and natriuresis that are associated with modest increases in the glomerular filtration rate *(43)*. Ang-(1–7) induces vasodilation of afferent arterioles through a NO-dependent pathway *(90)*. Indeed, immunocytochemical staining for the Ang-(1–7) receptor *mas* is evident in the afferent arteriole, as well as throughout the proximal tubules of the renal cortex providing biochemical support for the functional actions of the peptide *(87)*. Ang-(1–7) and its metabolite Ang-(3–7) are potent inhibitors of Na^+, K^+-ATPase activity in the renal epithelium *(91–93)*. Ang-(1–7) also inhibits the transcellular flux of sodium, which was associated with activation of phospholipase A_2 (PLA_2) *(94)*. Ang-(1–7) dependent inhibition of sodium transport is potentiated by ACE inhibition suggesting a shift toward the formation and protection of Ang-(1–7) within the proximal tubules. The chronic and pronounced diuresis following omapatrilat treatment was associated with large increases in urinary excretion of Ang-(1–7) and enhanced immunocytochemical staining of the peptide in the kidney *(32)*. Recent studies have revealed that Ang-(1–7) abolished the Ang II-dependent stimulation of the Na^+-ATPase activity in ovine kidney *(95,96)*. Furthermore, intrarenal administration of Ang-(1–7) blocked the antinatriuretic actions of Ang II *(97)*. These studies emphasize that the actions of Ang-(1–7) within the kidney may be particularly relevant in the setting of an activated RAS. Moreover, the discrete localization of Ang-(1–7), ACE2, and the *mas* receptor provides evidence for an alternative RAS within the proximal tubule epithelium that may antagonize the actions of Ang II in this renal compartment.

4.5. Ang-(1–7) in Gestation and Pregnancy

Pregnancy is a physiological condition characterized by increased RAS activity *(98)* that does not manifest in increased blood pressure *(99)*. Merrill et al. *(100)* evaluated the effect of pregnancy on Ang-(1–7) in nulliparous preeclamptic patients and in third trimester normotensive pregnant controls (3rd T; matched for parity, race, and gestational age). Plasma Ang-(1–7) was increased by 34% ($p < 0.05$), whereas plasma Ang II was increased by 50% ($p < 0.05$). In preeclampsia subjects plasma Ang-(1–7) was reduced (13 ± 2 pg/mL, $p < 0.05$ vs third T); plasma Ang II was also reduced (32 ± 4 pg/mL, preeclamptic vs 3rd trimester normal pregnant, $p < 0.05$), but remained elevated as compared to nonpregnant subjects and 50% higher than plasma Ang-(1–7). Other components of the RAS, with the exception of ACE, were reduced in preeclamptic subjects. Assessment of the relationship between Ang-(1–7) and blood pressure revealed a negative correlation of Ang-(1–7) with systolic ($r = -0.4$, $p < 0.02$) and diastolic ($r = -0.5$, $p < 0.02$) blood pressures. These data suggested a potential role for reduced production of Ang-(1–7) contributing to the elevated blood pressure. In preeclampsia, the decreased levels of plasma Ang-(1–7) in the presence of persistent elevated plasma Ang II are consistent with the development of hypertension.

Additionally, a 24-h urinary excretion of Ang-(1–7) and Ang II was evaluated during the ovulatory menstrual cycle, single normotensive pregnancies, and their subsequent lactation *(101)*. No significant differences in urinary Ang-(1–7) were observed between the follicular and luteal phase of the normal menstrual cycle. There was a progressive rise of urinary Ang-(1–7) throughout normal human gestation, attaining levels that are 10-fold greater than that of the normal menstrual cycle. Urinary Ang II showed a similar pattern reaching levels that were 25-fold higher than the values at the menstrual cycle. At 35 wk of gestation, Ang-(1–7) was the predominant angiotensin peptide in the urine, reaching levels that were sixfold higher than Ang II. The urinary excretion levels may reflect local kidney production of peptides. Thus, increases in renal Ang-(1–7) levels may play a role in the vasodilatory adaptations of mid and late human pregnancies.

To understand the contribution of the RAS during pregnancy, studies were conducted in pregnant rats at late gestation (19th day) and compared to virgin female rats at diestrus phase of the estrous cycle. Twenty-four hour urinary excretion of the angiotensin peptides was significantly increased in pregnant animals by 93% (Ang I), 44% (Ang II), and 60% [Ang-(1–7)] of values found in virgin rats. Kidney Ang I and Ang-(1–7) concentrations were significantly increased by seven- and fivefold, respectively ($p < 0.05$) in pregnant animals as compared to virgin females. In contrast, there was no significant change in renal Ang II concentrations of pregnant and virgin females. These studies provide evidence that urinary excretion of angiotensin peptides reflect local kidney content of angiotensins during pregnancy. The potential contribution of Ang-(1–7) to vascular control in pregnancy was also documented from increased vasodilator responses to the local application of the peptide in isolated small mesenteric arteries obtained from pregnant rats *(102)*. In alignment with this interpretation, Ang-(1–7) and ACE2 staining in the kidney of 19 d pregnant Sprague–Dawley rats showed higher intensity when compared with virgin rats *(103)*.

5. ANG-(1–7) RECEPTOR MECHANISMS

Ang-(1–7) is a poor competitor at pharmacologically defined AT_1 or AT_2 receptors *(104–107)*. Santos et al. *(62)* designed a selective antagonist for the Ang-(1–7) receptor by replacing the a-proline at position 7 of Ang-(1–7) with D-alamine [D-Ala[7]]–Ang-(1–7). In initial studies, [D-Ala[7]]–Ang-(1–7) blocked hemodynamic and renal effects of

Ang-(1–7), did not compete for binding at rat adrenal AT_1 or AT_2 receptors, and did not attenuate pressor or contractile responses to Ang II, demonstrating selectivity for Ang-(1–7). We identified Ang-(1–7) binding sites on bovine aortic endothelial cells (BAEC), canine coronary artery rings, and rat blood vessels that are sensitive to [D-Ala^7]–Ang-(1–7) *(108–110)*. In addition, a multitude of physiological responses to Ang-(1–7) are selectively blocked by [D-Ala^7]–Ang-(1–7) or the sarcosine analogs of Ang II, but not by AT_1 or AT_2 receptor antagonists, including the depressor response to Ang-(1–7) in the pithed rat and the lowering of blood pressure in hypertensive rats *(33,40,111)*. Collectively, these results demonstrate that the hypotensive response to Ang-(1–7) is mediated by a non-AT_1, non-AT_2, [D-Ala^7]–Ang-(1–7)-sensitive receptor. We refer to this receptor as the $AT_{(1-7)}$ receptor, as defined by its sensitivity to Ang-(1–7), its antagonism by [Sar^1–Thr^8]-Ang II and [D-Ala^7]–Ang-(1–7), and its lack of response to AT_1 or AT_2 receptor antagonists, either functionally or in competition for binding.

Identification of an $AT_{(1-7)}$ receptor is confounded by reports of responses to Ang-(1–7) that are sensitive to AT_1 or AT_2 receptor antagonists or both. Some of the renal and central effects of Ang-(1–7) are mediated by a losartan-sensitive receptor *(64,91,112)*. Arachidonic acid release from rabbit VSMCs and hypothalamic norepinephrine release were blocked by both [D-Ala^7]–Ang-(1–7) and the AT_2 antagonist PD123319 *(113,114)*. Additional responses to Ang-(1–7) in brain and heart are blocked by both AT_1 and AT_2 receptor antagonists *(74,115)*. These results provide evidence for additional subtypes of the $AT_{(1-7)}$ receptor that are sensitive to losartan and/or PD123319 or suggest an interaction with the AT_1 and/or the AT_2 receptor.

Many of the physiological and cellular responses that are mediated by the $AT_{(1-7)}$ receptor are linked to the production of prostaglandins. Ang-(1–7) stimulates prostaglandin production in endothelial cells, VSMCs, astrocytes, and renal tubular epithelial cells *(74,94,104–107,115)*. In addition, physiological responses to Ang-(1–7) are dependent on prostanoid production, based on the studies using the cyclooxygenase inhibitor indomethacin (Fig. 4).

Recently, Santos et al. *(65)* reported that the orphan G protein-coupled receptor *mas* is an Ang-(1–7) receptor. Ang-(1–7) bound with high affinity to cells transfected with the *mas* receptor, which was blocked by [D-Ala^7]–Ang-(1–7), and renal or depressor responses to Ang-(1–7) were lost in *mas*-depleted mice. We recently showed that antisense oligonucleotides or siRNAs to *mas* prevent the Ang-(1–7)-mediated inhibition of growth in VSMCs, which is also blocked by [D-Ala^7]–Ang-(1–7) *(116)*. These results suggest that the *mas* receptor serves as a selective Ang-(1–7) binding site. Fig. 4 shows the signal transduction pathway by which Ang-(1–7) activates the G protein-coupled *mas* receptor to increase the production of NO and prostacyclin (PGI_2) via increases in cGMP and cAMP, respectively. Ang-(1–7) also reduces the mitogen-activated protein kinases (MAPKs) by either increasing MAPK phosphatases or reducing the MAPK kinase MEK. The increase in cAMP and cGMP and the decrease in MAPK activity cause vasodilation and inhibit cell growth. The *mas* receptor is predominantly expressed in the testis and the hippocampus and amygdala of the mammalian forebrain with minimal levels in the rodent heart and kidney. This tissue distribution differs from previous reports of Ang-(1–7) binding and functional responses, suggesting the existence of other $AT_{(1-7)}$ receptors.

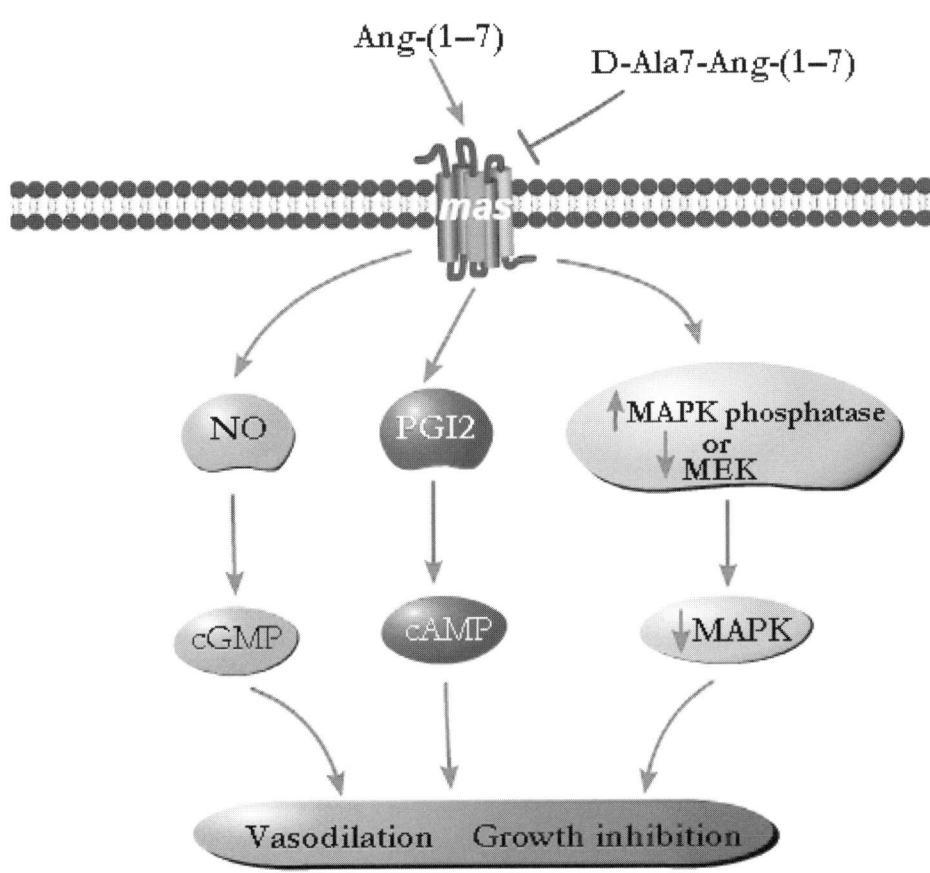

Fig. 4. The major signal transduction pathways for Ang-(1–7). Ang-(1–7) activates the G protein-coupled *mas* receptor to increase the production of nitric oxide (NO) and prostacyclin (PGI$_2$) to increase cGMP and cAMP, respectively. Ang-(1–7) also reduces the mitogen-activated protein kinases (MAPKs) by either increasing MAPK phosphatases or reducing the MAPK kinase MEK. The increase in cAMP and cGMP and the decrease in MAPK activity cause vasodilation and inhibit cell growth. (*See* color version of this figure on color plates.)

6. SUMMARY

Ang-(1–7), a product of both Ang I and Ang II metabolisms, functions to antagonize the actions of Ang II by acting primarily through binding to a non-AT$_1$/AT$_2$ receptor and also the *mas* receptor. Ang-(1–7) stimulates vasodilation through increased production of vasodilator prostaglandins and NO, as well as amplifying the intrinsic actions of bradykinin. In the kidney, Ang-(1–7) promotes natriuresis and diuresis through an effect on transport mechanisms involved in water and electrolyte absorption within the renal tubules and collecting ducts. In addition, Ang-(1–7) modulates the actions of tubular vasopressin via an effect on its V2 receptor. In the heart, Ang-(1–7) counteracts the hypertrophic, pro-fibrotic, and pro-thrombotic effects of Ang II as well as increases myocardial blood flow.

Ang-(1–7) contributes to the antihypertensive effects of ACE inhibitors and Ang II antagonists by several mechanisms *(84,117,118,119)*. Inhibition of ACE increases blood and tissue concentrations of Ang-(1–7) by preventing ACE-mediated Ang-(1–7) degradation and increasing substrate (Ang I) availability. In contrast, blockade of Ang II receptors increases blood and tissue levels of Ang-(1–7) by: (i) increasing Ang I substrate availability through the dis-inhibition of Ang II-mediated renin release, and (ii) augmenting the rate of Ang II conversion into Ang-(1–7) via increased ACE2 expression and activity. Both ACE and ACE2 represent critical steps at which modulation of angiotensin peptide functions are precisely regulated, the specific mechanisms of which need further investigation. Genomic studies are also urgently needed to determine whether polymorphisms in the ACE2 gene or the genes for Ang-(1–7)-forming enzymes exist.

ACKNOWLEDGMENTS

The study described in this review was supported in part by grants from the National Heart, Lung and Blood Institute of the National Institutes of Health (HL-51952, HL-068258, and HL-56973, HL-67363, HL-42631), and the American Heart Association (AHA 151521). An unrestricted grant from the Unifi Corporation (Greensboro, NC) is also acknowledged.

REFERENCES

1. Schiavone, M. T., Santos, R. A., Brosnihan, K. B., Khosla, M. C., and Ferrario, C. M. (1988) Release of vasopressin from the rat hypothalamo-neurohypophysial system by angiotensin-(1–7) heptapeptide. *Proc. Natl Acad. Sci. USA* **85(11)**, 4095–4098.
2. Bumpus, F. M. Schwarz, H., and Page, I. H. (1957) Synthesis and pharmacology of the octapeptide angiotonin. *Science* **125(3253)**, 886–887.
3. Ferrario, C. M., Brosnihan, K. B., Diz, D. I. et al. (1991) Angiotensin-(1–7): a new hormone of the angiotensin system. *Hypertension* **18(5)**, III126–III133.
4. Kohara, K., Brosnihan, K. B., Chappell, M. C., Khosla, M. C., and Ferrario, C. M. (1991) Angiotensin-(1–7). A member of circulating angiotensin peptides. *Hypertension* **17(2)**, 131–138.
5. Welches, W. R., Santos, R. A., Chappell, M. C., Brosnihan, K. B., Greene, L. J., and Ferrario, C. M. (1991) Evidence that prolyl endopeptidase participates in the processing of brain angiotensin. *J. Hypertens.* **9(7)**, 631–638.
6. Santos, R. A., Brosnihan, K. B., Jacobsen, D. W., DiCorleto, P. E., and Ferrario, C. M. (1992) Production of angiotensin-(1–7) by human vascular endothelium. *Hypertension* **19(2)**, II56–II61.
7. Chappell, M. C., Welches, W. R., Brosnihan, K. B., and Ferrario, C. M. (1992) Inhibition of angiotensin converting enzyme by the metalloendopeptidase 3.4.24.15 inhibitor c-phenylpropyl-alanyl-alanyl-phenylalanyl-p-aminobenzoate. *Peptides* **13**, 943–946.
8. Allred, A. J., Diz, D. I., Ferrario, C. M., and Chappell, M. C. (2000) Pathways for angiotensin-(1–7) metabolism in pulmonary and renal tissues. *Am. J. Physiol.* **279(5)**, F841–F850.
9. Chappell, M. C., Allred, A. J., and Ferrario, C. M. (2001) Pathways of angiotensin-(1–7) metabolism in the kidney. *Nephrol. Dial. Transplant.* **16(1)**, 22–26.
10. Chappell, M. C., Pirro, N. T., Sykes, A., and Ferrario, C. M. (1998) Metabolism of angiotensin-(1–7) by angiotensin converting enzyme. *Hypertension* **31(1)**, 362–367.
11. Chappell, M. C., Gomez, M. N., Pirro, N. T., and Ferrario, C. M. (2000) Release of angiotensin-(1–7) from the rat hindlimb: influence of angiotensin-converting enzyme inhibition. *Hypertension* **35(1)**, 348–352.
12. Yamada, K., Iyer, S. N., Chappell, M. C., Ganten, D., and Ferrario, C. M. (1998) Converting enzyme determines plasma clearance of angiotensin-(1–7). *Hypertension* **32(3)**, 496–502.
13. Iyer, S. N., Chappell, M. C., Averill, D. B., Diz, D. I., and Ferrario, C. M. (1998) Vasodepressor actions of angiotensin-(1–7) unmasked during combined treatment with lisinopril and losartan. *Hypertension* **31(2)**, 699–705.

14. Iyer, S. N., Ferrario, C. M., and Chappell, M. C. (1998) Angiotensin-(1–7) contributes to the antihypertensive effects of blockade of the renin-angiotensin system. *Hypertension* **31(1),** 356–361.
15. Donoghue, M., Hsieh, F., Baronas, E., et al. (2000) A novel angiotensin-converting enzyme-related carboxypeptidase (ACE2) converts angiotensin I to angiotensin 1–9. *Circ. Res.* **87(5),** E1–E9.
16. Turner, A. J., Tipnis, S. R., Guy, J. L., Rice, G., and Hooper, N. M. (2002) ACEH/ACE2 is a novel mammalian metallocarboxypeptidase and a homologue of angiotensin-converting enzyme insensitive to ACE inhibitors. *Can. J. Physiol. Pharmacol.* **80(4),** 346–353.
17. Turner, A. J. and Hooper, N. M. (2002) The angiotensin-converting enzyme gene family: genomics and pharmacology. *Trends Pharmacol. Sci.* **23(4),** 177–183.
18. Vickers, C., Hales, P., Kaushik, V., et al. (2002) Hydrolysis of biological peptides by human angiotensin-converting enzyme-related carboxypeptidase. *J. Biol. Chem.* **277(17),** 14,838–14,843.
19. Tipnis, S. R., Hooper, N. M., Hyde, R., Karran, E., Christie, G., and Turner, A. J. (2000) A human homolog of angiotensin-converting enzyme. Cloning and functional expression as a captopril-insensitive carboxypeptidase. *J. Biol. Chem.* **275(43),** 33,238–33,243.
20. Donoghue, M., Wakimoto, H., Maguire, C. T., et al. (2003) Heart block, ventricular tachycardia, and sudden death in ACE2 transgenic mice with downregulated connexins. *J. Mol. Cell. Cardiol.* **35(9),** 1043–1053.
21. Prabakaran, P., Xiao, X., and Dimitrov, D. S. (2004) A model of the ACE2 structure and function as a SARS-CoV receptor. *Biochem. Biophys. Res. Commun.* **314(1),** 235–241.
22. Dimitrov, D. S. (2003) The secret life of ACE2 as a receptor for the SARS virus. *Cell* **115(6),** 652–653.
23. Li, W., Moore, M. J., Vasilieva, N., et al. (2003) Angiotensin-converting enzyme 2 is a functional receptor for the SARS coronavirus. *Nature* **426(6965),** 450–454.
24. Turner, A. J., Hiscox, J. A., and Hooper, N. M. (2004) ACE2: from vasopeptidase to SARS virus receptor. *Trends Pharmacol. Sci.* **25(6),** 291–294.
25. Xiao, X., Chakraborti, S., Dimitrov, A. S., Gramatikoff, K., and Dimitrov, D. S. (2003) The SARS-CoV S glycoprotein: expression and functional characterization. *Biochem. Biophys. Res. Commun.* **312(4),** 1159–1164.
26. Block, C. H., Santos, R. A., Brosnihan, K. B., and Ferrario, C. M. (1988) Immunocytochemical localization of angiotensin-(1–7) in the rat forebrain. *Peptides* **9(6),** 1395–1401.
27. Krob, H. A., Vinsant, S. L., Ferrario, C. M., and Friedman, D. P. (1998) Angiotensin-(1–7) immunoreactivity in the hypothalamus of the (mRen-2d)27 transgenic rat. *Brain Res.* **798(1–2),** 36–45.
28. Calka, J. and Block, C. H. (1993) Angiotensin-(1–7) and nitric oxide synthase in the hypothalamo-neurohypophysial system. *Brain Res. Bull.* **30(5–6),** 677–685.
29. Zucker, I. H. (2002) Brain angiotensin II: new insights into its role in sympathetic regulation. *Circ. Res.* **90(5),** 503–505.
30. Averill, D. B., Ishiyama, Y., Chappell, M. C., and Ferrario, C. M. (2003) Cardiac angiotensin-(1–7) in ischemic cardiomyopathy. *Circulation* **108(17),** 2141–2146.
31. Loot, A. E., Roks, A. J., Henning, R. H., et al. (2002) Angiotensin-(1–7) attenuates the development of heart failure after myocardial infarction in rats. *Circulation* **105(13),** 1548–1550.
32. Ferrario, C. M., Averill, D. B., Brosnihan, K. B., et al. (2002) Vasopeptidase inhibition and Ang-(1–7) in the spontaneously hypertensive rat. *Kidney Int.* **62(4),** 1349–1357.
33. Benter, I. F., Diz, D. I., and Ferrario, C. M. (1993) Cardiovascular actions of angiotensin (1–7). *Peptides* **14(4),** 679–684.
34. Brosnihan, K. B., Li, P., and Ferrario, C. M. (1996) Angiotensin-(1–7) dilates canine coronary arteries through kinins and nitric oxide. *Hypertension* **27(3),** 523–528.
35. Brosnihan, K. B. (1998) Effect of the angiotensin-(1–7) peptide on nitric oxide release. *Am. J. Cardiol.* **82(10A),** 17S–19S.
36. Porsti, I., Bara, A. T., Busse, R., and Hecker, M. (1994) Release of nitric oxide by angiotensin-(1–7) from porcine coronary endothelium: implications for a novel angiotensin receptor. *Br. J. Pharmacol.* **111(3),** 652–654.
37. Meng, W. and Busija, D. W. (1993) Comparative effects of angiotensin-(1–7) and angiotensin II on piglet pial arterioles. *Stroke* **24(12),** 2041–2044.
38. Neves, L. A., Averill, D. B., Ferrario, C. M., et al. (2003) Characterization of angiotensin-(1–7) receptor subtype in mesenteric arteries. *Peptides* **24(3),** 455–462.
39. Kohara, K., Brosnihan, K. B., and Ferrario, C. M. (1993) Angiotensin-(1–7) in the spontaneously hypertensive rat. *Peptides* **14(5),** 883–891.

40. Iyer, S. N., Averill, D. B., Chappell, M. C., Yamada, K., Allred, A. J., and Ferrario, C. M. (2000) Contribution of angiotensin-(1–7) to blood pressure regulation in salt-depleted hypertensive rats. *Hypertension* **36(3),** 417–422.

41. Nakamoto, H., Ferrario, C. M., Fuller, S. B., Robaczwski, D. L., Winicov, E., and Dean, R. H. (1995) Angiotensin-(1–7) and nitric oxide interaction in renovascular hypertension. *Hypertension* **25,** 796–802.

42. Ueda, S., Masumori-Maemoto, S., Wada, A., Ishii, M., Brosnihan, K. B., and Umemura, S. (2001) Angiotensin-(1–7) potentiates bradykinin-induced vasodilatation in man. *J. Hypertens.* **19(11),** 2001–2009.

43. Ferrario, C. M., Averill, D. B., Brosnihan, K. B., et al. (2004) Angiotensin-(1–7): its contributions to arterial pressure control mechanisms. In: *Handbook of Experimental Pharmacology: Angiotensin* (Unger, T. and Scholkens, B. A., eds.), Vol. 1, Springer, Heidelberg, pp. 478–518.

44. Santos, R. A., Campagnole-Santos, M. J., and Andrade, S. P. (2000) Angiotensin-(1–7): an update. *Regul. Pept.* **91(1–3),** 45–62.

45. Chappell, M. C., Brosnihan, K. B., Diz, D. I., and Ferrario, C. M. (1989) Identification of angiotensin-(1–7) in rat brain. Evidence for differential processing of angiotensin peptides. *J. Biol. Chem.* **264(28),** 16,518–16,523.

46. Massi, M., Saija, A., Polidori, C., et al. (1991) The hypothalamic paraventricular nucleus is a site of action for the central effect of tachykinins on plasma vasopressin. *Brain Res. Bull.* **26(1),** 149–154.

47. Moriguchi, A., Tallant, E. A., Matsumura, K., et al. (1995) Opposing actions of angiotensin-(1–7) and angiotensin II in the brain of transgenic hypertensive rats. *Hypertension* **25(6),** 1260–1265.

48. Perfumi, M., Sajia, A., Costa, G., Massi, M., and Polidori, C. (1988) Vasopressin release induced by intracranial injection of eledoisin is mediated by central angiotensin II. *Pharmacol. Res. Commun.* **20(9),** 811–826.

49. Diz, D. I., Fantz, D. L., Benter, I. F., and Bosch, S. M. (1997) Acute depressor actions of angiotensin II in the nucleus of the solitary tract are mediated by substance P. *Am. J. Physiol.* **273(1),** R28–R34.

50. Kawabe, H., Husain, A., Khosla, M. C., Smeby, R. R., Bumpus, F. M., and Ferrario, C. M. (1986) Characterization of receptors for angiotensin-induced drinking and blood pressure responses in conscious rats using angiotensin analogs extended at the N-terminal. *Neuroendocrinology* **42(4),** 289–295.

51. Mahon, J. M., Carr, R. D., Nicol, A. K., and Henderson, I. W. (1994) Angiotensin-(1–7) is an antagonist at the type 1 angiotensin II receptor. *J. Hypertens.* **12(12),** 1377–1381.

52. Mahon, J. M., Allen, M., Herbert, J., and Fitzsimons, J. T. (1995) The association of thirst, sodium appetite and vasopressin release with c-fos expression in the forebrain of the rat after intracerebroventricular injection of angiotensin II, angiotensin-(1–7) or carbachol. *Neuroscience* **69(1),** 199–208.

53. Campagnole-Santos, M. J., Diz, D. I., and Ferrario, C. M. (1990) Actions of angiotensin peptides after partial denervation of the solitary tract nucleus. *Hypertension* **15(2),** I34–I39.

54. Averill, D. B. and Diz, D. I. (2000) Angiotensin peptides and baroreflex control of sympathetic outflow: pathways and mechanisms of the medulla oblongata. *Brain Res. Bull.* **51(2),** 119–128.

55. Diz, D. I., Jessup, J. A., Westwood, B. M., et al. (2002) Angiotensin peptides as neurotransmitters/ neuromodulators in the dorsomedial medulla. *Clin. Exp. Pharmacol. Physiol.* **29(5–6),** 473–482.

56. Sakima, A., Averill, D. B., Oden, S. D., et al. (2004) Reduced baroreflex sensitivity and diminished role for endogenous angiotensin-(1–7) at the nucleus tractus solitarii in older rats may reflect reduced formation of the peptide. *Hypertension* **44(4),** 521–522.

57. Sakima, A., Averill, D. B., Oden, S. D., Ganten, D., Ferrario, C. M., and Diz, D. I. (2004) Glial versus non-glial angiotensin II and angiotensin-(1–7) in the nucleus tractus solitarii independently modulate control of the circulation. *Hypertension* **44(4),** 522.

58. Baltatu, O., Fontes, M. A., Campagnole-Santos, M. J., et al. (2001) Alterations of the renin–angiotensin system at the RVLM of transgenic rats with low brain angiotensinogen. *Am. J. Physiol. Regul. Integr. Comp. Physiol.* **280(2),** R428–R433.

59. Fontes, M. A., Baltatu, O., Caligiorne, S. M., et al. (2000) Angiotensin peptides acting at rostral ventrolateral medulla contribute to hypertension of TGR(mREN2)27 rats. *Physiol. Genomics* **2(3),** 137–142.

60. Lima, C. V., Paula, R. D., Resende, F. L., Khosla, M. C., and Santos, R. A. (1997) Potentiation of the hypotensive effect of bradykinin by short-term infusion of angiotensin-(1–7) in normotensive and hypertensive rats. *Hypertension* **30(3),** 542–548.

61. Santos, R. A. and Campagnole-Santos, M. J. (1994) Central and peripheral actions of angiotensin-(1–7). *Braz. J. Med. Biol. Res.* **27(4),** 1033–1047.
62. Santos, R.A, Campagnole-Santos, M. J., Baracho, N. C., et al. (1994) Characterization of a new angiotensin antagonist selective for angiotensin-(1–7): evidence that the actions of angiotensin-(1–7) are mediated by specific angiotensin receptors. *Brain Res. Bull.* **35(4),** 293–298.
63. Jackson, L., Sakima, A., Averill, D. B., and Diz, D. I. (2004) Characterization of the receptors mediating the actions of angiotensin-(1–7) in the nucleus tractus solitarri. *FASEB J.* **18(4),** A663.
64. Potts, P. D., Horiuchi, J., Coleman, M. J., and Dampney, R. A. (2000) The cardiovascular effects of angiotensin-(1–7) in the rostral and caudal ventrolateral medulla of the rabbit. *Brain Res.* **877(1),** 58–64.
65. Santos, R. A., Simoes E., Silva, A. C., Maric, C., et al. (2003) Angiotensin-(1–7) is an endogenous ligand for the G protein-coupled receptor Mas. *Proc. Natl Acad. Sci. USA* **100(14),** 8258–8263.
66. Von Bohlenund, H. O., Walther, T., Bader, M., and Albrecht, D. (2000) Interaction between Mas and the angiotensin AT1 receptor in the amygdala. *J. Neurophysiol.* **83(4),** 2012–2021.
67. Neves, L. A., Almeida, A. P., Khosla, M. C., and Santos, R. A. (1995) Metabolism of angiotensin I in isolated rat hearts. Effect of angiotensin converting enzyme inhibitors. *Biochem. Pharmacol.* **50(9),** 1451–1459.
68. Santos, R. A., Brum, J. M., Brosnihan, K. B., and Ferrario, C. M. (1990) The renin–angiotensin system during acute myocardial ischemia in dogs. *Hypertension* **15(2),** I121–I127.
69. Wei, C. C., Ferrario, C. M., Brosnihan, K. B., et al. (2002) Angiotensin peptides modulate bradykinin levels in the interstitium of the dog heart in vivo. *J. Pharmacol. Exp. Ther.* **300,** 324–329.
70. Ferreira, A. J., Santos, R. A., Almeida, A. P. (2001) Angiotensin-(1–7): cardioprotective effect in myocardial ischemia/reperfusion. *Hypertension* **38(3),** 665–668.
71. Ferreira, A. J., Santos, R. A., and Almeida, A. P. (2002) Angiotensin-(1–7) improves the post-ischemic function in isolated perfused rat hearts. *Braz. J. Med. Biol. Res.* **35(9),** 1083–1090.
72. Neves, L. A., Almeida, A. P., Khosla, M. C., Campagnole-Santos, M. J., and Santos, R. A. (1997) Effect of angiotensin-(1–7) on reperfusion arrhythmias in isolated rat hearts. *Braz. J. Med. Biol. Res.* **30(6),** 801–809.
73. Roks, A. J., van Geel, P. P., Pinto, Y. M., et al. (1999) Angiotensin-(1–7) is a modulator of the human renin–angiotensin system. *Hypertension* **34(2),** 296–301.
74. Gironacci, M. M., Adler-Graschinsky, E., Pena, C., and Enero, M. A. (1994) Effects of angiotensin II and angiotensin-(1–7) on the release of [^{3}H]norepinephrine from rat atria. *Hypertension* **24(4),** 457–460.
75. Ishiyama, Y., Gallagher, P. E., Averill, D. B., Tallant, E. A., Brosnihan, K. B., and Ferrario, C. M. (2004) Upregulation of angiotensin-converting enzyme 2 after myocardial infarction by blockade of angiotensin II receptors. *Hypertension* **43(5),** 970–976.
76. Zisman, L. S., Meixell, G. E., Bristow, M. R., and Canver, C. C. (2003) Angiotensin-(1–7) formation in the intact human heart: in vivo dependence on angiotensin II as substrate. *Circulation* **108(14),** 1679–1681.
77. Ferrario, C. M., Richmond, R. S., Smith, R., Levy, P., Strawn, W. B., and Kivlighn, S. (2004) Renin–angiotensin system as a therapeutic target in managing atherosclerosis. *Am. J. Ther.* **11(1),** 44–53.
78. Strawn, W. B., Ferrario, C. M., Tallant, E. A. (1999) Angiotensin-(1–7) reduces smooth muscle growth after vascular injury. *Hypertension* **33(1),** 207–211.
79. Strawn, W. B., Chappell, M. C., Dean, R. H., Kivlighn, S., and Ferrario, C. M. (2000) Inhibition of early atherogenesis by losartan in monkeys with diet-induced hypercholesterolemia. *Circulation* **101(13),** 1586–1593.
80. Strawn, W. B. and Ferrario, C. M. (2002) Mechanisms linking angiotensin II and atherogenesis. *Curr. Opin. Lipidol.* **13(5),** 505–512.
81. Strawn, W. B., Richmond, R. S., Ann, T. E., Gallagher, P. E., and Ferrario, C. M. (2004) Renin–angiotensin system expression in rat bone marrow haematopoietic and stromal cells. *Br. J. Haematol.* **126(1),** 120–126.
82. Campbell, D. J., Alexiou, T., Xiao, H. D., et al. (2004) Effect of reduced angiotensin-converting enzyme gene expression and angiotensin-converting enzyme inhibition on angiotensin and bradykinin peptide levels in mice. *Hypertension* **43(4),** 854–859.
83. Crackower, M. A., Sarao, R., Oudit, G. Y., et al. (2002) Angiotensin-converting enzyme 2 is an essential regulator of heart function. *Nature* **417(6891),** 822–828.

84. Ferrario, C. M., Smith, R. D., Brosnihan, B., et al. (2002) Effects of omapatrilat on the renin–angiotensin system in salt-sensitive hypertension. *Am. J. Hypertens.* **15(6),** 557–564.
85. Chappell, M. C. (2001) Evidence for the formation of angiotensin-(1–7) and the inhibitory actions of the peptide on Na$^+$, K$^+$-ATPase activity in rat proximal tubules. *Hypertension* **38,** 523 (P186).
86. Chappell, M. C., Jung, F., Gallagher, P. E., et al. (2002) Omapatrilat treatment is associated with increased ACE-2 and angiotensin-(1–7) in spontaneously hypertensive rats. *Hypertension* **40,** 409.
87. Chappell, M. C., Modrall, J. G., Diz, D. I., and Ferrario, C. M. (2004) Novel aspects of the renal renin–angiotensin system: angiotensin-(1–7), ace2 and blood pressure regulation. In: *Kidney and Blood Pressure Regulation* (Suzuki, H. and Saruta, T., eds.) Karger, Basel, pp. 77–89.
88. Navar, L. G., Harrison-Bernard, L. M., Nishiyama, A., and Kobori, H. (2002) Regulation of intrarenal angiotensin II in hypertension. *Hypertension* **39(2),** 316–322.
89. Navar, L. G. and Nishiyama, A. (2004) Why are angiotensin concentrations so high in the kidney? *Curr. Opin. Nephrol. Hypertens.* **13(1),** 107–115.
90. Ren, Y., Garvin, J. L., and Carretero, O. A. (2002) Vasodilator action of angiotensin-(1–7) on isolated rabbit afferent arterioles. *Hypertension* **39(3),** 799–802.
91. Handa, R. K., Ferrario, C. M., and Strandhoy, J. W. (1996) Renal actions of angiotensin-(1–7): in vivo and in vitro studies. *Am. J. Physiol.* **270(1),** F141–F147.
92. Handa, R. K. (1999) Angiotensin-(1–7) can interact with the rat proximal tubule AT(4) receptor system. *Am. J. Physiol.* **277(1),** F75–F83.
93. Handa, R. K., Handa, S. E., and Elgemark, M. K. (2001) Autoradiographic analysis and regulation of angiotensin receptor subtypes AT(4), AT(1), and AT(1–7) in the kidney. *Am. J. Physiol. Renal. Physiol.* **281(5),** F936–F947.
94. Andreatta-van, L. S., Romero, M. F., Khosla, M. C., and Douglas, J. G. (1993) Modulation of phospholipase A$_2$ activity and sodium transport by angiotensin-(1–7). *Kidney Int.* **44(5),** 932–936.
95. Caruso-Neves, C., Lara, L. S., Rangel, L. B., Grossi, A. L., and Lopes, A. G. (2000) Angiotensin-(1–7) modulates the ouabain-insensitive Na$^+$-ATPase activity from basolateral membrane of the proximal tubule. *Biochim. Biophys. Acta* **1467(1),** 189–197.
96. Lara, L. S., Bica, R. B., Sena, S. L., et al. (2002) Angiotensin-(1–7) reverts the stimulatory effect of angiotensin II on the proximal tubule Na(+)-ATPase activity via a A779-sensitive receptor. *Regul. Pept.* **103(1),** 17–22.
97. Burgelova, M., Kramer, H. J., Teplan, V., et al. (2002) Intrarenal infusion of angiotensin-(1–7) modulates renal functional responses to exogenous angiotensin II in the rat. *Kidney Blood Press Res.* **25(4),** 202–210.
98. Alhenc-Gelas, F., Tache, A., Saint-Andre, J. P., et al. (1986) *The Renin–Angiotensin System in Pregnancy and Parturition,* Year Book Medical Publishers, Chicago, pp. 25–33.
99. Chesley, L. C. (1999) *Chesley's Hypertensive Disorders in Pregnancy,* 2nd edn, Appleton & Lange, Stamford, CT.
100. Merrill, D. C., Karoly, M., Chen, K., Ferrario, C. M., and Brosnihan, K. B. (2002) Angiotensin-(1–7) in normal and preeclamptic pregnancy. *Endocrine* **18(3),** 239–245.
101. Valdes, G., Germain, A. M., Corthorn, J., et al. (2001) Urinary vasodilator and vasoconstrictor angiotensins during menstrual cycle, pregnancy, and lactation. *Endocrine* **16(2),** 117–122.
102. Neves, L. A., Williams, A. F., Averill, D. B., Ferrario, C. M., Walkup, M. P., and Brosnihan, K. B. (2003) Pregnancy enhances the angiotensin (Ang)-(1–7) vasodilator response in mesenteric arteries and increases the renal concentration and urinary excretion of Ang-(1–7). *Endocrinology* **144(8),** 3338–3343.
103. Brosnihan, K. B., Neves, L. A., Joyner, J., et al. (2003) Enhanced renal immunocytochemical expression of Ang-(1–7) and ACE2 during pregnancy. *Hypertension* **42(4),** 749–753.
104. Jaiswal, N., Diz, D. I., Tallant, E. A., Khosla, M. C., and Ferrario, C. M. (1991) Characterization of angiotensin receptors mediating prostaglandin synthesis in C6 glioma cells. *Am. J. Physiol.* **260(5),** R1000–R1006.
105. Jaiswal, N., Jaiswal, R. K., Tallant, E. A., Diz, D. I., and Ferrario, C. M. (1993) Alterations in prostaglandin production in spontaneously hypertensive rat smooth muscle cells. *Hypertension* **21(6),** 900–905.
106. Jaiswal, N., Tallant, E. A., Jaiswal, R. K., Diz, D. I., and Ferrario, C. M. (1993) Differential regulation of prostaglandin synthesis by angiotensin peptides in porcine aortic smooth muscle cells: subtypes of angiotensin receptors involved. *J. Pharmacol. Exp. Ther.* **265(2),** 664–673.

107. Tallant, E. A., Jaiswal, N., Diz, D. I., and Ferrario, C. M. (1991) Human astrocytes contain two distinct angiotensin receptor subtypes. *Hypertension* **18(1),** 32–39.
108. Ferrario, C. M., Chappell, M. C., Tallant, E. A., Brosnihan, K. B., and Diz, D. I. (1997) Counterregulatory actions of angiotensin-(1–7). *Hypertension* **30(3),** 535–541.
109. Iyer, S. N., Yamada, K., Diz, D. I., Ferrario, C. M., and Chappell, M. C. (2000) Evidence that prostaglandins mediate the antihypertensive actions of angiotensin-(1–7) during chronic blockade of the renin-angiotensin system. *J. Cardiovasc. Pharmacol.* **36(1),** 109–117.
110. Tallant, E. A., Lu, X., Weiss, R. B., Chappell, M. C., and Ferrario, C. M. (1997) Bovine aortic endothelial cells contain an angiotensin-(1–7) receptor. *Hypertension* **29(1),** 388–393.
111. Widdop, R. E., Sampey, D. B., and Jarrott, B. (1999) Cardiovascular effects of angiotensin-(1–7) in conscious spontaneously hypertensive rats. *Hypertension* **34(4),** 964–968.
112. Garcia, N. H. and Garvin, J. L. (1994) Angiotensin-(1–7) has a biphasic effect on fluid absorption in the proximal straight tubule. *J. Am. Soc. Nephrol.* **5(4),** 1133–1138.
113. Gironacci, M. M., Vatta, M., Rodriguez-Fermepin, M., Fernandez, B. E., and Pena, C. (2000) Angiotensin-(1–7) reduces norepinephrine release through a nitric oxide mechanism in rat hypothalamus. *Hypertension* **35(6),** 1248–1252.
114. Muthalif, M. M., Benter, I. F., Uddin, M. R., Harper, J. L., and Malik, K. U. (1998) Signal transduction mechanisms involved in angiotensin-(1–7)-stimulated arachidonic acid release and prostanoid synthesis in rabbit aortic smooth muscle cells. *J. Pharm. Exp. Ther.* **284(1),** 388–398.
115. Ambuhl, P., Felix, D., Imboden, H., Khosla, M. C., and Ferrario, C. M. (1992) Effects of angiotensin analogues and angiotensin receptor antagonists on paraventricular neurones. *Regul. Pept.* **38,** 111–120.
116. Gironacci, M. M., Adler-Graschinsky, E., Pena, C., and Enero, M. A. (1994) Effects of angiotensin II and angiotensin-(1–7) on the release of [^{3}H] norepinephrine from rat atria. *Hypertension* **24,** 457–460.
117. Tallant, E. A., Chappell, M. C., Ferrario, C. M., and Gallagher, P. E. (2004) Inhibition of MAP kinase activity by angiotensin-(1–7) in vascular smooth muscle cells is mediated by the mas receptor. *Hypertension* **43,** 1348.
118. Ferrario, C. M., Martell, N., Yunis, C., et al. (1998) Characterization of angiotensin-(1–7) in the urine of normal and essential hypertensive subjects. *Am. J. Hypertens.* **11(2),** 137–146.
119. Luque, M., Martin, P., Martell, N., Fernandez, C., Brosnihan, K. B., and Ferrario, C. M. (1996) Effects of captopril related to increased levels of prostacyclin and angiotensin-(1–7) in essential hypertension. *J. Hypertens.* **14(6),** 799–805.

4

Angiotensin IV Binding Site
The AT$_4$ Receptor or Insulin-Regulated Aminopeptidase

T. A. Jenkins, F. A. O. Mendelsohn, A. L. Albiston, and S. Y. Chai

CONTENTS

1. INTRODUCTION

Angiotensin IV (Ang IV) is a hexapeptide fragment corresponding to amino acids 3–8 (VYIHPF) of angiotensin II (Ang II) that is formed by consecutive actions of aminopeptidase A and aminopeptidase N *(1)* (Fig. 1). Ang IV acts as a weak agonist at the Ang II AT$_1$ receptor, and was generally believed to have no physiological role because of its ineffectiveness in the regulation of blood pressure, fluid balance, or adrenal steroid secretion. However, in 1988, specific actions were discovered for Ang IV in the brain—the peptide was found to facilitate memory retention and retrieval *(2)*. A specific, high-affinity binding site was subsequently described in bovine adrenal membranes, which bound Ang IV saturably, reversibly, and with nanomolar affinity *(3,4)*. This binding site was termed as the angiotensin AT$_4$ receptor by an IUPHAR nomenclature committee *(5)*. This AT$_4$ receptor site is pharmacologically distinct from both Ang II AT$_1$ and AT$_2$ receptors, and bound Ang II at only micromolar affinity.

2. LIGANDS OF AT$_4$ RECEPTOR

Structure–activity studies conducted on Ang IV revealed that the N-terminal domain of the peptide is critical for receptor binding. In bovine adrenal membranes, Ang IV displays a K_i of 2.6 nM in competing for ^{125}I-Ang IV binding. Peptides containing mono-substitutions

From: *Contemporary Endocrinology: Hypertension and Hormone Mechanisms*
Edited by: R. M. Carey © Humana Press Inc., Totowa, NJ

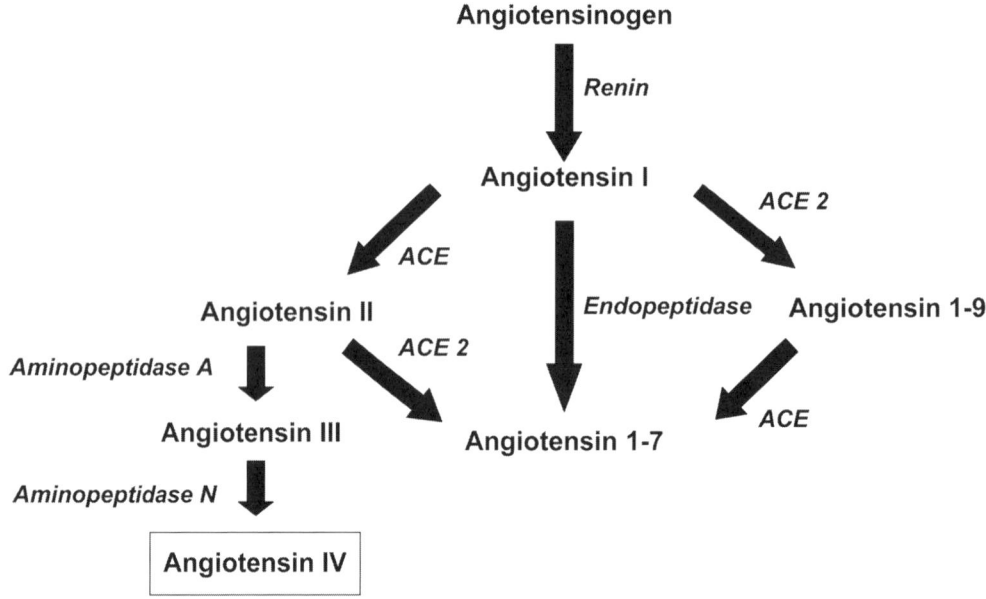

Fig. 1. Schematic diagram of the angiotensin system leading to the formation of angiotensin IV.

with glycine or the corresponding D-amino acid at positions 1, 2, or 3 possessed a K_i of greater than 100 nM. On the contrary, substitutions at positions 4, 5, and 6 had little effect *(6)*. Elongation of the N-terminal of Ang IV to yield Ang I, II, or III result in marked reductions in the affinity *(6)*.

Two N-terminally modified analogs of Ang IV have high affinities for the AT_4 receptor. These are Nle[1]-Ang IV and norleucinal Ang IV that exhibit *agonist* properties of Ang IV *(7)*. An AT_4 receptor antagonist was generated by the replacement of Ile[3] with Val[3], and the amide bonds connecting Val[1] and Tyr[2], as well as Val[3] and His[4] with methylene peptide bond isosteres to yield divalinal Ang IV, exhibit binding affinity similar to Ang IV *(8)*.

A structurally distinct peptide ligand, LVV–hemorphin-7, (LVVYPWTQRF/LVV-H7) was isolated by our group from sheep cerebral cortex based on its ability to bind to the AT_4 receptor *(9)*. This peptide competes for ^{125}I-Ang IV binding with nanomolar affinity *(9)*, and binds to the same sites as ^{125}I-Ang IV *(9)*. The first two N-terminal residues of LVV-H7 are not critical for binding but Val[3] is. The minimum requirement for binding to the AT_4 receptor is the V[3]Y[4]P[5]W[6]. The C-terminal domain appears to play only a minor role *(10)*.

3. AT_4 RECEPTOR IS INSULIN-REGULATED AMINOPEPTIDASE

We have purified the AT_4 receptor from bovine adrenal membranes and identified it as insulin-regulated aminopeptidase (IRAP) *(11)*. To verify that the AT_4 receptor is indeed identical to IRAP, we sought to (1) reconstitute [125]I-[Nle[1]]Ang IV binding site and investigate its biochemical properties by expression of IRAP cDNA, and (2) compare the distribution of the [125]I-[Nle[1]]Ang IV binding in brain with IRAP mRNA and protein expression. Using HEK 293T cells transfected with the full-length cDNA for human IRAP, we observed abundant high-affinity binding for [125]I-[Nle[1]]Ang IV with a pharmacological profile identical to the endogenous human AT$_4$ receptor *(12)*. In addition, membranes from cells transfected with human IRAP crosslinked with a radiolabeled analog of Ang IV expressed a major band at 165 kDa, which was displaced by 1 μ*M* Ang IV and is identical with our previous characterization of the native AT$_4$ receptor *(11,12)*. Cellular expression of both IRAP mRNA and protein closely paralleled the distribution of the AT$_4$ receptor in brain *(11)* (Fig. 2). We have therefore conclusively demonstrated that the specific high-affinity binding site for Ang IV/AT$_4$ receptor is the enzyme IRAP.

IRAP was described as an aminopeptidase colocalized in specialized intracellular vesicles with the glucose transporter, GLUT4, in insulin-responsive tissues, adipose, skeletal muscle, and cardiac muscle *(13)*. IRAP is a member of the M1 family of the zinc-dependent metallopeptidases, and is also known as placental leucine aminopeptidase (P-LAP), or oxytocinase *(14)*.

This review focuses on the IRAP/AT$_4$ receptor distribution and function in the cardiovascular system and brain. The AT$_4$ receptor was first described in bovine adrenal membranes *(3)*. Subsequently, it was shown to be widely distributed in many tissues including kidney, heart, spleen and brain in a number of different species. Although this protein was known as (1) the AT$_4$ receptor/^{125}I-Ang IV binding site (in most of the literature published about the kidney, adrenal, cardiovascular, and central nervous systems prior to 2002), (2) IRAP/vp165 (in insulin-responsive tissues), or (3) oxytocinase/P-LAP (in the placenta), in this review the protein will be referred to in the historical context according to the name given in the published literature.

3.1. Blood Vessels

3.1.1. DISTRIBUTION

In blood vessels, IRAP/AT$_4$ receptor was identified in cultures of bovine aortic smooth muscle cells *(15)* and bovine aortic *(16)*, coronary venular *(17)*, porcine aortic *(18)*, and pulmonary artery endothelial cells *(19)*. Using in vitro autoradiography, we localized ^{125}I-Ang IV binding in rabbit carotid arteries to the media, with weaker binding in the vasa vasorum of the adventitia. Little to no binding was observed in the endothelial layer *(20)*. After endothelial denudation of the carotid artery by balloon catheter, ^{125}I-Ang IV binding was increased in the media, neointima and regenerating endothelium *(20)*, indicating that this protein is upregulated during damage.

3.1.2. FUNCTION

Ang IV mediates vasodilation in blood vessels under certain conditions—this effect is thought to be mediated by the AT$_4$ receptor. Infusions of Ang IV or Nle[1]-Ang IV into the rat carotid artery in anesthetized rats increased cerebral blood flow by 25% and 32%, respectively *(21)*. Pretreatment with the nitric oxide synthetase (NOS) inhibitor blocked this vasodilatory effect. Infusion of Ang IV into the rat cerebral artery *(4)* or renal artery *(3)* also increased blood flow. In support for a role of nitric oxide (NO) in the vasodilatory effect of Ang IV, Patel et al. reported that Ang IV induced an endothelium-dependent relaxation of precontracted porcine pulmonary arterial rings, an effect blocked by an NOS inhibitor, L-NAME *(19)*. Moreover, after subarachnoid hemorrhage, Ang IV increased cerebral blood flow, but in this study. The effect did not appear to be mediated by NO *(22)*.

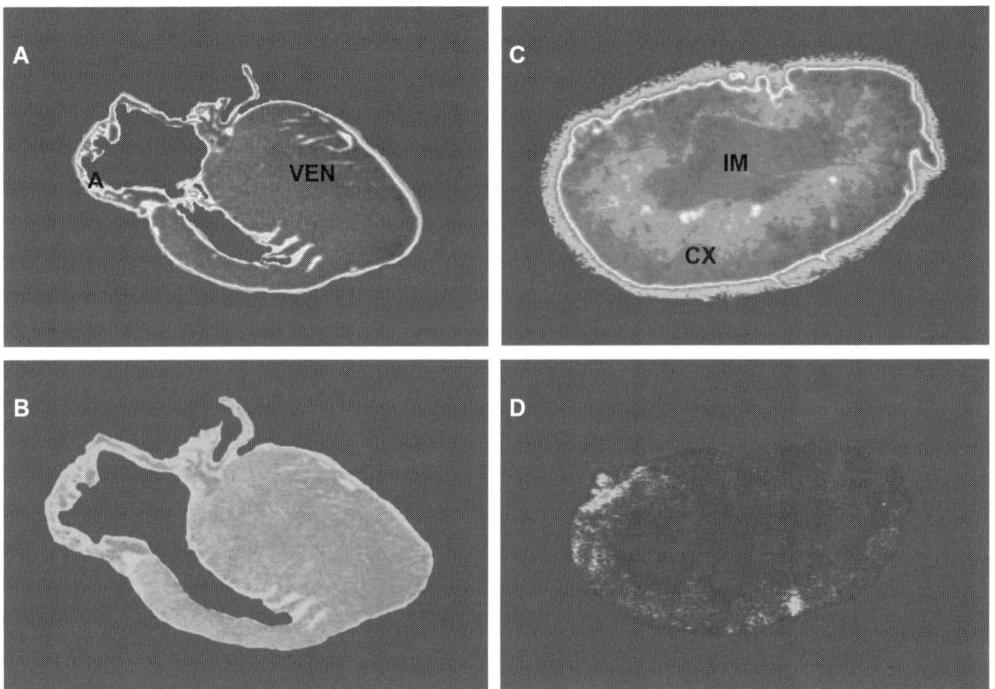

Fig. 2. Pseudocolor images of ^{125}I-[Nle^1]Ang IV binding in mouse heart and kidney demonstrating high levels of specific binding throughout the heart and in the inner medulla of the kidney. (**A**) Total ^{125}I-[Nle^1]Ang IV binding in mouse heart. (**B**) Nonspecific binding in the presence of 1 μ*M* Ang IV in mouse heart. (**C**) Total ^{125}I-[Nle^1]Ang IV binding in mouse kidney and (**D**) Nonspecific binding in the presence of 1 μM Ang IV in mouse kidney. Abbreviations: VEN, ventricle; A, atria; IM, inner medulla; CX, cortex.

At high concentrations, Ang IV also acts as an agonist at the angiotensin AT$_1$ receptor, and this underlies its weak vasoconstrictor action. For example, the effect of Ang IV in inducing vasocontriction in rat mesenteric artery *(23)*, aorta *(24)*, and pulmonary circulation *(25)* is blocked by AT$_1$ receptor antagonists, indicating involvement of the AT$_1$ receptor subtype.

In porcine pulmonary artery endothelial cells, Ang IV increased 5-bromo-2′-deoxy uridine incorporation into newly synthesized DNA in a concentration- and time-dependent manner *(26)*. Increased DNA synthesis by Ang IV stimulation was also observed in cultured bovine endothelial cells *(17)*.

3.1.3. SIGNALING

Activation of a number of signaling pathways by Ang IV has been reported in cultured blood vessel preparations. In porcine pulmonary artery endothelial cells, Ang IV was reported to induce the activation of phosphatidylinositol 3-kinase (PI3K), phosphatidy-linositide (PI)-dependent kinase-1, Erk 1 and 2, protein kinase B-α/Akt, and p70 ribosomal S6 kinase *(26)*. It was proposed that the activation of these multiple signaling pathways resulted in increase in DNA synthesis in these cells as selective inhibition of these kinases resulted in attenuation of Ang IV-mediated cellular proliferation *(26)*.

In a different study in porcine pulmonary artery endothelial cells, Ang IV stimulated cyclic guanosine monophosphate (cGMP) production and increased intracellular Ca^{2+} concentration *(27,28)*. The latter effect was blocked by divalinal Ang IV, G protein inhibitor, and phospholipase C and PI3K inhibitors, and regulated by PI3K and ryanodine-sensitive Ca^{2+} stores *(27)*. Chen et al. suggest that the endothelium-dependent relaxation observed in pulmonary artery is the result of the action of Ang IV on increased intra-cellular Ca^{2+} concentration via a G protein–phospholipase C–PI3K signaling mechanism.

Ang IV also stimulated plasminogen-activator inhibitor-1 (PAI-1) production in human coronary artery endothelial cells *(29)*, human adipocytes *(30)*, and cultured bovine endothelial cells *(31)*. There is a dispute concerning whether this effect on PAI-1 is mediated by IRAP/AT_4 receptor or by the angiotensin AT_1 receptor.

3.2. Heart

3.2.1. DISTRIBUTION

A specific binding site for ^{125}I-Ang IV has been described in membrane preparations of guinea pig and rabbit heart, with K_D values of 1.33 and 1.70 n*M*, respectively *(32)*. This binding site is localized in blood vessels, epicardium, and endocardium *(32)*. A relatively large level (1.2 pmol/mg protein) of ^{125}I-Ang IV binding sites has been detected in bovine cardiac membranes *(33)*. In the mouse heart, ^{125}I-[Nle[1]]Ang IV binding was detected throughout the ventricles and atria (Fig. 3A).

3.2.2. FUNCTION

In an isolated rabbit heart preparation, Nle[1]-Ang IV was reported to modulate left ventricular systolic function by reducing pressure-generating capability and enhancing the sensitivity of pressure development to volume change *(34)*. In rabbit cardiac fibro-blasts, Ang IV was reported to stimulate DNA and RNA synthesis *(35)*, which contrasts with an earlier report that Ang IV inhibited the effect of Ang II to increase protein synthesis in chick myocytes whereas having no effect alone *(36)*.

It is interesting to note that mice with targeted deletion of the IRAP gene exhibited no abnormal growth, except an enlarged heart *(37)*. This phenotypic abnormality could be resulting from the association of IRAP with GLUT4 in cardiac myocytes because cardiac hypertrophies have also been observed in mice with decreased levels or total absence of the insulin-responsive glucose transporter *(38–40)*.

3.2.3. SIGNALING

Treatment with Nle[1]-Ang IV decreased the mechanical load-induced increases in *c-fos* and *egr-1* mRNA expression in the isolated rabbit heart *(41)*. An increase in *PAI-1* gene expression was reported in the left ventricle of the rat heart after a 2-wk infusion of Ang IV, with no alteration in blood pressure *(42)*.

3.3. Kidney

3.3.1. DISTRIBUTION

In the rat kidney, ^{125}I-Ang IV binding sites have been localized to the cell body and apical membrane of convoluted and straight proximal tubules in the cortex and outer stripe of the outer medulla *(43–45)*. However, the distribution in the rat kidney contrasts with the binding in other species—high levels of the ^{125}I-Ang IV or ^{125}I-[Nle[1]]Ang IV

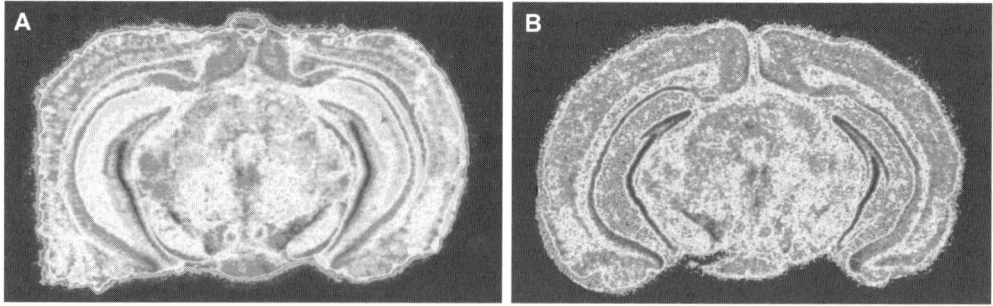

Fig. 3. Parallel distribution of ^{125}I-[Nle^1]Ang IV binding and IRAP gene expression on adjacent mouse brain sections. (**A**) Total ^{125}I-[Nle^1]Ang IV. Method described previously *(64)*. (**B**) IRAP mRNA determined by in situ hybridization *(11)*.

binding were found in the medullary rays and also in the inner medulla of the sheep, guinea-pig, rabbit, mouse, and human kidney, whereas moderate levels were detected in the collecting ducts, proximal and distal tubules, over the glomeruli and in the renal vasculature *(46)* (Fig. 3C). In the rabbit renal cortex, ^{125}I-Ang IV binding sites were detected in isolated apical and basolateral membrane preparations *(47)*. In the human kidney cortex, using an antibody to P-LAP, specific immunostaining was detected in distal tubules *(48)*. In the same study, P-LAP positive immunoreactivity was detected in the distal tubules and in the collecting duct of Wistar–Kyoto (WKY) rats *(48)*.

In cultured renal cell lines, ^{125}I-Ang IV binding sites were detected in human *(49)* and rabbit *(50)* collecting duct cells, in rat mesangial cells *(51)*, opossum proximal tubule OK7A cells *(52)*, the Mardin–Darby bovine kidney epithelial cells *(53)*, and HK2 human proximal tubular cells *(54)*. In the rat tubular epithelial NRK52E cells, P-LAP immuno-staining was found predominantly in the cytoplasm, as punctate staining in the perinuclear region *(48)*. This vesicular P-LAP was responsive to the activation of the vasopressin V$_2$ receptor by arginine–vasopressin, translocating to the basolateral plasma membrane *(48)*.

3.3.2. Function

Infusion of Ang IV into the renal artery of anesthetized rats increased renal cortical blood flow and urinary Na$^+$ secretion, without altering glomerular filtration rate, urine volume, or mean arterial pressure *(45,55)*. Pretreatment with divalinal Ang IV completely blocked the Ang IV-induced elevations in blood flow *(45,55)*, as did the NO inhibitor, N^G-monomethyl-L-arginine *(45)*, suggesting that the Ang IV-induced increases in blood flow may be mediated by NO in response to altered tubular Na$^+$ reabsorption. In isolated rat proximal tubules, Ang IV elicited a dose-dependent decrease in energy-dependent Na$^+$ transport, as measured by proximal tubule oxygen consumption, which was blocked by divalinal Ang IV and ouabain pre-treatment, suggesting involvement of ouabain-sensitive Na$^+$, K$^+$-ATPase activity *(43)*.

In a separate study, intrarenal infusion of Ang IV into anesthetized rats did not produce vasodilatation, but an AT$_1$ receptor-mediated vasoconstrictor effect that was blocked by the AT$_1$ receptor antagonist, losartan *(56)*. In isolated perfused hydronephrotic rat kidney, small preglomerular and postglomerular vessels constricted with high concentrations of Ang IV, an effect that was blocked by losartan *(57)*. These observations confirm that the vasoconstrictor effects of Ang IV in various vascular beds are mediated by the AT$_1$ receptor.

WKY and spontaneously hypertensive (SHR) rats fed on a 1% salt diet (normal) were shown to have similar distributions and levels of ^{125}I-Ang IV binding sites in the kidney. However, these binding sites were increased by 28% in the WKY on an 8% high-salt diet, but remained unchanged in the SHRs *(58)*.

A role of Ang IV in nephrogenesis has also been suggested. Papillary atrophy observed in angiotensinogen null mice is markedly attenuated by Ang IV on administration to neonates *(59)*.

3.3.3. SIGNALING

In OK7A opossum proximal tubule cells, Ang IV induced a Ca^{2+} influx, which was partially through voltage-sensitive Ca^{2+} channels *(52)*. In collecting duct cell membranes in humans, Ang IV was reported to stimulate cyclic adenosine monophosphate (cAMP) production in the presence of forskolin, but not under basal conditions *(49)*. A concentration-dependent biphasic rise in Ca^{2+} was observed in epithelial HK-2 human proximal tubular cell line after treatment with Ang IV, along with an intracellular rise in Na$^+$, and increased activation of Erk-1 and -2, and p38 kinase *(54)*. This result was also observed with divalinal Ang IV, the AT$_4$ receptor antagonist *(54)*. A time- and dose-dependent increase in PAI-1 mRNA expression was also observed in these cells after Ang IV stimulation *(60)*. Moreover, in the LLC-PK$_1$/Cl$_4$ cells, a proximal tubular epithelial cell line from pig kidney, Ang IV induced dose-dependent phosphorylation of two focal adhesion-associated proteins, p125-focal adhesion kinase (p125-FAK) and paxillin *(61)*.

3.4. Adrenal

The specific high-affinity binding site for ^{125}I-Ang IV was discovered in bovine adrenal membranes *(3)* in which it occurred in the glomerulosa and fasiculata/reticularis layers of the cortex, as well as cells in the medulla and in the blood vessels *(8)*.

3.5. Brain

3.5.1. DISTRIBUTION

The distribution of ^{125}I-Ang IV binding site in the brain is widely conserved across species. First described in guinea-pig brain *(62)*, it has since been mapped in rat *(63)*, mouse *(64)*, sheep *(65)*, macaque *(66)*, and humans *(67)*. In all cases, high levels of ^{125}I-Ang IV/[Nle^1]Ang IV binding sites were found in the CA1 to CA3 pyramidal layer of Ammon's horn of the hippocampus, in the basal nucleus of Meynert, and throughout the layers IV/V of the neocortex (Fig. 2). High levels were also observed in motor cortex, ventral lateral thalamic nucleus, cerebellum, motor neurons in the brain stem and ventral horn of the spinal cord. This pattern of binding corresponded closely to the distribution of cholinergic neurons and their projections.

3.5.2. FUNCTION

The most striking effects of Ang IV in the central nervous system were on enhancing learning and memory. When infused into the cerebral ventricles of rats, Ang IV was reported to improve the acquisition of conditioned avoidance responses *(2)* and to improve recall in the passive avoidance paradigm *(2,68)*. Chronic infusion of Nle^1-Ang IV facilitated acquisition in a hippocampal-dependent spatial learning task, the swim maze *(69)*, whereas chronic infusion of divalinal Ang IV produced a detrimental effect on acquisition *(69)*. However, a single central injection of Ang IV before training on the first day had no effect on acquisition rates in the water maze *(70)*. In another spatial memory task, the Barnes circular maze, a single intracerebroventricular dose of Nle[1]-Ang IV, or the structurally unrelated AT_4 ligand, LVV-H7, dramatically accelerated spatial learning *(71)*. Concurrent delivery of divalinal Ang IV prevented this increased rate of acquisition *(71)*.

An acute injection of Nle[1]-Ang IV or LVV-H7 reversed scopolamine-induced performance deficit assessed in the water maze or passive avoidance tasks *(72,73)*. This effect of Nle[1]-Ang IV was blocked by pre-treatment with Nle[1] Leual[3]-Ang IV *(74)*. A single intracerebral injection of the norleucinal Ang IV, administered prior to the training trial each day, reversed the deficit in spatial learning induced by bilateral knife-cuts of the perforant pathway in the rat *(69)*.

A role of AT_4 ligands on long-term potentiation (LTP), a cellular mechanism of memory, has also been reported. In hippocampal slices, application of Nle[1]-Ang IV stimulated synaptic transmission during low-frequency test pulses and increased tetanus-induced LTP by 63% in the CA1 region *(75)*. It was further shown to overcome ethanol-induced suppression of LTP *(76)*. Moreover, in anesthetized rats, Ang IV and norleucinal Ang IV enhanced LTP dose- and time-dependently in the dentate gyrus, whereas divalinal Ang IV blocked the enhancement of normal LTP *(77)*.

Because acetylcholine plays a role in modulating memory and learning, we investigated the effect of AT_4 ligands on acetylcholine release from hippocampal slices. Both Ang IV and LVV-H7 potentiated depolarization-induced [^{3}H]-acetylcholine release from the rat hippocampus in a concentration-dependent manner, 45% and 96% above control, respectively, an effect that was attenuated by divalinal Ang IV *(78)*.

In addition to their effects on memory, AT_4 ligands may also have trophic effects. Ang IV inhibited neurite outgrowth in cultured embryonic chicken sympathetic neurons *(79,80)* and both Ang IV and LVV-H7 stimulated DNA synthesis in a human neuroblastoma SKNMC cell line *(12)*.

A recent study reported that chronic overexpression of Ang IV in the brain resulted in a significant rise in systolic blood pressure *(81)*. Surprisingly, treatment with an AT_1 receptor antagonist, candersartan, and not with the angiotensin-converting enzyme (ACE) inhibitor, captopril, normalized the blood pressure increases in these transgenic mice *(81)*. The investigators postulated that this effect may be because of an allosteric interaction of Ang IV with the AT_1 receptor. It would therefore be interesting to determine whether the blood pressure in the IRAP knockout mouse is abnormal.

4. IMPLICATIONS OF AT_4 RECEPTOR AS IRAP ENZYME

IRAP belongs to the M1 family of zinc metallopeptidases that also includes aminopeptidases A, N, and B. It was initially identified as a marker protein for a special class of vesicles in adipose and skeletal muscle cells that contain the insulin-responsive glucose transporter, GLUT4 *(13)* but was also cloned from human placental cDNA library as oxytocinase *(14)*. If the AT_4 receptor is an enzyme, what happens when AT_4 ligands bind to the protein? Our group has shown that all the peptide AT_4 ligands, including Ang IV, Nle[1]-Ang IV, divalinal Ang IV, and LVV-H7, are potent inhibitors of the catalytic activity of IRAP, binding to its active site *(11,82)*. In contrast to our studies describing the competitive binding of Ang IV to the catalytic site of IRAP *(82)*, Caron et al. suggest that Ang IV binds to a juxtamembrane domain of the enzyme, distinct from its active site *(33)*.

The mechanisms of how AT$_4$ ligands mediate their effects by acting on IRAP are unclear. We propose that ligand binding to IRAP have at least three different possible actions: (1) inhibition of neuropeptide degradation by IRAP, leading to increased neuro-peptide levels that have been shown to potentiate memory; (2) altered trafficking of GLUT4 leading to changes in glucose uptake; and (3) direct signaling. These possibilities are discussed in more detail in the following sections.

4.1. Substrates of IRAP

IRAP mediates the degradation of a number of small peptides in vitro, including Lys-bradykinin, vasopressin, met- and leu-enkephalin, dynorphin A, somatostatin, CCK-8, and neurokinin A *(82–85)*. A number of the known substrates of IRAP, including vasopressin, cholecystokinin, and somatostatin, are capable of facilitating learning in passive avoidance and spatial memory tasks (for review, *see* ref. *86*). We postulate that the facilitation of memory by AT$_4$ ligands may be a consequence of inhibition of the enzymatic activity of IRAP, thereby protecting its peptide substrates from degradation. Memory enhancement by blockade of peptidases has been demonstrated previously. ACE inhibitors improve memory in passive avoidance paradigms and in models of cognitive impairment (for review, *see* ref. *87*). Moreover, inhibition of prolyl endopeptidase results in improvement in memory in aged *(88)* and scopolamine-treated *(89)* rats.

4.2. Regulation of GLUT4

IRAP and GLUT4 are colocalized in the basal state, located in post-endosomal vesicles and the *trans*-Golgi network in insulin-responsive cells. Under insulin stimulation, IRAP and GLUT4 rapidly translocate to the plasma membrane in which the GLUT4 mediates insulin-stimulated glucose release (for review, *see* ref. *90*). IRAP is the only member of the aminopeptidase family with an amino-terminus intracellular domain comprising more than 100 amino acids. This intracellular domain contains specific con-sensus sequences (dileucine motifs and acidic clusters) that are thought to be involved in protein trafficking and sorting *(13)*. Injection of this domain into differentiated adipocytes resulted in the translocation of GLUT4 vesicles to the cell surface suggesting that the amino terminus of IRAP may play a role in the intracellular retention or sorting of GLUT4 vesicles *(91)*.

GLUT4 mRNA and protein has recently been identified in the brain, and is found predominantly in the hippocampus, neocortex, and motor areas *(92,93)*, regions known to contain high levels of ^{125}I-Ang IV/[125]I-[Nle[1]]Ang IV binding *(62,64–67)*. The preliminary data we have suggest that GLUT4 and IRAP are colocalized in the same neurons of the brain. If this is the case then AT$_4$ ligands upon binding to IRAP may alter the intracellular distribution of GLUT4 vesicles, resulting in more GLUT4 at the cell surface and increased glucose uptake into neurons. The memory enhancing effect of exogenous glucose is well established in both humans and animals (for review, *see* ref. *94*). In animal studies, it has been shown that raising blood glucose levels can acutely facilitate memory, in part by increasing cholinergic activity (for review, *see* ref. *95*).

4.3. Direct Signaling

As reviewed in Section 3, a number of signaling events have been associated with the binding of Ang IV or its analogs to the AT$_4$ receptor/IRAP. It is difficult to conclude whether the effects of Ang IV on the different signaling pathways are via direct actions on IRAP. The enzyme has a 109-amino-acid intracellular tail with major phosphorylation sites at Ser[80] and Ser[91] *(96)*. It is possible that the binding of an AT$_4$ ligand to IRAP could lead to the direct stimulation of a signaling pathway. This has recently been demonstrated with ACE inhibitors or bradykinin binding to ACE in endothelial cells. The cytoplasmic tail of ACE, 28 amino acid in length, contains four serine residues, one of which (Ser[1270]) is phosphorylated by casein kinase 2 (CK2) leading to increased retention of ACE in the plasma membrane *(97)*. Binding of the ACE inhibitors, perindoprilat and ramiprilat, and the substrate bradykinin to ACE enhanced the activity of CK2, resulting in the activation of c-Jun N-terminal kinase and MAP kinase kinase 7. These results provide evidence that extracellular ligand binding of ACE results in the direct activation intracellular signaling pathways *(98)*.

5. CONCLUSION

It is clear that Ang IV and its analogs elicit effects, which are distinct from the traditional actions of the renin–angiotensin system that are mediated by the angiotensin AT$_1$ and AT$_2$ receptors. We propose that the effects of Ang IV and other AT$_4$ ligands are owing to their actions on IRAP. In light of the fact that the AT$_4$ receptor is not a G protein-coupled or tyrosine kinase receptor but the enzyme IRAP, much of the literature, particularly on the signaling pathways has to be re-evaluated.

Our identification of the AT$_4$ receptor as IRAP reveals previously unsuspected role(s) of IRAP and potentially GLUT4 in the brain and also provides the necessary tools to investigate the function of IRAP in insulin-responsive tissues.

REFERENCES

1. Zini, S., Fournie-Zaluski, M. C., Chauvel, E., Roques, B. P., Corvol, P., and Llorens-Cortes, C. (1996) Identification of metabolic pathways of brain angiotensin II and III using specific aminopeptidase inhibitors: predominant role of angiotensin III in the control of vasopressin release. *Proc. Natl Acad. Sci. USA* **93,** 11,968–11,973.
2. Braszko, J. J., Kupryszewski, G., Witczuk, B., and Wisniewski, K. (1988) Angiotensin II-(3–8)-hexa-peptide affects motor activity, performance of passive avoidance and a conditioned avoidance response in rats. *Neuroscience* **27,** 777–783.
3. Swanson, G. N., Hanesworth, J. M., Sardinia, M. F., et al. (1992) Discovery of a distinct binding site for angiotensin II (3–8), a putative angiotensin IV receptor. *Regul. Pept.* **40,** 409–419.
4. Wright, J. W., Krebs, L. T., Stobb, J. W., and Harding, J. W. (1995) The angiotensin IV system: functional implications. *Front Neuroendocrinol.* **16,** 23–52.
5. de Gasparo, M., Husain, A., Alexander, W., et al. (1995) Proposed update of angiotensin receptor nomenclature. *Hypertension* **25,** 924–927.
6. Sardinia, M. F., Hanesworth, J. M., Krebs, L. T., and Harding, J. W. (1993) AT4 receptor binding characteristics: D-amino acid- and glycine-substituted peptides. *Peptides* **14,** 949–954.
7. Sardinia, M. F., Hanesworth, J. M., Krishnan, F., and Harding, J. W. (1994) AT4 receptor structure-binding relationship: N-terminal-modified angiotensin IV analogues. *Peptides* **15,** 1399–1406.
8. Krebs, L. T., Kramar, E. A., Hanesworth, J. M., et al. (1996) Characterization of the binding properties and physiological action of divalinal-angiotensin IV, a putative AT4 receptor antagonist. *Regul. Pept.* **67,** 123–130.

9. Moeller, I., Lew, R. A., Mendelsohn, F. A., et al. (1997) The globin fragment LVV–hemorphin-7 is an endogenous ligand for the AT4 receptor in the brain. *J. Neurochem.* **68**, 2530–2537.

10. Lee, J. H., Mustafa, T., McDowall, S. G., et al. (2003) Structure–activity study of LVV–hemorphin-7: angiotensin AT4 receptor ligand and inhibitor of insulin-regulated aminopeptidase (IRAP). *J. Pharmacol. Exp. Ther.* **305**, 205–211.

11. Albiston, A. L., McDowall, S. G., Matsacos, D., et al. (2001) Evidence that the angiotensin IV (AT4) receptor is the enzyme insulin regulated aminopeptidase. *J. Biol. Chem.* **276**, 48,263–48,266.

12. Mustafa, T., Chai, S. Y., Mendelsohn, F. A., Moeller, I., and Albiston, A. L. (2001) Characterization of the AT(4) receptor in a human neuroblastoma cell line (SK-N-MC). *J. Neurochem.* **76**, 1679–1687.

13. Keller, S. R., Scott, H. M., Mastick, C. C., Aebersold, R., and Lienhard, G. E. (1995) Cloning and characterization of a novel insulin-regulated membrane aminopeptidase from Glut4 vesicles. *J. Biol. Chem.* **270**, 23,612–23,618.

14. Rogi, T., Tsujimoto, M., Nakazato, H., Mizutani, S., and Tomoda, Y. (1996) Human placental leucine aminopeptidase/oxytocinase. A new member of type II membrane-spanning zinc metallopeptidase family. *J. Biol. Chem.* **271**, 56–61.

15. Hall, K. L., Hanesworth, J. M., Ball, A. E., Felgenhauer, G. P., Hosick, H. L., and Harding, J. W. (1993) Identification and characterisation of a novel angiotensin binding site in cultured vascular smooth muscle cells that is specific for the hexapeptide (3–8) fragment of angiotensin II, angiotensin IV. *Regul. Pept.* **44**, 225–232.

16. Bernier, S. G., Servant, G., Boudreau, M., Fournier, A., and Guillemette, G. (1995) Characterization of a binding site for angiotensin IV on bovine aortic endothelial cells. *Eur. J. Pharmacol.* **291**, 191–200.

17. Hall, K. L., Venkateswaran, S., Hanesworth, J. M., Schelling, M. E., and Harding, J. W. (1995) Characterization of a functional angiotensin IV receptor on coronary microvascular endothelial cells. *Regul. Pept.* **58**, 107–115.

18. Riva, L. and Galzin, A. M. (1996) Pharmacological characterization of a specific binding site for angiotensin IV in cultured porcine aortic endothelial cells. *Eur. J. Pharmacol.* **305**, 193–199.

19. Patel, J. M., Martens, J. R., Li, Y. D., Gelband, C. H., Raizada, M. K., and Block, E. R. (1998) Angiotensin IV receptor-mediated activation of lung endothelial NOS is associated with vasorelaxation. *Am. J. Physiol.* **275**, L1061–L1068.

20. Moeller, I., Clune, E. F., Fennessy, P. A., et al. (1999) Up regulation of AT4 receptor levels in carotid arteries following balloon injury. *Regul. Pept.* **83**, 25–30.

21. Kramar, E. A., Krishnan, R., Harding, J. W., and Wright, J. W. (1998) Role of nitric oxide in angiotensin IV-induced increases in cerebral blood flow. *Regul. Pept.* **74**, 185–192.

22. Naveri, L., Stromberg, C., and Saavedra, J. M. (1994) Angiotensin IV reverses the acute cerebral blood flow reduction after experimental subarachnoid hemorrhage in the rat. *J. Cereb. Blood Flow Metab.* **14**, 1096–1099.

23. Loufrani, L., Henrion, D., Chansel, D., Ardaillou, R., and Levy, B. I. (1999) Functional evidence for an angiotensin IV receptor in rat resistance arteries. *J. Pharmacol. Exp. Ther.* **291**, 583–588.

24. Li, Q., Zhang, J., Pfaffendorf, M., and Zwieten, P. Av. (1995) Comparative effects of angiotensin II and its degradation products angiotensin III and angiotensin IV in rat aorta. *Br. J. Pharmacol.* **116**, 2963–2970.

25. Nossaman, B. D., Feng, C. J., Kaye, A. D., and Kadowitz, P. J. (1995) Analysis of responses to ANG IV: effects of PD-123319 and DuP-753 in the pulmonary circulation of the rat. *Am. J. Physiol.* **268**, L302–L308.

26. Li, Y. D., Block, E. R., and Patel, J. M. (2002) Activation of multiple signaling modules is critical in angiotensin IV-induced lung endothelial cell proliferation. *Am. J. Physiol.* **263**, L707 L716.

27. Chen, S., Patel, J. M., and Block, E. R. (2000) Angiotensin IV-mediated pulmonary artery vasorelaxation is due to endothelial intracellular calcium release. *Am. J. Physiol. Lung Cell. Mol. Physiol.* **279**, L849–L856.

28. Patel, J. M., Li, Y. D., Zhang, J., Gelband, C. H., Raizada, M. K., and Block, E. R. (1999) Increased expression of calreticulin is linked to ANG IV-mediated activation of lung endothelial NOS. *Am. J. Physiol.* **277**, L794–L801.

29. Mehta, J., Li, D. Y., Yang, H., and Raizada, M. K. (2002) Angiotensin II and IV stimulate expression and release of plasminogen activator inhibitor-1 in cultured human coronary artery endothelial cells. *J. Cardiovasc. Pharmacol.* **39**, 789–794.

30. Skurk, T., Lee, Y. M., and Hauner, H. (2001) Angiotensin II and its metabolites stimulate PAI-1 protein release from human adipocytes in primary culture. *Hypertension* **37**, 1336–1340.

31. Kerins, D. M., Hao, Q., and Vaughan, D. E. (1995) Angiotensin induction of PAI-1 expression in endothelial cells is mediated by the hexapeptide angiotensin IV. *J. Clin. Investig.* **96**, 2515–2520.

32. Hanesworth, J. M., Sardinia, M. F., Krebs, L. T., Hall, K. L., and Harding, J. W. (1993) Elucidation of a specific binding site for angiotensin II(3–8), angiotensin IV, in mammalian heart membranes. *J. Pharmacol. Exp. Ther.* **266**, 1036–1042.

33. Caron, A. Z., Arguin, G., and Guillemette, G. (2003) Angiotensin IV interacts with a juxtamembrane site on AT(4)/IRAP suggesting an allosteric mechanism of membrane modulation. *Regul. Pept.* **113**, 9–15.

34. Slinker, B. K., Wu, Y., Brennan, A. J., Campbell, K. B., and Harding, J. W. (1999) Angiotensin IV has mixed effects on left ventricle systolic function and speeds relaxation. *Cardiovasc. Res.* **42**, 660–669.

35. Wang, L., Eberhard, M., and Erne, P. (1995) Stimulation of DNA and RNA synthesis in cultured rabbit cardiac fibroblasts by angiotensin IV. *Clin. Sci. (Colch)* **88**, 557–562.

36. Baker, M. F. and Aceto, F. J. (1990) Angiotensin II stimulation of protein synthesis and cell growth in chick heart cells. *Am. J. Physiol. Heart Cir. Physiol.* **259(28)**, H610–H618.

37. Keller, S. R., Davis, A. C., and Clairmont, K. B. (2002) Mice deficient in the insulin-regulated membrane aminopeptidase show substantial decreases in glucose transporter GLUT4 levels but maintain normal glucose homeostasis. *J. Biol. Chem.* **277**, 17,677–17,686.

38. Katz, E. B., Stenbit, A. E., Hatton, K., DePinho, R., and Charron, M. J. (1995) Cardiac and adipose tissue abnormalities but not diabetes in mice deficient in GLUT4. *Nature* **377**, 151–155.

39. Stenbit, A. E., Tsao, T. S., Li, J., et al. (1997) GLUT4 heterozygous knockout mice develop muscle insulin resistance and diabetes. *Nature Medicine* **3**, 1096–1101.

40. Abel, E. D., Kaulbach, H. C., Tian, R, et al. (1999) Cardiac hypertrophy with preserved contractile function after selective deletion of GLUT4 from the heart. *J. Clin. Investig.* **104**, 1703–1714.

41. Yang, Q., Hanesworth, J. M., Harding, J. W., and Slinker, B. K. The AT4 receptor agonist [Nle1]-angiotensin IV reduces mechanically induced immediate-early gene expression in the isolated rabbit heart. *Regul. Pept.* **71**, 175–183.

42. Abrahamsen, C. T., Pullen, M. A., Schnackenberg, C. G., et al. (2002) Effect of angiotensins II and IV on blood pressure, renal function, and PAI-1 expression in the heart and kidney of the rat. *Pharmacology* **66**, 26–30.

43. Handa, R. K., Krebs, L. T., Harding, J. W., and Handa, S. E. (1998) Angiotensin IV AT4-receptor system in the rat kidney. *Am. J. Physiol.* **274**, F290–F299.

44. Harding, J. W., Wright, J. W., Swanson, G. N., Hanesworth, J. M., and Krebs, L. T. (1994) AT4 receptors: specificity and distribution. *Kidney Int.* **46**, 1510–1512.

45. Coleman, J. K., Krebs, L. T., Hamilton, T. A., et al. (1998) Autoradiographic identification of kidney angiotensin IV binding sites and angiotensin IV-induced renal cortical blood flow changes in rats. *Peptides* **19**, 269–277.

46. Chai, S. Y., Mendelsohn, F. A., Lee, J., Mustafa, T., McDowall, S. G., and Albiston, A. L. (2004) Angiotensin AT4 receptor. In: *Handbook of Experimental Pharmacology: Angiotensin* (Unger, T. and Schölkens, B., eds.), Vol. 163, Springer, Amsterdam, pp. 519–538.

47. Dulin, N. O., Ernsberger, P., Suciu, D. J., and Douglas, J. G. (1994) Rabbit renal epithelial angiotensin II receptors. *Am. J. Physiol.* **267**, F776–F782.

48. Masuda, S., Hattori, A., Matsumoto, H., et al. (2003) Involvement of the V2 receptor in vasopressin-stimulated translocation of placental leucine aminopeptidase/oxytocinase in renal cells. *Eur. J. Biochem.* **270**, 1988–1994.

49. Czekalski, S., Chansel, D., Vandermeersch, S., Ronco, P., and Ardaillou, R. (1996) Evidence for angiotensin IV receptors in human collecting duct cells. *Kidney Int.* **50**, 1125–1131.

50. Garreau, I., Chansel, D., Vandermeersch, S., Fruitier, I., Piot, J. M., and Ardaillou, R. (1998) Hemorphins inhibit angiotensin IV binding and interact with aminopeptidase N. *Peptides* **19**, 1339–1348.

51. Chansel, D., Czekalski, S., Vandermeersch, S., Ruffet, E., Fournie-Zaluski, M. C., and Ardaillou, R. (1998) Characterization of angiotensin IV-degrading enzymes and receptors on rat mesangial cells. *Am. J. Physiol.* **275**, F535–F542.

52. Dulin, N., Madhun, Z. T., Chang, C. H., Berti-Mattera, L., Dickens, D., and Douglas, J. G. (1995) Angiotensin IV receptors and signaling in opossum kidney cells. *Am. J. Physiol.* **269**, F644–F652.

53. Handa, R. K., Harding, J. W., and Simasko, S. M. (1999) Characterization and function of the bovine kidney epithelial angiotensin receptor subtype 4 using angiotensin IV and divalinal angiotensin IV as receptor ligands. *J. Pharmacol. Exp. Ther.* **291**, 1242–1249.

54. Handa, R. K. (2001) Characterization and signaling of the AT(4) receptor in human proximal tubule epithelial (HK-2) cells. *J. Am. Soc. Nephrol.* **12**, 440–449.

55. Hamilton, T. A., Handa, R. K., Harding, J. W., and Wright, J. W. (2001) A role for the angiotensin IV/AT4 system in mediating natriuresis in the rat. *Peptides* **22**, 935–944.

56. Fitzgerald, S. H., Evans, R. G., Bergstrom, G., and Anderson, W. P. (1999) Renal hemodynamic responses to intrarenal infusion of ligands for the putative angiotensin IV receptor in anesthetized rats. *J. Cardiovasc. Pharmacol.* **34**, 206–211.

57. van Rodijnen, W. F., van Lambalgen, T. A., van Wijhe, M. H., Tangelder, G.-J., and Ter Wee, P. M. (2002) Renal microvascular actions of angiotensin II fragments. *Am. J. Physiol.* **283**, F82–F92.

58. Grove, K. L. and Deschepper, C. F. (1999) High salt intake differentially regulates kidney angiotensin IV AT4 receptors in Wistar–Kyoto and spontaneously hypertensive rats. *Life Sci.* **64**, 1811–1818.

59. Kakinuma, S., Sugiyama, F., Taniguchi, K., et al. (1999) Developmental stage-specific involvement of angiotensin in murine nephrogenesis. *Pediatr. Nephrol.* **13**, 792–797.

60. Gesualdo, L., Ranieri, E., Monno, R., et al. (1999) Angiotensin IV stimulates plasminogen activator inhibitor-1 expression in proximal tubular epithelial cells. *Kidney Int.* **56**, 461–470.

61. Chen, J. K., Zimpelmann, J., Harris, R. C., and Burns, K. D. (2001) Angiotensin IV induces tyrosine phosphorylation of focal adhesion kinase and paxillin in proximal tubule cells. *Am. J. Physiol. Renal. Physiol.* **280**, F980–F988.

62. Miller-Wing, A. V., Hanesworth, J. M., Sardinia, M. F., et al. (1993) Central angiotensin IV binding sites: distribution and specificity in guinea pig brain. *J. Pharmacol. Exp. Ther.* **266**, 1718–1726.

63. Roberts, K. A., Krebs, L. T., Kramar, E. A., Shaffer, M. J., Harding, J. W., and Wright, J. W. (1995) Autoradiographic identification of brain angiotensin IV binding sites and differential c-Fos expression following intracerebroventricular injection of angiotensin II and IV in rats. *Brain Res.* **682**, 13–21.

64. Chai, S. Y., Lee, J. H., Matscos, D., et al. (2001) Angiotensin AT4 receptor distribution in mouse brain and its possible role in facilitation of spatial memory. *J. Neurochem.* **78**, 15.

65. Moeller, I., Chai, S. Y., Oldfield, B. J., McKinley, M. J., Casley, D., and Mendelsohn, F. A. (1995) Localization of angiotensin IV binding sites to motor and sensory neurons in the sheep spinal cord and hindbrain. *Brain Res.* **701**, 301–306.

66. Moeller, I., Paxinos, G., Mendelsohn, F. A., Aldred, G. P., Casley, D., and Chai, S. Y. (1996) Distribution of AT4 receptors in the Macaca fascicularis brain. *Brain Res.* **712**, 307–324.

67. Chai, S. Y., Bastias, M. A., Clune, E. F., et al. (2000) Distribution of angiotensin IV binding sites (AT(4) receptor) in the human forebrain, midbrain and pons as visualised by in vitro receptor autoradiography. *J. Chem. Neuroanat.* **20**, 339–348.

68. Wright, J. W., Miller-Wing, A. V., Shaffer, M. J., et al. (1993) Angiotensin II(3–8) (ANG IV) hippocampal binding: potential role in the facilitation of memory. *Brain Res. Bull.* **32**, 497–502.

69. Wright, J. W., Stubley, L., Pederson, E. S., Kramar, E. A., Hanesworth, J. M., and Harding, J. W. (1999) Contributions of the brain angiotensin IV-AT4 receptor subtype system to spatial learning. *J. Neurosci.* **19**, 3952–3961.

70. Holownia, A. and Braszko, J. J. (2003) Effect of angiotensin IV on the acquisition of the water maze task and ryonodine channel function. *Pharmacol. Biochem. Behav.* **76**, 85–91.

71. Lee, J., Albiston, A. L., Allen, A. M., et al. (2004) Effect of intracerebroventricular injection of AT4 receptor ligands, Nle1-angiotensin IV and LVv–hemorphin 7, on spatial learning in rats. *Neuroscience* **124**, 341–349.

72. Pederson, E. S., Harding, J. W., and Wright, J. W. (1998) Attenuation of scopolamine-induced spatial learning impairments by an angiotensin IV analog. *Regul. Pept.* **74**, 97–103.

73. Albiston, A. L., Pederson, E. S., Burns, P., et al. (2004) Reversal of scopolamine-induced memory deficits by LVV–hemorphin 7 in rats in the passive avoidance and Morris water maze paradigms. *Behav. Brain Res.* **154**, 239–243.

74. Pederson, E. S., Krishnan, R., Harding, J. W., and Wright, J. W. (2001) A role for the angiotensin AT4 receptor subtype in overcoming scopolamine-induced spatial memory deficits. *Regul. Pept.* **102**, 147–156.

75. Kramar, E. A., Armstrong, D. L., Ikeda, S., Wayner, M. J., Harding, J. W., and Wright, J. W. (2001) The effects of angiotensin IV analogs on long-term potentiation within the CA1 region of the hippocampus in vitro. *Brain Res.* **897**, 114–121.

76. Wright, J. W., Kramar, E. A., Myers, E. D. T., Davis, C. J., and Harding, J. W. (2003) Ethanol-induced suppression of LTP can be attenuated with an angiotensin IV analog. *Peptides* **113**, 49–56.

77. Wayner, M. J., Armstrong, D. L., Phelix, C. F., Wright, J. W., and Harding, J. W. (2001) Angiotensin IV enhances LTP in rat dentate gyrus in vivo. *Peptides* **22**, 1403–1414.

78. Lee, J., Chai, S. Y., Mendelsohn, F. A., Morris, M. J., and Allen, A. M. (2001) Potentiation of cholinergic transmission in the rat hippocampus by angiotensin IV and LVV–hemorphin-7. *Neuropharmacology* **40,** 618–623.

79. Moeller, I., Albiston, A. L., Lew, R. A., Mendelsohn, F. A., and Chai, S. Y. (1999) A globin fragment, LVV–hemorphin-7, induces [^{3}H]thymidine incorporation in a neuronal cell line via the AT4 receptor. *J. Neurochem.* **73,** 301–308.

80. Reed, G., Moeller, I., Mendelsohn, F. A., and Small, D. H. (1996) A novel action of angiotensin peptides in inhibiting neurite outgrowth from isolated chick sympathetic neurons in culture. *Neurosci. Lett.* **210,** 209–212.

81. Lochard, N., Thibault, G., Silversides, D. W., Touyz, R. M., and Reudelhuber, T. L. (2004) Chronic production of angiotensin IV in the brain leads to hypertension that is reversible with an angiotensin II AT1 receptor antagonist. *Circ. Res.* **94,** 1451–1457.

82. Lew, R. A., Mustafa, T., Ye, S., McDowall, S. G., Chai, S. Y., and Albiston, A. L. (2003) Angiotensin AT4 ligands are potent, competitive inhibitors of insulin regulated aminopeptidase (IRAP). *J. Neurochem.* **86,** 344–350.

83. Herbst, J. J., Ross, S. A., Scott, H. M., et al. (1997) Insulin stimulates cell surface aminopeptidase activity toward vasopressin in adipocytes. *Am. J. Physiol.* **272,** E600–E606.

84. Matsumoto, H., Rogi, T., Yamashiro, K., et al. (2000) Characterization of a recombinant soluble form of human placental leucine aminopeptidase/oxytocinase expressed in Chinese hamster ovary cells. *Eur. J. Biochem.* **267,** 46–52.

85. Matsumoto, H., Nagasaka, T., Hattori, A., et al. (2001) Expression of placental leucine aminopeptidase/oxytocinase in neuronal cells and its action on neuronal peptides. *Eur. J. Biochem.* **268,** 3259–3266.

86. Kovacs, G. L. and De Wied, D. (1994) Peptidergic modulation of learning and memory processes. *Pharmacol. Rev.* **46,** 269–291.

87. Gard, P. R. (2004) Amgiotensin as a target for the treatment of Alzheimer's disease, anxiety and depression. *Exp. Opin. Ther. Targets* **8,** 1–8.

88. Toide, K., Shinoda, M., Iwamoto, Y., Fujiwara, T., Okamiya, K., and Uemura, A. (1997) A novel prolyl endopeptidase inhibitor, JTP-4819, with potential for treating Alzheimer's disease. *Behav. Brain Res.* **83,** 147–151.

89. Toide, K., Iwamoto, Y., Fujiwara, T., and Abe, H. (1995) JTP-4819: a novel prolyl endopeptidase inhibitor with potential as a cognitive enhancer. *J. Pharmacol. Exp. Ther.* **274,** 1370–1378.

90. Bryant, N. J., Govers, R., and James, D. E. (2002) Regulated transport of the glucose transporter GLUT4. *Nat. Rev. Mol. Cell. Biol.* **3,** 267–277.

91. Waters, S. B., D'Auria, M., Martin, S. S., Nguyen, C., Kozma, L. M., and Luskey, K. L. (1997) The amino terminus of insulin-responsive aminopeptidase causes Glut4 translocation in 3T3-L1 adipocytes. *J. Biol. Chem.* **272,** 23,323–23,327.

92. El Messari, S., Leloup, C., Quignon, M., Brisorgueil, M. J., Penicaud, L., and Arluison, M. (1998) Immunocytochemical localization of the insulin-responsive glucose transporter 4 (Glut4) in the rat central nervous system. *J. Comp. Neurol.* **399,** 492–512.

93. El Messari, S., Ait-Ikhlef, A., Ambroise, D.-H., Penicaud, L., and Arluison, M. (2002) Expression of insulin-responsive glucose trnasporter GLUT4 mRNA in the rat brain and spinal cord: an in situ hybridization study. *J. Chem. Neuroanatomy* **24,** 225–242.

94. Messier, C. (2004) Glucose improvement of memory: a review. *Eur. J. Pharmacol.* **490,** 33–57.

95. Watson, G. S. and Craft, S. (2004) Modulation of memory by insulin and glucose: neuropsychological observations in Alzheimer's disease. *Eur. J. Pharmacol.* **490,** 97–113.

96. Ryu, J., Hah, J. S., Park, J. S., Lee, W., Rampal, A. L., and Jung, C. Y. (2002) Protein kinase C-zeta phosphorylates insulin-responsive aminopeptidase in vitro at Ser-80 and Ser-91. *Arch. Biochem. Biophys.* **403,** 71–82.

97. Kohlstedt, K., Shoghi, F., Muller-Esterl, W., Busse, R., and Fleming, I. (2002) CK2 phosphorylates the angiotensin-converting enzyme and regualtes its retention in the endothelial cell plasma membrane. *Circ. Res.* **91,** 749–756.

98. Kohlstedt, K., Brandes, R. P., Muller-Esterl, W., Busse, R., and Fleming, I. (2004) Angiotensin-converting enzyme is involved in outside-in signaling in endothelial cells. *Circ. Res.* **94,** 60–67.

5

Angiotensin AT_2 Receptors in Blood Pressure Regulation

Robert M. Carey and Helmy M. Siragy

CONTENTS

1. INTRODUCTION

The renin–angiotensin system (RAS) is a major physiological regulator of body fluid volume, electrolyte balance, and blood pressure (BP). The mechanisms by which these actions occur remain incompletely understood in spite of intensive study over decades. Prior to the late-1980s, it was thought that the major RAS effector peptide, angiotensin II (Ang II), acted by binding to a single Ang II receptor *(1–4)*. However, this principle was disproved when highly specific nonpeptide Ang II receptor antagonists revealed two distinct receptor subtypes, termed AT_1 and AT_2 *(1–6)*. AT_1 receptors were defined as those selectively inhibited by biphenylimidazoles (prototype losartan), whereas AT_2 receptors were blocked with tetrahydroimidazopyridines (prototype PD-123319) *(5,6)*.

In the first half of the 1990s, the vast majority of the biological properties of Ang II were characterized as acting via the AT_1 receptor *(7)*. These included Ang II-induced cardiovascular effects, such as vasoconstriction/pressor activity, renal sodium (Na^+) retention, aldosterone secretion, inhibition of renin secretion, sympathetic nervous system stimulation, and growth-promoting effects leading to cardiac and vascular hypertrophy and remodeling *(7)*. The understanding of Ang II receptors was greatly facilitated in 1991 with the cloning of the AT_1 receptor *(8)*, followed closely by AT_2 receptor cloning in 1993 *(9)*. Since that time, increasing evidence has suggested that

From: *Contemporary Endocrinology: Hypertension and Hormone Mechanisms*
Edited by: R. M. Carey © Humana Press Inc., Totowa, NJ

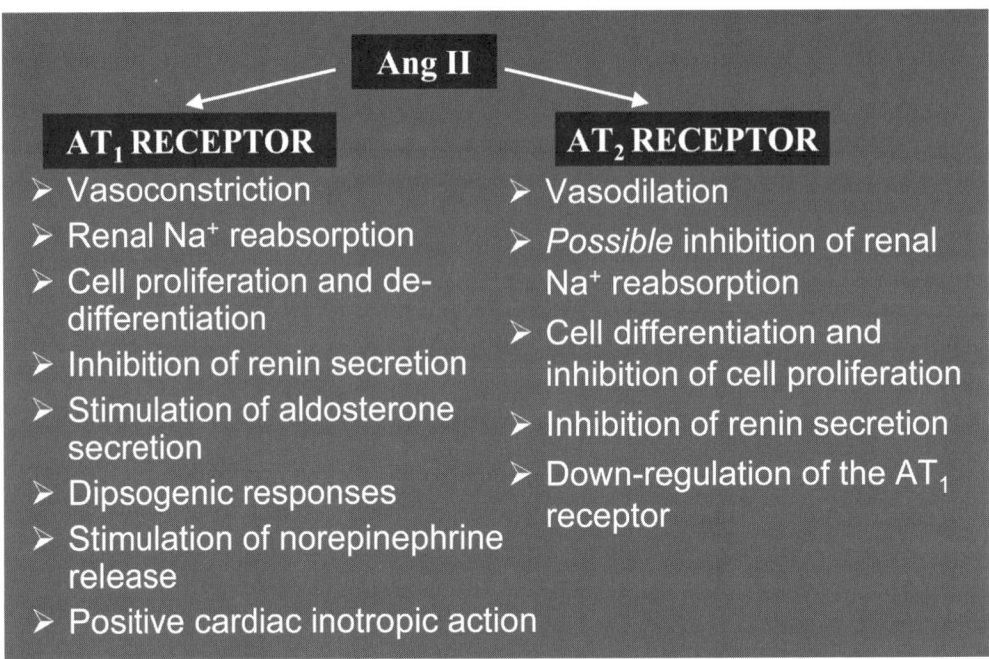

Fig. 1. Actions of Ang II via its two major G protein-coupled 7-transmembrane receptors, AT_1 and AT_2.

the AT_2 receptor is involved in a variety of cardiovascular actions, including vasodilatation, natriuresis, antigrowth effects, and contributions to the beneficial efficacy of AT_1 receptor antagonists *(10–16)*.

This chapter will focus on the AT_2 receptor, the physiological actions of which were obscure until the mid-1990s, when studies began to elucidate novel physiological actions of Ang II via AT_2 receptors. It is now apparent that many, but not all, of the cardiovascular and renal actions of Ang II at AT_2 receptors are counter-regulatory to those of Ang II via AT_1 receptors (Fig. 1) *(10–16)*.

2. GENERAL CONSIDERATIONS OF AT_2 RECEPTORS

The molecular structure of the AT_2 receptor is consistent with the super-family of G protein-coupled receptors containing 7-transmembrane domains *(17,18)*. The gene encoding the AT_2 receptor is localized on human chromosome Xq22-q2, rat chromosome Xq3, and mouse chromosome X *(7)*. The open-reading frame of the AT_2 receptor cDNA encodes a 363 amino acid protein with a molecular weight of 41,220 Da that has 93% sequence identity between rat and mouse and 72% identity between rat and human *(7)*. The homology resides mainly in the transmembrane hydrophilic domains. The gene for the AT_2 receptor has three exons but the entire coding region is on the third exon *(19)*.

The AT_2 receptor shares only 34% sequence homology with the AT_1 receptor. Almost complete divergence between AT_1 and AT_2 receptors has been observed in the third extracellular loop, and extensive differences have also been found in the intracellular carboxy-terminal tail of these receptors *(7)*.

Promoter activity of the rat AT$_2$ receptor gene is regulated by a number of cis-regulatory domains *(19)*. The AT$_2$ receptor protein contains five potential glycosylation sites in its extracellular N-terminal tail. Among the many differences in amino acid sequence, the AT$_2$ receptor, but not the AT$_1$ receptor, has a conserved LYS[199], which is important for ligand–receptor interactions. There is also a potential protein kinase C phosphorylation site in the second intracellular loop and there are three consensus sequences for phosphorylation by protein kinase C and one phosphorylation site for cyclic adenosine monophosphate-dependent protein kinase in the C-terminal cytoplasmic tail of the receptor *(2)*.

3. DISTRIBUTION OF AT$_2$ RECEPTORS

In fetal tissues, the AT$_2$ receptor is highly expressed and indeed predominates over the expression of AT$_1$ receptors *(7,20,21)*. However, shortly after birth, AT$_2$ receptor expression diminishes rapidly leaving the AT$_1$ receptor predominant in adult life. Although the AT$_2$ receptor is a low-copy receptor with barely detectable levels of mRNA in most tissues during adulthood, the AT$_2$ receptor protein is easily detectable by Western blot in heart, blood vessels, and kidney in adults. In this respect, AT$_2$ receptor expression resembles that of the dopamine D$_1$ receptor with very low mRNA but readily detectable protein *(22)*. Although there is a relatively low level of AT$_2$ receptor expression in adult tissues, the AT$_2$ receptor predominates at certain tissue sites, including uterus, ovary, adrenal zona glomerulosa and medulla, and in distinct areas of the brain *(7,23,24)*. The distribution of AT$_2$ receptors in the cardiovascular and renal systems is briefly reviewed as follows.

AT$_2$ receptors are detectable in the adult kidney with the most reliable method being Western blot analysis to detect the protein. AT$_2$ receptor protein is distributed throughout tubules and vascular segments of the renal cortex and medulla *(25,26)*. There is also variable receptor expression in the glomerulus *(25–27)*. The AT$_2$ receptor is particularly well-expressed in the proximal tubule *(25–27)*. The renal AT$_2$ receptor is upregulated by Na$^+$ depletion *(25)* and is downregulated in the ischemic kidney from 2-kidney, 1-clip hypertensive rats *(27)*. Furthermore, Ang II infusion does not alter AT$_2$ receptor expression, suggesting that receptor regulation is model-specific *(27)*. The AT$_2$ receptor is also downregulated in kidneys of stroke-prone spontaneously hypertensive rats (SHR-SP) compared with Wistar–Kyoto (WKY) control rats, and growth-factor-induced AT$_2$ receptors are upregulated in cultured mesangial cells from WKY but not from SHR-SP rats *(28)*. The AT$_2$ receptor is markedly upregulated in renal failure *(29)*.

AT$_2$ receptors have been localized in blood vessels at relatively low levels *(7,12)*. AT$_2$ receptors have been detected in small resistance arterioles in the mesenteric and uterine circulations as well as in large capacitance vessels such as the aorta *(30–36)*. Vascular AT$_2$ receptors are developmentally regulated in contrast to the AT$_1$ receptor that maintains constant expression throughout life *(7,37,38)*. AT$_2$ receptors are also expressed in the renal vasculature *(26)*. AT$_2$ receptors are present on both endothelial and vascular smooth muscle cells of small resistance arteries in the rat and also in coronary microarteries in mouse, pig, and human *(31,39–43)*. Vascular AT$_2$ receptors are upregulated by tissue injury and during the process of wound healing *(38,44,45)*. Ang II administration increases AT$_2$ receptor expression in mesenteric-resistance arteries *(46)* but downregulates the receptor in uterine arteries *(34)*. Interestingly, vascular AT_1 receptors are upregulated in AT_2 receptor–null (AT_2–null) mice *(47)*, but vascular overexpression of the AT_2 receptor does not alter the level of AT_1 receptor expression *(48)*. AT_2 receptor expression is increased in SHR compared with control WKY rats *(32,49)*.

In the heart, AT_2 receptors are expressed in cardiomyocytes of the atrial and ventricular myocardium as well as in coronary blood vessels *(7,12,50)*. Interestingly, in the normal heart in humans, in contrast to rodents, AT_2 receptor expression predominates over AT_1 receptor expression *(20,51–53)*. AT_2 receptor expression in the heart can be decreased, increased, or unchanged in animal models with cardiac dysfunction.

4. AT_2 RECEPTOR SIGNALING

4.1. Kinase–Phosphatase Interactions

AT_2 receptor signal transduction mechanisms are substantially different from those of the AT_1 receptor. AT_2 receptor activation in multiple cell lines stimulates protein phosphatases, which directly inhibit the protein kinase pathways mediated by the AT_1 receptor *(7,12)*. Although the cell signaling mechanisms of the AT_2 receptor are not as completely understood as those of the AT_1 receptor, studies performed to date demonstrate that AT_2 receptor activation stimulates tyrosine and/or serine–threonine phosphatases. These phosphatases serve to counter-regulate the cell proliferative and growth promoting effects mediated by protein kinases in response to AT_1 receptor activation *(7,12)*.

Some of the earliest studies of AT_2 receptor signaling were conducted in PC12W cells, a cultured pheochromocytoma cell line that expresses only AT_2 and not AT_1 receptors. In PC12W cells, Ang II induces the activation of protein tyrosine phosphatase (PTPase), which dephophorylates tyrosine residues *(54,55)*. Regarding the specific PTPases involved following AT_2 receptor activation, the vast majority of studies have demonstrated the inhibition of phosphorylation of certain members of the mitogen-activated protein kinase (MAP kinase) family, extracellular signal-related kinases (ERK) 1 and 2 (p42 and p44 MAP kinases), which are stimulated by AT_1 receptor activation *(38,56–60)*. Although there is ample evidence that the AT_2 receptor inhibits ERK phosphorylation in various cell lines, whether this mechanism accounts for AT_2 receptor signaling in vivo remains open to explore. However, transgenic mice over-expressing the AT_2 receptor in the heart have been reported to have reduced cardiac ERK activity, suggesting that ERK inhibition may indeed be modified by the AT_2 receptor in vivo *(61)*.

SH2-domain containing phosphatase-1 (SHP-1) is a soluble PTPase, which is involved in the terminal signaling of various cytokines and growth factors. Now, there is a substantial evidence that SHP-1 is an early transducer of AT_2 receptor signaling *(60,62–64)*. In both PC12W cells and in rat fetal vascular smooth muscle cells, AT_2 receptor-induced apoptosis appears to be mediated via SHP-1 activation *(62,63)*.

Serine–threonine phosphatase (PP2A) is also involved in AT_2 receptor signaling PP2A dephosphorylates phosphothreonine, thereby inactivating MAP kinases *(65)*. In neurons cultured from neonatal rat hypothalamus and brain stem, the AT_2 receptor activates PP2A, inhibiting AT_1 receptor-mediated MAP kinase activation and inducing apoptosis *(59,66,67)*.

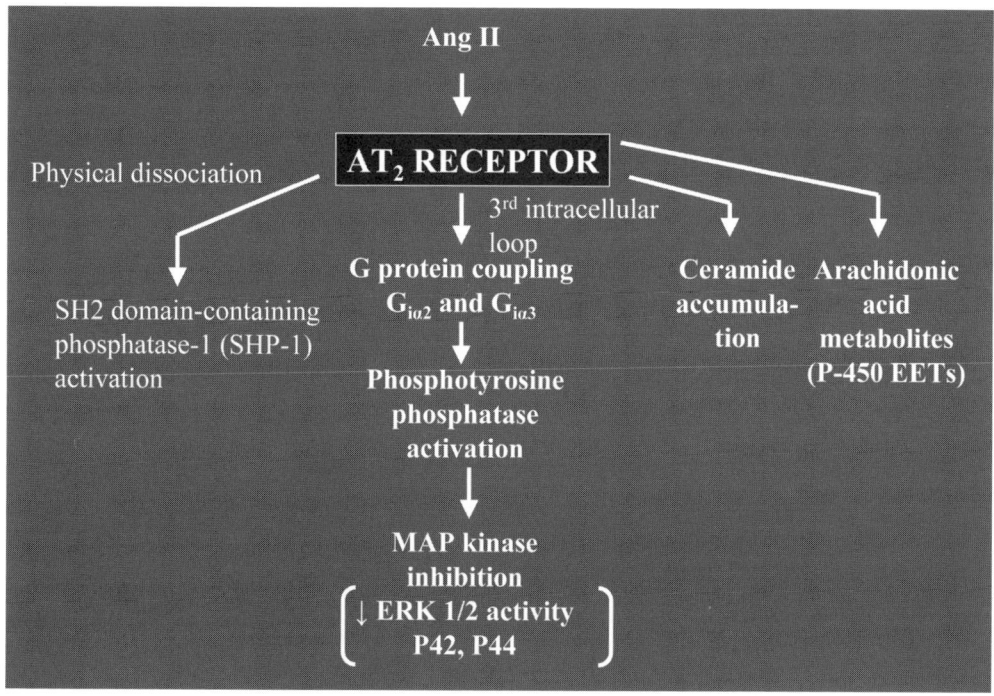

Fig. 2. Cell signaling mechanisms mediated by the AT$_2$ receptor.

In addition to the inhibition of the MAP kinase pathway, AT$_2$ receptors are capable of inducing the dephophorylation of other protein–kinase pathways. For example, Janus kinases (JAK) and signal transducers and activators of transcription (STAT) represent important pathways of AT$_1$ receptor-mediated vascular smooth muscle cell proliferation *(7,68)*. AT$_2$ receptor activation has been demonstrated to reduce AT$_1$ receptor-mediated tyrosine phosphorylation of STAT 1–3 and to inhibit the effects of growth factors, epidermal growth factor (EGF) and platelet-derived growth factor (PGDF), on STAT 1 activity *(69)*. Ceremide, which is linked to phosphatase activation, has also been proposed as a second messenger in AT$_2$ receptor-mediated apoptosis *(11)*. Therefore, the AT$_2$ receptor inhibits growth factor signaling pathways that are stimulated by the AT$_1$ receptor.

The major intracellular signaling pathways mediated by the AT$_2$ receptor are summarized diagrammatically in Fig. 2.

4.2. Bradykinin–Nitric Oxide–Cyclic GMP Pathway

Perhaps the major AT$_2$ receptor signaling pathway is the bradykinin (BK)–nitric oxide (NO)–cyclic guanosine 3', 5'-monophosphate (cGMP) pathway, which has been demonstrated as the major vasodilator pathway counter-regulating AT$_1$ receptor-mediated vasoconstriction (Fig. 3). The AT$_2$ receptor was first demonstrated to stimulate BK, NO, and cGMP production in 1996–1997 *(70–72)*. The AT$_2$ receptor-mediated vasodilator cascade constitutes a cell-to-cell (paracrine) communication mechanism that begins with AT$_2$ receptor induction of cellular acidification via the amiloride-sensitive Na$^+$ channel, resulting in kininogenase activation in vascular smooth muscle cells *(48)*.

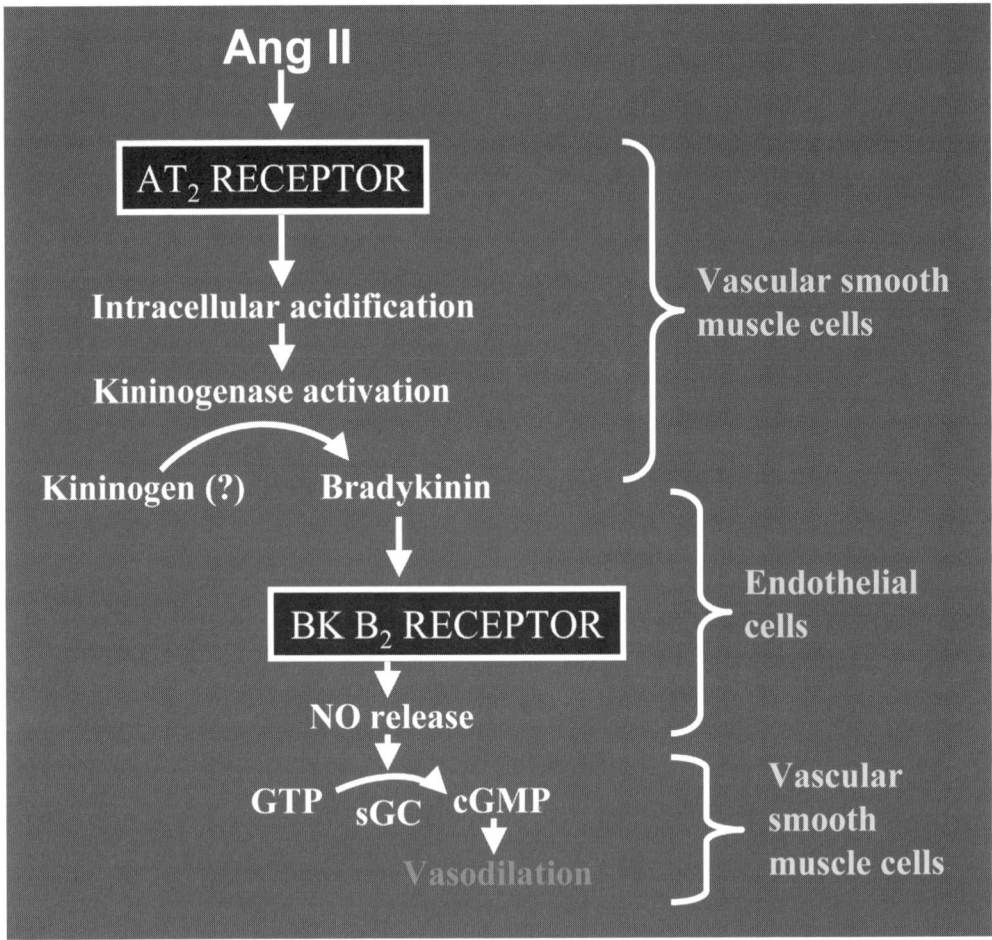

Fig. 3. Extracellular signaling mechanism of the AT$_2$ receptor involving the BK–NO–cGMP vasodilator cascade.

Kininogenase activation probably converts kininogen to the potent vasodilator BK, which acts at BK B$_2$ receptors on endothelial cells. B$_2$ receptor activation stimulates nitric oxide synthase (NOS) to form NO, which diffuses back into vascular smooth muscle cells to stimulate soluble guanylyl cyclase, with the intracellular production of cGMP, a potent vasodilator signaling module. Thus, the BK–NO–cGMP pathway has been demonstrated to be the major signaling pathway mediating vasodilatation both in vitro and in vivo in experimental animals *(7,10–12,73)*.

Since the time of its first demonstration, a multitude of studies have confirmed that the AT$_2$ receptor mediates its vasodilator action via the BK–NO–cGMP pathway *(7,10–12,73)*. Subsequent studies have revealed that both endogenous Ang II (increased by dietary Na$^+$ restriction) and exogenously infused Ang II stimulate an increase in cGMP, an effect abolished by pharmacological AT$_2$ receptor blockade and AT$_2$ receptor antisense oligodeoxynucleotide administration, as well as by BK B$_2$ receptor blockade and NOS inhibition *(70–72,74,75)*. In normal rats as well as a renal-wrap model of experimental hypertension, Ang II infusion induced an AT$_2$ receptor-mediated increase in BK, confirming a direct link between AT$_2$ receptor activation and BK synthesis *(76)*. Genetic studies involving targeted disruption of the AT$_2$ receptor gene *(77)* or over-expression of the AT$_2$ receptor in vascular smooth muscle cells of transgenic mice *(48)* provided direct support for the link between AT$_2$ receptor-mediated vasodilation and BK–NO–cGMP production. AT$_2$ receptor–null mice exhibited markedly reduced tissue levels of BK and cGMP and were hypersensitive to the pressor and antinatriuretic actions of Ang II compared with their wild-type litter-mates *(77)*. Although the exaggerated vascular reactivity to Ang II in AT$_2$ receptor–null mice might be attributable to upregulation of the AT$_1$ receptor *(47)*, this would not account for the reduced BK and cGMP tissue levels observed *(77)*. Conversely, AT$_2$ receptor over-expression in vascular smooth muscle cells unmasked an Ang II-induced increase in aortic cGMP, which was abolished by AT$_2$ or B$_2$ receptor antagonism or NOS inhibition *(48)*. The increase in aortic cGMP was associated with complete abrogation of the pressure response to Ang II which was restored with the same inhibitors *(48)*. Furthermore, in SHR-SP, Ang II increased aortic cGMP content via an AT$_2$ receptor mechanism involving BK, B$_2$ receptors and NO *(78)*.

Collectively, the evidence indicates that AT$_2$ receptors in the cardiovascular and renal system—albeit at low levels of expression—mediate vasodilation via a BK–NO–cGMP pathway. Recently, it was shown that the NO–cGMP mechanisms of AT$_2$ receptor action may be BK-dependent or -independent and that the receptor may stimulate NO production directly without involving BK *(79)*.

4.3. Heterodimer Formation

Recent studies have suggested that the AT$_2$ receptor may inhibit the actions of the AT$_1$ receptor directly by a ligand-independent process involving heterodimer formation *(80)*. Simultaneous activation of AT$_2$ and B$_2$ receptors led to a 70% increase in NO production, suggesting potentiation between these two receptors *(79)*. Indeed, the mechanism of this potentiation appears to be the production of an AT$_2$–B$_2$ receptor heterodimer, recently demonstrated in PC12W cells *(81)*. The rate of AT$_2$–B$_2$ receptor heterodimer formation is largely a function of the degree of AT$_2$ and B$_2$ receptor membrane expression. The physical association between these receptors initiates changes in intracellular phospho-protein signaling leading to the phosphorylation of JNK and PTP and dephosphorylation of ERK and p38 MAP kinases and STAT3 with marked enhancement of NO and cGMP formation *(81)*.

5. AT$_2$ RECEPTOR-MEDIATED VASODILATION

Results during the late 1990s through 2002 suggested that the AT$_2$ receptor might serve as a vasodilator counter-force to AT$_1$ receptor-mediated vasoconstriction *(7,10–12)*. However, vasorelaxation was difficult to elicit because of the relatively low level of AT$_2$ receptor expression and because of the predominant vasoconstrictor action of Ang II via the AT$_2$ receptor. In order to unmask the vasodilator action of the AT$_2$ receptor, experimental focus was changed to pharmacological reduction of AT$_1$ receptor action with AT$_1$ receptor blockers before and during AT$_2$ receptor stimulation with Ang II and related peptides. These studies clearly demonstrated that AT$_2$ receptor activation dilates blood vessels and reduces blood pressure *(82,83)*. Studies also showed that at least part of the acute depressor action of AT_1 receptor blockade is mediated by concurrent AT_2 receptor stimulation *(74,76)*. The vasodilator action of Ang II via the AT_2 receptor was easier to elicit when the renin–angiotensin system was upregulated, such as during Na^+ restriction, Ang II infusion or in renovascular hypertension *(10,74,76)*. The majority of studies endorsed the role of BK, NO, and cGMP in mediating the observed AT_2 receptor vasodilator action *(10–12)*.

Recently, several additional studies have confirmed the vasodilator action of the AT_2 receptor. AT_2 receptors were reported to mediate vasodilation in the uterine artery, in which the Ang II increased arterial cGMP, and vasodilation was blocked by AT_2 receptor antagonist PD-123319 (PD), BK B_2 receptor antagonist icatibant or NOS inhibitor N-nitro-L-arginine *(84)*. In addition, the AT_2 receptor was shown to dilate mesenteric arterioles under flow conditions by a BK-dependent mechanism *(85,86)*. Taken altogether, the available information suggests that resistance microvessels are a major site of AT_2 receptor-mediated vasodilation. However, recent evidence also demonstrates a vasodilatory role of AT_2 receptors in large capacitance vessels, such as the aorta. AT_2 receptor-mediated vasodilation is present in the pressure-overloaded rat thoracic aorta because of suprarenal aortic banding *(35,36)*. In this model, a counter-regulatory feedback loop may have been established in which the AT_1 receptor-induced vasoconstriction is counter-balanced by AT_2 receptor upregulation and vasodilation *(35,36)*. The mechanisms of AT_2 receptor-induced vasodilation in the capacitance vessels were demonstrated to be BK–NO–cGMP *(35,36)*.

AT_2 receptor-mediated vasodilation has also been demonstrated in the coronary circulation *(41,87)*. In normal and failing rat hearts, chronic candesartan-induced coronary vasodilation is abolished by AT_2 receptor blocker PD or by NOS inhibitor N^G-nitro-L-arginine methyl ester (L-NAME) *(87)*. Thus, AT_1 receptor blockade induced endothelium-dependent coronary vasodilation that was mediated by Ang II stimulation of the AT_2 receptor. Similarly, in human coronary resistance microvessels, functional AT_2 receptors mediated vasodilation via a BK–NO–cGMP signaling mechanism *(41)*. Because AT_1 and AT_2 receptor expression is quantitatively similar in the human coronary artery *(41)*, AT_2 receptors may constitute a legitimate therapeutic target for coronary ischemia.

Mechanisms other than BK–NO–cGMP have been proposed for the demonstrated renal vasodilator action of the AT_2 receptor. In the rabbit afferent arteriole, AT_2 receptor-mediated, endothelium-dependent relaxation occurs via a cytochrome P-450-dependent, NO-independent pathway, which likely involves the production of epoxyeicosatetranoic acid and the opening of large conductance, Ca^{2+}-activated K^+ (BK_{Ca}) channels *(88)*. Also, in preglomerular vascular smooth muscle cells from SHR kidneys, AT_2 receptors inhibited the ability of Ang II to activate phospholipase D via AT_1 receptors *(89)*. In addition, AT_2 receptor activation counteracted both AT_1 receptor-mediated vasoconstriction in the renal cortex and AT_1 receptor-mediated vasodilation in the renal medulla *(90)*. Thus, the actions and signaling mechanisms of the AT_2 receptor are especially complex within the kidney. Similarly, in mesenteric vessels, AT_2 receptor activation causes the opening of BK_{Ca} channels leading to membrane repolarization and vasodilation *(91)*.

Ang (1–7) is a recently discovered Ang N-heptapeptide fragment of Ang II with a range of central and peripheral actions, including vasodilation (*see* Chap. 3). Although Ang (1–7) may act at its own receptor (the *mas* oncogene), recent evidence suggests that Ang (1–7) may induce vasodilation through activation of the AT_2 receptor in the

Table 1
Vascular Sites and Mechanisms of AT$_2$ Receptor-Mediated Vasodilation

Site	Vasodilation	Mechanism
Mesenteric arterioles	Yes	BK–NO–cGMP
		BK$_{Ca}$ channels
Uterine arterioles	Yes	BK–NO–cGMP
Coronary arterioles	Yes	BK–NO–cGMP
Renal arterioles		
Cortical afferent arterioles	Yes	Phospholipase D
		Cytochrome P-450
		metabolites
		BK$_{Ca}$ channels
Medullary arterioles	No	–
Aorta	Yes	BK–NO–cGMP

presence of partial AT$_1$ receptor blockade *(92)*. This vasodepressor action involves the BK–NO–cGMP cascade *(92)*. Additionally, recent studies suggest a role of the AT$_2$ receptor in hypertension, as the receptor is downregulated in resistance arteries of SHR and nonspecific correction of the hypertension restores AT$_2$ receptor expression and vasodilator function *(93)*.

In summary, although a few exceptions exist, a multitude of studies have demonstrated that the AT$_2$ receptor mediates vasodilation in small resistance arteries, including the mesenteric, uterine, and coronary circulation. AT$_2$ receptors also dilate large capacitance vessels such as the aorta. The predominant cell signaling mechanism mediating vasodilation is the BK–NO–cGMP cascade. At least some of the beneficial vasodilation engendered by AT$_1$ receptor blockade appear to be mediated by AT$_2$ receptor stimulation. However, most of the available evidence come from acute studies, and the chronic vasodilator action of the AT$_2$ receptor requires further investigation. The vascular beds in which the AT$_2$ receptor has been shown to be a dilator mediator are shown in Table 1.

6. AT$_2$ RECEPTOR-MEDIATED NATRIURESIS

As discussed earlier, the majority of Ang II actions are believed to occur via the AT$_1$ receptor, including antinatriuresis *(7)*. Indeed, studies involving AT$_2$ receptors in the regulation of Na$^+$ excretion have been limited to only a few observations. In vitro studies have demonstrated that AT$_2$ receptors may reduce bicarbonate reabsorption in the proximal tubule via stimulation of phospholipase A$_2$ and arachidonic acid release *(94)*. In vivo studies in AT$_2$–null mice have demonstrated a shift-to-the-right (less sensitive) in the pressure–natriuresis curve and antinatriuretic hypersensitivity to Ang II *(77,95)*. However, as mentioned earlier, the AT$_1$ receptor is upregulated in AT$_2$–null mice, which could account for at least some of the aforementioned pressure–natriuresis and antinatriuresis effects, respectively *(47)*.

Recently, the AT$_2$ receptor has been demonstrated to mediate natriuresis and the heptapeptide fragment of Ang II, des-Aspartyl[1]-Ang II (Ang III) has been shown to be the preferential agonist *(95)*. In order to unmask natriuretic effects mediated by the AT$_2$ receptor, it was necessary to block the AT$_1$ receptor in vivo selectively within the kidney in normal rats. Intrarenal AT_1 receptor blockade with candesartan increased Na^+ excretion, and this effect was abolished by intrarenal AT_2 receptor blockade with PD. In the presence of systemic AT_1 receptor blockade with candesartan, but not in its absence, intrarenal Ang III infusion induced a significant natriuresis that was abolished with concurrent intrarenal administration of PD *(96)*. However, similar experiments with intrarenal Ang II administration at equimolar or higher infusion rates did not demonstrate a natriuretic effect. Collectively, these studies demonstrated for the first time that the beneficial effect of natriuresis induced by AT_1 receptor blockade is mediated, at least in part, by AT_2 receptor stimulation *(96)*. This study also demonstrated that Ang III is the preferential agonist for this response. Although the mechanism(s) of Ang III induction of natriuresis via the AT_2 receptor is (are) not clear, these results identify the AT_2 receptor as a potential therapeutic target for hypertension.

In conceptual agreement with these studies, it has recently been shown that systemic AT_2 receptor blockade with PD abolished candesartan-induced natriuresis/diuresis in obese Zucker rats to a greater degree than in lean rats *(97)*. In this study, direct AT_2 receptor stimulation with CGP-42112A induced a greater diuresis/natriuresis in obese than in lean rats *(98)*. In addition, AT_2 receptor-induced natriuresis has been demonstrated in streptozotocin-induced diabetic rats *(98)*. Furthermore, recent studies in normal rat proximal tubules suggest that activation of the AT_2 receptor via stimulation of the NO–cGMP pathway causes inhibition of Na^+, K^+-ATPase activity that is reversed with PD *(99)*.

In summary, there is recent substantial evidence that the AT_2 receptor mediates natriuresis in the normal rat and that Ang III is likely to be the preferential endogenous ligand. It is also evident that AT_2 receptor-mediated natriuresis is exaggerated in diabetic and obese models. The role of the AT_2 receptor in the antinatriuresis observed in early hypertension awaits further investigation.

7. AT_2 RECEPTOR-MEDIATED INHIBITION OF RENIN BIOSYNTHESIS AND SECRETION

The AT_2 receptor is expressed in renal juxtaglomerular (JG) cells. AT_1 receptors on JG cells inhibit renin biosynthesis and secretion, providing a short-loop negative feedback mechanism to retard Ang II production *(100)*. Angiotensin-converting enzyme (ACE) inhibition and/or AT_1 receptor blockade unmasks this short-loop mechanism resulting in increased renin and Ang I production. Recent evidence suggests that, unlike the AT_2 vasodilator and natriuretic actions that oppose AT_1 receptor effects, the AT_2 receptor behaves similarly to the AT_1 receptor in suppressing renin production and release directly at the JG cell. AT_1 receptor blockade can inhibit prorenin processing in JG cells via the activation of AT_2 receptors *(101)*. Furthermore, in conscious rats both circulating active renin and renal tissue levels of Ang II are increased by direct renal cortical administration of AT_1 receptor blocker valsartan or AT_2 receptor blocker PD *(102)*. Both receptor blockers independently increased renal renin mRNA and renin concentration. In response to valsartan and PD, renal renin immunoreactivity was markedly increased in both JG and tubule cells *(102)*. Therefore, renin biosynthesis and secretion are inhibited by a novel short-loop AT_2 receptor negative feedback mechanism in parallel with that of AT_1 receptors in JG cells. Further studies are necessary to determine the physiological and possible pathophysiological significance of AT$_2$ receptor-mediated renin suppression.

8. CONCLUSIONS

The AT$_2$ receptor is now firmly established as a vasodilator receptor with the vast majority of studies pointing to the BK–NO–cGMP signal cascade in its vasorelaxant action. The AT$_2$ receptor is counter-regulatory to the vasoconstrictor actions of Ang II via the AT$_1$ receptor. Indeed, AT$_2$ receptor stimulation may provide a substantial fraction of the antihypertensive benefit of AT$_1$ receptor blockade in hypertension. The AT$_2$ receptor is a vasodilator not only in small resistance arteries but also in large capacitance vessels. Future studies should focus on whether the AT$_2$ receptor mediates vasodilation chronically and in humans. If so, the AT$_2$ receptor is a candidate for design of nonpeptide agonist compounds for the treatment of hypertension.

Recent studies have demonstrated two novel actions of the AT$_2$ receptor, natriuresis and renin suppression. Regarding natriuresis, Ang III, not Ang II, appears to be the preferential ligand. Future studies should address the role of Ang III, a less-studied peptide, on renal function and the interactions of the renal AT$_2$ receptor with other natriuretic receptors. The role of the AT$_2$ receptor in the antinatriuresis of hypertension awaits further study. Similarly, the involvement of the AT$_2$ receptor in short-loop negative feedback suppression of renin and its potential role in the pathophysiology of hypertension require further study. Although the past decade has brought enhanced understanding of the AT$_2$ receptor and its functions, much more remain to be learned.

REFERENCES

1. Goodfriend, T. L., Elliott, M. E., and Catt, K. J. (1996) Angiotensin receptors and their antagonists. *N. Engl. J. Med.* **334,** 1649–1654.
2. Griendling, K. K., Lassegue, B., and Alexander, R. W. (1996) Angiotensin receptors and their therapeutic implications. *Annu. Rev. Pharmacol. Toxicol.* **36,** 281–306.
3. Matsukawa, T. and Ichikawa, I. (1997) Biological functions of angiotensin and its receptors. *Ann. Rev. Physiol.* 395–412.
4. Ardaillou, R. (1999) Angiotensin II receptors. *J. Am. Soc. Nephrol.* **10(Suppl 11),** S30–S39.
5. Chiu, A. T., McCall, D. E., Price, W. A., et al. (1990) Nonpeptide angiotensin II receptor antagonists. VII. Cellular and biochemical pharmacology of DuP 753, an orally active antihypertensive agent. *J. Pharmacol. Exp. Ther.* **252,** 711–718.
6. Timmermans, P. B., Wong, P. C., Chiu, A. T., et al. (1993) Angiotensin II receptors and angiotensin II receptor antagonists. *Pharmacol. Rev.* **45,** 205–251.
7. de Gasparo, M., Catt, K. J., Inagami, T., Wright, J. W., and Unger, T. (2000) International union of pharmacology. XXIII. The angiotensin II receptors. *Pharmacol. Rev.* **52,** 415–472.
8. Murphy, T. J., Alexander, R. W., Griendling, K. K., Runge, M. S., and Bernstein, K. E. (1991) Isolation of a cDNA encoding the vascular type-1 angiotensin II receptor. *Nature* **351,** 233–236.
9. Kambayashi, Y., Bardhan, S., Takahashi, K., et al. (1993) Molecular cloning of a novel angiotensin II receptor isoform involved in phosphotyrosine phosphatase inhibition. *J. Biol. Chem.* **268,** 24,543–24,546.
10. Carey, R. M., Wang, Z. Q., and Siragy, H. M. (2000) Role of the angiotensin type 2 receptor in the regulation of blood pressure and renal function. *Hypertension* **35,** 155–163.
11. Berry, C., Touyz, R., Dominiczak, A. F., Webb, R. C., and Johns, D. G. (2001) Angiotensin receptors: signaling, vascular pathophysiology, and interactions with ceramide. *Am. J. Physiol. Heart Circ. Physiol.* **281,** H2337–H2365.
12. Widdop, R. E., Jones, E. S., Hannan, R. E., and Gaspari, T. A. (2003) Angiotensin AT2 receptors: cardiovascular hope or hype? *Br. J. Pharmacol.* **140,** 809–824.

13. Carey, R. M. and Siragy, H. M. (2003) Newly recognized components of the renin–angiotensin system: potential roles in cardiovascular and renal regulation. *Endocrinol. Rev.* **24,** 261–271.

14. Carey, R. M. (2005) Update on the role of the AT2 receptor. *Curr. Opin. Nephrol. Hypertens.* **14,** 67–71.

15. Carey, R. M. (2005) Cardiovascular and renal regulation by the angiotensin type 2 receptor: the AT2 receptor comes of age. *Hypertension* **45,** 840–844.

16. Carey, R. M. (2005) Angiotensin type-2 receptors and cardiovascular function: are angiotensin type-2 receptors protective? *Curr. Opin. Cardiol.* **20,** 264–269.

17. Inagami, T. (1999) Molecular biology and signaling of angiotensin receptors: an overview. *J. Am. Soc. Nephrol.* **10(Suppl 11),** S2–S7.

18. Lazard, D., Briend-Sutren, M. M., Villageois, P., Mattei, M. G., Strosberg, A. D., and Nahmias, C. (1994) Molecular characterization and chromosome localization of a human angiotensin II AT2 receptor gene highly expressed in fetal tissues. *Receptors Channels* **2,** 271–280.

19. Ichiki, T. and Inagami, T. (1995) Expression, genomic organization, and transcription of the mouse angiotensin II type 2 receptor gene. *Circ. Res.* **76,** 693–700.

20. Matsubara, H. (1998) Pathophysiological role of angiotensin II type 2 receptor in cardiovascular and renal diseases. *Circ. Res.* **83,** 1182–1191.

21. Horiuchi, M., Akishita, M., and Dzau, V. J. (1999) Recent progress in angiotensin II type 2 receptor research in the cardiovascular system. *Hypertension* **33,** 613–621.

22. Carey, R. M. (2001) Theodore Cooper Lecture: Renal dopamine system: paracrine regulator of sodium homeostasis and blood pressure. *Hypertension* **38,** 297–302.

23. Zhuo, J., Allen, A. M., Alcorn, D., Aldred, G. P., MacGregor, D. P., and Mendelsohn, F. A. (1995) The distribution of angiotensin II receptors. *Hypertens. Pathophysiol. Diagn. Manag.* 1739–1762.

24. Roulston, C. L., Lawrence, A. J., Jarrott, B., and Widdop, R. E. (2003) Localization of AT(2) receptors in the nucleus of the solitary tract of spontaneously hypertensive and Wistar Kyoto rats using [^{125}I] CGP42112: upregulation of a non-angiotensin II binding site following unilateral nodose ganglionectomy. *Brain Res.* **968,** 139–155.

25. Ozono, R., Wang, Z. Q., Moore, A. F., Inagami, T., Siragy, H. M., and Carey, R. M. (1997) Expression of the subtype 2 angiotensin (AT2) receptor protein in rat kidney. *Hypertension* **30,** 1238–1246.

26. Miyata, N., Park, F., Li, X. F., and Cowley, A. W., Jr. (1999) Distribution of angiotensin AT1 and AT2 receptor subtypes in the rat kidney. *Am. J. Physiol.* **277,** F437–F446.

27. Wang, Z. Q., Millatt, L. J., Heiderstadt, N. T., Siragy, H. M., Johns, R. A., and Carey, R. M. (1999) Differential regulation of renal angiotensin subtype AT1A and AT2 receptor protein in rats with angiotensin-dependent hypertension. *Hypertension* **33,** 96–101.

28. Goto, M., Mukoyama, M., Sugawara, A., et al. (2002) Expression and role of angiotensin II type 2 receptor in the kidney and mesangial cells of spontaneously hypertensive rats. *Hypertens. Res.* **25,** 125–133.

29. Bautista, R., Sanchez, A., Hernandez, J., Oyekan, A., and Escalante, B. (2001) Angiotensin II type AT(2) receptor mRNA expression and renal vasodilatation are increased in renal failure. *Hypertension* **38,** 669–673.

30. Matrougui, K., Levy, B. I., and Henrion, D. (2000) Tissue angiotensin II and endothelin-1 modulate differently the response to flow in mesenteric resistance arteries of normotensive and spontaneously hypertensive rats. *Br. J. Pharmacol.* **130,** 521–526.

31. Matrougui, K., Loufrani, L., Heymes, C., Levy, B. I., and Henrion, D. (1999) Activation of AT(2) receptors by endogenous angiotensin II is involved in flow-induced dilation in rat resistance arteries. *Hypertension* **34,** 659–665.

32. Touyz, R. M., Endemann, D., He, G., Li, J. S., and Schiffrin, E. L. (1999) Role of AT2 receptors in angiotensin II-stimulated contraction of small mesenteric arteries in young SHR. *Hypertension* **33,** 366–372.

33. Burrell, J. H. and Lumbers, E. R. (1997) Angiotensin receptor subtypes in the uterine artery during ovine pregnancy. *Eur. J. Pharmacol.* **330,** 257–267.

34. McMullen, J. R., Gibson, K. J., Lumbers, E. R., and Burrell, J. H. (2001) Selective down-regulation of AT2 receptors in uterine arteries from pregnant ewes given 24-h intravenous infusions of angiotensin II. *Regul. Pept.* **99,** 119–129.

35. Yayama, K., Horii, M., Hiyoshi, H., et al. (2004) Up-regulation of angiotensin II type 2 receptor in rat thoracic aorta by pressure-overload. *J. Pharmacol. Exp. Ther.* **308,** 736–743.

36. Hiyoshi, H., Yayama, K., Takano, M., and Okamoto, H. (2004) Stimulation of cyclic GMP production via AT2 and B2 receptors in the pressure-overloaded aorta after banding. *Hypertension* **43,** 1258–1263.

37. Viswanathan, M., Tsutsumi, K., Correa, F .M., and Saavedra, J. M. (1991) Changes in expression of angiotensin receptor subtypes in the rat aorta during development. *Biochem. Biophys. Res. Commun.* **179,** 1361–1367.

38. Nakajima, M., Hutchinson, H. G., Fujinaga, M., et al. (1995) The angiotensin II type 2 (AT2) receptor antagonizes the growth effects of the AT1 receptor: gain-of-function study using gene transfer. *Proc. Natl Acad. Sci. USA* **92,** 10,663–10,667.

39. Nora, E. H., Munzenmaier, D. H., Hansen-Smith, F. M., Lombard, J. H., and Greene, A. S. (1998) Localization of the ANG II type 2 receptor in the microcirculation of skeletal muscle. *Am. J. Physiol.* **275,** H1395–H1403.

40. Zhang, C., Hein, T. W., Wang, W., and Kuo, L. (2003) Divergent roles of angiotensin II AT1 and AT2 receptors in modulating coronary microvascular function. *Circ. Res.* **92,** 322–329.

41. Batenburg, W. W., Garrelds, I. M., Bernasconi, C. C., et al. (2004) Angiotensin II type 2 receptor-mediated vasodilation in human coronary microarteries. *Circulation* **109,** 2296–2301.

42. Wu, L., Iwai, M., Nakagami, H., et al. (2002) Effect of angiotensin II type 1 receptor blockade on cardiac remodeling in angiotensin II type 2 receptor null mice. *Arterioscler. Thromb. Vasc. Biol.* **22,** 49–54.

43. Akishita, M., Horiuchi, M., Yamada, H., et al. (2000) Inflammation influences vascular remodeling through AT2 receptor expression and signaling. *Physiol. Genom.* **2,** 13–20.

44. Viswanathan, M. and Saavedra, J. M. (1992) Expression of angiotensin II AT2 receptors in the rat skin during experimental wound healing. *Peptides* **13,** 783–786.

45. Kimura, B., Sumners, C., and Phillips, M. I. (1992) Changes in skin angiotensin II receptors in rats during wound healing. *Biochem. Biophys. Res. Commun.* **187,** 1083–1090.

46. Bonnet, F., Cooper, M. E., Carey, R. M., Casley, D., and Cao, Z. (2001) Vascular expression of angiotensin type 2 receptor in the adult rat: influence of angiotensin II infusion. *J. Hypertens.* **19,** 1075–1081.

47. Tanaka, M., Tsuchida, S., Imai, T., et al. (1999) Vascular response to angiotensin II is exaggerated through an upregulation of AT1 receptor in AT2 knockout mice. *Biochem. Biophys. Res. Commun.* **258,** 194–198.

48. Tsutsumi, Y., Matsubara, H., Masaki, H., et al. (1999) Angiotensin II type 2 receptor overexpression activates the vascular kinin system and causes vasodilation. *J. Clin. Invest.* **104,** 925–935.

49. Otsuka, S., Sugano, M., Makino, N., Sawada, S., Hata, T., and Niho, Y. (1998) Interaction of mRNAs for angiotensin II type 1 and type 2 receptors to vascular remodeling in spontaneously hypertensive rats. *Hypertension* **32,** 467–472.

50. Busche, S., Gallinat, S., Bohle, R. M., et al. (2000) Expression of angiotensin AT(1) and AT(2) receptors in adult rat cardiomyocytes after myocardial infarction. A single-cell reverse transcriptase-polymerase chain reaction study. *Am. J. Pathol.* **157,** 605–611.

51. Brink, M., Erne, P., de Gasparo, M., et al. (1996) Localization of the angiotensin II receptor subtypes in the human atrium. *J. Mol. Cell. Cardiol.* **28,** 1789–1799.

52. Wharton, J., Morgan, K., Rutherford, R. A., et al. (1998) Differential distribution of angiotensin AT2 receptors in the normal and failing human heart. *J. Pharmacol. Exp. Ther.* **284,** 323–336.

53. Tsutsumi, Y., Matsubara, H., Ohkubo, N., et al. (1998) Angiotensin II type 2 receptor is upregulated in human heart with interstitial fibrosis, and cardiac fibroblasts are the major cell type for its expression. *Circ. Res.* **83,** 1035–1046.

54. Bottari, S. P., King, I. N., Reichlin, S., Dahlstroem, I., Lydon, N., and de Gasparo, M. (1992) The angiotensin AT2 receptor stimulates protein tyrosine phosphatase activity and mediates inhibition of particulate guanylate cyclase. *Biochem. Biophys. Res. Commun.* **183,** 206–211.

55. Brechler, V., Reichlin, S., De Gasparo, M., and Bottari, S. P. (1994) Angiotensin II stimulates protein tyrosine phosphatase activity through a G protein independent mechanism. *Receptors Channels* **2,** 89–98.

56. Yamada, T., Horiuchi, M, and Dzau, V. J. (1996) Angiotensin II type 2 receptor mediates programmed cell death. *Proc. Natl Acad. Sci. USA* **93,** 156–160.

57. Horiuchi, M., Hayashida, W., Kambe, T., Yamada, T., and Dzau, V. J. (1997) Angiotensin type 2 receptor dephosphorylates Bcl-2 by activating mitogen-activated protein kinase phosphatase-1 and induces apoptosis. *J. Biol. Chem.* **272,** 19,022–19,026.

58. Duff, J. L., Marrero, M. B., Paxton, W. G., et al. (1993) Angiotensin II induces 3CH134, a protein-tyrosine phosphatase, in vascular smooth muscle cells. *J. Biol. Chem.* **268**, 26,037–26,040.

59. Huang, X. C., Richards, E. M., and Sumners, C. (1996) Mitogen-activated protein kinases in rat brain neuronal cultures are activated by angiotensin II type 1 receptors and inhibited by angiotensin II type 2 receptors. *J. Biol. Chem.* **271**, 15,635–15,641.

60. Bedecs, K., Elbaz, N., Sutren, M., et al. (1997) Angiotensin II type 2 receptors mediate inhibition of mitogen-activated protein kinase cascade and functional activation of SHP-1 tyrosine phosphatase. *Biochem. J.* **325(2)**, 449–454.

61. Masaki, H., Kurihara, T., Yamaki, A., et al. (1998) Cardiac-specific overexpression of angiotensin II AT2 receptor causes attenuated response to AT1 receptor-mediated pressor and chronotropic effects. *J. Clin. Invest.* **101**, 527–535.

62. Lehtonen, J. Y., Daviet, L., Nahmias, C., Horiuchi, M., and Dzau, V. J. (1999) Analysis of functional domains of angiotensin II type 2 receptor involved in apoptosis. *Mol. Endocrinol.* **13**, 1051–1060.

63. Cui, T., Nakagami, H., Iwai, M., et al. (2001) Pivotal role of tyrosine phosphatase SHP-1 in AT2 receptor-mediated apoptosis in rat fetal vascular smooth muscle cell. *Cardiovasc. Res.* **49**, 863–871.

64. Feng, Y. H., Sun, Y., and Douglas, J. G. (2002) Gβγ–independent constitutive association of Gαs with SHP-1 and angiotensin II receptor AT2 is essential in AT2-mediated ITIM-independent activation of SHP-1. *Proc. Natl Acad. Sci. USA* **99**, 12,049–12,054.

65. Gallinat, S., Busche, S., Raizada, M. K., and Sumners, C. (2000) The angiotensin II type 2 receptor: an enigma with multiple variations. *Am. J. Physiol. Endocrinol. Metab.* **278**, E357–E374.

66. Huang, X. C., Richards, E. M., and Sumners, C. (1995) Angiotensin II type 2 receptor-mediated stimulation of protein phosphatase 2A in rat hypothalamic/brainstem neuronal cocultures. *J. Neurochem.* **65**, 2131–2137.

67. Shenoy, U. V., Richards, E. M., Huang, X. C., and Sumners, C. (1999) Angiotensin II type 2 receptor-mediated apoptosis of cultured neurons from newborn rat brain. *Endocrinology* **140**, 500–509.

68. Marrero, M. B., Schieffer, B., Paxton, W. G., et al. (1995) Direct stimulation of Jak/STAT pathway by the angiotensin II AT1 receptor. *Nature* **375**, 247–250.

69. Horiuchi, M., Hayashida, W., Akishita, M., et al. (1999) Stimulation of different subtypes of angiotensin II receptors, AT1 and AT2 receptors, regulates STAT activation by negative crosstalk. *Circ. Res.* **84**, 876–882.

70. Siragy, H. M. and Carey, R. M. (1996) The subtype-2 (AT2) angiotensin receptor regulates renal cyclic guanosine 3′, 5′-monophosphate and AT1 receptor-mediated prostaglandin E2 production in conscious rats. *J. Clin. Invest.* **97**, 1978–1982.

71. Siragy, H. M., Jaffa, A. A., Margolius, H. S., and Carey, R. M. (1996) Renin–angiotensin system modulates renal bradykinin production. *Am. J. Physiol.* **271**, R1090–R1095.

72. Siragy, H. M. and Carey, R. M. (1997) The subtype 2 (AT2) angiotensin receptor mediates renal production of nitric oxide in conscious rats. *J. Clin. Invest.* **100**, 264–269.

73. Carey, R. M., Jin, X. H., and Siragy, H. M. (2001) Role of the angiotensin AT2 receptor in blood pressure regulation and therapeutic implications. *Am. J. Hypertens.* **14**, 98S–102S.

74. Siragy, H. M., de Gasparo, M., and Carey, R. M. (2000) Angiotensin type 2 receptor mediates valsartan-induced hypotension in conscious rats. *Hypertension* **35**, 1074–1077.

75. Moore, A. F., Heiderstadt, N. T., Huang, E., et al. (2001) Selective inhibition of the renal angiotensin type 2 receptor increases blood pressure in conscious rats. *Hypertension* **37**, 1285–1291.

76. Siragy, H. M. and Carey, R. M. (1999) Protective role of the angiotensin AT2 receptor in a renal wrap hypertension model. *Hypertension* **33**, 1237–1242.

77. Siragy, H. M., Inagami, T., Ichiki, T., and Carey, R. M. (1999) Sustained hypersensitivity to angiotensin II and its mechanism in mice lacking the subtype-2 (AT2) angiotensin receptor. *Proc. Natl Acad. Sci. USA* **96**, 6506–6510.

78. Gohlke, P., Pees, C., and Unger, T. (1998) AT2 receptor stimulation increases aortic cyclic GMP in SHRSP by a kinin-dependent mechanism. *Hypertension* **31**, 349–355.

79. Abadir, P. M., Carey, R. M., and Siragy, H. M. (2003) Angiotensin AT2 receptors directly stimulate renal nitric oxide in bradykinin B2-receptor-null mice. *Hypertension* **42**, 600–604.

80. AbdAlla, S., Lother, H., Abdel-tawab, A. M., and Quitterer, U. (2001) The angiotensin II AT2 receptor is an AT1 receptor antagonist. *J. Biol. Chem.* **276**, 39,721–39,726.

81. Abadir, P., Periasamy, A., Carey, R. M., and Siragy, H. M. (2006) Angiotensin AT$_2$ receptor-bradykinin B$_2$ receptor functional heterodimerization. *Hypertension* **48**, 316–322.

82. Carey, R., Howell, N. L., Jin, X.-H., and Siragy, H. M. (2002) Angiotensin type-2 receptor-mediated hypotension in angiotensin type-1 receptor-blocked rats. *Hypertension* **40,** 516–520.

83. Widdop, R. E., Matrougui, K., Levy, B. I., and Henrion, D. (2002) AT2 receptor-mediated relaxation is preserved after long-term AT1 receptor blockade. *Hypertension* **40,** 516–520.

84. Hannan, R. E., Davis, E. A., and Widdop, R. E. (2003) Functional role of angiotensin II AT2 receptor in modulation of AT1 receptor-mediated contraction in rat uterine artery: involvement of bradykinin and nitric oxide. *Br. J. Pharmacol.* **140,** 987–995.

85. Katada, J. and Majima, M. (2002) AT(2) receptor-dependent vasodilation is mediated by activation of vascular kinin generation under flow conditions. *Br. J. Pharmacol.* **136,** 484–491.

86. Bergaya, S., Hilgers, R. H., Meneton, P., et al. (2004) Flow-dependent dilation mediated by endogenous kinins requires angiotensin AT2 receptors. *Circ. Res.* **94,** 1623–1629.

87. Thai, H., Wollmuth, J., Goldman, S., and Gaballa, M. (2003) Angiotensin subtype 1 receptor (AT1) blockade improves vasorelaxation in heart failure by up-regulation of endothelial nitric-oxide synthase via activation of the AT2 receptor. *J. Pharmacol. Exp. Ther.* **307,** 1171–1178.

88. Arima, S., Endo, Y., Yaoita, H., et al. (1997) Possible role of P-450 metabolite of arachidonic acid in vasodilator mechanism of angiotensin II type 2 receptor in the isolated microperfused rabbit afferent arteriole. *J. Clin. Invest.* **100,** 2816–2823.

89. Anderson, B., Romaro, G. G., and Jackson, E. K. (2003) AT$_2$ receptors attenuate AT$_1$ receptor-induced phospholipase D activation in vascular smooth muscle cells. *J. Pharmacol. Exp. Ther.* 425–431.

90. Duke, L. M., Eppel, G. A., Widdop, R. E., and Evans, R. G. (2003) Disparate roles of AT2 receptors in the renal cortical and medullary circulations of anesthetized rabbits. *Hypertension* **42,** 200–205.

91. Dimitropoulou, C., White, R. E., Fuchs, L., Zhang, H., Catravas, J. D., and Carrier, G. O. (2001) Angiotensin II relaxes microvessels via the AT(2) receptor and Ca(2+)-activated K(+) (BK(Ca)) channels. *Hypertension* **37,** 301–307.

92. Walters, P. E., Gaspari, T. A., and Widdop, R. E. (2005) Angiotensin-(1–7) acts as a vasodepressor agent via angiotensin II type 2 receptors in conscious rats. *Hypertension* **45,** 960–966.

93. You, D., Loufrani, L., Baron, C., Levy, B. I., Widdop, R. E., and Henrion, D. (2005) High blood pressure reduction reverses angiotensin II type 2 receptor-mediated vasoconstriction into vasodilation in spontaneously hypertensive rats. *Circulation* **111,** 1006–1011.

94. Haithcock, D., Jiao, H., Cui, X. L., Hopfer, U., and Douglas, J. G. (1999) Renal proximal tubular AT2 receptor: signaling and transport. *J. Am. Soc. Nephrol.* **10(Suppl 11),** S69–S74.

95. Gross, V., Schunck, W. H., Honeck, H., et al. (2000) Inhibition of pressure natriuresis in mice lacking the AT2 receptor. *Kidney Int.* **57,** 191–202.

96. Padia, S. H., Howell, N. L., Siragy, H. M., and Carey, R. M. (2006) Renal angiotensin type 2 receptors mediate natriuresis via angiotensin III in the angiotensin II type 1 receptor-blocked rat. *Hypertension* **47,** 537–544.

97. Hakam, A. C. and Hussain, T. (2005) Renal angiotensin II type-2 receptors are upregulated and mediate the candesartan-induced natriuresis/diuresis in obese Zucker rats. *Hypertension* **45,** 270–275.

98. Hakam, A. C., Siddiqui, A. H., and Hussain, T. (2006) Renal angiotensin II AT2 receptors promote natriuresis in streptozotocin-induced diabetic rats. *Am. J. Physiol. Renal. Physiol.* **290,** F503–F508.

99. Hakam, A. and Hussein, T. (2006) Angiotensin II AT$_2$ receptors inhibit proximal tubular Na$^+$-K$^+$-ATPase activity via a NO/cGMP-dependent pathway. *Am. J. Physiol. Renal. Physiol.* **290,** F1430–F1436.

100. Johns, D. W., Peach, M. J., Gomez, R. A., Inagami, T., and Carey, R. M. (1990) Angiotensin II regulates renin gene expression. *Am. J. Physiol.* **259,** F882–F887.

101. Ichihara, A., Hayashi, M., Hirota, N., et al. (2003) Angiotensin II type 2 receptor inhibits prorenin processing in juxtaglomerular cells. *Hypertens. Res.* **26,** 915–921.

102. Siragy, H., Xue, C., Abadir, P., and Carey, R. M. (2005) Angiotensin type-2 receptors inhibit renin biosynthesis and angiotensin II formation. *Hypertension* **45,** 1–5.

6 Angiotensin II and Inflammation

Rhian M. Touyz and Ernesto L. Schiffrin

CONTENTS

1. INTRODUCTION

The renin-angiotensin system (RAS) was originally described as a hemodynamic regulator that increases blood pressure acutely by vasoconstriction and chronically through aldosterone-mediated extracellular volume expansion *(1)*. It is now clear that a tissue-based RAS exists, which is independently controlled from the circulation *(2)*. Elevated tissue levels of components of the RAS including Ang II, the effector peptide of the RAS, have been demonstrated in numerous diseases independently of blood pressure elevation, such as hypertension, atherosclerosis, myocardial infarction, cardiac failure, diabetes, and renal disease *(2,3)*.

Ang II, which mediates its cardiovascular and renal effects primarily through the Ang II type 1 receptor (AT_1R) subtype, has pleiotropic actions in multiple organ systems. In the vasculature, Ang II induces contraction, cell growth, migration, and differentiation and is pro-fibrotic *(4,5)*. In addition, compelling evidence indicates that Ang II has important proinflammatory properties in the vascular wall, stimulating the generation of reactive oxygen species (ROS) and the production of inflammatory cytokines and adhesion molecules through the cytoplasmic transcription factor nuclear factor-κB (NF-κB) *(5,6)*. Through these actions, Ang II augments vascular inflammation and promotes endothelial dysfunction and structural remodeling.

Inflammation is a complex set of interactions among soluble factors and cells that can arise in any tissue in response to pathogenic stimuli. Normally, the process leads to

From: *Contemporary Endocrinology: Hypertension and Hormone Mechanisms*
Edited by: R. M. Carey © Humana Press Inc., Totowa, NJ

recovery, healing, and scar formation. However, if repair is uncontrolled, inflammation can result in persistent tissue damage by leukocytes, lymphocytes, or collagen (7). The magnitude of inflammation is critical: insufficient reactions lead to immunodeficiency, which can result in infection and cancer, whereas excessive responses cause morbidity and mortality in diseases such as atherosclerosis, myocardial infarction, and diabetes (8). Homeostasis is restored when inflammation is limited by anti-inflammatory responses that are rapid, reversible, localized, and adaptive. Independent of the etiology of the primary insult, the inflammatory response characteristically involves three processes: (1) alterations in vascular permeability, (2) leukocyte extravasation (adhesion, transmigration, and chemotaxis), and (3) tissue repair and cell growth (9). The RAS, particularly Ang II, has been implicated in all of these processes (Fig. 1) and is increasingly being recognized as a major contributor in the inflammatory response in many organs, including the kidney, heart, liver, brain, and ovaries. Here we will discuss the role of Ang II as a pro-inflammatory mediator, focusing specifically on the vasculature, and implications in cardiovascular disease.

2. ANG II AND VASCULAR PERMEABILITY

The initial phase of inflammation is associated with a local increase in vascular permeability with consequent cell infiltration and protein-rich fluid exudation (9). Ang II influences vascular permeability indirectly via pressure-mediated mechanical injury to the endothelium particularly in hypertension, and locally through hemodynamic-independent processes (10) (Fig. 1). Local mechanisms underlying these events involve Ang II-elicited production of second mediators, specifically prostaglandins (leukotriene C4, prostaglandin E2, prostaglandin 12) and vascular endothelial cell growth factor (VEGF). Ang II stimulates production of PGE2 and thromboxane and increases generation of cytochrome P450 metabolites of arachidonic acid (11–13). These effects occur through AT_1R-dependent processes (14), because losartan, a selective AT_1R blocker, prevents thromboxane A2-mediated increase in vascular permeability.

The VEGF family (VEGF-A, VEGF-B, VEGF-C, and VEGF-D) and their corresponding receptor tyrosine kinases (VEGFR-1 [Flt-1], VEGFR-2 [Flk-1, KDR], and VEGFR-3 [Flt-4]) are important in inducing vascular permeability and in stimulating endothelial cell growth (15). VEGF, also called vascular permeability factor (16), is a key regulator of physiological vasculogenesis and has been implicated in pathological angiogenesis, vascular leakage, and inflammation (17). These processes are influenced by Ang II. In vitro studies demonstrated that Ang II stimulates secretion and/or expression of VEGF by vascular smooth muscle cells (VSMC) (18), endothelial cells (19,20), cardiac myofibroblasts (21), and mesangial cells (22). This action is mediated primarily by the AT_1R (18,19) although the AT_2R has also been implicated in retinal and renal cells (23,24). Ang II upregulates VEGF mRNA expression through transcriptional regulation by NADPH oxidase-mediated, redox-sensitive processes (25,26). Ang II also influences VEGF-mediated signal transduction or post-transcriptional regulation of VEGFR-2 (27,28). The importance of VEGF in Ang II-induced vascular inflammation and remodeling, independently of hemodynamic changes, was demonstrated in Ang II-infused mice, in which VEGF was inhibited. VEGF blockade by soluble VEGF receptor 1 (sFlt-1) gene transfer attenuated Ang II-mediated inflammation

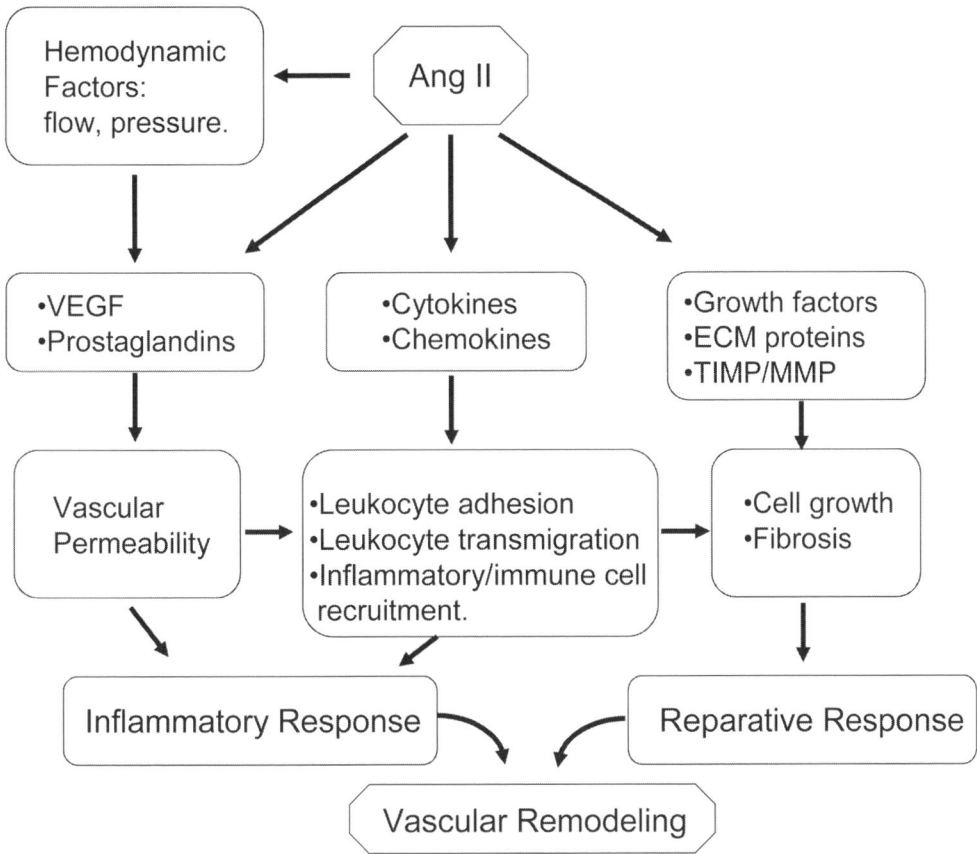

Fig. 1. Pro-inflammatory processes of Ang II in the vasculature. Ang II influences vascular perme-ability through direct and indirect (hemodynamic changes) mechanisms by increasing production of VEGF and prostaglandins. Ang II-induced activation of chemokines, cytokines, and growth factors results in leukocyte recruitment, cell growth and fibrosis. These events constitute the inflammatory-reparative response, leading to vascular injury and structural remodeling in cardiovascular disease. ECM, extracellular matrix; MMP, matrix metalloproteinase; TIMP, tissue inhibitor of matrix metallo-proteinase; VEGF, vascular endothelial cell growth factor.

and remodeling without influencing Ang II-induced arterial hypertension and cardiac hypertrophy.

Some of the pathological processes that are associated with changes in vascular permeability and inflammation in response to Ang II-induced effects mediated by VEGF include diabetic retinopathy *(29,30)* and tubulointerstitial damage leading to proteinuria. Ang II is a potent stimulus for ocular VEGF expression, as it increases VEGFR-2 expression in bovine retinal microcapillary endothelial cells and retinal pericytes, an effect that is inhibited by AT_1R blockers *(27,28)*. In diabetic rats, angiotensin-converting enzyme (ACE) inhibitors normalize diabetes-associated changes of VEGF expression and vascular permeability *(31)* whereas Ang II potentiates VEGF-induced endothelial cell growth and tube formation *(27,28)*. Patients with diabetic retinopathy have increased vitreous fluid Ang II and VSGF levels, and increased retinal vasopermeability and neovascularization *(29)*. ACE inhibitors prevent retinal neovascularization in retinopathy of prematurity, an effect accompanied by reduced VEGF and VEGFR-2 expression, indicating a retinoprotective effect of RAS blockade *(32)*.

The association between Ang II and diabetic retinopathy is particularly important in relation to hypertension. The Wisconsin Epidemiologic Study of Diabetic Retinopathy (WESDR) demonstrated that diastolic blood pressure is a significant predictor of progression to diabetic retinopathy in patients with type 1 diabetes *(33)*, whereas the UK Prospective Diabetes Study (UKPDS) group showed that in type 2 diabetes, the incidence of diabetic complications is associated with systolic blood pressure *(34)*. A series of large clinical trials (UKPDS; Controlled Trial of Lisinopril in Insulin Dependent Diabetes Mellitus, EUCLID; Diabetic Retinpathy Candesartan Trials, DIRECT) further support a role for Ang II in diabetic retinopathy, by which it was demonstrated that ACE inhibitors or AT_1R blockers not only reduce blood pressure in diabetic patients but also decrease progression of diabetic retinopathy *(29,33–35)*.

Ang II effects on vascular permeability are especially important in the kidneys, in which enhanced glomerular capillary permeability and inflammation lead to tubulo-interstitial damage and proteinuria. Ang II promotes glomerular hyperpermeability through its pressor action and through direct mechanisms, probably by altering cytoskeletal arrangement of glomeular epithelial cells *(36)*. Based on data from large clinical trials, it is clear that microalbuminuria is a renal signal that cardiovascular risk is increased and that vascular responses are altered. The risk of cardiovascular events and mortality is estimated to be 2–8 times higher when microalbuminuria is present in patients with diabetes and hypertension *(37,38)*. Interruption of the RAS with ACE inhibitors or AT_1 receptor blockers decreases proteinuria in patients with hypertension, diabetes, and renal disease *(39,40)*. These effects have been attributed, in part, to direct improvement of glomerular permeability and reduced renovascular inflammation, independently of blood pressure lowering *(41)*.

3. ANG II EFFECTS ON LEUKOCYTES: CELL ADHESION AND CHEMOTAXIS IN THE VASCULATURE

A fundamental process in inflammation is extravasation or recruitment of leukocytes from the vascular lumen to the interstitial tissue *(9)*. This phenomenon involves three basic steps: (1) cell rolling, (2) cell adhesion, and (3) transendothelial migration and chemotaxis (movement toward chemotactic stimuli) (Fig. 2).

Adhesion and transendothelial migration of leukocytes into the vessel wall involve sequential interaction of distinct receptors on the surface of leukocytes and endothelial cells. Cellular adhesion molecules, especially members of the selectin family and immuno-globulin superfamily, are involved in leukocyte recruitment to sites of inflammation. Selectins, which are lectin-like molecules expressed on leukocytes (L-selectin), endothelial cells (E-selectin, P-selectin), and platelets (P-selectin), mediate initial contact between circulating leukocytes and vascular endothelium *(42,43)*. Selectins stimulate leukocyte rolling on endothelial cells and promote platelet-leukocyte aggregation. P-selectin is stored in specific granules present in platelets (α-granules) and endothelial cells (Weibel–Palade bodies) from which it can be rapidly recruited to the cell surface after stimulation *(44)*. Rolling leukocytes encounter activated stimuli that trigger activation-dependent adhesion

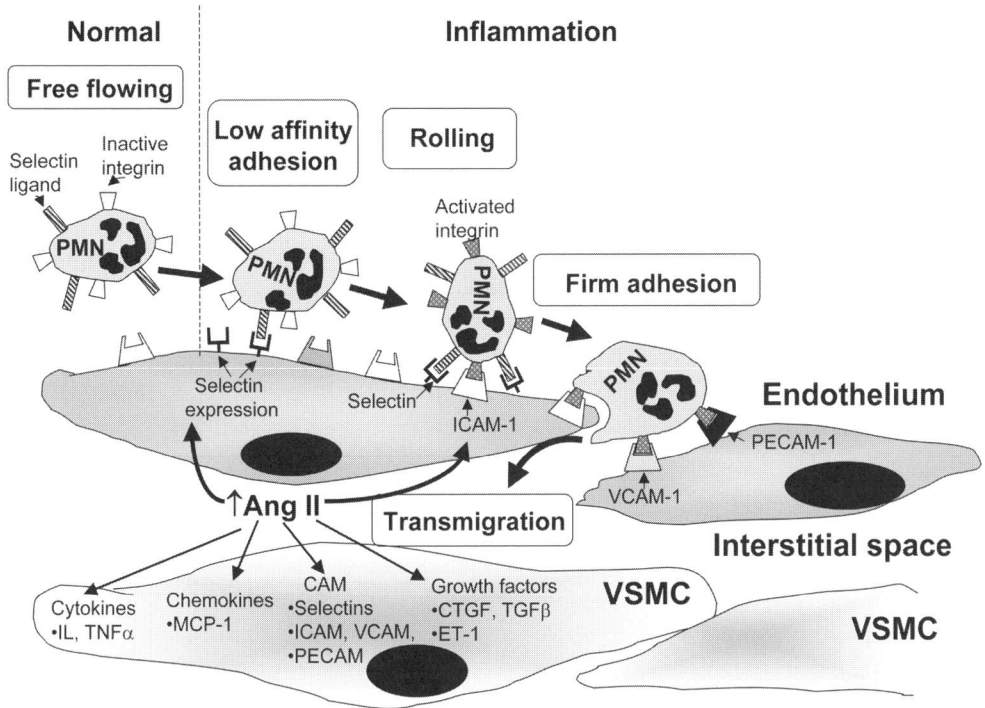

Fig. 2. Ang II-mediated processes in vascular leukocyte recruitment. Normally, leukocytes and endothelial cells do not interact. In physiological conditions, leukocytes possess inactive integrins and selectin-binding sites (ligands), but these are unbound, as endothelial cells do not express selectins. Following a pathogenic stimulus, such as increased Ang II levels, endothelial cells are activated and selectin-binding sites are expressed. This results in leukocyte–endothelial cell interaction through weak adhesion (low affinity binding), followed by leukocyte rolling along the endothelium. Subsequent leukocyte activation promotes leukocyte integrins to bind with Ig-supergene family glycoproteins, including ICAM-1 and VCAM-1, resulting in firm adhesion. This is followed by transendothelial migration, which is facilitated by additional Ig-supergene family member expression, including endothelial PECAM-1. Ang II further contributes to the inflammatory process by stimulating synthesis of cytokines, chemokines, and growth factors by VSMCs. CAM, cell adhesion molecules; CTGF, connective tissue growth factor; ICAM-1, intercellular cell adhesion molecule, MCP-1, monocyte chemoattractant protein-1; PECAM, platelet-endothelial cell adhesion molecule; PMN, polymorphonuclear leukocytes; TGF-β, transforming growth factor-β; VCAM, vascular cell adhesion molecule.

necessary for integrin-mediated arrest. The integrin family includes heterodimeric proteins composed of noncovalently linked α and β subunits. To date at least 15 α- and 8 β-chains have been identified. Ligand specificity of integrins is based on the α-subunit and comprises two groups: extracellular matrix proteins and cell surface molecules of the immunoglobulin supergene family. Extracellular matrix proteins of importance include fibronectin, thrombospondin, vitronectin, and fibrinogen *(44)*. Important Ig-supergene family members include: intercellular cell adhesion molecules-1 and -2 (ICAM-1, ICAM-2), which bind CD11a/CD18 (LFA-1) and CD11b/CD18 (Mac-1); vascular cell adhesion molecule-1 (VCAM-1), which binds VLA-4, platelet-endothelial cell adhesion molecule-1 (PECAM-1); and the mucosal address in cell adhesion molecule-2 (MAsCAM-1). ICAM-1 is expressed mainly on endothelial cells *(45)*. VCAM-1, which exhibits low expression on unstimulated endothelial cells, is upregulated by cytokines, and mediates adhesion of lymphocytes and monocytes in inflamed vascular beds *(44)*. PECAM-1 is constitutively expressed on platelets, leukocytes, and endothelial cells *(46)*, and MAdCAM-1 is mainly expressed on mucosal endothelial venules *(47)*.

Establishment of an adhesive interaction between endothelial cells and circulating leukocytes involves movement from flowing blood toward the vessel wall *(44)*. Selectins, particularly L-selectin and their ligands, mediate initial weak (low-affinity) adhesive interactions manifested as leukocyte rolling *(48)*. Rolling leukocytes are exposed to low concentrations of chemoattractants or inflammatory mediators resulting in leukocyte activation, which induces leukocyte integrins to bind with Ig-supergene family glyco-proteins, such as ICAM-1 and VCAM-1, permitting firm adhesion. This is associated with downregulation (shedding) of L-selectin *(44)*. Transendothelial migration is mediated by additional Ig-supergene family members, like PECAM-1 and occurs when adherent leukocytes move toward the endothelial cell-cell junctions. During this process, the cell steadily establishes new adhesive contacts at the migration pole, while reducing adhesive interactions at the tail. Leukocytes then migrate into tissues by a chemoattractant gradient. Chemokines are a superfamily of small proteins with chemoattractant properties for specific types of leukocytes. In general, CXC chemokines (α-subfamily) play a role in acute inflammation through neutrophil activation, whereas CC chemokines (β-subfamily) are involved in chronic inflammation through monocytes and lymphocytes *(49)*. Many Ang II-dependent forms of cardiovascular disease, including atherosclerosis, hypertension, cardiac failure, and diabetes, are characterized by vascular monocyte-macrophage infiltration *(49–51)*.

Ang II regulates multiple steps in leukocyte recruitment into the vessel wall. It stimulates production of many pro-inflammatory molecules (Table 1), enhances adhesion of monocytes-neutrophils to endothelial cells by influencing cell adhesion molecules, and promotes transendothelial migration through cytokines and chemokines *(51)*. These effects appear to be independent of pressor actions. Intravital microscopy of rat mesenteric postcapillary venules demonstrated that Ang II infusion increases leukocyte rolling, adhesion, and migration without any vasoconstrictor activity *(52)*. Both AT_1R and AT_2R appear to play a role in this process, because Ang II-induced effects were abolished by the combination therapy of AT_1R and AT_2R antagonists *(52)*. In endothelial cells, Ang II upregulates expression of VCAM-1, ICAM-1, and E-selectin through pathways involving ROS *(53–55)*. In VSMCs, Ang II stimulates production of VCAM-1, chemokine monocyte chemotactic protein-1 (MCP-1), interleukin (IL)-6, IL-8, and osteopontin in a time- and dose-dependent manner *(56–59)*. These effects are mediated via AT_1R and involve RhoA-dependent and redox-sensitive processes *(57)*.

IL-6, a 26-kDa glycoprotein, is a pro-inflammatory cytokine that induces synthesis of acute phase proteins, such as C-reactive protein (CRP), cytokines, and growth factors *(60,61)*. It also activates platelets, has procoagulant activity, and is mitogenic for VSMCs *(60–62)*. IL-8, also called CXCL8 because of a potent neutrophil chemotactic factor *(63)*, induces VSMC proliferation and migration *(64)*. MCP-1 is a small (8–10 kDa) CC type chemokine that specifically attracts monocytes and memory T lymphocytes

Table 1
Summary of Cytokines, Chemokines, Growth Factors, and Other Pro-
Inflammatory Mediators Synthesized in Response to Ang II Stimulation

Cytokines
- IL-1
- IL-6
- IL-18
- GM-CSF
- TNF-α

Chemokines
- IL-8
- MCP-1
- MIP1
- RANTES

Growth factors
- ET-1
- TGFβ
- CTGF
- bFGF
- PDGF
- EGF
- VEGF

Other immune modulators
- IFN
- Tissue factor
- PAI-1

Abbreviations: bFGF, basic fibroblast growth factor; CTGF, connective tissue growth factor; EGF, epidermal growth factor; ET-1, endothelin-1; GM-CSF, granulocyte-macrophage colony stimulating factor; IFN, interferon; IL, interleukin; MCP-1, monocyte chemoattractant protein-1; MIP, macrophage inflammatory protein; PDGF, platelet-derived growth factor; RANTES, regulated on activation, normal T cell expressed and secreted; TGF-β, transforming growth factor-β; TNF-α, tumor necrosis factor α; VEGF, vascular endothelial cell growth factor.

expressing the CC chemokine receptor 2 (CCR2). MCP-1 functions locally in the vessel wall by establishing a chemical gradient to attract adherent monocytes and T-lymphocytes. It is among the most important chemokines regulating migration and infiltration of monocytes-macrophages in the vessel wall *(65)* and has been implicated to play an essential role in hypertension-induced vascular inflammation and remodeling *(66)*. MCP-1–CCR2 interactions are important in atherosclerosis, because hyperlipidemic-atherosclerotic-prone mice, made genetically deficient in MCP-1 or CCR2, exhibit decreased vascular macrophages with fewer atherosclerotic plaques than control counterparts *(67,68)*. MCP-1–CCR2 is also important in vascular remodeling in Ang II-induced hypertension *(69)*. Osteopontin is a macrophage chemotactic and adhesion molecule, and has been associated with monocyte-macrophage infiltration in atherosclerosis and vascular remodeling with Ang II-mediated hypertension *(59)*. The capacity of Ang II to stimulate regulated expression of adhesion molecules, cytokines, and chemokines promotes recruitment of mononuclear leukocytes into the vessel wall and contributes to the pro-inflammatory properties of this peptide.

Direct Ang II vascular inflammatory effects have also been demonstrated in studies in vivo. Ang II infusion increases expression of vascular ICAM-1 and VCAM-1 through AT_1 receptors. These processes occur independently of blood pressure changes and involve activation of redox-dependent, mitogen-activated protein (MAP) kinase-regulated pathways (9). To confirm a role of endogenous Ang II in vascular inflammation, studies in apoE–/– mice treated with irbesartan decreased MCP-1 expression in atherosclerotic lesions (70). In hyperlipidemic rabbits, losartan reduced aortic intimal proliferation and induced a significant reduction in expression of P-selectin and MCP-1 (71). Moreover, recent studies from our laboratory demonstrated that the mice lacking macrophage colony-stimulating factor (m-CSF) developed less endothelial dysfunction, vascular remodeling and oxidative stress induced by Ang II than wild-type littermates, further supporting a critical role of pro-inflammatory mediators in Ang II-induced vascular injury (72). In human studies, irbesartan reduced serum levels of VCAM-1 and tumor necrosis factor (TNF)-α in patients with premature atherosclerosis (73); and in hypertensive patients, candesartan decreased plasma levels of MCP-1, TNF-α, and plasminogen activator inhibitor type 1 (PAI-1) (74). In atherosclerotic plaques and in atherectomy specimens of patients with unstable angina, IL-6 and Ang II colocalized with macrophages, further suggesting a role of local Ang II in the recruitment of macrophages in atherogenesis (75). Also, in patients with cardiovascular disease, plasma elevation of MCP-1 was reduced by ACE inhibitors and AT_1R blockers (76).

4. EFFECTS OF ANG II ON VASCULAR REPAIR

As part of the inflammatory response, tissues undergo repair. This process involves cell growth and fibrosis, both of which are modulated by Ang II (Fig. 1). Ang II influences cell growth by stimulating hyperplasia, hypertrophy, and apoptosis (77). In cultured VSMC through the AT_1R, Ang II induces hyperplasia (increase in cell number associated with DNA synthesis) or hypertrophy (increased protein synthesis and/or increased intracellular cell water volume). These effects are partially mediated through transactivation of EGFR, PDGFR, and IGFR and involve activation of growth-signaling pathways including c-Src and MAP kinases (78–80). Vascular cell hyperplasia and hypertrophy contribute to remodeling associated with vascular injury and inflammation (81,82). Ang II also has antigrowth and pro-apoptotic actions, mediated primarily through AT_2R (83–85). These effects are particularly important in pathological conditions associated with vascular inflammation in which AT_2R may be upregulated, such as in aortic banding-induced hypertension (86), renal injury (87), myocardial infarction (88), and in human atherosclerotic coronary arteries (89).

Vascular fibrosis, an important component in the inflammatory-reparative process, involves accumulation of extracellular matrix proteins, particularly collagen and fibronectin, in the vascular media and contributes to structural remodeling and scar formation. Ang II is critically involved in fibrosis. In cultured VSMCs, fibroblasts and cardiac cells, Ang II stimulates profibrotic signaling pathways and stimulates production of vascular collagen and fibronectin (77,90–92). Systemic infusion of Ang II leads to cardiac, vascular, and renal fibrosis, which is prevented by AT$_1$R blockade *(93)*. Studies in AT$_1$R-deficient mice further confirm the importance of Ang II in cardiovascular fibrosis *(94,95)*. In addition to stimulating collagen production, Ang II influences extracellular matrix composition by inducing collagen degradation by attenuating interstitial matrix metalloproteinase (MMP) activity and by enhancing tissue inhibitor of metalloproteinase (TIMP)-1 production *(96)*. In young SHR, activity of MMP1 and MMP3 is reduced *(52)*, whereas in adult SHR, MMP2 activity is decreased *(96)*. These effects promote accumulation of fibronectin, proteoglycans, and collagen, which contribute to remodeling in hypertension. AT$_1$R blockade normalized TIMP-1 expression and collagenase activity, supporting the role for Ang II in these processes *(96)*.

Ang II-elicited growth and profibrotic effects are modulated by the endogenous production of various mitogenic factors, such as TGF-β, PDGF, and ET-1 *(97–101)*. Of these, TGF-β, a multifunctional cytokine, appears to be particularly important. TGF-β increases extracellular matrix biosynthesis, downregulates matrix degradative enzymes and influences integrin receptors *(102)*. TGF-β is synthesized by macrophages, lymphocytes, fibroblasts, VSMCs, and renal cells *(102)*. Vascular and renal injury induced by hypertension, diabetes and/or the RAS appear to be mediated by overexpression and conversion of TGF-β$_1$ from its latent form to its active form *(103)*. Activation of latent TGF-β$_1$ is preceded by overexpression of thrombospondin-1 *(104)*, an extracellular matrix protein responsible for its activation. Invading monocytes expressing TGF-β$_1$ also contribute to vascular TGF-β$_1$ overexpression. TGF-β$_1$ elicits its effects by interacting with two cell surface membrane signaling receptors, a type II TGF-β receptor and a type I receptor (ALK-5). Signals from the activated TGF-β receptor complex are transduced to the nucleus by Smad proteins, a family of transcription factors recently implicated as intracellular mediators of inflammation *(105)*. Key downstream profibrogenic mediators of TGF-β include p38MAP kinase and connective tissue growth factor (CTGF). CTGF mediates Ang II-stimulated cardiac fibroblast activation in heart failure and is a potent inducer of vascular and renal fibrosis *(106–108)*. Furthermore, Ang II increases CTGF mRNA expression and production *(9,106,109,110)*. TGF-β is negatively regulated by unique proto-oncoproteins, Ski, and SnoN *(111)*. It is clear that TGF-β is a fundamental pathogenic cytokine that is consistently overexpressed in many cardiovascular and renal disorders associated with activation of the RAS. In support of this, inhibition of the RAS with ACE inhibitors or AT$_1$R blockers is closely correlated with the suppression of TGF-β production and amelioration of fibrosis *(103,112)*.

5. MOLECULAR MECHANISMS OF ANG II-MEDIATED VASCULAR INFLAMMATION

5.1. Role of NF-κB and Other Transcription Factors

Expression of genes involved in the inflammatory response is controlled by activation of transcription factors, including NF-κB, AP-1, and HIF-1, which are activated by Ang II *(113,114)* (Fig. 3). NF-κB is particularly important in vascular inflammation, as many pro-inflammatory genes are under NF-κB control, including adhesion molecules (VCAM-1, ICAM-1), chemokines (MCP-1, RANTES), and cytokines (IL-6) *(9)*. NF-κB also regulates Ang II and angiotensinogen gene expression thereby amplifying the

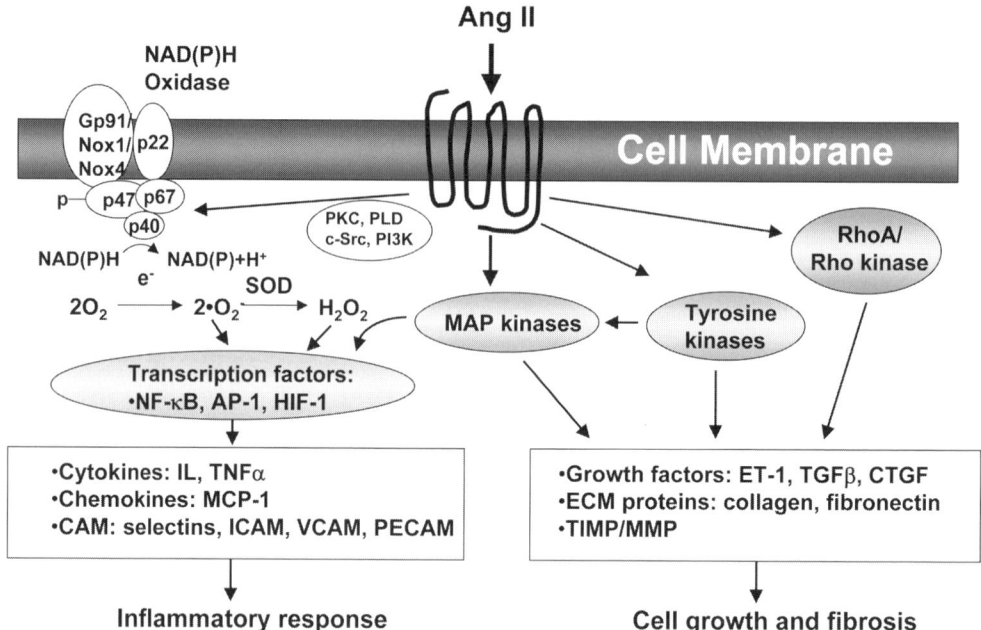

Fig. 3. Molecular mechanisms whereby Ang II induces inflammatory-reparative responses in the vascular wall. Ang II is a potent stimulator of NAD(P)H oxidase, which generates reactive oxygen species (ROS), such as $\bullet O_2^-$ and H_2O_2. These effects are mediated through PKC, PLD, and c-Src. Increased intracellular ROS formation stimulates activation of redox-sensitive transcription factors, including NF-κB, AP-1, and HIF-1, which in turn activate pro-inflammatory genes to produce cytokines and chemokines and to induce expression of cell adhesion molecules. Ang II also activates MAP kinases, tyrosine kinases, and RhoA/Rho kinase, which stimulate cell growth and fibrogenic pathways. AP-1, activator protein-1; CAM, cell adhesion molecules; CTGF, connective tissue growth factor; e⁻, electron; HIF-1, hypoxia inducible factor-1; ICAM-1, intercellular cell adhesion molecule; IL, interleukin; MAP, mitogen-activated protein; MCP-1, monocyte chemoattractant protein-1; NF-κB, nuclear factor κB; PECAM, platelet-endothelial cell adhesion molecule; PKC, protein kinase C; PLD, phospholipase D; TGF-β, transforming growth factor-β; TNF-α, tumor necrosis factor α; VCAM, vascular cell adhesion molecule.

Ang II-mediated inflammatory cascade *(115,116)*. NF-κB is a family of highly inducible DNA-binding proteins regulated by protein processing and by association with the cytoplasmic inhibitor, IκB *(117)*. Ang II influences the NF-κB activation pathway at multiple levels in VSMCs *(117)*. It stimulates translocation to the nucleus, DNA-binding, transcription of a NF-κB reporter gene and IκB degradation *(114,117)*. Presence of other inflammatory mediators, such as IL-1β, may be necessary for Ang II to fully activate NF-κB in VSMCs *(118)*.

The importance of NF-κB to inflammatory molecule expression is evidenced by in vitro studies demonstrating that the inhibition of NF-κB activation prevents Ang II-induced expression of IL-6, VCAM-1 and MCP-1 *(114,115)*. NF-κB activation is also essential for Ang II-dependent proliferation and migration of VSMCs, because SN50, selective NF-κB inhibitor; phenethyl caffeinate, inhibitor of NF-κB nuclear translocation; and Bay 11-7085, inhibitor of IκB phosphorylation effectively arrest Ang II-dependent DNA synthesis and migration *(119)*. Both AT_1R and AT_2R have been implicated in these processes.

In Ang II-infused animals, NF-κB activation is increased and expression of cytokines (TNF-α, IL-6) and chemokines (MCP-1) is augmented *(120)*. In experimental models of atherosclerosis, renal injury, and in pulmonary hypertension, ACE inhibitors reduce tissue NF-κB activity, decrease cytokine and chemokine expression, and prevent vascular and renal inflammation *(121–123)*. In a model of Ang II-dependent severe hypertension with end-organ damage, leukocyte infiltration in the vascular wall accompanies vascular PAI-1, MCP-1, iNOS, and Tissue Factor overexpression, and NF-κB activation *(124)*. These effects were directly associated with NF-κB activation, because NF-κB inhibition by pyrrolidine dithiocarbamate decreased blood pressure, reduced cardiac hypertrophy, and ameliorated vascular injury in small renal and cardiac vessels *(124)*. These findings suggest that NF-κB is a major inducer of Ang II-mediated upregulation of adhesion molecules and cytokine expression.

Ang II regulation of NF-κB involves ROS, since antioxidants interfere with its activation by Ang II *(125,126)*. ROS-induced NF-κB activation probably occurs through redox modification of reactive cysteines *(127)*. Upstream kinase(s) and/or phosphatase(s) prone to thiolation or oxidation of SH groups are possible candidates mediating redox regulation. In particular, thioredoxin and Redox-factor-1 (Ref-1) are important activators of NF-κB *(128)*.

5.2. Role of Reactive Oxygen Species

Reactive oxygen species (ROS) play an important role in the modulation of inflammatory reactions (Fig. 3). Major ROS produced within vascular cells include superoxide anion ($•O_2^-$), hydrogen peroxide (H_2O_2), hydroxyl radical ($•OH$), nitric oxide (NO), and peroxynitrite (ONOO–) *(126)*. ROSs are implicated at virtually every stage in the inflammatory response, including vascular permeability, leukocyte adhesion and transmigration, chemotaxis, cell growth, and fibrosis *(126,129)*. These processes are mediated via multiple Ang II-stimulated redox-sensitive signaling pathways, including intracellular Ca^{2+} mobilization, activation of JAK/STAT, Akt/PKB, MAP kinase and RhoA/Rho kinase pathways, and inhibition of protein tyrosine phosphatases *(130–134)*. ROS also influence transcription factor activity and thereby modulate expression of many other mediators of inflammation.

Among the many generators of ROS, including leakage from the mitochondrial electron transport chain, cyclooxygenase, lipoxygenase, heme oxygenase, cytochrome P450 monooxygenase, and xanthine oxidase, the membrane-associated nicotinamide adenine dinucleotide phosphate (reduced form; NAD(P)H) oxidases have been demonstrated to be of major importance in vascular cells *(135)*. Vascular ROS are produced in endothelial, adventitial and VSMCs, and derived predominantly from NAD(P)H oxidase, a multisubunit enzyme *(136–138)* that catalyzes the production of $•O_2^-$ by the one electron reduction of oxygen using NAD(P)H as the electron donor: $2O_2 + NAD(P)H \rightarrow 2O_2^- + NAD(P)H + H^+$. The prototypical NAD(P)H oxidase is that found in phagocytes, which comprises five components (phox, *PH*agocyte *OX*idase): p47phox, p67phox, p40phox, p22phox, and gp91phox (babior), and the small G proteins Rac 1/2. Unlike phagocytic NAD(P)H oxidase, which is activated only on stimulation and which generates $•O_2^-$ in a burst-like manner extracellulary, vascular oxidases are constitutively active, produce $•O_2^-$ intracellulary in a slow and sustained fashion and act as intracellular signaling molecules, influencing not only transcription factors, but also other molecules involved in inflammation, such as MAP kinases, tyrosine kinases and protein phosphatases *(136,139)*. All of the phagocytic NAD(P)H oxidase subunits are expressed, to varying degrees, in vascular cells *(135–139)*. The newly discovered gp91phox (nox2) homologs, nox1 and nox4 (Nox, *N*AD(P)H *ox*idase), implicated in atherogenesis, have also been detected in the vasculature *(136,140,141)*.

Ang II is a potent stimulator of vascular NAD(P)H oxidase *(137,139)*. It induces activation of the enzyme, it increases expression of NAD(P)H oxidase subunits, and it stimulates ROS production in cultured VSMC and intact arteries *(135,137,139)*. Mechanisms linking Ang II to the enzyme and upstream signaling molecules modulating NAD(P)H oxidase in vascular cells have not been fully elucidated, but PLD, PKC, c-Src, PI3K, and Rac may be important *(136,142)*. The significance of these molecular events is evidenced by findings from several models of vascular injury, including athero-sclerosis, hypertension, diabetes, and renal disease, demonstrating that Ang II-mediated ROS production is a major participant in the inflammatory response *(129,143)*.

6. MARKERS OF INFLAMMATION IN CARDIOVASCULAR DISEASE

In otherwise healthy individuals, cytokines that are generated by injured or athero-sclerotic vessels do not produce systemic manifestations typically associated with inflammation *(115)*. However, systemic effects are detectable biochemically. Numerous markers of inflammation, such as CRP, IL-1, IL-6, IL-18, serum amyloid A (SAA), TNF-α, soluble adhesion molecules (sICAM, sVCAM, sE-selectin, and sP-selectin), myeloperoxidase, CD 40 ligand, and macrophage inhibitory cytokine-1 are now being considered as predictors of clinical risk *(144,145)*. Of these, high-sensitivity (hs) CRP is the most stable and powerful inflammatory marker of future cardiovascular risk.

CRP is an acute-phase reactant, initially considered to be a simple marker of vascular inflammation *(146)*. However, increasing evidence indicates that CRP directly partici-pates in the inflammatory response. CRP activates endothelial cells to produce ICAM-1, VCAM-1, and E-selectin *(146)*. CRP also stimulates MCP-1 production, induces monocyte release of IL-6 and TNF-α, and decreases eNOS expression and bioactivity *(146–148)*. Hence CRP can directly activate the entire inflammatory recruitment cascade. For these reasons, the role of CRP as a predictor of cardiovascular events has been extensively investigated.

Prospective studies reported that CRP is an independent predictor of risks of future myocardial infarction, stroke, and peripheral vascular disease *(144,149–151)*. In a recent study, a cohort from the Framingham Heart Study, in which the participants were free of cardiovascular disease, the relationship between CRP and coronary calcification was evaluated *(152)*. The authors found that CRP levels were associated with epicardial coronary calcification, even after adjustment for age and the traditional risk factors. The clinical utility of CRP has also been assessed to predict future risk of sudden cardiac death in apparently healthy men who have no clinical evidence of coronary heart disease *(144,149,151)*. In addition to its predictive value for cardiovascular events, CRP has been associated with the development of type II diabetes, metabolic syndrome, and hypertension *(153–155)*. Taken together, these clinical data further support a role for inflammation in cardiovascular disease and reinforce the hypothesis that inflammatory markers, such as CRP, can improve methods of global cardiovascular risk assessment.

7. CONCLUSIONS

Over the recent past, our views of Ang II have changed from being a simple vasocon-strictor mediated through increased intracellular free Ca^{2+} concentration, to a sophisticated growth factor mediated through complex signaling pathways involving MAP kinases, tyrosine kinases, proto-oncogene expression, and cell cycle modulation. More recently, it has become clear that Ang II is also a key player in vascular inflammation. Through increased generation of ROS and activation of redox-sensitive transcription factors, Ang II promotes expression of cell adhesion molecules and induces synthesis of pro-inflammatory mediators and growth factors. These processes facilitate increased vascular permeability, leukocyte recruitment, and vascular fibrosis leading to vascular injury and structural remodeling. In addition, Ang II-mediated vascular inflammation elicits local and systemic effects, resulting in production of acute-phase reactants, such as CRP, that may be important in further amplifying the inflammatory process. These Ang II-dependent events play a major role in cardiovascular disease associated with vascular injury.

ACKNOWLEDGMENTS

Studies performed by the authors were supported by grants 57786 and 44018 (RMT), 13570 and 37917 (ELS), and by a grant to the Multidisciplinary Research Group on Hypertension, all from the Canadian Institutes of Health Research.

REFERENCES

1. Wolf, G., Butzmann, U., and Wenzel, U. O. (2003) The renin–angiotensin system and progression of renal disease: from hemodynamics to cell biology. *Nephron Physiol.* **93(1),** 3–13.
2. Stock, P., Liefeldt, L., Paul, M., and Ganten, D. (1995) Local renin–angiotensin systems in cardio-vascular tissues: localization and functional role. *Cardiology* **86,** 2–8.
3. Re, R. N. (2004) Tissue renin angiotensin systems. *Med. Clin. North Am.* **88(1),** 19–38.
4. Touyz, R. M. and Schiffrin, E. L. (2000) Signal transduction mechanisms mediating the physiological and pathophysiological actions of angiotensin II in vascular smooth muscle cells. *Pharmacol. Rev.* **52,** 639–672.
5. Schiffrin, E. L. and Touyz R. M. (2003) Multiple actions of angiotensin II in hypertension: benefits of AT_1 receptor blockade. *J. Am. Coll. Cardiol.* **42(5),** 911–913.
6. Wolf, G., Wenzel, U., Burns, K. D., Harris, R. C., Stahl, R. A., and Thaiss, F. (2002) Angiotensin II activates nuclear transcription factor-kappa B through AT1 and AT2 receptors. *Kidney Int.* **61(6),** 1986–1995.
7. Nathan, C. (2002) Points of control in inflammation. *Nature* **420,** 846–853.
8. Tracey, K. J. (2002) The inflammatory reflex. *Nature* **420,** 853–860.
9. Suzuki, Y., Ruiz-Ortega, M., Lorenzo, O., Ruperez, M., Esteban, V., and Egido, J. (2003) Inflammation and angiotensin II. *Int. J. Biochem. Cell. Biol.* **35(6),** 881–900.
10. Gruden, G., Thomas, S., Burt, D., et al. (1999) Interaction of angiotensin II and mechanical stretch on vascular endothelial growth factor production by human mesangial cells. *J. Am. Soc. Nephrol.* **10(4),** 730–737.
11. Reddy, H. K., Sigusch, H., Zhou, G., Tyagi, S. C., Janicki, J. S., and Weber, K. T. (1995) Coronary vascular hyperpermeability and angiotensin II. *J. Lab. Clin. Med.* **126(3),** 307–315.
12. Schlondorff, D., Perez, J., and Satriano, J. A. (1985) Differential stimulation of PGE2 synthesis in mesangial cells by angiotensin and A23187. *Am. J. Physiol.* **248(1),** C119–C126.
13. Chu, Z. M., Croft, K. D., Kingsbury, D. A., Falck, J. R., Reddy, K. M., and Beilin, L. J. (2000) Cytochrome P450 metabolites of arachidonic acid may be important mediators in angiotensin II-induced vasoconstriction in the rat mesentery in vivo. *Clin. Sci.* **98(3),** 277–282.

14. Valentin, J. P., Jover, B., Maffre, M., Bertolino, F., Bessac, A. M., and John, G. W. (1997) Losartan prevents thromboxane A2/prostanoid (TP) receptor mediated increase in microvascular permeability in the rat. *Am. J. Hypertens.* **10,** 1058–1063.

15. Ruhrberg, C. (2003) Growing and shaping the vascular tree: multiple roles for VEGF. *Bioessays* **25(11),** 1052–1060.

16. Dvorak, H. F. (2000) VPF/VEGF and the angiogenic response. *Semin. Perinatol.* **24(1),** 75–78.

17. Ferrara, N., Gerber, H. P., and LeCouter, J. (2003) The biology of VEGF and its receptors. *Nat. Med.* **9(6),** 669–676.

18. Williams, B., Baker, A. Q., Gallacher, B., and Lodwick, D. (1995) Angiotensin II increases vascular permeability factor gene expression by human vascular smooth muscle cells. *Hypertension* **25(5),** 913–917.

19. Chua, C. C., Hamdy, R. C., and Chua, B. H. (1998) Upregulation of vascular endothelial growth factor by angiotensin II in rat heart endothelial cells. *Biochim. Biophys. Acta* **1401(2),** 187–194.

20. Fujiyama, S., Matsubara, H., Nozawa, Y., et al. (2001) Angiotensin AT(1) and AT(2) receptors differentially regulate angiopoietin-2 and vascular endothelial growth factor expression and angiogenesis by modulating heparin binding-epidermal growth factor (EGF)-mediated EGF receptor transactivation. *Circ. Res.* **88(1),** 22–29.

21. Chintalgattu, V., Nair, D. M., and Katwa, L. C. (2003) Cardiac myofibroblasts: a novel source of vascular endothelial growth factor (VEGF) and its receptors Flt-1 and KDR. *J. Mol. Cell. Cardiol.* **35(3),** 277–286.

22. Pupilli, C., Lasagni, L., Romagnani, P., et al. (1999) Angiotensin II stimulates the synthesis and secretion of vascular permeability factor/vascular endothelial growth factor in human mesangial cells. *J. Am. Soc. Nephrol.* **10(2),** 245–255.

23. Zhang, X., Lassila, M., Cooper, M. E., and Cao, Z. (2004) Retinal expression of vascular endothelial growth factor is mediated by angiotensin type 1 and type 2 receptors. *Hypertension* **43(2),** 276–281.

24. Rizkalla, B., Forbes, J. M., Cooper, M. E., and Cao, Z. (2003) Increased renal vascular endothelial growth factor and angiopoietins by angiotensin II infusion is mediated by both AT1 and AT2 receptors. *J. Am. Soc. Nephrol.* **14(12),** 3061–3071.

25. Yamagishi, S., Amano, S., Inagaki, Y., et al. (2003) Angiotensin II-type 1 receptor interaction upregulates vascular endothelial growth factor messenger RNA levels in retinal pericytes through intracellular reactive oxygen species generation. *Drugs Exp. Clin. Res.* **29(2),** 75–80.

26. Brandes, R. P., Miller, F. J., Beer, S., et al. (2002) The vascular NADPH oxidase subunit p47phox is involved in redox-mediated gene expression. *Free Radic. Biol. Med.* **32(11),** 1116–1122.

27. Otani, A., Takagi, H., Oh, H., et al. (2000) Angiotensin II-stimulated vascular endothelial growth factor expression in bovine retinal pericytes. *Investig. Ophthalmol. Vis. Sci.* **41(5),** 1192–1199.

28. Otani, A., Takagi, H., Suzuma, K., and Honda, Y. (1998) Angiotensin II potentiates vascular endothelial growth factor-induced angiogenic activity in retinal microcapillary endothelial cells. *Circ. Res.* **82(5),** 619–628.

29. Funatsu, H. and Yamashita, H. (2003) Pathogenesis of diabetic retinopathy and the renin–angiotensin system. *Ophthal. Physiol. Opt.* **23(6),** 495–501.

30. Lee, E. Y., Shim, M. S., Kim, M. J., Hong, S. Y., Shin, Y. G., and Chung, C. H. (2004) Angiotensin II receptor blocker attenuates overexpression of vascular endothelial growth factor in diabetic podocytes. *Exp. Mol. Med.* **36(1),** 65–70.

31. Gilbert, R. E., Kelly, D. J., Cox, A. J., et al. (2003) Angiotensin converting enzyme inhibition reduces retinal overexpression of vascular endothelial growth factor and hyperpermeability in experimental diabetes. *Diabetologia* **43(11),** 1360–1367.

32. Moravski, C. J., Skinner, S. L., Stubbs, A. J., et al. (2003) The renin–angiotensin system influences ocular endothelial cell proliferation in diabetes: transgenic and interventional studies. *Am. J. Pathol.* **162(1),** 151–160.

33. Klein, R., Klein, B. E., Moss, S. E., and Cruickshanks, K. J. (1998) The Wisconsin Epidemiologic Study of Diabetic Retinopathy: XVII. The 14-year incidence and progression of diabetic retinopathy and associated risk factors in type 1 diabetes. *Ophthalmology* **105(10),** 1801–1815.

34. UK Prospective Diabetes Study Group. (1998) Tight blood pressure control and risk of macrovascular and microvascular complications in type 2 diabetes. (UKPDS 38). *BMJ* **317,** 703–713.

35. Chaturvedi, N., Sjolie, A. K., Stephenson, J. M., et al. (1998) Effect of lisinopril on progression of retinopathy in normotensive people with type 1 diabetes. The EUCLID Study Group. EURODIAB Controlled Trial of Lisinopril in Insulin-Dependent Diabetes Mellitus. *Lancet* **351,** 28–31.

36. Clavant, S. P., Forbes, J. M., Thallas, V., Osicka, T. M., Jerums, G., and Comper, W. D. (2003) Reversible angiotensin II-mediated albuminuria in rat kidneys is dynamically associated with cytoskeletal organization. *Nephron. Physiol.* **93(2)**, 51–60.

37. Park, H. Y., Schumock, G. T., Pickard, A. S., and Akhras, K. (2003) A structured review of the relationship between microalbuminuria and cardiovascular events in patients with diabetes mellitus and hypertension. *Pharmacotherapy* **23(12)**, 1611–1616.

38. Garg, J. P. and Bakris, G. L. (2002) Microalbuminuria: marker of vascular dysfunction, risk factor for cardiovascular disease. *Vasc. Med.* **7(1)**, 35–43.

39. Arnold, J. M., Yusuf, S., Young, J., et al. (2003) Prevention of Heart Failure in Patients in the Heart Outcomes Prevention Evaluation (HOPE) Study. *Circulation* **107(9)**, 1284–1290.

40. Gaede, P., Vedel, P., Larsen, N., Jensen, G. V., Parving, H. H., and Pedersen, O. (2003) Multifactorial intervention and cardiovascular disease in patients with type 2 diabetes. *N. Engl. J. Med.* **348(5)**, 383–393.

41. Ranieri, G., Andriani, A., Lamontanara, G., and De Cesaris, R. (1994) Effects of lisinopril and amlodipine on microalbuminuria and renal function in patients with hypertension. *Clin. Pharmacol. Ther.* **56(3)**, 323–330.

42. Ley, K. (2003) The role of selectins in inflammation and disease. *Trends Mol. Med.* **9(6)**, 263–268.

43. Blann, A. D., Nadar, S. K., and Lip, G. Y. (2003) The adhesion molecule P-selectin and cardiovascular disease. *Eur. Heart J.* **24(24)**, 2166–2179.

44. Krieglstein, C. F. and Granger, D. N. (2001) Adhesion molecules and their role in vascular disease. *Am. J. Hypertens.* **14**, 44S–54S.

45. Henninger, D. D., Panes, J., Eppihimer, M., et al. (1997) Cytokine-induced VCAM-1 and ICAM-1 expression in different organs of the mouse. *J. Immunol.* **158(4)**, 1825–1832.

46. Sun, J., Paddock, C., Shubert, J., et al. (2000) Contributions of the extracellular and cytoplasmic domains of platelet-endothelial cell adhesion molecule-1 (PECAM-1/CD31) in regulating cell-cell localization. *J. Cell. Sci.* **113**, 1459–1469.

47. Wang, J. and Springer, T. A. (1998) Structural specializations of immunoglobulin superfamily members for adhesion to integrins and viruses. *Immunol. Rev.* **163**, 197–215.

48. Takano-Ishikawa, Y., Goto, M., and Yamaki, K. (2004) Analysis of leukocyte rolling and migration—using inhibitors in the undisturbed microcirculation of the rat mesentery—on inflammatory stimulation. *Mediators Inflamm.* **13(1)**, 33–37.

49. Wenzel, U. O. and Abboud, H. E. (1995) Chemokines and renal disease. *Am. J. Kidney Dis.* **26(6)**, 982–994.

50. Ross, R. (1999) Atherosclerosis: an inflammatory disease. *N. Engl. J. Med.* **340**, 115–126.

51. Ruiz-Ortega, M., Lorenzo, O., Suzuki, Y., Ruperez, M., and Egido, J. (2001) Proinflammatory actions of angiotensins. *Curr. Opin. Nephrol. Hypertens.* **10(3)**, 321–329.

52. Piqueras, L., Kubes, P., Alvarez, A., et al. (2000) Angiotensin II induces leukocyte-endothelial cell interactions in vivo via AT(1) and AT(2) receptor-mediated P-selectin upregulation. *Circulation* **102(17)**, 2118–2123.

53. Pastore, L., Tessitore, A., Martinotti, S., et al. (1999) Angiotensin II stimulates intercellular adhesion molecule-1 (ICAM-1) expression by human vascular endothelial cells and increases soluble ICAM-1 release in vivo. *Circulation* **100(15)**, 1646–1652.

54. Diep, Q. N., Amiri, F., Touyz, R. M., et al. (2002) PPARalpha activator effects on Ang II-induced vascular oxidative stress and inflammation. *Hypertension* **40(6)**, 866–871.

55. Grafe, M., Auch-Schwelk, W., Zakrzewicz, A., et al. (1997) Angiotensin II-induced leukocyte adhesion on human coronary endothelial cells is mediated by E-selectin. *Circ. Res.* **81(5)**, 804–811.

56. Ito, T., Ikeda, U., Yamamoto, K., and Shimada, K. (2002) Regulation of interleukin-8 expression by HMG-CoA reductase inhibitors in human vascular smooth muscle cells. *Atherosclerosis* **165(1)**, 51–55.

57. Funakoshi, Y., Ichiki, T., Ito, K., and Takeshita, A. (1999) Induction of interleukin-6 expression by angiotensin II in rat vascular smooth muscle cells. *Hypertension* **34(1)**, 118–125.

58. Funakoshi, Y., Ichiki, T., Shimokawa, H., et al. (2001) Rho-kinase mediates angiotensin II-induced monocyte chemoattractant protein-1 expression in rat vascular smooth muscle cells. *Hypertension* **38(1)**, 100–104.

59. deBlois, D., Lombardi, D. M., Su, E. J., Clowes, A. W., Schwartz, S. M., and Giachelli, C. M. (1996) Angiotensin II induction of osteopontin expression and DNA replication in rat arteries. *Hypertension* **28(6)**, 1055–1063.

60. Rattazzi, M., Puato, M., Faggin, E., Bertipaglia, B., Zambon, A., and Pauletto, P. (2003) C-reactive protein and interleukin-6 in vascular disease: culprits or passive bystanders? *J. Hypertens.* **21(10),** 1787–1803.

61. Kanda, T. and Takahashi, T. (2004) Interleukin-6 and cardiovascular diseases. *Jpn. Heart J.* **45(2),** 183–193.

62. Ikeda, U., Ikeda, M., Oohara, T., et al. (1991) Interleukin 6 stimulates growth of vascular smooth muscle cells in a PDGF-dependent manner. *Am. J. Physiol.* **260(5),** H1713–H1717.

63. Mukaida, N. (2003) Pathophysiological roles of interleukin-8/CXCL8 in pulmonary diseases. *Am. J. Physiol. Lung Cell. Mol. Physiol.* **284(4),** L566–L577.

64. Yue, T. L., Wang, X., Sung, C. P., et al. (1994) Interleukin-8. A mitogen and chemoattractant for vascular smooth muscle cells. *Circ. Res.* **75(1),** 1–7.

65. Egashira, K. (2003) Molecular mechanisms mediating inflammation in vascular disease: special reference to monocyte chemoattractant protein-1. *Hypertension* **41(3),** 834–841.

66. Ishibashi, M., Hiasa, K., Zhao, Q., et al. (2004) Critical role of monocyte chemoattractant protein-1 receptor CCR2 on monocytes in hypertension-induced vascular inflammation and remodeling. *Circ. Res.* **94(9),** 1203–1210.

67. Boring, L., Gosling, J., Cleary, M., and Charo, I. F. (1998) Decreased lesion formation in CCR2–/– mice reveals a role for chemokines in the initiation of atherosclerosis. *Nature* **394(6696),** 894–897.

68. Gosling, J., Slaymaker, S., Gu, L., et al. (1999) MCP-1 deficiency reduces susceptibility to atherosclerosis in mice that overexpress human apolipoprotein B. *J. Clin. Investig.* **103(6),** 773–778.

69. Bush, E., Maeda, N., Kuziel, W. A., et al. (2000) CC chemokine receptor 2 is required for macrophage infiltration and vascular hypertrophy in angiotensin II-induced hypertension. *Hypertension* **36(3),** 360–363.

70. Martin, G., Dol, F., Mares, A. M., et al. (2004) Lesion progression in apoE-deficient mice: implication of chemokines and effect of the AT1 angiotensin II receptor antagonist irbesartan. *J. Cardiovasc. Pharmacol.* **43(2),** 191–199.

71. Chen, H. J., Li, D. Y., Saldeen, T., Phillips, M. I., and Mehta, J. L. (2001) Attenuation of tissue P-selectin and MCP-1 expression and intimal proliferation by AT(1) receptor blockade in hyperlipidemic rabbits. *Biochem. Biophys. Res. Commun.* **282(2),** 474–479.

72. De Ciuceis, C., Amiri, F., Endemann, D. H., Touyz, R. M., and Schiffrin, E. L. (2005) Reduced vascular remodeling, endothelial dysfunction and oxidative stress in resistance arteries of angiotensin II-infused macrophage colony-stimulating factor-deficient mice: Evidence for a role in inflammation in angiotensin-induced vascular injury. [Abstract]. *Arterioscl. Thromb. Vasc. Biol.* **25(10),** 2106–2113.

73. Navalkar, S., Parthasarathy, S., Santanam, N., and Khan, B. V. (2001) Irbesartan, an angiotensin type 1 receptor inhibitor, regulates markers of inflammation in patients with premature atherosclerosis. *J. Am. Coll. Cardiol.* **37(2),** 440–444.

74. Koh, K. K., Ahn, J. Y., Han, S. H., et al. (2003) Pleiotropic effects of angiotensin II receptor blocker in hypertensive patients. *J. Am. Coll. Cardiol.* **42(5),** 905–910.

75. Schieffer, B., Schieffer, E., Hilfiker-Kleiner, D., et al. (2000) Expression of angiotensin II and interleukin 6 in human coronary atherosclerotic plaques: potential implications for inflammation and plaque instability. *Circulation* **101(12),** 1372–1378.

76. Rahman, S. T., Lauten, W. B., Khan, Q. A., Navalkar, S., Parthasarathy, S, and Khan, B. V. (2002) Effects of eprosartan versus hydrochlorothiazide on markers of vascular oxidation and inflammation and blood pressure (renin–angiotensin system antagonists, oxidation, and inflammation). *Am. J. Cardiol.* **89(6),** 686–690.

77. Touyz, R. M., He, G., El Mabrouk, M., and Schiffrin, E. L. (2001) p38 Map kinase regulates vascular smooth muscle cell collagen synthesis by angiotensin II in SHR but not in WKY. *Hypertension* **37,** 574–580.

78. Touyz, R. M., He, G., Wu, X. H., Park, J. B., Mabrouk, M. E., and Schiffrin, E. L. (2001) Src is an important mediator of extracellular signal-regulated kinase 1/2-dependent growth signaling by angiotensin II in smooth muscle cells from resistance arteries of hypertensive patients. *Hypertension* **38(1),** 56–64.

79. Touyz, R. M., Cruzado, M., Tabet, F., Yao, G., Salomon, S., and Schiffrin, E. L. (2003) Redox-dependent MAP kinase signaling by Ang II in vascular smooth muscle cells: role of receptor tyrosine kinase transactivation. *Can J. Physiol. Pharmacol.* **81(2),** 159–167.

80. Kelly, D. J., Cox, A. J., Gow, R. M., Zhang, Y., Kemp, B. E., and Gilbert, R. E. (2004) Platelet-derived growth factor receptor transactivation mediates the trophic effects of angiotensin II in vivo. *Hypertension* **44(2)**, 195–202.

81. Ezaki, T., Baluk, P., Thurston, G., La Barbara, A., Woo, C., and McDonald, D. M. (2001) Time course of endothelial cell proliferation and microvascular remodeling in chronic inflammation. *Am. J. Pathol.* **158(6)**, 2043–2055.

82. Touyz, R. M. (2003) The role of angiotensin II in regulating vascular structural and functional changes in hypertension. *Curr. Hypertens. Rep.* **5(2)**, 155–164.

83. Tea, B. S., Der Sarkissian, S., Touyz, R. M., Hamet, P., and deBlois, D. (2000) Proapoptotic and growth-inhibitory role of angiotensin II type 2 receptor in vascular smooth muscle cells of spontaneously hypertensive rats in vivo. *Hypertension* **35(5)**, 1069–1073.

84. Suzuki, J., Iwai, M., Nakagami, H., et al. (2002) Role of angiotensin II-regulated apoptosis through distinct AT1 and AT2 receptors in neointimal formation. *Circulation* **106(7)**, 847–853.

85. Diep, Q. N., Li, J. S., and Schiffrin, E. L. (1999) In vivo study of AT(1) and AT(2) angiotensin receptors in apoptosis in rat blood vessels. *Hypertension* **34(4)**, 617–624.

86. Hiyoshi, H., Yayama, K., Takano, M., and Okamoto, H. (2004) Stimulation of cyclic GMP production via AT2 and B2 receptors in the pressure-overloaded aorta after banding. *Hypertension* **43(6)**, 1258–1263.

87. Ruiz-Ortega, M., Esteban, V., Suzuki, Y., et al. (2003) Renal expression of angiotensin type 2 (AT2) receptors during kidney damage. *Kidney Int.* **86**, S21–S26.

88. Sandmann, S., Yu, M., Kaschina, E., et al. (2001) Differential effects of angiotensin AT1 and AT2 receptors on the expression, translation and function of the Na^+-H^+ exchanger and $Na^+-HCO_3^-$ symporter in the rat heart after myocardial infarction. *J. Am. Coll. Cardiol.* **37(8)**, 2154–2165.

89. Katugampola, S. D. and Davenport, A. P. (2000) Changes in ET(A)-, AT1- and AT2-receptors in the phenotypically transformed intimal smooth muscle layer of human atherosclerotic coronary arteries. *J. Cardiovasc. Pharmacol.* **36**, S395–S396.

90. Gonzalez, A., Lopez, B., and Diez, J. (2004) Fibrosis in hypertensive heart disease: role of the renin–angiotensin–aldosterone system. *Med. Clin. North Am.* **88(1)**, 83–97.

91. Schuttert, J. B., Liu, M. H., Gliem, N., et al. (2003) Human renal fibroblasts derived from normal and fibrotic kidneys show differences in increase of extracellular matrix synthesis and cell proliferation upon angiotensin II exposure. *Pflugers Arch.* **446(3)**, 387–393.

92. Ruiz-Ortega, M., Lorenzo, O., Ruperez, M., et al. (2000) Angiotensin II activates nuclear transcription factor kappaB through AT(1) and AT(2) in vascular smooth muscle cells: molecular mechanisms. *Circ. Res.* **86**, 1266–1272.

93. Lombardi, D. M., Viswanathan, M., Vio, C. P., Saavedra, J. M., Schwartz, S. M., and Johnson, R. J. (2001) Renal and vascular injury induced by exogenous angiotensin II is AT1 receptor-dependent. *Nephron* **87(1)**, 66–74.

94. Brede, M. and Hein, L. (2001) Transgenic mouse models of angiotensin receptor subtype function in the cardiovascular system. *Regul. Pept.* **96(3)**, 125–132.

95. Ruiz-Ortega, M., Ruperez, M., Lorenzo, O., et al. (2002) Angiotensin II regulates the synthesis of proinflammatory cytokines and chemokines in the kidney. *Kidney Int. Suppl.* **82**, 12–22.

96. Intengan, H. D. and Schiffrin, E. L. (2001) Vascular remodeling in hypertension: roles of apoptosis, inflammation, and fibrosis. *Hypertension* **38**, 581–587.

97. Sarkar, S., Vellaichamy, E., Young, D., and Sen, S. (2004) Influence of cytokines and growth factors in Ang II-mediated collagen upregulation by fibroblasts in rats: role of myocytes. *Am. J. Physiol. Heart Circ. Physiol.* **287(1)**, H107–H117.

98. Satoh, C., Fukuda, N., Hu, W. Y., Nakayama, M., Kishioka, H., and Kanmatsuse, K. (2001) Role of endogenous angiotensin II in the increased expression of growth factors in vascular smooth muscle cells from spontaneously hypertensive rats. *J. Cardiovasc. Pharmacol.* **37(1)**, 108–118.

99. Deguchi, J., Makuuchi, M., Nakaoka, T., Collins, T., and Takuwa, Y. (1999) Angiotensin II stimulates platelet-derived growth factor-B chain expression in newborn rat vascular smooth muscle cells and neointimal cells through Ras, extracellular signal-regulated protein kinase, and c-Jun N-terminal protein kinase mechanisms. *Circ. Res.* **85(7)**, 565–574.

100. Jesmin, S., Sakuma, I., Hattori, Y., and Kitabatake, A. (2003) Role of angiotensin II in altered expression of molecules responsible for coronary matrix remodeling in insulin-resistant diabetic rats. *Arterioscler. Thromb. Vasc. Biol.* **23(11)**, 2021–2026.

101. Moreau, P., d'Uscio, L. V., Shaw, S., Takase, H., Barton, M., and Luscher, T. F. (1997) Angiotensin II increases tissue endothelin and induces vascular hypertrophy: reversal by ET(A)-receptor antagonist. *Circulation* **96(5)**, 1593–1597.

102. Azhar, M., Schultz Jel, J., Grupp, I., et al. (2003) Transforming growth factor beta in cardiovascular development and function. *Cytokine Growth Factor Rev.* **14(5)**, 391–407.

103. Bobik, A. (2004) Hypertension, transforming growth factor-β, angiotensin II and kidney disease. *J. Hypertens.* **22(7)**, 1265–1267.

104. Hugo, C., Kang, D. H., and Johnson, R. J. (2002) Sustained expression of thrombospondin-1 is associated with the development of glomerular and tubulointerstitial fibrosis in the remnant kidney model. *Nephron* **90**, 460–470.

105. ten Dijke, P. and Hill, C. S. (2004) New insights into TGF-beta-Smad signalling. *Trends Biochem. Sci.* **29(5)**, 265–273.

106. Dai, C., Yang, J., and Liu, Y. (2003) Transforming growth factor-beta1 potentiates renal tubular epithelial cell death by a mechanism independent of Smad signaling. *J. Biol. Chem.* **278**, 12,537–12,545.

107. Ruperez, M., Lorenzo, O., Blanco-Colio, L. M., Esteban, V., Egido, J., and Ruiz-Ortega, M. (2003) Connective tissue growth factor is a mediator of angiotensin II-induced fibrosis. *Circulation* **108(12)**, 1499–1505.

108. Ahmed, M. S., Oie, E., Vinge, L. E., et al. (2004) Connective tissue growth factor—a novel mediator of angiotensin II-stimulated cardiac fibroblast activation in heart failure in rats. *J. Mol. Cell. Cardiol.* **36(3)**, 393–404.

109. Ruiz-Ortega, M. and Egido, J. (1997) Angiotensin II modulates cell growth-related events and synthesis of matrix proteins in renal interstitial fibroblasts. *Kidney Int.* **52(6)**, 1497–1510.

110. Liu, B. C., Sun, J, Chen, Q., Ma, K. L., Ruan, X. Z., and Phillips, A. O. (2003) Role of connective tissue growth factor in mediating hypertrophy of human proximal tubular cells induced by angiotensin II. *Am. J. Nephrol.* **23(6)**, 429–437.

111. Luo, K. (2004) Ski and SnoN: negative regulators of TGF-beta signaling. *Curr. Opin. Genet Dev.* **14(1)**, 65–70.

112. Shin, G. T., Kim, S. J., Ma, K. A., Kim, H. S., and Kim, D. (2000) ACE inhibitors attenuate expression of renal transforming growth factor-beta1 in humans. *Am. J. Kidney Dis.* **36**, 894–902.

113. Viedt, C., Fei, J., Krieger-Brauer, H. I., et al. (2004). Role of p22phox in angiotensin II and platelet-derived growth factor AA induced activator protein 1 activation in vascular smooth muscle cells. *J. Mol. Med.* **82(1)**, 31–38.

114. Brasier, A. R., Jamaluddin, M., Han, Y., Patterson, C., and Runge, M. S. (2000) Angiotensin II induces gene transcription through cell-type-dependent effects on the nuclear factor-kappaB (NF-kappaB) transcription factor. *Mol. Cell. Biochem.* **212(1–2)**, 155–169.

115. Brasier, A. R., Recinos, A. 3rd, and Eledrisi, M. S. (2002) Vascular inflammation and the renin–angiotensin system. *Arterioscler. Thromb. Vasc. Biol.* **22(8)**, 1257–1266.

116. Muller, D. N., Fiebeler, A., Park, J. K., Dechend, R., and Luft, F. C. (2003) Angiotensin II and endothelin induce inflammation and thereby promote hypertension-induced end-organ damage. *Clin. Nephrol.* **60**, S2–S12.

117. Han, Y., Runge, M. S., and Brasier, A. R. (1999) Angiotensin II induces interleukin-6 transcription in vascular smooth muscle cells through pleiotropic activation of nuclear factor-kappa B transcription factors. *Circ. Res.* **84(6)**, 695–703.

118. Jiang, B., Xu, S., Hou, X., Pimentel, D. R., and Cohen, R. A. (2004) Angiotensin II differentially regulates interleukin-1-β-inducible NO synthase (iNOS) and vascular cell adhesion molecule-1 (VCAM-1) expression. Role of p38 MAPK. *J. Biol. Chem.* **279(19)**, 20,363–20,368.

119. Zahradka, P., Werner, J. P., Buhay, S., Litchie, B., Helwer, G., and Thomas, S. (2002) NF-kappaB activation is essential for angiotensin II-dependent proliferation and migration of vascular smooth muscle cells. *J. Mol. Cell. Cardiol.* **34(12)**, 1609–1621.

120. Ruiz-Ortega, M., Lorenzo, O., and Egido, J. (2000) Angiotensin III increases MCP-1 and activates NF-kappaB and AP-1 in cultured mesangial and mononuclear cells. *Kidney Int.* **57(6)**, 2285–2298.

121. Ortiz, L. A., Champion, H. C., Lasky, J. A., et al. (2002) Enalapril protects mice from pulmonary hypertension by inhibiting TNF-mediated activation of NF-kappaB and AP-1. *Am. J. Physiol. Lung Cell. Mol. Physiol.* **282(6)**, L1209–L1212.

122. Amann, B., Tinzmann, R., and Angelkort, B. (2003) ACE inhibitors improve diabetic nephropathy through suppression of renal MCP-1. *Diabetes Care* **26(8)**, 2421–2425.

123. Hernandez-Presa, M. A., Bustos, C., Ortego, M., Tunon, J., Ortega, L., and Egido, J. (1998) ACE inhibitor quinapril reduces the arterial expression of NF-kappaB-dependent proinflammatory factors but not of collagen I in a rabbit model of atherosclerosis. *Am. J. Pathol.* **153(6)**, 1825–1837.

124. Theuer, J., Dechend, R., Muller, D. N., et al. (2002) Angiotensin II induced inflammation in the kidney and in the heart of double transgenic rats. *BMC Cardiovasc. Disord.* **2(1)**, 3–7.

125. Costanzo, A., Moretti, F., Burgio, V. L., et al. (2003) Endothelial activation by angiotensin II through NFkappaB and p38 pathways: Involvement of NFkappaB-inducible kinase (NIK), free oxygen radicals, and selective inhibition by aspirin. *J. Cell. Physiol.* **195(3)**, 402–410.

126. Guzik, T. J., Korbut, R., and Adamek-Guzik, T. (2003) Nitric oxide and superoxide in inflammation and immune regulation. *J. Physiol. Pharmacol.* **54(4)**, 469–487.

127. Haddad, J. J. (2002) Antioxidant and prooxidant mechanisms in the regulation of redox(y)-sensitive transcription factors. *Cell. Signal.* **14(11)**, 879–897.

128. Fritz, G. (2002) Human APE/Ref-1 protein, *Int. J. Biochem. Cell. Biol.* **32(9)**, 925–929.

129. Harrison, D., Griendling, K. K., Landmesser, U., Hornig, B., and Drexler, H. (2003) Role of oxidative stress in atherosclerosis. *Am. J. Cardiol.* **91(3A)**, 7–11.

130. Touyz, R. M., Tabet, F., and Schiffrin, E. L. (2003) Redox-dependent signalling by angiotensin II and vascular remodelling in hypertension. *Clin. Exp. Pharmacol. Physiol.* **30(11)**, 860–866.

131. Melillo, G. (2004) HIF-1: a target for cancer, ischemia and inflammation—too good to be true? *Cell Cycle* **3(2)**, 154–155.

132. El Bekay, R., Alvarez, M., Monteseirin, J., et al. (2003) Oxidative stress is a critical mediator of the angiotensin II signal in human neutrophils: involvement of mitogen-activated protein kinase, calcineurin, and the transcription factor NF-kappaB. *Blood* **102(2)**, 662–671.

133. Seshiah, P. N., Weber, D. S., Rocic, P., Valppu, L., Taniyama, Y., and Griendling, K. K. (2002) Angiotensin II stimulation of NAD(P)H oxidase activity. Upstream mediators. *Circ. Res.* **9**, 406–413.

134. Kataoka, C., Egashira, K., Inoue, S., et al. (2003) Important role of Rho-kinase in the pathogenesis of cardiovascular inflammation and remodeling induced by long-term blockade of nitric oxide synthesis in rats. *Hypertension* **39(2)**, 245–250.

135. Griendling, K. K., Minieri, C. A., Ollerenshaw, J. D., and Alexander, R. W. (1994) Angiotensin II stimulates NADH and NADPH oxidase activity in cultured vascular smooth muscle cells, *Circ. Res.* **74(6)**, 1141–1148.

136. Lassegue, B. and Clempus, R. E. (2003) Vascular NAD(P)H oxidases: specific features, expression, and regulation. *Am. J. Physiol. Regul. Integr. Comp. Physiol.* **285(2)**, R277–R297.

137. Rey, F. E. and Pagano, P. J. (2002) The reactive adventitia: fibroblast oxidase in vascular function. *Arterioscler. Thromb. Vasc. Biol.* **22(12)**, 1962–1971.

138. Babior, B. M., Lambeth, J. D., and Nauseef, W. (2002) The neutrophil NADPH oxidase. *Arch. Biochem. Biophys.* **397**, 342–344.

139. Touyz, R. M., Chen, X., He, G., Quinn, M. T., and Schiffrin, E. L. (2002) Expression of a gp91phox-containing leukocyte-type NADPH oxidase in human vascular smooth muscle cells—modulation by Ang II. *Circ. Res.* **90**, 1205–1213.

140. Lambeth, J. D. (2004) NOX enzymes and the biology of reactive oxygen. *Nat Rev Immunol.* **4(3)**, 181–189.

141. Heidari, Y., Shah, A. M., and Gove, C. (2004) NOX-2S is a new member of the NOX family of NADPH oxidases. *Gene* **335**, 133–140.

142. Touyz, R. M., Yao, G., and Schiffrin, E. L. (2003) c-Src induces phosphorylation and translocation of p47phox: role in superoxide generation by angiotensin II in human vascular smooth muscle cells. *Arterioscler. Thromb. Vasc. Biol.* **23(6)**, 981–987.

143. Virdis, A., Neves, M. F., Amiri, F., Touyz, R. M., and Schiffrin, E. L. (2004) Role of NAD(P)H oxidase on vascular alterations in angiotensin II-infused mice. *J. Hypertens.* **22(3)**, 535–542.

144. Willerson, J. T. and Ridker, P. M. (2004) Inflammation as a cardiovascular risk factor. *Circulation* **109**, 2–10.

145. Brennan, M. L., Penn, M. S., Van Lente, F., et al. (2003) Prognostic value of myeloperoxidase in patients with chest pain. *N Engl. J. Med.* **349(17)**, 1595–1604.

146. Yeh, E. T. (2004) CRP as a mediator of disease. *Circulation* **109**, II11– II14.

147. Pasceri, V., Cheng, J. S., and Willerson, J. T. (2001) Modulation of C-reactive protein-mediated monocyte chemoattractant protein-1 induction in human endothelial cells by anti-atherosclerosis drugs. *Circulation* **103**, 2531–2534.

148. Venugopal, S. K., Devaraj, S., and Yuhuanna, I. (2002) Demonstration that C-reactive protein decreases eNOS expression and bioactivity in human aortic endothelial cells. *Circulation* **106,** 1439–1441.

149. Ridker, P. M., Cushman, M., Stampfer, M. J., Tracy, R. P., and Hennekens, C. H. (1997) Inflammation, aspirin, and the risk of cardiovascular disease in apparently healthy men. *N. Engl. J. Med.* **336(14),** 973–979.

150. Blake, G. J. and Ridker, P. M. (2001) Novel clinical markers of vascular wall inflammation. *Circ. Res.* **89,** 763–771.

151. Libby, P., Willerson, J. T., and Braunwald, E. (2004) C-reactive protein and coronary heart disease. *N. Engl. J. Med.* **351(3),** 295–298.

152. Wang, T. J., Larson, M. G., and Levy, D. (2002) C-reactive protein is associated with subclinical epicardial coronary calcification in men and women: the Framingham Heart Study. *Circulation* **106,** 1189–1191.

153. Pradhan, A. D., Manson, J. E., Meigs, J. B., et al. (2003) Insulin, proinsulin, proinsulin:insulin ratio, and the risk of developing type 2 diabetes mellitus in women. *Am. J. Med.* **114(6),** 438–444.

154. Ridker, P. M., Buring, J. E., Cook, N. R., and Rifai, N. (2003) C-reactive protein, the metabolic syndrome, and risk of incident cardiovascular events: an 8-year follow-up of 14 719 initially healthy American women. *Circulation* **107(3),** 391–397.

155. Sesso, H. D., Buring, J. E., Rifai, N., Blake, G. J., Gaziano, J. M., and Ridker, P. M. (2003) C-reactive protein and the risk of developing hypertension. *JAMA* **290(22),** 2945–2951.

7 Aldosterone and Vascular Damage

Hylton V. Joffe, Gordon H. Williams, and Gail K. Adler

1. INTRODUCTION

Aldosterone, the final product of the renin–angiotensin–aldosterone system (RAAS), is traditionally viewed as a regulator of renal sodium and potassium handling, extracellular volume, and blood pressure *(1)*. Until a few years ago, the adverse vascular effects of the RAAS have been attributed to angiotensin II (Ang II) *(2,3)*. However, Ang II is a potent aldosterone secretagogue, and recent human and animal studies suggest that aldosterone also has adverse cardiovascular effects, including microvascular damage, vascular inflammation, oxidative stress, and endothelial dysfunction. This chapter focuses on the adverse effects of aldosterone on the cardiovascular system, kidney, and brain in humans and animals, and describes our current understanding of the underlying mechanisms for this injury.

2. MINERALOCORTICOID RECEPTOR

The mineralocorticoid receptor (MR), a member of the steroid nuclear receptor superfamily, is expressed in a wide range of tissues throughout the body, including the heart, blood vessels, colon, kidney, liver, and brain *(4–7)*. After ligand binds to the MR,

From: *Contemporary Endocrinology: Hypertension and Hormone Mechanisms*
Edited by: R. M. Carey © Humana Press Inc., Totowa, NJ

the MR–ligand complex translocates to the nucleus, binds specific sites on DNA, and regulates gene transcription *(7)*. Activation of the MR by aldosterone also has rapid effects such as activation of the protein kinase C pathway and stimulation of sodium, potassium, and calcium ion fluxes *(8,9)*. These effects are thought to be mediated by non-genomic actions of aldosterone because they are not blocked by protein synthesis inhibitors and occur too rapidly (within minutes) to be mediated by changes in transcription and translation *(10)*.

The MR has similar in vitro affinity for aldosterone and cortisol. In many tissues, including the kidneys and vasculature, 11β-hydroxysteroid dehydrogenase-2 (11β-HSD2) is found in association with the MR. This enzyme converts cortisol to cortisone, thereby preventing the activation of the MR by glucocorticoids *(11)*. In humans, inactivating mutations of 11β-HSD2 or consumption of licorice containing the 11β-HSD2 inhibitor glycyrrhetinic acid leads to hypertension, volume expansion, and hypokalemia because of the cortisol activation of the renal MR *(12)*.

3. ALDOSTERONE: CONTEMPORARY VIEW

The Randomized Aldactone Evaluation Study (RALES) *(13)* is a landmark study that prompted a dramatic shift in our understanding of aldosterone. In this study, more than 1600 patients with moderate or severe congestive heart failure (CHF) on standard medical therapy were randomized to a low dose of the MR antagonist spironolactone (mean dose, 26 mg) or placebo. Most subjects were also receiving angiotensin-converting enzyme (ACE) inhibitors. After a mean follow-up of 2 yr, the spironolactone group had a 30% reduction in the risk of death and a 35% lower frequency of hospitalization for worsening heart failure, even though spironolactone did not significantly alter blood pressure (Fig. 1).

Results similar to those found in RALES were reported by the Eplerenone Post-Acute Myocardial Infarction Heart Failure Efficacy and Survival Study (EPHESUS) *(14)*. This study randomized more than 6600 patients with acute myocardial infarction complicated by left ventricular dysfunction and CHF to either a low dose of the selective MR antagonist eplerenone (25–50 mg daily, approx equivalent to 50–100 mg spironolactone daily) or placebo. Again, subjects were already receiving optimal medical therapy, including ACE inhibitors, angiotensin II receptor blockers (ARBs), beta-blockers, diuretics, and reperfusion therapy. During a mean follow-up of 16 mo, the eplerenone group had significant reductions in the risk of death and hospitalization compared to the placebo group.

4. ACE INHIBITORS AND ALDOSTERONE SUPPRESSION

Although ACE inhibitors acutely lower plasma aldosterone concentrations, this effect is not sustained over a long term *(15–17)*. Mechanisms of aldosterone breakthrough are poorly understood, but may include insufficient inhibition of ACE activity, Ang II synthesis through non-ACE pathways, and increases in the serum potassium concentration, which is a potent stimulus for aldosterone production independent of the renin–angiotensin feedback loop *(17)*. This lack of chronic aldosterone suppression may contribute to the progression of cardiovascular and renal injury in patients already receiving ACE inhibitor therapy *(16,18)*.

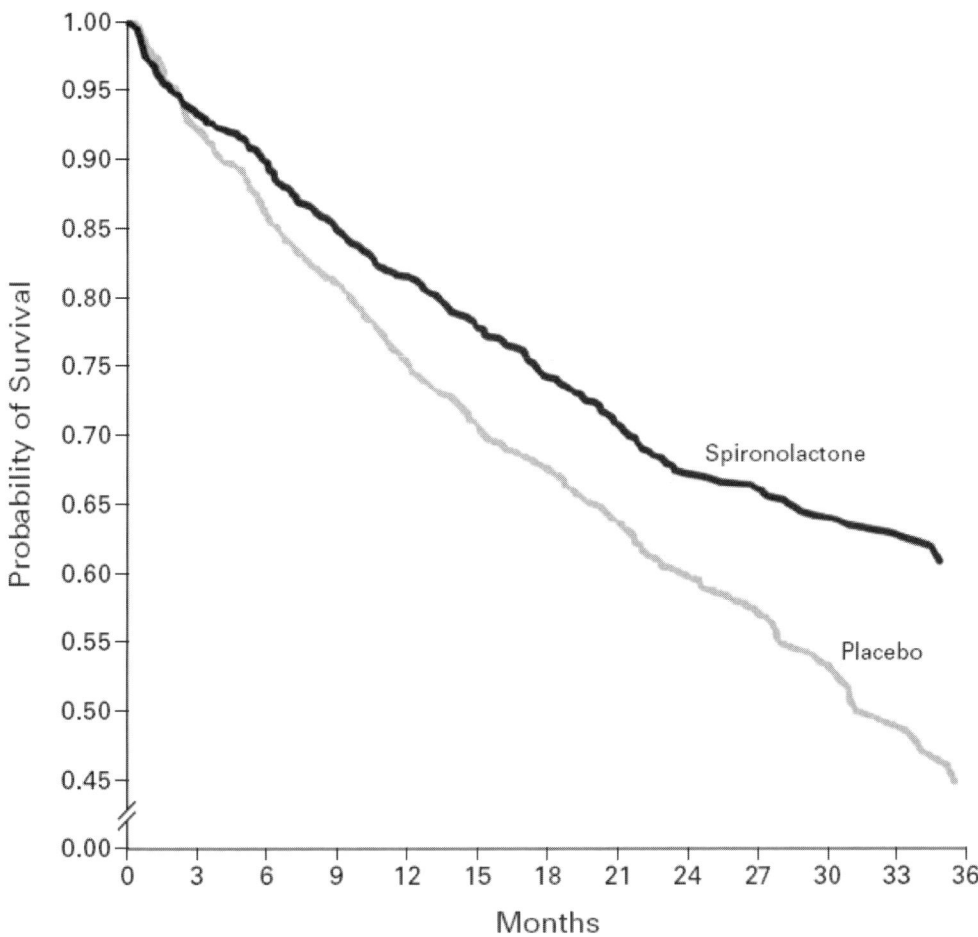

Fig. 1. Survival curves for congestive heart failure patients treated with spironolactone or placebo in addition to standard medical therapy. (From ref. *13* with permission.)

5. PRIMARY ALDOSTERONISM: A REAPPRAISAL

Patients with primary aldosteronism have excess aldosterone production, which causes sodium retention, volume expansion, and suppression of renin and Ang II. This patient population provides a unique opportunity for studying the cardiovascular effects of aldosterone in the relative absence of its primary secretagogue, Ang II. Patients with primary aldosteronism have high rates of left ventricular hypertrophy (LVH), proteinuria, retinopathy, and stroke *(19–22)*. There is an excess of LVH and proteinuria in these patients when compared to patients with a similar degree and duration of essential hypertension. Furthermore, patients with primary aldosteronism who are treated with surgical resection of an aldosterone-producing tumor appear to have more LVH regression than patients treated with medical therapy despite similar reductions in blood pressure *(22)*. Myocardial damage (estimated by thallium myocardial scintigraphy) is more severe in primary aldosteronism than in essential hypertension, despite a similar severity of LVH *(23)*. In one study, exercise-induced moderate myocardial ischemic defects were also more frequent in patients with primary aldosteronism than in those with essential hypertension, even though the essential hypertensive patients had a higher prevalence of significant coronary lesions *(24)*. Finally, aldosterone levels are associated with reduced arterial compliance in patients with primary aldosteronism *(25)*. These data suggest that aldosterone has adverse cardiovascular effects that cannot be fully attributed to elevations in blood pressure.

6. EFFECTS OF ALDOSTERONE ON TARGET ORGANS

In humans, the adverse effects of aldosterone are not limited to patients with primary aldosteronism or CHF. Recent studies suggest that aldosterone can contribute to LVH, diastolic dysfunction, albuminuria, and strokes in various clinical settings, as described below.

6.1. Heart: Left Ventricular Hypertrophy

MR blockade causes regression of LVH in individuals with essential hypertension. In the 4E-LVH Study *(26)*, patients with hypertension and LVH were tapered off their blood pressure medications, then randomized to 9 mo of enalapril, eplerenone, or combination therapy. Hydrochlorothiazide and/or amlodipine were added if diastolic blood pressure remained above 90 mmHg. As a result, blood pressure reductions were similar in the monotherapy groups and only slightly greater in the combination group. Eplerenone was as effective as enalapril in reducing LVH, and the combination therapy was twice as effective as either drug alone. It is unlikely that these results are fully explained by the systolic blood pressure differences of 4–5 mmHg observed between the monotherapy and combination treatment groups.

6.2. Heart: Diastolic Dysfunction

MR antagonists may improve diastolic dysfunction in patients with essential hypertension. In a prospective study, patients already receiving ACE inhibitors and calcium channel blockers were randomized to an MR antagonist or no additional therapy *(27)*. Based on echocardiographic findings, the MR antagonist group had significantly better improvement in diastolic dysfunction despite similar reductions in blood pressure and left ventricular mass.

6.3. Kidney: Albuminuria

MR blockade reduces albuminuria in patients with essential hypertension, diabetes, or isolated systolic hypertension of the elderly *(28–31)*. This beneficial effect is not solely attributable to blood pressure reduction. For example, despite similar reductions in blood pressure, eplerenone was found to reduce microalbuminuria to a much greater extent than does amlodipine in a randomized study of older patients with widened pulse pressure hypertension *(28)*. Similarly, eplerenone controlled blood pressure as effectively as titration-to-blood-pressure in an effect study of patients with mild-to-moderate essential hypertension *(29)*. However, the eplerenone-treated patients had a greater reduction in microalbuminuria (−62% vs −26%). Furthermore, in patients with chronic renal disease or diabetic nephropathy with persistent proteinuria despite ACE inhibitor therapy, the addition of an MR antagonist further reduces proteinuria without changing blood pressure *(18,30)*. Finally, in a large trial of patients with diabetes and albuminuria,

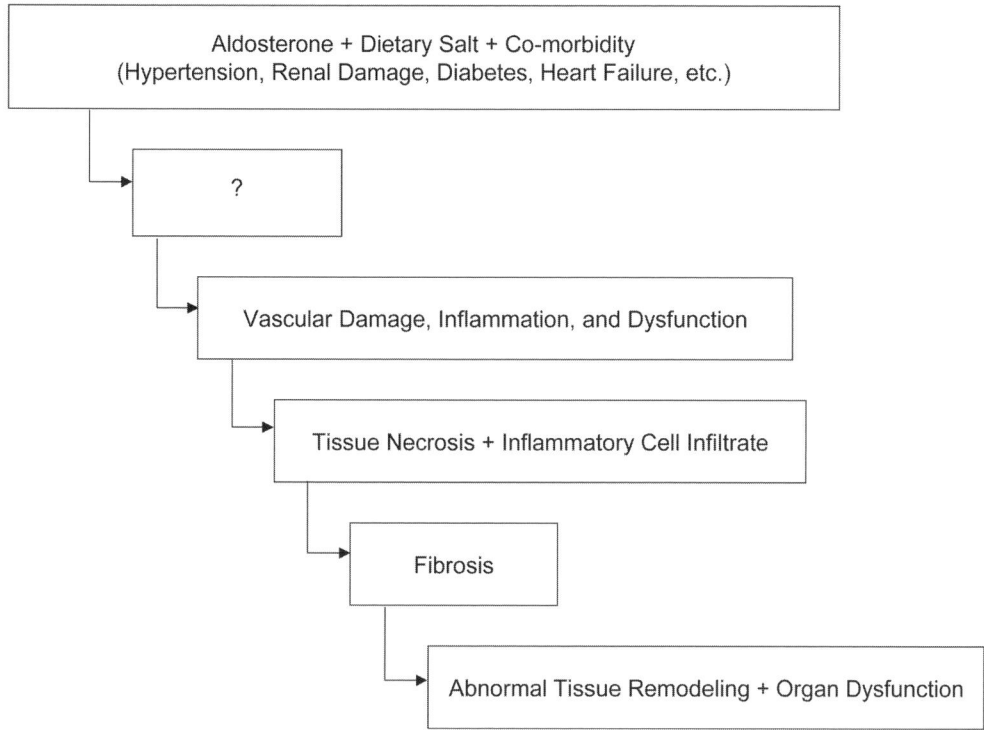

Fig. 2. Working model for aldosterone-induced cardiovascular injury. (Revised and adapted from ref. *1* with permission.)

combination therapy with an MR antagonist and an ACE inhibitor more effectively reduces proteinuria than ACE inhibitor monotherapy *(31)*.

6.4. Brain: Strokes

Glucocorticoid-remediable aldosteronism, a genetic cause of excess aldosterone, is associated with hemorrhagic stroke at an early age, and patients with primary aldosteronism also have high stroke rates *(19,32)*.

7. MECHANISMS OF ALDOSTERONE-MEDIATED VASCULAR DAMAGE

For the most part, animal models have been used to study mechanisms that may explain the detrimental effects of aldosterone on the cardiovascular system in humans. Our current understanding of these mechanisms is explained below, and a working model of aldosterone's adverse cardiovascular effects is summarized in Fig. 2.

7.1. Heart: Myocardial Necrosis, Vascular Inflammation, and Fibrosis

The N^{ω}-nitro-L-arginine methyl ester (L-NAME)/Ang II rodent model is characterized by hypertension, increased Ang II, and suppressed nitric oxide production *(33)*. Rodents consume a moderately high-sodium diet, receive L-NAME for 14 d (which causes chronic nitric oxide synthase inhibition) and are given an Ang II infusion for 3–7 d. This regimen causes hypertension and cardiac hypertrophy. Histological examination of the heart reveals multiple areas of micro-infarction in both ventricles with organizing myocardial necrosis, a mixed inflammatory infiltrate, loose collagen deposition, and neo-vascularization (Fig. 3). There is also intimal thickening around the coronary vessels, often frank vascular wall necrosis, and the formation of surrounding granulation tissue (Fig. 4) *(34)*. Decreasing aldosterone levels by adrenalectomy or blocking the actions of aldosterone by administering a MR antagonist markedly reduces this injury without lowering systolic blood pressure *(33,34)*. The protective effect of adrenalectomy is lost when aldosterone is infused into the adrenalectomized rats.

Short-term subcutaneous administration of mineralocorticoids induces inflammation of the coronary vessels in the uninephrectomized rat fed a high-salt diet *(35)*. These animals develop inflammation around the coronary arteries with associated ischemic and necrotic lesions of the adjacent myocardium. MR antagonists prevent this damage.

In the aldosterone-infused uninephrectomized rat, prolonged aldosterone exposure (8–12 wk) is associated with myocardial fibrosis, which may result from the reparative response to the inflammatory and necrotic injury, although direct effects of aldosterone on fibrosis are possible *(36,37)*. In a RALES follow-up analysis, the benefits of spirono-lactone occurred predominantly in patients with the highest levels of cardiac collagen synthesis markers *(38)*. These markers were reduced by spironolactone, suggesting that limitation of excessive extracellular matrix turnover is a mechanism by which MR antagonists improve outcomes in patients with CHF.

7.2. Kidneys: Renal Vascular Inflammation

Animals given L-NAME, Ang II, and a moderately high-sodium diet develop severe renal arteriopathy with fibrinoid necrosis of the vascular wall, medial thickening, proliferation of the perivascular connective tissue, perivascular inflammation, focal thrombosis in glomeruli, and proteinuria (Fig. 5) *(33)*. This injury is significantly reduced by MR antagonists or adrenalectomy but recurs when aldosterone is infused into adrenalectomized animals. Similarly, aldosterone-infused uninephrectomized rats fed a high-salt diet develop severe hypertension, renal inflammation and injury, albuminuria, and elevated expression of several proinflammatory molecules *(39)*. These effects are attenuated with MR antagonists. In both these models, the protective effects of MR antagonism do not appear to be mediated by changes in blood pressure.

7.3. Brain: Stroke and Inflammation

Stroke-prone spontaneously hypertensive rats fed a high-salt diet develop inflammation of the vasculature in the brain and kidney leading to stroke, proteinuria, and death. MR antagonists reduce this injury *(40)*.

7.4. Vasculature: Endothelial Dysfunction

In a rat model of CHF, the addition of spironolactone to ACE inhibitor therapy normalized nitric oxide-mediated endothelial relaxation by beneficially modulating the balance of nitric oxide and superoxide anion formation *(41)*. In the New Zealand rabbit, eplerenone improved endothelial function and reduced free radical stress in early atherosclerosis *(42)*. In vitro studies suggest that aldosterone causes non-genomic vasoconstriction of rabbit pre-glomerular afferent arterioles via the protein kinase C and inositol (1,4,5)-triphosphate (IP_3) pathways *(9)*. This effect of aldosterone, which

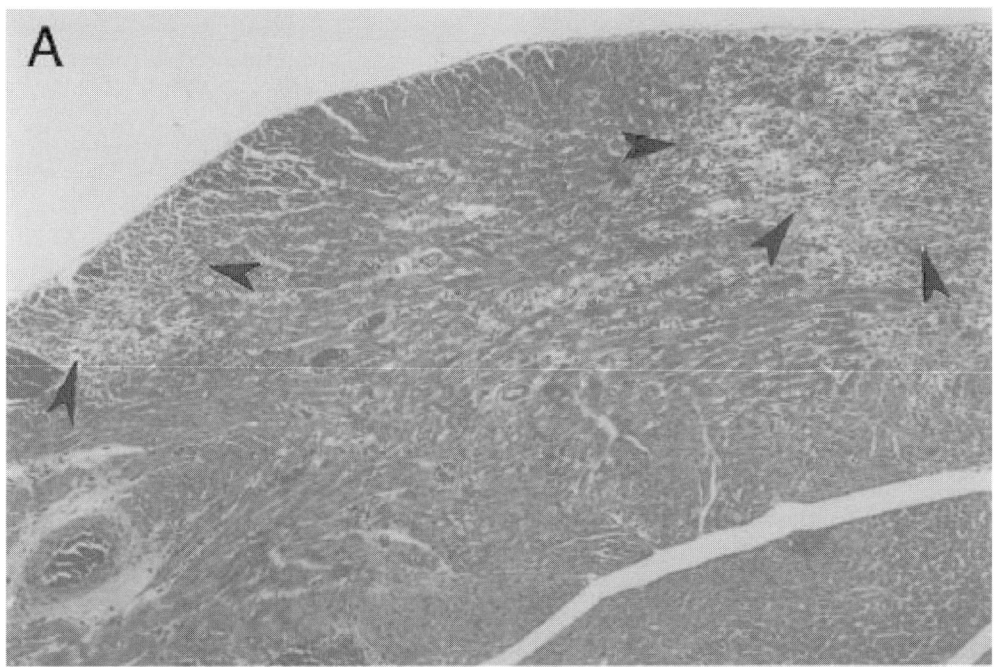

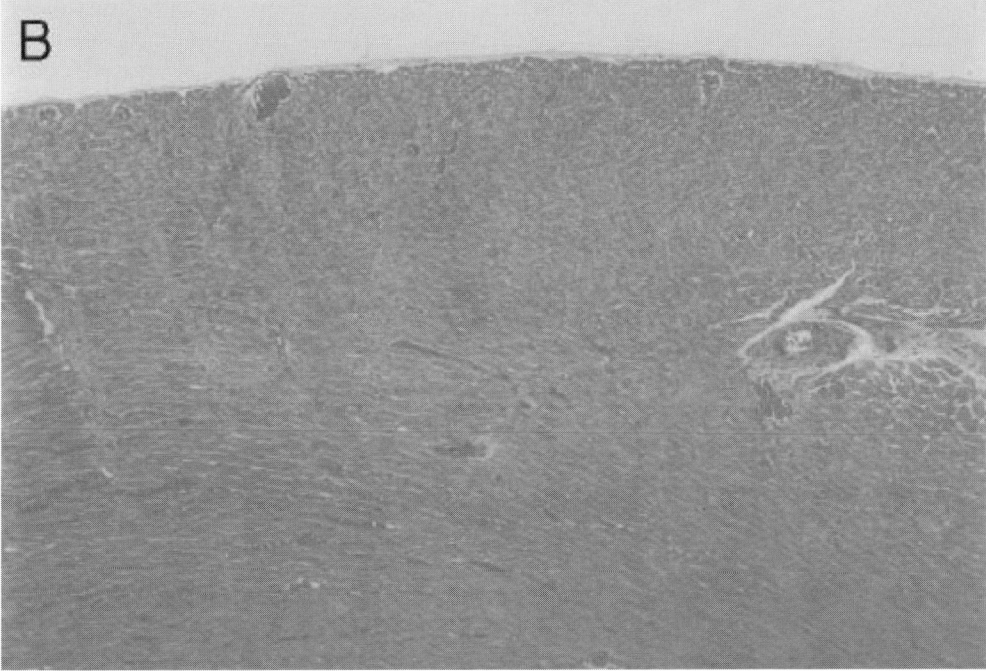

Fig. 3. Aldosterone-mediated cardiac damage. (**A**) Myocardial necrotic lesions (arrowheads) develop in rats treated with a high-salt diet, Ang II, and the nitric oxide synthase inhibitor L-NAME. (**B**) Necrotic lesions are markedly reduced when these animals are adrenalectomized or are simultaneously receiving the mineralocorticoid receptor antagonist eplerenone. Panel B is also representative of histological sections from control animals fed a high-salt diet (HSE; magnification, ×340). (Reproduced from ref. *33* with permission.)

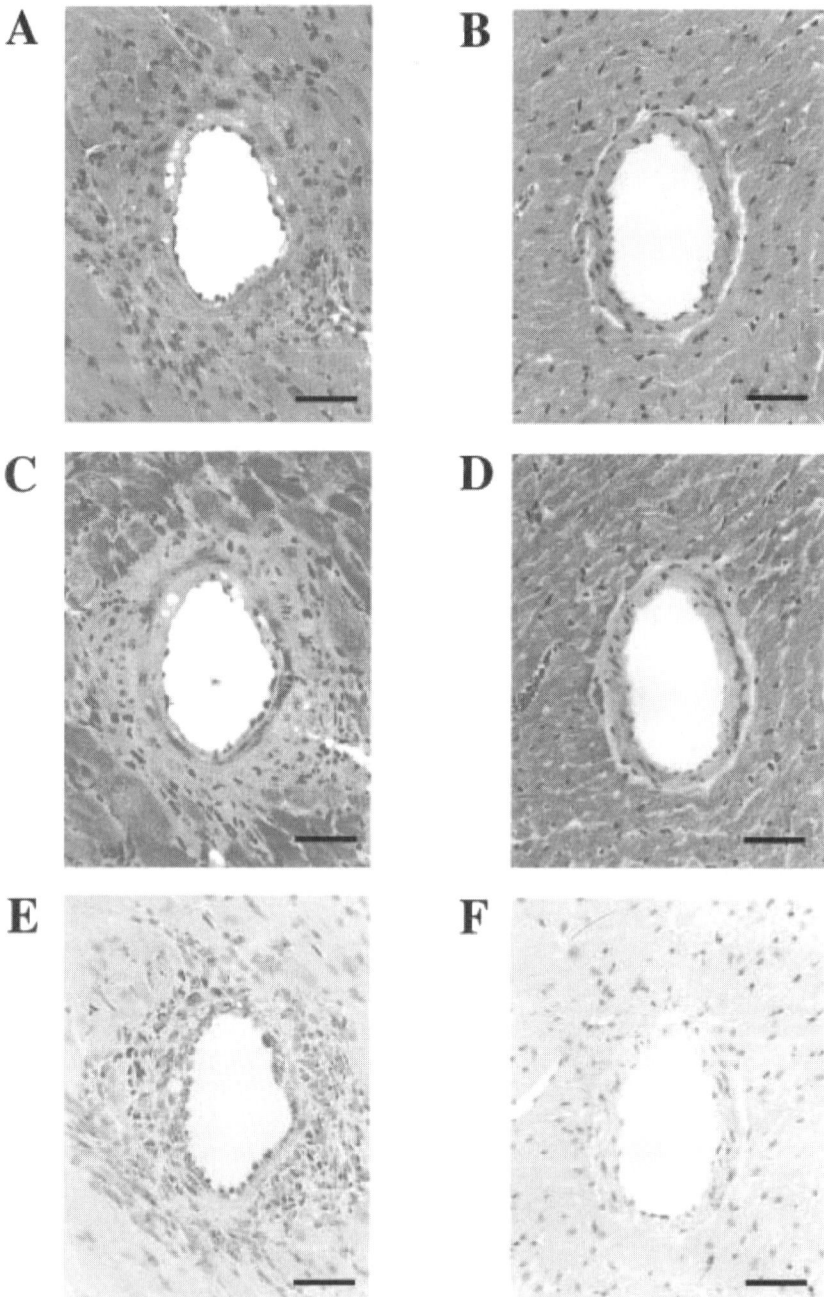

Fig. 4. Aldosterone-mediated coronary artery injury. Coronary arteries from mice treated with Ang II and L-NAME (**A,C,E**) and control animals (**B,D,F**). The Ang II/L-NAME animals develop fibrinoid necrosis of the vessel wall with intimal thickening, a mixed inflammatory response, and PAI-1 immunostaining. (A and B) H&E; (C and D) Masson's trichrome; (E and F) PAI-1 H135 antibody staining. Magnification, ×225; bars = 50 μm. (Reproduced from ref. *34* with permission.)

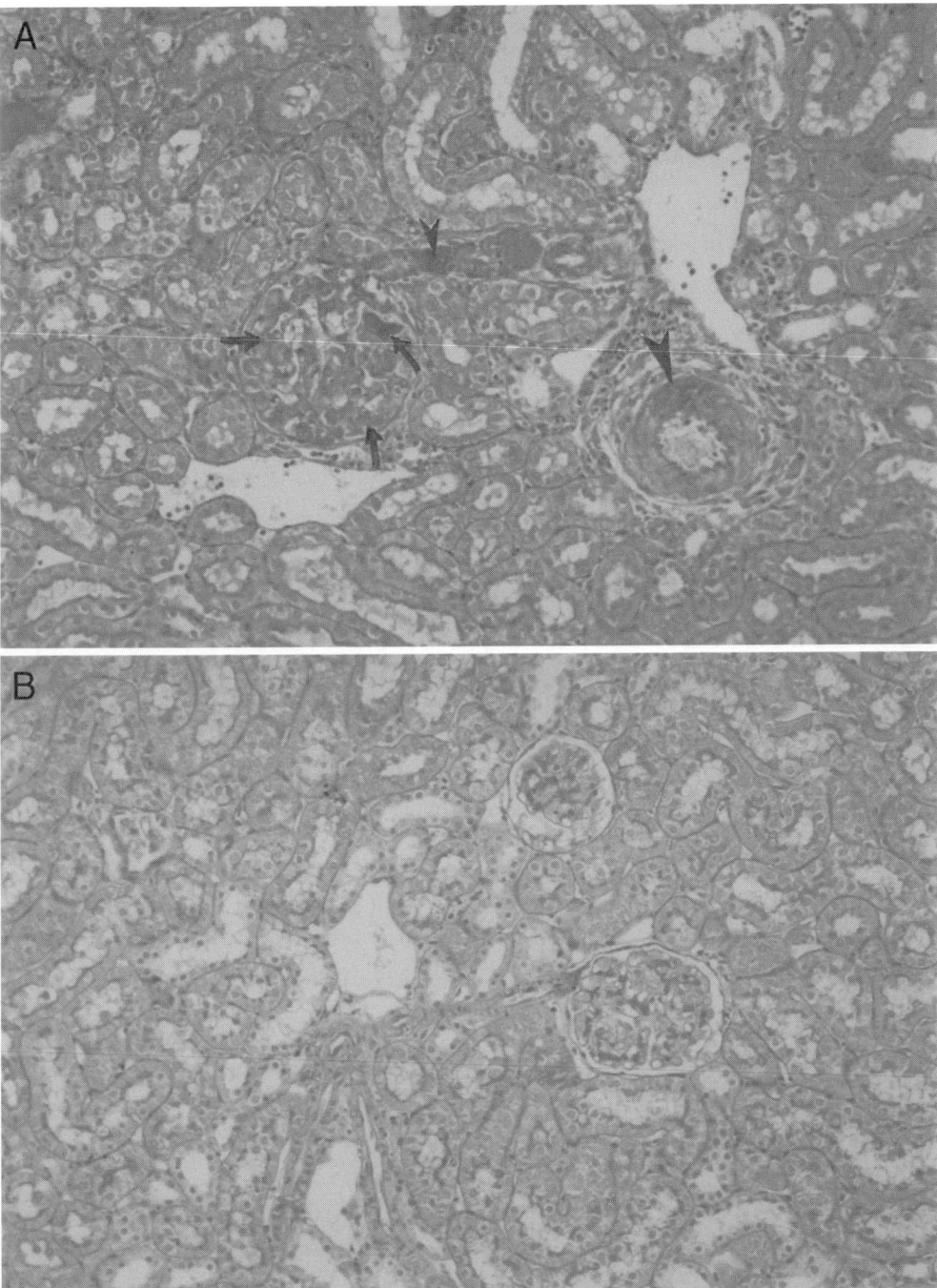

Fig. 5. Aldosterone-mediated renal damage. (**A**) Arterial myointimal proliferation and transmural fibrinoid necrosis (arrowheads) and glomerular thrombosis (arrows) with obliteration of the capillary lumen in rats treated with a high-salt diet, Ang II, and the nitric oxide synthase inhibitor, L-NAME. (**B**) Necrotic lesions are markedly reduced when these animals are adrenalectomized or are simultaneously receiving the mineralocorticoid receptor antagonist, eplerenone. Panel B is also representative of histological sections from control animals fed a high-salt diet (periodic acid, Schiff; magnification, ×340). (Reproduced from ref. *33* with permission.)

appears to be modulated by endothelium-derived nitric oxide, has been postulated to contribute to hypertension by elevating renal vascular resistance in cardiovascular diseases associated with endothelium dysfunction.

Aldosterone also causes endothelial dysfunction in humans. For example, a 4-h systemic aldosterone infusion in young healthy volunteers induces endothelial dysfunction (43). In patients with CHF, treatment with an MR antagonist for 4 wk improved endothelial function, increased nitric oxide bioactivity, and further inhibited vascular angiotensin I/Ang II conversion in the presence of chronic ACE inhibition (44).

7.5. Autonomic Nervous System

Aldosterone can also adversely affect the autonomic nervous system. Baroreflex dysfunction occurs in patients with primary aldosteronism and when aldosterone is infused into healthy volunteers (25,45). Among CHF patients, spironolactone increases cardiac norepinephrine uptake, reduces heart rate, and improves heart rate variability and QT dispersion (46–48). Aldosterone-mediated autonomic dysfunction has been postulated to contribute to cardiac arrhythmias and sudden cardiac death in CHF patients (48).

7.6. Aldosterone, Inflammation, Oxidative Stress, and Vascular Injury

The primary insult caused by aldosterone in susceptible individuals and animals has not yet been identified. In the aldosterone-infused uninephrectomized rat model, an increase in mRNA expression of proinflammatory molecules, including cyclooxygenase-2, macrophage chemoattractant protein-1, interleukin-6, and osteopontin in renal and coronary vessels precedes monocyte and macrophage infiltration (35,39). In these animals, aldosterone increases vascular oxidative stress and reactive oxygen species generation (49,50). The leukocytes invading the myocardium also have increased oxidative stress as well as activation of nuclear transcription factor-κB which regulates the expression of many genes involved in inflammation (50). Activation of circulating peripheral blood mononuclear cells by aldosterone appears to be initiated by reduction in the cytosolic-free magnesium concentration and oxidative stress, which precede the inflammation and focal myocardial ischemic and necrotic changes (51).

8. PREREQUISITES FOR ALDOSTERONE-MEDIATED CARDIOVASCULAR INJURY

8.1. Aldosterone, Dietary Sodium, and Vascular Injury

Development of aldosterone-mediated vascular injury appears to require the combination of a moderately high salt intake and an underlying co-morbidity, such as hypertension, CHF, or renal disease. Control animals fed a high-salt diet do not develop cardiovascular injury (52). Animals given L-NAME/Ang II in the presence of sodium restriction also do not develop cardiovascular damage, despite a 10-fold increase in plasma aldosterone levels compared to animals on a high-salt diet (Fig. 6) (53). Rather, injury occurs in L-NAME/Ang II animals on a high-salt diet with low-to-normal plasma aldosterone levels and can be prevented by an MR antagonist. The influence of dietary sodium on the adverse effects of aldosterone in vivo raises concerns regarding the applicability of in vitro studies of aldosterone's actions.

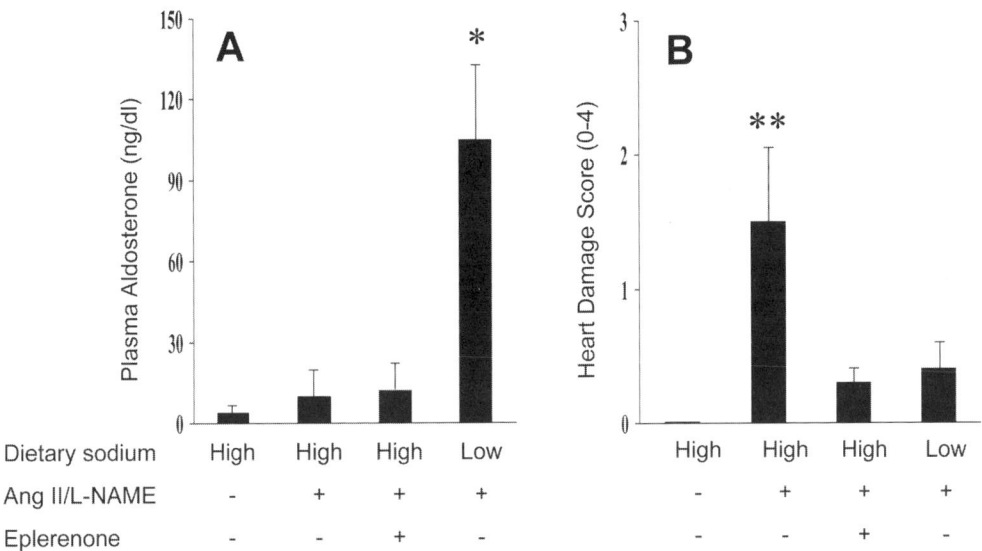

Fig. 6. (**A**) Mean plasma aldosterone concentrations in rats given various interventions including a low- or high-salt diet, L-NAME and Ang II, and eplerenone. (**B**) Corresponding mean semiquantitative histopathological scores for myocardial necrosis from 0 to 4, with 0 representing no damage and 4 representing damage to more than 50% of the myocardium. Heart damage is not correlated with circulating aldosterone levels. *$p < 0.05$, **$p < 0.001$ vs all other groups. (Revised and adapted from ref. *53* with permission.)

8.2. Aldosterone, Hypertension, and Vascular Injury

The adverse effects of aldosterone are not entirely explained by changes in blood pressure. For example, in the L-NAME/Ang II animal model aldosterone blockade reduces cardiovascular injury without significantly lowering blood pressure *(33,34,53)*. Spironolactone markedly reduces strokes and cerebrovascular lesions in stroke-prone spontaneously hypertensive rats despite no difference in blood pressure compared to animals given placebo *(40)*. Intracerebral administration of an MR antagonist in the aldosterone-infused uninephrectomized rat prevents blood pressure elevation, but cardiac fibrosis and hypertrophy still occur *(36)*. Finally, in humans with CHF, MR antagonists reduce morbidity and mortality without significantly altering blood pressure *(13)*.

8.3. Aldosterone, Plasminogen Activator Inhibitor-1, and Vascular Injury

The role of plasminogen activator inhibitor (PAI)-1 in aldosterone-mediated cardiovascular injury has been studied. PAI-1, the major physiological inhibitor of fibrinolysis, is associated with cardiovascular events and is stimulated by Ang II and aldosterone *(54–56)*. Animals given L-NAME have increased PAI-1 immunoreactivity in the endothelium and media of the aorta and coronary arteries. Furthermore, this induction of PAI-1 precedes the development of vascular injury, and both processes are prevented by ACE inhibition *(57)*. PAI-1 expression is also increased in areas of cardiac damage in the L-NAME/Ang II model. However, MR blockade, but not PAI-1 deficiency, is protective in these animals, suggesting that PAI-1 is not causative in L-NAME/Ang II-mediated myocardial injury, but may be generated in response to damage and might play a role in repair *(34)*.

8.4. Aldosterone, Dietary Potassium, and Vascular Injury

In the L-NAME/Ang II animal model, eplerenone, but not dietary potassium supplementation, prevented the development of cardiac damage, suggesting that the beneficial effects of MR antagonists are not mediated by increases in body potassium stores *(53)*. Similarly, potassium supplementation did not reduce cardiovascular injury in the aldosterone-infused uninephrectomized rat *(36)*.

9. AREAS OF FUTURE RESEARCH

There are gaps in our understanding of the function of MR in the cardiovascular system. Although many of the adverse effects of aldosterone appear to be mediated by changes in the vasculature, direct effects on target organs are also possible. Future research should explore not only the specific mechanisms by which aldosterone causes vascular damage and dysfunction, but also the mechanisms by which high-salt intake contributes to this injury.

Cardiovascular damage does not necessarily correlate with absolute plasma aldosterone levels. Therefore, tissue levels of aldosterone may contribute to the injury in the heart and vasculature *(58)*. Although there is minimal aldosterone production in the normal heart, cardiac aldosterone levels may be increased in patients with CHF or essential hypertension *(59–61)*. Both ACE activation and upregulation of the aldosterone synthase gene have been demonstrated in the hearts of CHF patients *(62)*. Cardiac aldosterone production is also increased in rats with hypertension or myocardial infarction and appears to be primarily mediated by tissue Ang II *(63,64)*. The relative importance of circulating aldosterone levels, local cardiac aldosterone production, and aldosterone uptake from the circulation remains to be determined.

Although MR antagonists are beneficial in CHF, the MR may play an important role in healthy cardiac function. Transgenic mice develop severe CHF when MR expression by the cardiomyocyte is reduced using a conditional MR antisense RNA; restoration of MR expression reverses the CHF *(65)*. Altering MR expression in the cardiomyocyte may have a different effect than activating MR in the vasculature. Furthermore, cardiomyocytes do not express 11β-HSD2. Therefore, cortisol may activate the MR in the heart. Transgenic mice that overexpress 11β-HSD2 in cardiomyocytes develop cardiac fibrosis that is reduced by MR antagonists *(66)*. Thus, it is possible that in cardiomyocytes, activation of MR by aldosterone has adverse effects whereas activation by cortisol has beneficial effects. Further studies are needed to better define the role of MR in cardiomyocytes and the vasculature. Finally, whether aldosterone contributes to injury and fibrosis in other organs, such as retinopathy, pulmonary fibrosis, and cirrhosis is speculative.

10. CONCLUSIONS

Although aldosterone has classically been considered a regulator of electrolyte homeostasis, blood volume, and blood pressure, MR activation is emerging as an important contributor to vascular inflammation, endothelial dysfunction, cardiovascular injury, cerebrovascular disease, and nephropathy. This damage occurs in susceptible individuals without primary aldosteronism and may be modified by dietary sodium intake.

Table 1
Potential Beneficial Effects of Mineralocorticoid Receptor Antagonists

Organ	Potential beneficial effects
Heart	↓ Vascular injury and inflammation
	↓ Myocardial necrosis and fibrosis
	↓ Left ventricular hypertrophy
	↓ Sudden death
	↓ Heart failure morbidity/mortality
Kidney	↓ Vascular injury and inflammation
	↓ Glomerulosclerosis
	↓ Proteinuria
Brain	↓ Vascular injury and inflammation
	↓ Stroke
Endothelium	↓ Endothelial dysfunction
	↓ Oxidative stress
Autonomic nervous system	↓ Baroreflex dysfunction
	↓ Impaired heart rate variability
	↓ Impaired QT dispersion

Several human and animal studies have shown that MR antagonists have beneficial effects on the heart, kidney, brain, vasculature, and autonomic nervous system (Table 1). Although MR antagonists are effective antihypertensive agents, these medications can reduce cardiovascular injury without lowering blood pressure. This suggests that there are mechanisms independent of blood pressure by which aldosterone causes tissue injury. Although ACE inhibitors acutely lower plasma aldosterone concentrations, these medications do not provide long-term aldosterone suppression. This breakthrough phenomenon may partly explain the additive beneficial effects of MR antagonists in patients with CHF, diabetic proteinuria, and LVH. This is an exciting time for aldosterone research. Future efforts will more precisely define the role of this hormone in common cardiovascular diseases.

REFERENCES

1. Williams, J. S. and Williams, G. H. (2003) 50th anniversary of aldosterone. *J. Clin. Endocrinol. Metab.* **88,** 2364–2372.
2. Dzau, V. J., Bernstein, K., Celermajer, D., et al. (2001) The relevance of tissue angiotensin-converting enzyme: manifestations in mechanistic and endpoint data. *Am. J. Cardiol.* **88,** 1L–20L.
3. Gavras, I. and Gavras, H. (2002) Angiotensin II as a cardiovascular risk factor. *J. Hum. Hypertens.* **16(Suppl 2),** S2–S6.
4. Zhou, M. Y., Gomez-Sanchez, C. E., and Gomez-Sanchez, E. P. (2000) An alternatively spliced rat mineralocorticoid receptor mRNA causing truncation of the steroid binding domain. *Mol. Cell. Endocrinol.* **159,** 125–131.
5. Takeda, Y., Miyamori, I., Inaba, S., et al. (1997) Vascular aldosterone in genetically hypertensive rats. *Hypertension* **29,** 45–48.
6. Lombes, M., Alfaidy, N., Eugene, E., Lessana, A., Farman, N., and Bonvalet, J. P. (1995) Prerequisite for cardiac aldosterone action. Mineralocorticoid receptor and 11 beta-hydroxysteroid dehydrogenase in the human heart. *Circulation* **92,** 175–182.
7. Rogerson, F. M., Brennan, F. E., and Fuller, P. J. (2003) Dissecting mineralocorticoid receptor structure and function. *J. Steroid Biochem. Mol. Biol.* **85,** 389–396.

8. Wehling, M. (1997) Specific, nongenomic actions of steroid hormones. *Annu. Rev. Physiol.* **59**, 365–393.

9. Arima, S., Kohagura, K., Xu, H. L., et al. (2004) Endothelium-derived nitric oxide modulates vascular action of aldosterone in renal arteriole. *Hypertension* **43**, 352–357.

10. Losel, R. M., Feuring, M., Falkenstein, E., and Wehling, M. (2002) Nongenomic effects of aldosterone: cellular aspects and clinical implications. *Steroids* **67**, 493–498.

11. Krozowski, Z. (1999) The 11beta-hydroxysteroid dehydrogenases: functions and physiological effects. *Mol. Cell Endocrinol.* **151**, 121–127.

12. Shimojo, M. and Stewart, P. M. (1995) Apparent mineralocorticoid excess syndromes. *J. Endocrinol. Investig.* **18**, 518–532.

13. Pitt, B., Zannad, F., Remme, W. J., et al. (1999) The effect of spironolactone on morbidity and mortality in patients with severe heart failure. Randomized aldactone evaluation study investigators. *N. Engl. J. Med.* **341**, 709–717.

14. Pitt, B., Remme, W., Zannad, F., et al. (2003) Eplerenone, a selective aldosterone blocker, in patients with left ventricular dysfunction after myocardial infarction. *N. Engl. J. Med.* **348**, 1309–1321.

15. Sato, A., Suzuki, Y., Shibata, H., and Saruta, T. (2000) Plasma aldosterone concentrations are not related to the degree of angiotensin-converting enzyme inhibition in essential hypertensive patients. *Hypertens. Res.* **23**, 25–31.

16. Sato, A. and Saruta, T. (2001) Aldosterone escape during angiotensin-converting enzyme inhibitor therapy in essential hypertensive patients with left ventricular hypertrophy. *J. Int. Med. Res.* **29**, 13–21.

17. Sato, A. and Saruta, T. (2003) Aldosterone breakthrough during angiotensin-converting enzyme inhibitor therapy. *Am. J. Hypertens.* **16**, 781–788.

18. Sato, A., Hayashi, K., Naruse, M., and Saruta, T. (2003) Effectiveness of aldosterone blockade in patients with diabetic nephropathy. *Hypertension* **41**, 64–68.

19. Nishimura, M., Uzu, T., Fujii, T., et al. (1999) Cardiovascular complications in patients with primary aldosteronism. *Am. J. Kidney Dis.* **33**, 261–266.

20. Rossi, G. P., Sacchetto, A., Pavan, E., et al. (1997) Remodeling of the left ventricle in primary aldosteronism due to Conn's adenoma. *Circulation* **95**, 1471–1478.

21. Halimi, J. M. and Mimran, A. (1995) Albuminuria in untreated patients with primary aldosteronism or essential hypertension. *J. Hypertens.* **13**, 1801, 1802.

22. Rossi, G. P., Sacchetto, A., Visentin, P., et al. (1996) Changes in left ventricular anatomy and function in hypertension and primary aldosteronism. *Hypertension* **27**, 1039–1045.

23. Abe, M., Hamada, M., Matsuoka, H., Shigematsu, Y., Sumimoto, T., and Hiwada, K. (1994) Myocardial scintigraphic characteristics in patients with primary aldosteronism. *Hypertension* **23**, 1164–1167.

24. Napoli, C., Di Gregorio, F., Leccese, M., et al. (1999) Evidence of exercise-induced myocardial ischemia in patients with primary aldosteronism: the cross-sectional primary aldosteronism and heart italian multicenter study. *J. Investig. Med.* **47**, 212–221.

25. Veglio, F., Molino, P., Cat Genova, G., et al. Impaired baroreflex function and arterial compliance in primary aldosteronism. *J. Hum. Hypertens.* **13**, 29–36.

26. Pitt, B., Reichek, N., Willenbrock, R., et al. (2003) Effects of eplerenone, enalapril, and eplerenone/enalapril in patients with essential hypertension and left ventricular hypertrophy: the 4E-left ventricular hypertrophy study. *Circulation* **108**, 1831–1838.

27. Grandi, A. M., Imperiale, D., Santillo, R., et al. (2002) Aldosterone antagonist improves diastolic function in essential hypertension. *Hypertension* **40**, 647–652.

28. White, W. B., Duprez, D., St Hillaire, R., et al. (2003) Effects of the selective aldosterone blocker eplerenone versus the calcium antagonist amlodipine in systolic hypertension. *Hypertension* **41**, 1021–1026.

29. Williams, G. H., Burgess, E., Kolloch, R. E., et al. (2004) Efficacy of eplerenone versus enalapril as monotheraply in systemic hypertension. *Am. J. Cardiol.* **93**, 990–996.

30. Chrysostomou, A. and Becker, G. (2001) Spironolactone in addition to ACE inhibition to reduce proteinuria in patients with chronic renal disease. *N. Engl. J. Med.* **345**, 925, 926.

31. Epstein, M., Williams, G. H., Weinberger, M., et al. (2006) Selective aldosterone blockade with eplerenone reduces albuminuria in patients with type 2 diabetes. *Clin. J. Am. Soc. Nephrol.* CJASN epress Published on July 19, 2006 as doi: 10.2215/CJN. 00240106.

32. Litchfield, W. R., Anderson, B. F., Weiss, R. J., Lifton, R. P., and Dluhy, R. G. (1998) Intracranial aneurysm and hemorrhagic stroke in glucocorticoid-remediable aldosteronism. *Hypertension* **31**, 445–450.

33. Rocha, R., Stier, C. T. Jr., Kifor, I., et al. (2000) Aldosterone: a mediator of myocardial necrosis and renal arteriopathy. *Endocrinology* **141,** 3871–3878.
34. Oestreicher, E. M., Martinez-Vasquez, D., Stone, J. R., et al. (2003) Aldosterone and not plasminogen activator inhibitor-1 is a critical mediator of early angiotensin II/NG-nitro-L-arginine methyl ester-induced myocardial injury. *Circulation* **108,** 2517–2523.
35. Rocha, R., Rudolph, A. E., Frierdich, G. E., et al. (2002) Aldosterone induces a vascular inflammatory phenotype in the rat heart. *Am. J. Physiol. Heart Circ. Physiol.* **283,** H1802–H1810.
36. Young, M., Head, G., and Funder, J. (1995) Determinants of cardiac fibrosis in experimental hypermincralocorticoid states. *Am. J. Physiol.* **269,** E657–E662.
37. Weber, K. T., Brilla, C. G., and Janicki, J. S. (1993) Myocardial fibrosis: functional significance and regulatory factors. *Cardiovasc. Res.* **27,** 341–348.
38. Zannad, F, Alla, F., Dousset, B., Perez, A., and Pitt, B. (2000) Limitation of excessive extracellular matrix turnover may contribute to survival benefit of spironolactone therapy in patients with congestive heart failure: insights from the randomized aldactone evaluation study (RALES). RALES Investigators. *Circulation* **102,** 2700–2706.
39. Blasi, E. R., Rocha, R., Rudolph, A. E., Blomme, E. A., Polly, M. L., and McMahon, E. G. (2003) Aldosterone/salt induces renal inflammation and fibrosis in hypertensive rats. *Kidney Int.* **63,** 1791–1800.
40. Rocha, R., Chander, P. N., Khanna, K., Zuckerman, A., and Stier, C. T. Jr. (1998) Mineralocorticoid blockade reduces vascular injury in stroke-prone hypertensive rats. *Hypertension* **31,** 451–458.
41. Bauersachs, J., Heck, M., Fraccarollo, D., et al. (2002) Addition of spironolactone to angiotensin-converting enzyme inhibition in heart failure improves endothelial vasomotor dysfunction: role of vascular superoxide anion formation and endothelial nitric oxide synthase expression. *J. Am. Coll. Cardiol.* **39,** 351–358.
42. Rajagopalan, S., Duquaine, D., King, S., Pitt, B., and Patel, P. (2002) Mineralocorticoid receptor antagonism in experimental atherosclerosis. *Circulation* **105,** 2212–2216.
43. Farquharson, C. A. and Struthers, A. D. (2002) Aldosterone induces acute endothelial dysfunction in vivo in humans: evidence for an aldosterone-induced vasculopathy. *Clin. Sci. (Lond)* **103,** 425–431.
44. Farquharson, C. A. and Struthers, A. D. (2000) Spironolactone increases nitric oxide bioactivity, improves endothelial vasodilator dysfunction, and suppresses vascular angiotensin I/angiotensin II conversion in patients with chronic heart failure. *Circulation* **101,** 594–597.
45. Yee, K. M. and Struthers, A. D. (1998) Aldosterone blunts the baroreflex response in man. *Clin. Sci. (Lond)* **95,** 687–692.
46. Barr, C. S., Lang, C. C., Hanson, J., Arnott, M., Kennedy, N., and Struthers, A. D. (1995) Effects of adding spironolactone to an angiotensin-converting enzyme inhibitor in chronic congestive heart failure secondary to coronary artery disease. *Am. J. Cardiol.* **76,** 1259–1265.
47. Yee, K. M., Pringle, S. D., and Struthers, A. D. (2001) Circadian variation in the effects of aldosterone blockade on heart rate variability and QT dispersion in congestive heart failure. *J. Am. Coll. Cardiol.* **37,** 1800–1807.
48. MacFadyen, R. J., Barr, C. S., and Struthers, A. D. (1997) Aldosterone blockade reduces vascular collagen turnover, improves heart rate variability and reduces early morning rise in heart rate in heart failure patients. *Cardiovasc. Res.* **35,** 30–34.
49. Virdis, A., Neves, M. F., Amiri, F., Viel, E., Touyz, R. M., and Schiffrin, E. L. (2002) Spironolactone improves angiotensin-induced vascular changes and oxidative stress. *Hypertension* **40,** 504–510.
50. Sun, Y., Zhang, J., Lu, L., Chen, S. S., Quinn, M. T., and Weber, K. T. (2002) Aldosterone-induced inflammation in the rat heart: role of oxidative stress. *Am. J. Pathol.* **161,** 1773–1781.
51. Gerling, I. C., Sun, Y., Ahokas, R. A., et al. (2003) Aldosteronism: an immunostimulatory state precedes proinflammatory/fibrogenic cardiac phenotype. *Am. J. Physiol. Heart Circ. Physiol.* **285,** H813–H821.
52. Rocha, R., Martin-Berger, C. L., Yang, P., Scherrer, R., Delyani, J., and McMahon, E. (2002) Selective aldosterone blockade prevents angiotensin II/salt-induced vascular inflammation in the rat heart. *Endocrinology* **143,** 4828–4836.
53. Martinez, D. V., Rocha, R., Matsumura, M., et al. (2002) Cardiac damage prevention by eplerenone: comparison with low sodium diet or potassium loading. *Hypertension* **39,** 614–618.
54. Kerins, D. M., Hao, Q., and Vaughan, D. E. (1995) Angiotensin induction of PAI-1 expression in endothelial cells is mediated by the hexapeptide angiotensin IV. *J. Clin. Investig.* **96,** 2515–2520.
55. Brown, N. J., Kim, K. S., Chen, Y. Q., et al. (2000) Synergistic effect of adrenal steroids and angiotensin II on plasminogen activator inhibitor-1 production. *J. Clin. Endocrinol. Metab.* **85,** 336–344.

56. Kohler, H. P. and Grant, P. J. (2000) Plasminogen-activator inhibitor type 1 and coronary artery disease. *N. Engl. J. Med.* **342,** 1792–1801.

57. Katoh, M., Egashira, K., Mitsui, T., Chishima, S., Takeshita, A., and Narita, H. (2000) Angiotensin-converting enzyme inhibitor prevents plasminogen activator inhibitor-1 expression in a rat model with cardiovascular remodeling induced by chronic inhibition of nitric oxide synthesis. *J. Mol. Cell. Cardiol.* **32,** 73–83.

58. Hatakeyama, H., Miyamori, I., Fujita, T., Takeda, Y., Takeda, R., and Yamamoto, H. (1994) Vascular aldosterone. Biosynthesis and a link to angiotensin II-induced hypertrophy of vascular smooth muscle cells. *J. Biol. Chem.* **269,** 24,316–24,320.

59. Mizuno, Y., Yoshimura, M., Yasue, H., et al. (2001) Aldosterone production is activated in failing ventricle in humans. *Circulation* **103,** 72–77.

60. Yamamoto, N., Yasue, H., Mizuno, Y., et al. (2002) Aldosterone is produced from ventricles in patients with essential hypertension. *Hypertension* **39,** 958–962.

61. Young, M. J., Clyne, C. D., Cole, T. J., and Funder, J. W. (2001) Cardiac steroidogenesis in the normal and failing heart. *J. Clin. Endocrinol. Metab.* **86,** 5121–5126.

62. Yoshimura, M., Nakamura, S., Ito, T., et al. (2002) Expression of aldosterone synthase gene in failing human heart: quantitative analysis using modified real-time polymerase chain reaction. *J. Clin. Endocrinol. Metab.* **87,** 3936–3940.

63. Silvestre, J. S., Heymes, C., Oubenaissa, A., et al. (1999) Activation of cardiac aldosterone production in rat myocardial infarction: effect of angiotensin II receptor blockade and role in cardiac fibrosis. *Circulation* **99,** 2694–2701.

64. Takeda, Y., Yoneda, T., Demura, M., Miyamori, I., and Mabuchi, H. (2000) Cardiac aldosterone production in genetically hypertensive rats. *Hypertension* **36,** 495–500.

65. Beggah, A. T., Escoubet, B., Puttini, S., et al. (2002) Reversible cardiac fibrosis and heart failure induced by conditional expression of an antisense mRNA of the mineralocorticoid receptor in cardiomyocytes. *Proc. Natl Acad. Sci. USA* **99,** 7160–7165.

66. Qin, W., Rudolph, A. E., Bond, B. R., et al. (2003) Transgenic model of aldosterone-driven cardiac hypertrophy and heart failure. *Circ. Res.* **93,** 69–76.

II THE SYMPATHO-ADRENAL SYSTEM IN HYPERTENSION

Neurogenic Human Hypertension

David Robertson, Andre Diedrich, and Italo Biaggioni

CONTENTS

1. INTRODUCTION

The autonomic nervous system exerts powerful control over human cardiovascular function through many delicate regulatory mechanisms that modulate blood pressure, heart rate (HR), cardiac output, and contractility in a highly specific and targeted manner (1,2). The arterial and cardiopulmonary reflex mechanisms converging on the brainstem (3,4) are perhaps the best studied systems, but others such as cortical, insular cortical, and amygdala centers, and renal and skeletal muscle afferents have important effects as well. Visceral sympathetic afferent reflexes may also contribute to pressor mechanisms (5).

In contrast to the well-appreciated role of the autonomic nervous system in the minute-by-minute regulation of these variables, the role of the sympathetic nervous system in producing chronic hypertension has remained controversial over many decades. Certainly there is little doubt that the sympathetic nervous system plays a contributory role in most hypertension, as evidenced by baroreflex resetting, but in some cases, here

From: *Contemporary Endocrinology: Hypertension and Hormone Mechanisms*
Edited by: R. M. Carey © Humana Press Inc., Totowa, NJ

Table 1
Some Presentations of Neurogenic Human Hypertension

Baroreflex failure
Medullary vascular compression
Severe paroxysmal hypertension
Alcohol withdrawal
Pheochromocytoma
Essential hypertension
Supine hypertension of autonomic failure
Obesity
Sleep apnea
Postural tachycardia syndrome

collectively termed as neurogenic hypertension, it seems to be the primary signal eliciting the effect.

Although there are many causes of neurogenic hypertension, the following are the best established and most widely studied entities proposed to be related to sympathetic mechanisms to date (Table 1): baroreflex failure, medullary vascular compression, severe paroxysmal hypertension, alcohol withdrawal, essential hypertension, obesity, sleep apnea, and postural tachycardia syndrome (POTS).

2. BAROREFLEX FAILURE

Perhaps the most dramatic form of neurogenic hypertension is baroreflex failure *(6,7)*. Baroreflex failure occurs when afferent IX and X cranial nerves are lost *(8)*. Although unilateral loss occasionally causes altered heart rate regulation *(9,10)*, it is more typically tolerated from a cardiovascular standpoint. On the other hand, bilateral loss results acutely in an important syndrome of accelerated hypertension *(11)* and even encephalopathy *(12)*. Baroreflex failure should be diagnosed when a patient initially presumed to have pheochromocytoma is found to have no tumor. Blood pressures in this condition can be among the highest found in human subjects. We have seen an acute pressure of 320/160 mmHg in a patient with baroreflex failure who was asymptomatic except for headache. In such patients, systolic blood pressures (SBP) of 260–300 mmHg are commonly observed during stress, requiring urgent admission to an intensive care unit for blood pressure control. Such pressures are most likely to be seen after acute baroreflex disruption by injury or by surgery *(13)*. However, over succeeding days and weeks, there is a moderation in the hypertension, and the episodes of normal or low blood pressures punctuate the elevated blood pressures. Eventually, some patients with baroreflex failure develop orthostatic hypotension.

Patients with baroreflex failure are exquisitely sensitive to the effects of α-2 agonists to lower blood pressure. There is often a 50-mmHg fall in systolic blood pressure within 1 h of oral administration of 0.1 mg of clonidine in this disorder *(14)*. Patients with baroreflex failure also often have excessive elevated blood pressures in response to the cold pressor test *(6)*. Benzodiazepines, which promote GABA transmission, also reduce hypertension in these individuals. It is likely that this model of neurogenic hypertension is the most susceptible to interventions involving biofeedback, though this has not been systematically tested. Over a period, many patients with baroreflex failure learn on their own how best to control their pressure by avoiding stressful situations and thoughts if they sense their blood pressure is rising.

The selective baroreflex failure (Jordan syndrome), a special disorder, has been described in ref. *(15)*. These patients differ from others in having retained at least some efferent control of heart rate by the vagus. Thus, in times of sedation or during sleep, profound bradycardia may occur. Pauses of 10 or 20 s in heartbeat have been noted (malignant vagotonia), causing patients to awaken with confusion and headache. The unusual regimen of cardiac pacemaker, guanethidine, and fludrocortisone has proven helpful to these patients.

3. MEDULLARY VASCULAR COMPRESSION

Peter Jannetta, in a series of studies over the last 25 yr, has implicated vascular compression in the left lateral medulla in eliciting hypertension *(16,17)*. The areas implicated in his studies lie close to several structures known to control autonomic mechanisms including the rostral ventrolateral medulla (RVLM) and the brain nuclei that closely associated with the IX and X cranial nerves. Jannetta et al. have argued that the pulsatile pressure of artery loops in the medulla may have a functional impact on autonomic cardiovascular control leading to hypertension, and seem to have elicited replication in a primate model *(18)*. When they have operated on patients and cushioned these loops, improvements in the hypertension have been seen. Unfortunately, there has been considerable divergence in results among studies attempting to confirm Jannetta's observations. Many investigators have reported generally the analogous results *(19,20)*, but others have failed to replicate the finding in all its particulars *(21,22)*. This important research area needs further clarification about the puzzling implication of selectively left-sided loop lateralization Jannetta has described (although he has maintained that right-sided loops may give rise to diabetes mellitus *(23,24)* rather than hypertension).

The early reports also suggested that left-sided vascular compression was almost universally associated with essential hypertension, and the decompression generally alleviated hypertension. It has seemed unlikely to many investigators that such decompression could result in normalization of blood pressure in more than 90% of individuals of whom it was undertaken, given the heterogeneity of essential hypertension. State-of-the-art imaging techniques, such as high-resolution functional magnetic resonance imaging, have offered a promise to determine the frequency of medullary vascular compression and its association with neurogenic forms of high blood pressure, but are still not perfect in detecting it *(25)*.

4. SEVERE PAROXYSMAL HYPERTENSION

There are some patients with severe paroxysmal hypertension in whom the baroreflex failure, pheochromocytoma, and medullary vascular compression all appear to be absent. Sometimes paroxysmal hypertension is seen in patients with renal artery stenosis, but this can usually be ruled out with standard diagnostic techniques. In other patients, the etiology is less clear, but certainly it is observed in rare conditions such as tumors in the fourth ventricle or in the ancillary structures *(26)*, Leigh's syndrome *(4)*, and "pseudopheochromocytoma," a poorly characterized nonepileptic disorder proposed to be related to abnormalities in dopamine function *(27)*.

5. ALCOHOL WITHDRAWAL

One of the most dramatic causes of acute and transient sympathetic activation in hypertension seen in ordinary clinical practice is severe alcohol withdrawal. In the most severely affected patients, fivefold elevations of plasma norepinephrine are by no means rare. Such patients typically have tachycardia and sometimes arrhythmias in association with these dramatic blood pressure elevations. In some cases, sympathetic excitation is a first stage in what later becomes delirium tremens. When these patients are treated with GABA-ergic or related agents, such as benzodiazepines, the blood pressure often declines toward normal, though high doses of benzodiazepines may be required.

6. PHEOCHROMOCYTOMA

Catecholamine-producing tumors such as pheochromocytoma can appear as episodic hypertension, sustained hypertension, or occasionally even as orthostatic hypotension. Although these tumors are rare in the general hypertensive population, it is important that they can be ruled out because of their therapeutic implications and by the new methods, pioneered by Graeme Eisenhofer et al. including plasma metanephrine, yield sensitive and relatively specific diagnostic information, which was previously unavailable.

7. ESSENTIAL HYPERTENSION

Athough a central role of the autonomic nervous system in essential hypertension remains controversial, evidence for a contributory role has been repeatedly documented, particularly in the early hyperkinetic phase of the disease (28). There is also evidence of enhanced norepinephrine spillover in essential hypertension (29) and enhanced sympathetic nerve traffic. However, because many genes that are recently shown to be involved in familial hypertension syndromes have included first and foremost gene products involved in volume regulation in some way, autonomic mechanisms must be viewed as a component rather than the sole player in the pathophysiological mosaic of essential hypertension.

Increased central sympathetic outflow, impaired baroreflex buffering, altered regulation of norepinephrine release, and reuptake can contribute to essential hypertension. The pathogenesis of the sustained or increased central sympathetic drive in essential hypertension is unclear. In the brainstem, noradrenergic neurotransmission inhibits central sympathetic outflow. In contrast, some suprabulbar noradrenergic projections to the hypothalamus and amygdala are sympathoexcitatory. Esler et al. (29,30) estimated norepinephrine turnover from these subcortical suprabulbar brain regions by measuring internal jugular vein overflow of norepinephrine and found it to be increased in patients with essential hypertension. Increased rates of sympathetic nerve firing and a reduction of cardiac neuronal norepinephrine reuptake contribute to essential hypertension. Central noradrenergic turnover correlated with systemic sympathetic activation, suggesting that this mechanism contributes to the sympathetic overactivity that is observed in essential hypertension.

Blood pressure and heart rate are kept within a relatively narrow range appropriate to physiological demands (exercise level or orthostatic stress) by autonomic baroreflex mechanisms. However, substantial variability from heart beat-to-heart beat is present and reflects both the presence of a variety of naturally occurring physiological perturbations to cardiovascular homeostasis and the dynamic response of the cardiovascular control systems to these pertubations *(31)*. Spectral analysis of cardiovascular rhythms has become an important tool in the investigation of autonomic contributions to hypertension. Continuous blood pressure fluctuations are caused by several factors. Respiration modulates blood pressure in the high frequency (HF) band of the breathing rate. Atropine abolishes HF oscillations of heart rate, whereas HF oscillations of systolic blood pressure remain constant. The hypothesis that the vagally mediated HR oscillations associated with respiration generate the respiratory oscillations in blood pressure can therefore be excluded *(32)*. Systolic blood pressure fluctuations with a 10-s periodicity, or low frequency band (LFSBP), which are also termed as "Traube–Hering–Mayer" waves, mainly reflect sympathetic-mediated changes in vasomotor tone *(33)*. Indeed, LFSBP is linked to low frequency oscillations in the activity of postganglionic sympathetic neurons *(34)*. A tight relationship between LFSBP and muscle sympathetic activity could be found in humans *(35)*. LFSBP is increased by maneuvers that induce sympathetic activation, such as upright posture *(36,37)*, lower body negative pressure *(38)*, or infusion of depressor substances *(39)*. LFSBP was similar or increased *(40)* in hypertensive patients as compared to normotensive subjects.

Ganglionic blockade has been quite valuable in studies that deal with sympathetic outflow in hypertension. Trimethaphan (Afronad) is an adrenergic, anticholinergic, antihypertensive, and ganglionic blocking agent, which for many years was marketed for intravenous therapy of hypertension in the United States. It prevents transmission in both adrenergic and cholinergic ganglia by blocking N_N postganglionic receptors (Fig. 1). It also has a minor direct peripheral arterial and venous vasodilatory effect and is a weak histamine releaser.

The contribution of the sympathetic nervous system in hypertension can be examined by gaging the decrease in blood pressure produced by acute sympathetic withdrawal during ganglionic blockade *(15,40,41)*. Studies with ganglionic blockade reveal that sympathetic nervous system contributes to essential hypertension, and severes supine hypertension in patients with multiple system atrophy (MSA) *(40)*.

8. SUPINE HYPERTENSION IN MSA

One of the most unexpected findings in recent years has been the constitutive role of sympathetic activity in the supine hypertension of autonomic failure. Supine hypertension is seen in approximately half of the patients with autonomic failure. The mechanism of supine hypertension in these patients is heterogeneous. In patients with MSA, also termed as Shy–Drager syndrome, blood pressure was uniformly and considerably reduced by ganglionic blockade. This implied that the residual sympathetic activity accounted for most of the hypertension in these subjects. In contrast, ganglionic blockade had little to no effect in patients with pure autonomic failure (PAF). This finding indicates that mechanisms other than sympathetic tone were responsible for hypertension in PAF patients *(41)*.

Differences in sympathetic tone between MSA and PAF patients are also reflected in the power spectrum of blood pressure variability. PAF patients had greatly reduced LFSBP, with no consistent change during trimethaphan infusion. In contrast, LFSBP power was high in patients with MSA, and was greatly reduced by trimethaphan

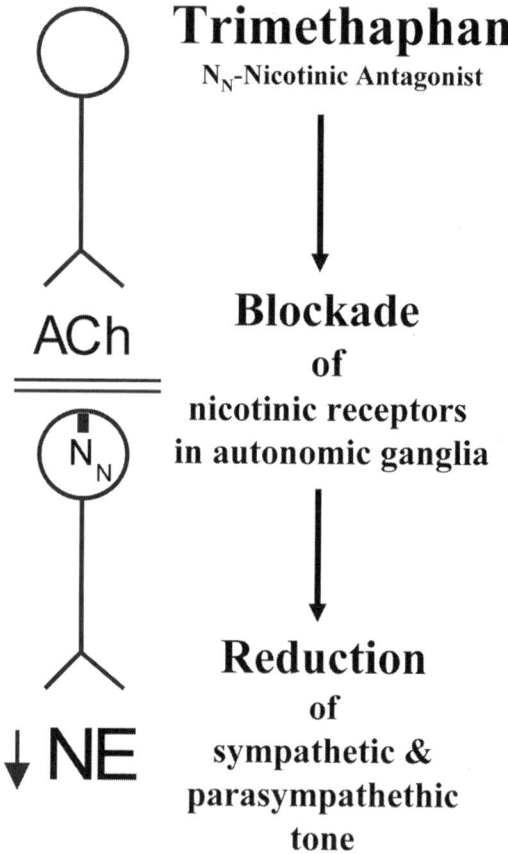

Fig. 1. Mechanism of ganglionic blocking agent trimethaphan (Afronad).

(Figs. 2 and 3). These observations contribute to our understanding of Mayer waves and their origin. Brief selective stimulation of arterial baroreceptors generates a damped oscillation in blood pressure in the low frequency (LF) range *(42)*. This observation has been evoked to propose that LFSBP oscillations result from loop properties of the baroreflex rather than originating from central sympathetic regulation. However, the results in MSA patients demonstrate that LFSBP is intact, and even increased, in the total absence of functional baroreflex mechanisms.

9. OBESITY

Strong evidence has been developed that autonomic control importantly and often crucially determines sodium and water homeostasis, and this autonomic control may have an important link with the hypertension of obesity. Ganglionic blockade with the combined analysis of blood pressure fall and changes in blood pressure variability is a unique utility to dissect autonomic mechanisms of hypertension. As an example, the majority of obese patients have high blood pressure that can be reduced to normal values by ganglionic blockade. Moreover, the initial power of low frequency oscillation is higher in obese patients than in healthy subjects. This indicates that hypertension in obese patients is mainly caused through neurogenic pathways.

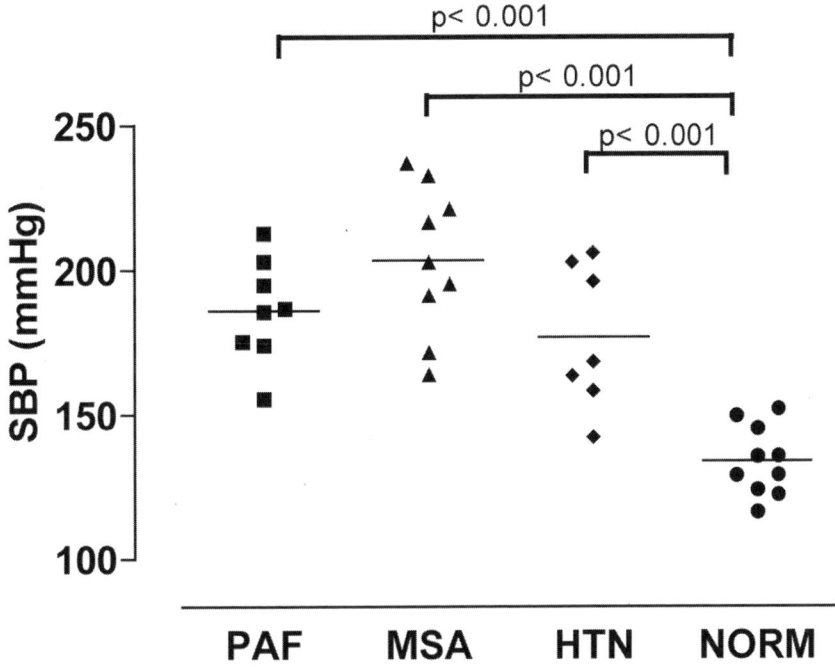

Fig. 2. Final intrinsic systolic blood pressure (SBP) produced by intravenous infusion of trimethaphan in patients with pure autonomic failure (PAF), multiple system atrophy (MSA), essential hypertension (HTN), and normal subjects (NORM).

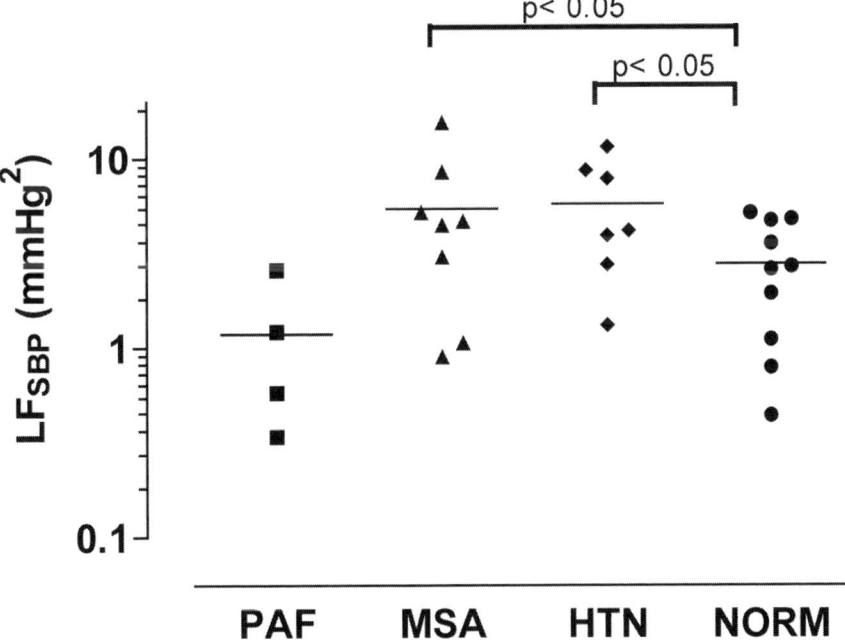

Fig. 3. Resting systolic blood pressure (SBP) variability in the low frequency range (LFSBP) in patients with pure autonomic failure (PAF), multiple system atrophy (MSA), essential hypertension (HTN), and normal subjects (NORM).

10. SLEEP APNEA

There is an increasing evidence that sleep apnea is one of the most common syndromes of neurally mediated hypertension. In many cases, there may be overlaps between this entity and the hypertension of obesity *(43–45)*.

11. POSTURAL TACHYCARDIA SYNDROME

In discussions of neurogenic hypertension, orthostatic disorders are rarely considered. Many orthostatic disorders are due to nonautonomic mechanisms, and there may sometimes be evidence of excessive sympathetic activation in some of the patients in response to the depressor pathophysiology, whatever it may be *(46)*. However, in one syndrome—orthostatic intolerance or POTS *(47)*, it is especially important to keep this potential relationship between an orthostatic abnormality and neurogenic hypertension firmly in mind. This syndrome is defined based on the evidence of sympathetic activation with upright posture and an absence of orthostatic hypotension. POTS has the dubious distinction of perhaps having the most names of any cardiovascular problem. Some of these names are listed in Table 2. Some of the most important and widely used ones include mitral valve prolapse syndrome, postural tachycardia syndrome, vasoregulatory asthenia, neurasthenia, and idiopathic hypovolemia. A large number of names are deserved by this syndrome because it has a very large number of etiologies. Unfortunately, because of the difficulty in accurately diagnosing these many different pathophysiologies in the clinic, the names are not used in any clear pathophysiological way and therefore constitute more of a barrier than a door to improved understanding. The situation is complicated even further by the fact that many patients with chronic fatigue syndrome also meet the hemodynamic criteria for POTS. Indeed, sometimes the name of the condition depends more on the kind of a specialist that a patient visits. The endocrinologist may be most struck by the hypovolemic aspect of the illness and term the problem as idiopathic hypovolemia. The cardiologist may be struck by physical findings of mitral prolapse and diagnose as mitral valve prolapse syndrome. The rheumatologist may call the problem chronic fatigue syndrome, and the neurologist may call the problem as partial dysautonomia or hyperadrenergic orthostatic intolerance. When a patient is examined in a hypertension center, the hyperadrenergic features and the relative youth of a typical patient may more likely lead to the diagnosis of labile hypertension. Because there are probably significant numbers of patients in this last category among those we now call pre-hypertension, it is important to consider features that might lead to this diagnosis.

Patients with orthostatic intolerance or POTS have symptoms while standing that resemble those elicited by inadequate cerebral blood flow. On standing, they have increased heart rates of at least 30 bpm with dizziness, palpitations, poor exercise tolerance, and pre-syncopal symptoms, although syncope itself is very infrequent. Blood pressure is usually slightly higher than average in these patients and may be much higher on standing than when lying down. The form of this syndrome most likely to be encountered in a hypertension clinic is hyperadrenergic POTS.

Early investigators observing the tachycardia and hyperkinetic heart in these patients generally assumed that enhanced sympathetic activation or β adrenal receptor hypersensitivity was somehow involved. Friesinger et al. reported that these patients often had

Table 2
Terms Used for Postural Tachycardia Syndrome

Postural tachycardia syndrome
Postural orthostatic tachycardia syndrome
Hyperadrenergia
Hyperadrenergic orthostatic intolerance
Orthostatic intolerance
Mitral valve prolapse syndrome
Neurocirculatory asthenia
Vasoregulatory asthenia
Hyperkinetic heart syndrome
Orthostatic tachycardia
Effort syndrome
Soldier's heart
Irritable heart
Labile hypertension

STT wave changes in the inferior electrocardiogram leads *(48)*. These changes were more significant after upright posture and may in some cases have been heart rate related. Similar hyperadrenergic symptoms are sometimes seen in patients with baroreflex failure and those having tumors involving the brainstem. Furthermore, destruction of the nuclei of the solitary tracts in rats yields a profoundly hyperadrenergic state that culminates in death within hours. This view was strengthened by the findings that plasma norepinephrine was often increased in POTS *(49)*, and that α-2 agonists, β antagonists, and phenobarbital attenuated the tachycardia or at least relieved some of the symptoms.

One of the most important evidence in support of a central etiology for hyperadrenergic POTS has emanated from studies in which both sympathetic and parasympathetic activities had been blocked by the N_N nicotinic antagonist trimethaphan. With this agent, patients with POTS had greater decreases in sympathetic activity than control subjects. Systolic blood pressure decreased by 17 mmHg in patients with POTS but only 4 mmHg in control subjects under similar supine circumstances. Among the patients with POTS, the half of them having the greatest decrease (26 mmHg) after trimethaphan had greater pretrimethaphan supine systolic blood pressures, and greater supine and upright plasma norepinephrine levels than those who had a lesser response. However, the supine and upright heart rates were similar in both POTS subgroups. Analysis of simultaneous peroneal sympathetic nerve traffic and heart rate variability in patients with POTS suggests a greater increase in sympathetic tone to the heart than to the vasculature *(50)*, a finding confirmed in studies of cardiac norepinephrine spillover, which is increased. The discordance seemed robust and may prove to be an important clue to the nature of the central pathophysiology of POTS. Currently, it is often impossible to identify patients with POTS likely to have enhanced central sympathetic outflow but some help is afforded by features noted in Tables 3 and 4. The use of such guidelines must however be approached cautiously because of our primitive understanding of the nature of POTS in most patients.

Recently, norepinephrine transporter dysfunction has been identified as a disorder presenting with tachycardia and mildly increased blood pressure in certain circumstances *(51)*. Abnormalities in norepinephrine transporter function have been identified

Table 3
Features of Hyperadrenergic and Neuropathic Postural Tachycardia Syndrome

Features suggestive of hyperadrenergic postural tachycardia syndrome
Plasma norepinephrine levels > 1000 pg/mL
Increased muscle sympathetic nerve activity
Increase in low-frequency/high-frequency ratio of heart rate variability
Symptomatic benefit with low-dose clonidine
Features suggestive of neuropathic postural tachycardia syndrome
Plasma norepinephrine levels of high normal to 800 pg/mL
Absent galvanic skin response or abnormal quantitative sudomotor axon reflex test
Other evidence of peripheral neuropathy
Poor response to low-dose clonidine

Table 4
Treatment of Hyperadrenergic Postural Tachycardia Syndrome

16 oz water; 2–3 times daily as needed (acts for ~1 h only)
10 g sodium diet
Support garment
Propranolol: 10–20 mg; 2–4 times daily
Clonidine: 0.05–0.10 mg; orally twice daily
Methyldopa: 125–250 mg; half strength or twice daily
Fludrocortisone: 0.05–0.30 mg; daily (attenuates tachycardia)
Midodrine: 2.5–10 mg; three times daily (reflexly attenuates tachycardia)
Phenobarbital: 30–100 mg; daily

in some individuals with hypertension, though it remains uncertain if this is a primary or secondary event. Mice with norepinephrine transporter knockout have exhibited similar effects, with chronic stress-evoked increases in both heart rate and blood pressure *(52)*. Furthermore, in response to the N_N-nicotinic receptor antagonist, trimethaphan, which interrupts autonomic ganglionic transmission, blood pressure falls more in hypertensive subjects than in normal subjects, confirming the substantial role of sympathetic mechanisms in blood pressure maintenance.

12. SUMMARY

Autonomic mechanisms play a pivotal role in the control of blood pressure. This effect is usually more pronounced in individuals with essential hypertension than in normotensive subjects. Many of the large amplitude gene effects in hypertension seem to relate to gene products involved in volume regulation. However, in the great majority of individuals with hypertension, autonomic perturbations seem to play an important role. There is a need for further research at the bedside to identify the role of polymorphisms in adrenoreceptors, catecholamine and acetylcholine synthesizing, metabolizing and transport mechanisms, and the analogous determinants of synthesis, fate and receptor and postreceptor actions of the nontraditional autonomic co-transmitters neuropeptide Y, adenosine and adenosine triphosphate (ATP), as well as the genetic basis of differences in central sympathetic outflow and its organ-specific targeting.

ACKNOWLEDGMENTS

Supported by grants from NIH 5 M01 RR00095, 5P01 HL56693, and 1R01 HL071784 and HL37232.

REFERENCES

1. Dickinson, C. J. (1981) Neurogenic hypertension revisited. *Clin. Sci.* **60,** 471–477.
2. Julius, S. (1990) Changing role of the autonomic nervous system in human hypertension. *J. Hypertens.* **8,** S59–S65.
3. Sved, A. F., Ito, S., and Sved, J. C. (2003) Brainstem mechanisms of hypertension: role of the rostral ventrolateral medulla. *Curr. Hypertens. Rep.* **5,** 262–268.
4. Biaggioni, I., Whetsell, W. O., Jobe, J., and Nadeau, J. H. (1994) Baroreflex failure in a patient with central nervous system lesions involving the nucleus tractus solitarii. *Hypertension* **23,** 491–495.
5. Jordan, J., Shannon, J. R., Black, B. K., et al. (2000) The presser response to water drinking in humans—a sympathetic reflex? *Circulation* **101,** 504–509.
6. Robertson, D., Hollister, A. S., Biaggioni, I., Netterville, J. L., Mosqueda-Garcia, R., and Robertson, R. M. (1993) The diagnosis and treatment of baroreflex failure. *N. Engl. J. Med.* **329,** 1449–1455.
7. Timmers, H. J. L. M., Wieling, W., Karemaker, J. M., and Lenders, J. W. M. (2003) Denervation of carotid baro- and chemoreceptors in humans. *J. Physiol. Lond.* **553,** 3–11.
8. Jardine, D. L., Melton, I. C., Bennett, S. I., Crozier, I. G., Donaldson, I. M., and Ikram, H. (2000) Baroreceptor denervation presenting as part of a vagal mononeuropathy. *Clin. Auton. Res.* **10,** 69–75.
9. Esteban, J. C. G., Boyero, S., Fernandez, C., et al. (2004) Baroreflex failure after chemodectoma resection. *Neurologia* **19,** 452–455.
10. Timmers, H. J. L. M., Buskens, F. G. M., Wieling, W., Karemaker, J. M., and Lenders, J. W. M. (2004) Long-term effects of unilateral carotid endarterectomy arterial baroreflex function. *Clin. Auton. Res.* **14,** 72–79.
11. Ketch, T., Biaggioni, I., Robertson, R., and Robertson, D. (2002) Four faces of baroreflex failure— hypertensive crisis, volatile hypertension, orthostatic tachycardia, and malignant vagotonia. *Circulation* **105,** 2518–2523.
12. Ille, O., Woimant, F., Pruna, A., Corabianu, O., Idatte, J. M., and Haguenau, M. (1995) Hypertensive encelphalopathy after bilateral carotid endarterectomy. *Stroke* **26,** 488–491.
13. De Toma, G., Nicolanti, V., Plocco, M., et al. (2003) Baroreflex failure syndrome after bilateral excision of carotid body tumors: an underestimated problem. *J. Vasc. Surg.* **31,** 806–810.
14. Robertson, D., Goldberg, M. R., Hollister, A. S., and Robertson, R. M. (1984) Baroreceptor dysfunction in humans. *Am. J. Med.* **76,** A58.
15. Jordan, J., Shannon, J. R., Black, B. K., et al. (1997) Malignant vagotonia due to selective baroreflex failure. *Hypertension* **30,** 1072–1077.
16. Jannetta, P. J., Segal, R., Dujovny, M., et al. (1981) Neurogenic hypertension. *Clin. Res.* **29,** A211.
17. Jannetta, P. J., Segal, R., and Wolfson, S. K. (1985) Neurogenic hypertension—etiology and surgical treatment. 1. Observations in 53 patients. *Ann. Surg.* **201,** 391–398.
18. Jannetta, P. J., Segal, R., Wolfson, S. K., Dujovny, M., Semba, A., and Cook, E. E. (1985) Neurogenic hypertension—etiology and surgical treatment. 2. Observations in an experimental nonhuman primate model. *Ann. Surg.* **202,** 253–261.
19. Akimura, T., Furutani, Y., Jimi, Y., et al. (1995) Essential hypertension and neurovascular compression at the ventrolateral medulla oblongata—Mr evaluation. *Am. J. Neuroradiol.* **16,** 401–405.
20. Anding, K., Bloss, H. G., Krummel, B., et al. (1998) Neurovascular decompression of the left ventro-lateral medulla as a treatment of hypertension in a patient with renal artery stenosis. *Nephrol. Dial. Transplant.* **13,** 3253–3257.
21. Colon, G. P., Quint, D. J., Dickinson, L. D., et al. (1998) Magnetic resonance evaluation of ventro-lateral medullary compression in essential hypertension. *J. Neurosurg.* **88,** 226–231.
22. Frank, H., Schobel, H. P., Heusser, K., Geiger, H., Fahlbusch, R., and Naraghi, R. (2001) Long-term results after microvascular decompression in essential hypertension. *Stroke* **32,** 2950–2954.
23. Jannetta, P. J. and Hollihan, L. (2004) Type 2 diabetes mellitus, etiology and possible treatment: preliminary report. *Surg. Neurol.* **61,** 422–428.

24. Hohenbleicher, H., Schmitz, S. A., Koennecke, H. C., et al. (2001) Neurovascular contact of cranial nerve IX and X root-entry zone in hypertensive patients. *Hypertension* **37,** 176–181.

25. Johnson, D. R., Coley, S. C., Brown, J., and Moseley, I. F. (2000) The role of MRI in screening for neurogenic hypertension. *Neuroradiology* **42,** 99–103.

26. Worner, B. A., Rahim, T., Lange, M., Fink, U., and Oeckler, R. (2002) Long-lasting improvement of arterial hypertension after surgical treatment of a foramen magnum meningioma—case report. *Surg. Neurol.* **58,** 189–193.

27. Kuchel, O. (1998) Increased plasma dopamine in patients presenting with the pseudopheochromocytoma quandary: retrospective analysis of 10 years' experience. *J. Hypertens.* **16,** 1531–1537.

28. Julius, S. and Nesbitt, S. (1996) Sympathetic overactivity in hypertension—a moving target. *Am. J. Hypertens.* **9,** S113–S120.

29. Esler, M. (2000) The sympathetic system and hypertension. *Am. J. Hypertens.* **3,** 99S–105S.

30. Esler, M. D., Jennings, G. L., and Lambert, G. W. (1988) Release of noradrenaline into the cerebrovascular circulation in patients with primary hypertension. *J. Hypertens. Suppl.* **6,** S494–S496.

31. Akselrod, S., Gordon, D., Madwed, J. B., Snidman, N. C., Shannon, D. C., and Cohen, R. J. (1985) Hemodynamic regulation: investigation by spectral analysis. *Am. J. Physiol.* **249,** H867–H875.

32. Elghozi, J. L., Laude, D., and Girard, A. (1991) Effects of respiration on blood pressure and heart rate variability in humans. *Clin. Exp. Pharmacol. Physiol.* **18,** 735–742.

33. Malliani, A., Pagani, M., Lombardi, F., and Cerutti, S. (1991) Cardiovascular neural regulation explored in the frequency domain. *Circulation* **84,** 482–492.

34. Polosa, C. (1984) Rhythms in the activity of the autonomic nervous system: their role in the generation of systemic arterial pressure waves. *Mechanisms of Blood Pressure Waves,* Springer, New York.

35. Pagani, M., Montano, N., Porta, A., et al. (1997) Relationship between spectral components of cardiovascular variabilities and direct measures of muscle sympathetic nerve activity in humans. *Circulation* **95,** 1441–1448.

36. Mukai, S. and Hayano, J. (1995) Heart rate and blood pressure variabilities during graded head-up tilt. *J. Appl. Physiol.* **78,** 212–216.

37. Lucini, D., Furlan, R., Villa, P., et al. (2004) Altered profile of baroreflex and autonomic responses to lower body negative pressure in chronic orthostatic intolerance. *J. Hypertens.* **22,** 1535–1542.

38. Lucini, D., Pagani, M, Mela, G. S., and Malliani, A. (1994) Sympathetic restraint of baroreflex control of heart period in normotensive and hypertensive subjects. *Clin. Sci. (Colch.)* **86,** 547–556.

39. Izdebska, E., Cybulska, I., Izdebskir, J., Makowiecka-Ciesla, M., and Trzebski, A. (2004) Effects of moderate physical training on blood pressure variability and hemodynamic pattern in mildly hypertensive subjects. *J. Physiol. Pharmacol.* **55,** 713–724.

40. Diedrich, A., Jordan, J., Tank, J., et al. (2003) The sympathetic nervous system in hypertension: assessment by blood pressure variability and ganglionic blockade. *J. Hypertens.* **21,** 1677–1686.

41. Shannon, J. R., Jordan, J., Black, B. K., et al. (1998) Complete N_N-nicotinic blockade to study the components of cardiovascular regulation in multiple system atrophy. *Parkinson Dis. Mov. Disord.* **13,** 178.

42. Leuzzi, S., Radaelli, A., Passino, C., Johnston J. A., and Sleight P. (1994) Low frequency spontaneous fluctuations of R–R interval and blood pressure in conscious humans: a baroreceptor or central phenomenon? *Clin. Sci. (Colch.)* **87,** 649–654.

43. Narkiewicz, K., van de Borne, P. J., Cooley, R. L., Dyken, M. E., and Somers, V. K. (1998) Sympathetic activity in obese subjects with and without obstructive sleep apnea. *Circulation* **98,** 772–776.

44. Ziegler, M. G. (2003) Sleep disorders and the failure to lower nocturnal blood pressure. *Curr. Opin. Nephrol. Hypertens.* **12,** 97–102.

45. Calhoun, D. A., Nishizaka, M. K., Zaman, M. A., and Harding, S. M. (2004) Aldosterone excretion among subjects with resistant hypertension and symptoms of sleep apnea. *Chest* **125,** 112–117.

46. Jacob, G., Costa, F., Shannon, J. R., et al. (2000) The neuropathic postural tachycardia syndrome. *N. Engl. J. Med.* **343,** 1008–1014.

47. Low, P. A., Opfer-Gehrking, T. L., Textor, S. C., et al. (1995) Postural tachycardia syndrome (POTS). *Neurology* **45,** S19–S25.

48. Friesinger, G. C., Biern, R. O., Likar I., and Mason, R. E. (1972) Exercise electrocardiography and vasoregulatory abnormalities. *Am. J. Cardiol.* **30,** 733–740.

49. Ali, Y. S., Daamen, N., Jacob, G., et al. (2000) Orthostatic intolerance: a disorder of young women. *Obstet. Gynecol. Surv.* **55,** 251–259.

50. Furlan, R., Jacob, G., Snell, M., et al. (1998) Chronic orthostatic intolerance—a disorder with discordant cardiac and vascular sympathetic control. *Circulation* **98,** 2154–2159.
51. Shannon, J. R., Flattem, N. L., Jordan, J., et al. (2000) Orthostatic intolerance and tachycardia associated with norepinephrine transporter deficiency. *N. Engl. J. Med.* **342,** 541–549.
52. Keller, N. R., Diedrich, A., Appalsamy, M., et al. (2004) Norepinephrine transporter-deficient mice exhibit excessive tachycardia and elevated blood pressure with wakefulness and activity. *Circulation* **110,** 1191–1196.

9   Calcitonin Gene-Related Peptide and Hypertension

Donald J. DiPette and Scott C. Supowit

CONTENTS

1. INTRODUCTION

Calcitonin gene-related peptide (CGRP) is the most potent endogenous vasodilator peptide known to date *(1–4)*. There are two forms of CGRP, α and β, which differ in only two amino acids in rats and three in humans. α-CGRP is derived from the tissue-specific splicing of the calcitonin/CGRP gene. Whereas calcitonin is produced mainly in the C cells of the thyroid, CGRP synthesis is limited almost exclusively to specific regions of the central and peripheral nervous systems. The β-CGRP gene that is located on the same chromosome as the calcitonin/α-CGRP gene does not produce calcitonin and is also synthesized primarily in neuronal tissues. α-CGRP is prevalent in the central nervous system and in the peripheral sensory neural network. β-CGRP is also prevalent in the central nervous system, but peripherally is common in intestinal neurons *(1–5)*. However, the biological activities of both peptides are similar in most vascular beds.

Immunoreactive CGRP (iCGRP) and its receptors are widely distributed in the nervous and cardiovascular systems *(1–5)*. In the peripheral sensory nervous system, prominent sites of CGRP synthesis are the dorsal root ganglia (DRG). These structures contain the cell bodies of sensory nerves that terminate peripherally on blood vessels and all other tissues innervated by sensory nerves and centrally in laminae I/II of the dorsal horn of the spinal cord *(6)*. A dense perivascular CGRP neural network is seen around the blood vessels in all vascular beds. In these vessels CGRP containing nerves are found at the junction of the adventitia and the media passing into the muscle layer *(2,4,7)*. It is thought that circulating CGRP is largely derived from these perivascular nerve terminals and represents a spillover phenomenon related to the release of these peptides to promote

From: *Contemporary Endocrinology: Hypertension and Hormone Mechanisms*
Edited by: R. M. Carey © Humana Press Inc., Totowa, NJ

vasodilation or other tissue functions *(2,7)*. Receptors for CGRP have been identified in the media and intima of resistance vessels as well as the endothelial layer.

2. STRUCTURE OF CGRP

Both forms of CGRP belong to a superfamily of closely related genes that include calcitonin, adrenomedullin (ADM), and amylin *(2,3,7)*. The α and β forms of CGRP, calcitonin, and ADM are all found on human chromosome 11, whereas amylin is located on chromosome 12. ADM, calcitonin, and amylin share structural and functional homology with CGRP although they are less potent. Moreover, all of these genes are further related to the insulin superfamily of peptides. The agonist properties of all of the calcitonin/ CGRP superfamily peptides reside at the N-terminal end (residues 1–8) and are dependent on a disulfide bridge between two cystein residues at positions 2 and 7 and an arginine at position 11, which is important for receptor interactions. The highest degree of homology of these proteins that have vasodilator activity (CGRP, ADM, and amylin) is found within the sequence 1–13. The C-terminal CGRP sequence 8–37 is a potent high affinity antagonist for the CGRP (and ADM) receptor and for years has been the primary antagonist used to characterize the functions of CGRP and its receptor(s). All members of the CGRP superfamily discovered to date interact with seven-transmembrane domain G protein receptors *(4)*.

2.1. CGRP Receptor(s)

CGRP has been shown to selectively dilate multiple vascular beds, with the coronary vasculature being a particularly sensitive target *(1,2,8,9)*. Systemic administration of CGRP decreases blood pressure (BP) in a dose-dependent manner in normotensive and hypertensive animals and humans *(2,9)*. The primary mechanism responsible for this reduction in BP is peripheral arterial dilation. The CGRP (and ADM) receptor(s) are coupled to G proteins and in a number of tissues, including vascular smooth muscle, CGRP increases intracellular cAMP. Other reports indicate that CGRP is capable of activating ATP-sensitive potassium (K-ATP) channels of vascular smooth muscle *(2,4,10)*. There is additional evidence that the vasodilator response evoked by CGRP is mediated, in part, by NO release and that various vascular beds differ in their dependence on the endothelium for the dilator response to CGRP. Therefore, CGRP can dilate blood vessels through endothelium-dependent and -independent mechanisms. Originally, two types of CGRP receptors were identified. The CGRP1 receptor was characterized by high affinity binding to the aforementioned CGRP antagonist $CGRP_{8-37}$, and the CGRP2 receptor was characterized by binding to the linear agonist analog diacetoaminomethylcysteine CGRP *(2,4)*.

The identification and characterization of the functional CGRP receptor(s) have since become very controversial, especially following the publication of the receptor activity modifying protein (RAMP) hypothesis *(11)*. This hypothesis states that both ADM and CGRP signal through the common receptor, calcitonin receptor-like receptor (CRLR). Ligand specificity is determined by the co-expression of either of two chaperone proteins RAMP1 (CGRP) or RAMP2 (ADM). Another RAMP (RAMP3) has also been postulated to confer ADM specificity to the CRLR. So far, three biological functions for RAMPs have been defined: they transport CRLR to the cell surface, define its pharmacology, and determine its glycosylation state. In light of the recent studies, it now appears that a functional CGRP (or ADM) receptor must include three proteins in a complex: the ligand binding, membrane-spanning protein (CRLR); a chaperone (RAMP1 or -2); and a third peptide, the receptor component protein (RCP), which couples the receptor to the cellular signal transduction pathway (12). The configuration of the CGRP receptor has been complicated further by the cloning of a canine orphan receptor (RDC-1) that was later identified as the putative CGRP1 receptor. Indeed, several pharmacological and functional studies suggest that there are additional CGRP and/or ADM receptors that have yet to be discovered (2,11,12).

2.2. Release of CGRP From Sensory Nerve Terminals

CGRP-rich nerve fibers are components of the primary afferent nervous system, comprising principally capsaicin-sensitive C- and Aδ-fiber nerves that respond to chemical, thermal, and mechanical stimuli (2,10,13). Although these nerves have traditionally been thought to "sense" stimuli in the periphery and transmit the information centrally, there was early evidence that they also have an efferent function. It is clear that DRG neuron-derived peptides are released at peripheral sensory nerve terminals in the absence of afferent nerve stimulation (13). The continuous release of peptides from DRG neurons may reflect a paracrine function implying that these neurons participate in the continuous regulation of blood flows and other tissue activities. Indeed, it has been postulated that some DRG neurons are specialized in controlling peripheral effector mechanisms, but have no role in sensation (13). Sensory nerve terminals can release CGRP in response to local factors including nerve growth factor (NGF) (10,14), vascular wall tension (10,13), bradykinin/prostaglandins (15,16), endothelin, and the sympathetic nervous system (17). Our laboratory has demonstrated that these same factors that alter the acute release of CGRP can also modulate the long-term production and release of this peptide. Using primary cultures of adult rat DRG neurons, we have reported that NGF or bradykinin/prostaglandins (15,16) can stimulate CGRP synthesis and release, whereas glucocorticoids (18) or α_2-adrenoreceptor agonists (14) inhibit the stimulatory effects of NGF on CGRP. Thus, alterations in these factors, some of which are known to occur in hypertension, may mediate any changes seen in CGRP expression.

3. ROLE OF CGRP IN HYPERTENSION

Although CGRP administration can markedly decrease high BP in humans (2,7), it is not clear what role CGRP plays in human hypertension. Data concerning circulating levels of iCGRP in hypertensive humans have been conflicting. These results have been attributed to several factors including the assay itself, heterogenity of the disease, severity and duration of the hypertension, the degree of end organ damage, and the variety of treatment regimens used in these patients. In contrast, a direct role for CGRP in experimental hypertension has now been established. Earlier reports demonstrate that CGRP can attenuate chronic hypoxic pulmonary hypertension (PH) (19) and we have, for the first time, demonstrated that CGRP acts as a compensatory depressor mechanism to partially attenuate the BP increase in three models of experimental hypertension: (1) deoxycorticosterone (DOC-salt; 20,21), (2) subtotal nephrectomy (SN-salt; 22), and (3) N^G-nitro-L-arginine methyl ester (L-NAME)-induced hypertension during pregnancy

(23). A similar role for CGRP has also been shown in the two-kidney one-clip model *(24)*. In contrast, in the spontaneously hypertensive rat (SHR) CGRP may contribute to the development and maintenance of high blood pressure in this genetic model of hypertension *(25)*. Because these studies were done acutely, the important question regarding the long-term participation of CGRP in hypertension is not known. We are currently using α-CGRP knockout (KO) mice to address this issue. Each of the different rat models as well as studies on the α-CGRP KO mice will be described in a separate section.

3.1. Role of CGRP in DOC-Salt-Induced Hypertension

The first evidence that CGRP plays a role in systemic hypertension was provided by studies using the DOC-salt rat *(20,21)*. For these studies, we used DOC-salt rats during the onset stage (4 wk after the initiation of the protocol) and four groups of normotensive rats to control for pellet implantation, uninephrectomy, and/or salt administration. In our initial studies, we demonstrated that CGRP mRNA accumulation was significantly increased in DRG, and correspondingly, iCGRP levels were elevated in laminae I/II of the spinal cord compared to the control groups. Furthermore, this increase in neuronal CGRP expression in the DOC-salt rats was specific for the DRG, because we did not observe any alterations in the brain or in the brainstem. In order to determine if these changes in CGRP were playing an important hemodynamic role, groups of rats had intravenous (for drug administration) and arterial (for continuous mean arterial pressure, MAP) catheters surgically placed and were studied in the conscious, unrestrained state. As shown in Fig. 1, injection of saline did not alter MAP in any of the five groups, and $CGRP_{8-37}$ (the CGRP receptor antagonist) administration did not significantly increase MAP in any of the four normotensive control groups. However, administration of the CGRP antagonist to the DOC-salt rats rapidly induced, in a dose-dependent manner, a further increase of the elevated MAP. The rapid onset of the hypertensive effects of $CGRP_{8-37}$ and because of the antagonist probably does not penetrate the central nervous system, it is likely that the pressor activity of $CGRP_{8-37}$ results from a direct interaction of the antagonist with vascular CGRP receptors. These data support the hypothesis that, in DOC-salt hypertension, CGRP is acting as a compensatory depressor to buffer the increased BP.

3.2. Role of CGRP in SN-Salt-Induced Hypertension

To determine if the compensatory depressor effect of CGRP could be observed in a second model of hypertension we, therefore, examined the effect of endogenous CGRP on blood pressure in SN-salt-induced hypertension, another type of low-renin, salt-dependent hypertension *(22)*. SN-salt and normotensive controls were instrumented and given saline or $CGRP_{8-37}$ as described earlier (Fig. 2). The effects of two doses of $CGRP_{8-37}$ in the control group were similar to those observed with saline, which did not significantly alter the MAP. In contrast, administration of the antagonist to the SN-salt rats produced a dose-dependent increase of the elevated MAP similar to what was observed in the DOC-salt rats. These results suggest that, in this setting, CGRP is also playing a compensatory depressor role. Surprisingly, when the CGRP mRNA and peptide levels were quantified in the DRG from hypertensive and control rats, there were no detectable differences. These results suggested a second mechanism by which CGRP exerts its counterregulatory action. As opposed to increased CGRP synthesis and release,

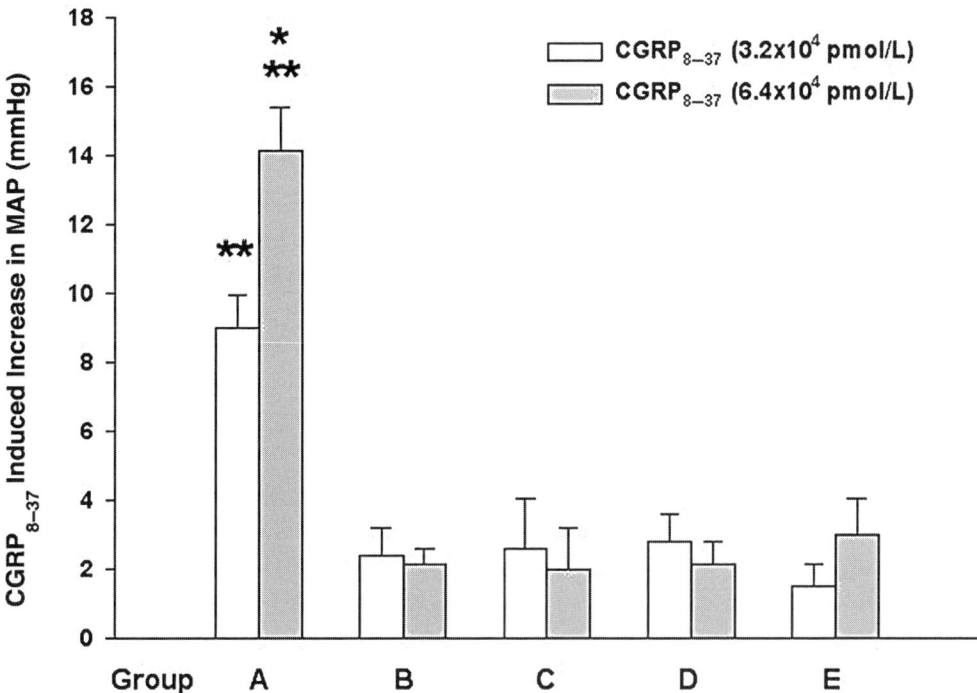

Fig. 1. $CGRP_{8-37}$ increases MAP in DOC-salt hypertensive rats but not in the controls. Rats were instrumented for continuous MAP recording and $CGRP_{8-37}$ administration. With the rats fully awake and unrestrained, bolus doses of the indicated amounts of the antagonist were given intravenously. $**p < 0.001$, DOC-salt (group A) vs each of the four control groups at both doses; $*p < 0.01$, higher vs lower dose of $CGRP_{8-37}$ in DOC-salt rats. MAP values are reported as the mean ± SEM.

this effect is mediated through an increase in vascular responsiveness to CGRP. This was shown in vivo where SN-salt hypertensive rats displayed a significantly greater dose-dependent depressor response (as a percent of baseline) to exogenous CGRP than did the controls (26). The hypertensive rats were also markedly more sensitive to the hypotensive effects of exogenous ADM than the control animals (unpublished observations). Furthermore, in vitro studies using isolated blood vessels from SN-salt and control rats showed that the vessel preparations from the hypertensive animals were much more sensitive to the dilator effect of CGRP compared to vessels from the normotensive control rats (26). The mechanism underlying the increased vascular responsiveness to CGRP (and ADM) in this setting is currently under investigation.

3.3. Role of CGRP in L-NAME-Induced Hypertension During Pregnancy

The purpose of this series of experiments was to determine the involvement of CGRP in the vascular adaptations that occur in normal pregnancy and its role in hypertensive L-NAME-treated female rats. Yallampalli et al. (27) has demonstrated that the inhibition of NO synthesis with L-NAME in pregnant rats causes hypertension, proteinuria, fetal growth retardation, and increased fetal mortality. The co-administration of CGRP with the L-NAME prevented the gestational, but not the postpartum hypertension and the proteinuria; and also significantly decreased pup mortality. Further studies revealed that this differential effect of CGRP on BP during gestation and postpartum is mediated

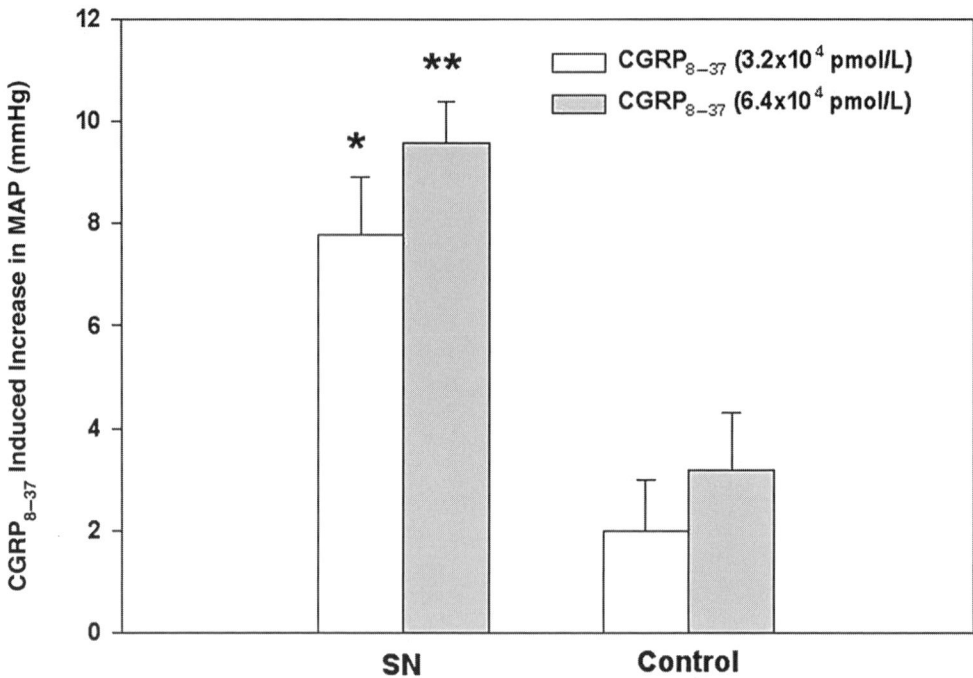

Fig. 2. CGRP$_{8-37}$ increases MAP in the SN-hypertensive rats but not in the controls. Rats were instrumented for continuous MAP recording and antagonist administration. With the rats fully awake and unrestrained, bolus doses of CGRP$_{8-37}$ were given intravenously. MAP values are reported as the mean ± SEM. *$p < 0.01$, SN-hypertensive rats vs control rats at the higher CGRP$_{8-37}$ dose.

by progesterone *(23)*. Similar to the findings in postpartum rats, CGRP reversed the hypertension in L-NAME-treated ovx rats receiving progesterone injections. Therefore, these studies suggest that CGRP is antihypertensive in L-NAME-treated pregnant and non-pregnant rats and that the vasodilator effects of CGRP are modulated by progesterone. To determine whether endogeneous CGRP participates in BP regulation in the L-NAME-treated pregnant rats, the treated (starting from day 17 of gestation) and control pregnant rats were instrumented and given the CGRP antagonist (Fig. 3). In summary, baseline BP was higher in the L-NAME-treated than the control rats on days 19, 20, and 21 of pregnancy and postpartum day 1. CGRP$_{8-37}$ did not change BP in the control groups. However, antagonist administration to the L-NAME-treated rats further increased BP on days 19, 20, and 21 of pregnancy but was without effect on postpartum day 1. Furthermore, CGRP mRNA and peptide levels in DRG were not different between the L-NAME-treated and control rats at any point of time studied. These data indicate that CGRP also plays a counterregulatory role in a salt-independent model. Although the mechanism by which this occurs has not been elucidated, it appears that the sensitivity of the vasculature to CGRP is enhanced in this model, and that this is mediated, at least in part, by progesterone.

3.4. Role of CGRP in the SHR

In contrast to the acquired models of hypertension described earlier, we observed a marked decrease in DRG CGRP expression in 12-wk-old SHRs compared to normotensive

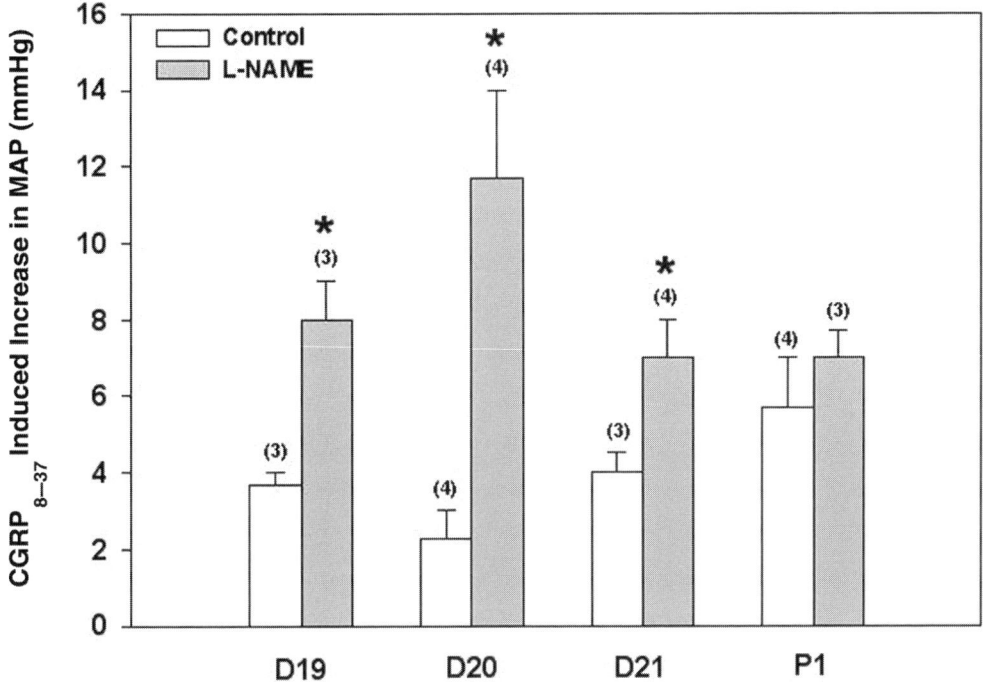

Fig. 3. CGRP$_{8-37}$ increases MAP in the L-NAME-treated pregnant rats. Animals were instrumented for continuous MAP recording and antagonist administration on days 19, 20, and 21 (D19–D21) of pregnancy and postpartum day 1 (P1). With the animals in a fully awake and unrestrained state, bolus doses of 100 μg CGRP$_{8-37}$ were given. Changes in MAP values are reported as the mean ± SEM. *$p < 0.05$.

Wistar Kyoto (WKY) rats *(25)*. Moreover, this reduction in neuronal CGRP was age related and correlated well with the increase in blood pressure that occurs between 5 and 12 wk of age *(2,7)*. These results suggested that the age-related decrease in neuronal CGRP expression in the SHRs could contribute to the elevated blood pressure through the loss of a potent vasodilator. We therefore proposed that NGF administration to SHR would decrease the blood pressure through the stimulation of CGRP synthesis in DRG *(25)*. NGF was administered by intraperitoneal injection to 12-wk-old SHRs. NGF was given once on days 1, 3, and 7. A separate group of control SHRs received vehicle only. At the end of each treatment period, the animals were instrumented for continuous MAP recording and infusion of saline or CGRP$_{8-37}$. After a single NGF treatment (day 1), the MAP was reduced by 21 ± 2 mmHg compared to the control SHRs. The MAP was still reduced by 22 ± 3 mmHg on day 3; however, by day 7 the MAP had returned to control levels. To determine whether any of the MAP reduction observed on days 1 and 3 was owing to CGRP, during the course of the MAP determinations each animal was treated (iv) with either saline or the CGRP receptor antagonist. Neither the saline in the controls or NGF-treated SHRs, nor the CGRP$_{8-37}$ in the control SHRs significantly changed the MAP. However, on days 1 and 3 of NGF treatment, CGRP$_{8-37}$ produced a 12.7 ± 2.2 and 11.6 ± 2.1 mmHg increase in MAP on these days, respectively. Unexpectedly, on day 7 when the MAP was back up to control levels, antagonist treatment still resulted in an 11.7 ± 2.4 mmHg increase in MAP. When we examined CGRP mRNA levels in DRG from the control and NGF-treated rats, there was a significant twofold increase on days 1, 3, and 7. CGRP peptide levels in DRG displayed a similar increase. Therefore, NGF treatment on days 1 and 3 produces a significant 21 mmHg decrease in MAP. About half of this MAP reduction is because of CGRP as determined by blockade of the CGRP receptor. This action of CGRP most likely results from the enhanced release and production of this peptide. These results (days 1 and 3) strongly suggest that the decreased production of CGRP that is observed in the SHRs could contribute to the elevated BP. After a week of NGF treatment, CGRP synthesis is still elevated. Antagonist administration indicates that CGRP is continuing to play a compensatory role, but the MAP has returned to control levels. The continued activity of $CGRP_{8-37}$ argues against downregulation of the CGRP receptor as the cause for the increase in MAP on day 7. One possibility is that the enhanced production of CGRP is acting to decrease the MAP on days 1, 3, and 7. However, by day 7, NGF may have stimulated a pressor system to counteract the depressor effects of CGRP and brought back the MAP up to control levels. The sympathetic nervous system and neuropeptide Y are the two candidates that are upregulated by NGF.

3.5. Role of CGRP in Two-Kidney, One-Clip Hypertension

Recently, the role of capsaicin-sensitive sensory nerves in two-kidney, one-clip (2K1C) renovascular hypertension has been investigated (24). Systolic blood pressure (measured by the tail-cuff method) was significantly elevated approx 25% in the 2K1C group compared to control rats 10 d following the initiation of the protocol. Treatment with capsaicin, which selectively depletes neuropeptides in sensory nerves, enhanced the hypertensive response to the procedure by another 20% at the same time period. A second injection of capsaicin produced an additional 25% increase in systolic blood pressure compared to the rats that had received a single injection at the second time point (30 d postoperative). The expression of α-CGRP mRNA in DRG, the level of CGRP in the plasma, and the density of CGRP immunoreactive fibers in mesenteric artery were all significantly increased in the 2K1C rats compared to the sham-operated controls. Treatment with capsaicin prevented the increase in CGRP expression in the hypertensive rats. Based on these results the authors concluded that in this model of renovascular hypertension the activity of capsaicin-sensitive sensory nerves is increased, via an upregulation of α-CGRP synthesis and release, as a compensatory response to partially counteract the increase in blood pressure.

3.6. Role of CGRP in Chronic Hypoxic Pulmonary Hypertension

As described previously, CGRP participates in the regulation of regional organ blood flows both under normal physiological conditions and in the pathophysiology of various disease states. For example, in the lung, CGRP plays a critical role in modulating local pulmonary vascular tone. An excellent review describing the role of CGRP and other endogenous lung neuropeptides in the regulation of the pulmonary circulation has been published (28). Indeed, to the best of our knowledge, the first report demonstrating a role for CGRP in hypertension of any type was a study showing that CGRP and somatostatin modulate PH. Two earlier clinical studies suggested that CGRP might be involved in the pathophysiology of this disease (29,30). However, for this review we focus on studies using rodent models of PH and the antihypertensive effects of CGRP. Chronic hypoxic PH, associated with increased pulmonary arterial pressure and right ventricular hypertrophy, correlates significantly with CGRP levels in lung and blood *(19,29,30)*. In this series of experiments CGRP, its antibody, and the CGRP receptor antagonist $CGRP_{8-37}$ were infused into the pulmonary circulation of hypobaric hypoxia rats on days 4, 8, and 16. Pulmonary arterial pressure was then measured in the right ventricle and in the main pulmonary artery. Chronic CGRP infusion prevented PH at all time points, whereas, immunoneutralization and receptor blockade exacerbated PH. Additional in vitro pharmacological studies demonstrated that CGRP exerts a receptor mediated nonadrenergic, nonmuscarinic vasodilator effect in the lung, which is independent of endothelium-derived relaxing factor and does not involve ATP-dependent potassium channels. Taken together, these data indicated that endogenous CGRP plays an important role in pulmonary pressure homeostasis during hypoxia, by directly dilating the pulmonary vasculature, thus attenuating the development of chronic hypoxic PH in rats.

More recent reports from this same group *(19)* as well as other investigators have confirmed these initial findings. For example, rats were pretreated with capsaicin to deplete stores of sensory neuropeptides, primarily CGRP and substance P, and placed in hypobaric hypoxia or normoxia for 16 d together with control animals *(31)*. Hypoxia increased PH, right ventricular hypertrophy, arterial medial thickness, elasticized capillaries, endothelial cell density, lung water, and hematocrit in control rats. Capsaicin augmented PH and right ventricular hypertrophy in hypoxia, and medial thickness and endothelial cell density in both normoxia and hypoxia. Because of the limited effects on these parameters by substance P and other capsacin-sensitive lung agents, these results demonstrated that a sensory nerve deficit of CGRP severely exacerbates hypoxic PH. In contrast, pulmonary overexpression of CGRP via in vivo gene transfer, in a mouse model of hypoxia-induced PH significantly attenuated pulmonary arterial pressure, right ventricular hypertrophy, and pulmonary vascular remodeling in chronically hypoxic mice *(32,33)*. These data provide additional evidence that CGRP plays an important role in maintaining low pulmonary vascular resistance.

4. STUDIES IN THE α-CGRP KO MICE

The mouse model lacking the α-CGRP/CT gene was created by replacing exons 2–5 of the mouse CT I gene with PGK neoBPA *(34)*. Homologous recombination was confirmed by Southern analysis with 5′ and 3′ probes. The homozygous α-CGRP (–/–) breeding pairs were derived from an inbred strain on a 129/C57 genetic background. The KO mice were generated and kindly provided by Robert F. Gagel (M.D. Anderson Cancer Center, University of Texas, Houston). The α-CGRP KO mice are born normally, are fertile, and have a normal life span *(34)*. As shown in Fig. 4, α-CGRP mRNA was not detectable; β-CGRP mRNA was reduced twofold; and substance P mRNA was unchanged as determined by Northern blot analysis of DRGRNA preparations from the KO mice. Likewise, immunohistological staining revealed the absence of α-CGRP peptide in laminae I/II of the dorsal horn of the spinal cord from the α-CGRP KO mice *(35)*.

Systolic blood pressure was significantly higher in the KO mice ($n = 9$; 160 ± 6.1 mmHg) compared to controls ($n = 10$; 125 ± 5 mmHg). To confirm this finding, previously instrumented KO ($n = 9$) and wild type (WT; $n = 9$) fully awake and unrestrained mice (25–30 g males) were studied. The MAP was significantly elevated in the KO mice

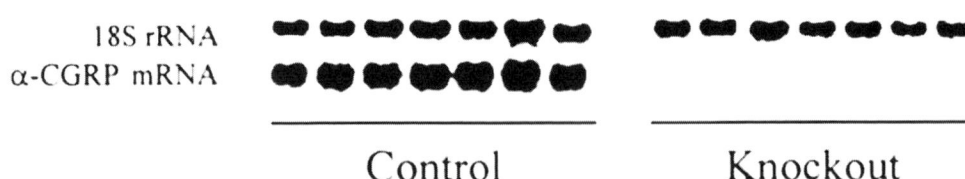

18S rRNA
α-CGRP mRNA

Control   Knockout

Fig. 4. Northern blot analysis of DRG RNA samples from α-CGRP KO and WT mice.

(139 ± 5 mmHg) compared to the controls (118 ± 4 mmHg). Because of serious concerns regarding the accuracy and reproducibility of acute blood pressure measurements in mice, it was necessary to confirm the blood pressure phenotype of these mice using long-term telemetric recording *(36)*. In agreement with our previous reports, telemetric MAP determination showed that basal average 24 h MAP was significantly higher in the α-CGRP KO mice (120 ± 3 mmHg, $n = 7$) compared to WT controls (107 ± 3 mmHg, $n = 7$) *(37)*. It should be noted that in order to delete the α-CGRP gene, it was also necessary to inactivate the calcitonin gene as well as katacalcin that is derived from the processing of the calcitonin peptide precursor *(2)*. It is important to note that it has been clearly demonstrated that endogenous calcitonin or katacalcin do not play a role in cardiovascular regulation *(2,7)*. A second KO mouse, specific for α-CGRP, has recently been generated, but on a different genetic background, by another investigator *(38)*. Interestingly these KO mice do not appear to display an increased baseline MAP. Another α-CGRP specific KO strain that has the same genetic background as the mice used in our study has been generated. In a recently published report, the CGRP null mice display a significantly elevated BP and heart rate compared to controls *(39)*. These latter results confirm our findings that basal MAP is elevated in the α-CGRP null mice.

4.1. Gross Postmortem and Histopathological Studies

Although the α-CGRP KO mice appear to have a normal phenotype *(34)* with the exception of an elevated basal MAP *(35)*, before using these animals for more extensive studies, a comprehensive pathological evaluation was performed to determine if there were any significant developmental or pathological changes in the absence of treatment *(40)*. No significant gross postmortem or histopathological alterations were detected in the body cavities, or integumentary, alimentary, respiratory, circulatory, urogenital, endocrine, hematopoetic, musculoskeletal, and nervous systems of the α-CGRP KO mice compared to their WT counterparts. In addition, there was no microscopic evidence of vascular alterations or vascular variations among the mice examined. The one exception to the results described above was that the heart to body weight ratio was increased approx 10% in the α-CGRP KO mice compared to the WT mice. This finding is consistent with data that we have published previously.

4.2. Role of CGRP in the Regulation of Coronary Blood Flow

In a seminal study concerning the nonadrenergic noncholinergic regulation of basal coronary flow, Yaoita et al. *(41)* clearly demonstrated that capsaicin-sensitive neuropeptides (primarily CGRP) in the rat's heart provide approx 30% of basal coronary flow modulation. To provide additional evidence that α-CGRP plays a critical role in the

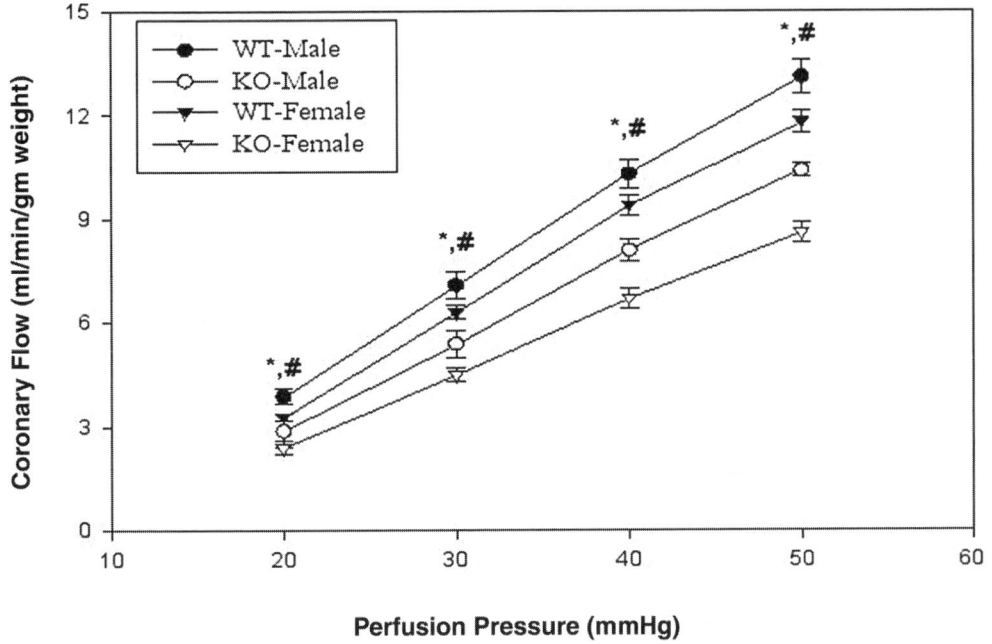

Fig. 5. Coronary flow rates are decreased in α-CGRP KO mice. Isolated perfused heart preparations were used to determine coronary flow rates at the indicated perfusion pressures. Data are expressed as the mean ± SEM. *$p < 0.05$ WT vs KO males and #$p < 0.05$ for WT vs KO females.

regulation of coronary blood flow, Langendorff-perfused heart preparations were used to compare coronary flow rates between α-CGRP KO and WT control mice under various pressure-loading conditions. Hearts from 33 mice (female, 6 KO and 9 WT; male, 8 KO and 10 WT) were used in this study. Deletion of the α-CGRP gene in both genders resulted in a significant reduction in the coronary flow at all pressures tested (Fig. 5). In addition, coronary flows for both strains of mice were consistently lower in female than in male mice. Therefore, these data suggest that CGRP is responsible for up to 30% of basal coronary blood flow. In addition, based on the histological analysis, there are no obvious structural or pathological alterations in the myocardium or coronary vasculature between the groups. Because blood vessel diameter is directly related to coronary flow, pilot studies were done to determine the range of blood vessel diameters (optical micrometer) in heart sections from the KO and WT mice. No detectable differences were observed between the two strains. Thus, the mechanism of this reduction in coronary flow is likely to decrease coronary vasodilation resulting from an ablation of α-CGRP from perivascular sensory nerve terminals.

4.3. CGRP is Protective Against Hypertension-Induced End Organ Damage

The results described above in Sections 4 and 4.2 demonstrate that the α-CGRP/CT deficient mice display a significant increase in basal blood pressure and a significant decrease in basal coronary flow rates. Hypertension-induced end organ damage is one of the most severe and common consequences of chronic increased blood pressure. Because CGRP has such potent biological effects on the heart and kidneys, and in light of several lines of indirect evidence suggesting that CGRP is an endogenous organ-protective agent

(42,43), the purpose of this study was to determine whether end organ damage is enhanced in the DOC-salt hypertensive α-CGRP KO mice compared to their hypertensive WT counterparts. After initiation of the DOC-salt protocol, the blood pressure, as determined by long-term telemetric recording, increased rapidly in both groups to final values of 166 ± 5 mmHg for the α-CGRP KO and 147 ± 4 mmHg for the WT mice *(36,44)*. When normalized to basal blood pressure this represents an approx 35% (and equal) increase in MAP for the two groups. The MAP was unchanged in the two control groups (unpublished observations). Both the α-CGRP KO and WT mice displayed a normal 24 h circadian rhythm, both before and after DOC-salt treatment, with the highest blood pressure and heart rate occurring near midnight and the lowest in the early afternoon.

At the conclusion of the blood pressure measurement studies, the mice were sacrificed and the hearts, kidneys, aortas, and femoral arteries were removed for histopathological examination *(44)*. As before, no changes were seen in the hearts and kidneys between the control α-CGRP KO and WT mice. Furthermore, no significant pathological changes were seen in the hearts and kidneys from the DOC-salt hypertensive WT mice compared to their normotensive controls. The only exception was that heart sections from both the DOC-salt hypertensive α-CGRP KO and WT mice displayed a marked increase in cardiac myocyte size. This result demonstrates left ventricular hypertrophy and is consistent with the increased heart-to-body weight ratios of the heats from the DOC-salt treated mice of both strains. In contrast, extensive damage was evident in the heart and kidney sections from the DOC-salt hypertensive α-CGRP KO mice. Marked (2+, in scale of 1+ to 4+) small vessel disease was seen in the heart sections from DOC-salt treated α-CGRP mice with thickening and inflammation of the vessel walls. Perivascular inflammation was also noted and the endothelial cells were prominent which is consistent with inflammation of this critical cell layer. In the myocardium, there were prominent 2+ myocarditis, myocardial necrosis, and foci of inflammation that extended to the epicardium. The kidneys of these mice showed marked 2+ glomerular changes including congestion of the capillary loops, focal mesangial proliferation, crescentic proliferation, and focal histocytic infiltration. Proteinaceous casts were also noted in a number of tubules.

These data demonstrate that deletion of the α-CGRP gene enhances hypertension-induced end organ damage in the heart and kidney. The mechanism of this increased tissue damage may be through the loss of CGRP-mediated vasodilator activity and/or to an increase in the local tissue production of reactive oxygen species. Indirect mechanisms such as activation of the sympathetic nervous system and/or the RAS system may also be involved. To our knowledge this is the first report of a sensory nerve-mediated cardio- and renal-protective effect against hypertension-induced end organ damage. Traditionally, sensory nerves were defined as purely afferent neurons that monitor changes in their chemical and physical environment and convey this information to the central nervous system. They also have the capacity to act in an efferent manner. This efferent function is mediated by the release of neuropeptides, including CGRP, from their peripheral terminals that regulate vasodilation and other tissue activities independently of sensation. Thus, this organ-protective activity of CGRP may reflect another significant function of the efferent arm of the sensory nervous system.

5. SUMMARY

In the four models of acquired hypertension that have been studied to date, CGRP appears to act as a compensatory vasodilator in an attempt to counteract the blood pressure increase. In the DOC-salt and 2K1C models, this activity appears to be mediated through a marked increase in the neuronal expression and release of this peptide. Likewise, in PH CGRP levels are elevated act to directly dilate the pulmonary vasculature, thus attenuating the development of chronic hypoxic PH in rats. The factors that cause this upregulation of CGRP have yet to be determined. The SN-salt and L-NAME models do not exhibit increases in CGRP expression, suggesting another mechanism by which this peptide could exert its antihypertensive effect. This second mechanism is enhanced sensitivity of the vasculature to CGRP that is likely regulated at the level of the vascular CGRP receptor complex. It is probable that CGRP is one of several counter-regulatory mechanisms that are stimulated in hypertension. In contrast, in genetic hypertension such as in the SHR, several studies demonstrate that there is a marked downregulation of CGRP. Although this decrease in CGRP expression is probably not the primary cause of hypertension in this model, the decrease in such a potent vasodilator could contribute to the elevated blood pressure.

The inability of $CGRP_{8-37}$ to alter blood pressure in control rats implies that CGRP does not participate in the regulation of basal systemic blood pressure in the normotensive state, but this does not rule out a role for CGRP in the modulation of regional organ blood flows under normal physiological conditions. CGRP participates in the modulation of blood flow in the gut and, as described previously, is responsible for approx 30% of basal coronary blood flow. Studies in the α-CGRP KO mice confirm the pivotal role of CGRP in the regulation of basal coronary flows. In addition, our laboratory has novel data showing a protective action of CGRP against hypertension-induced damage in the heart and kidney. Unlike the rat models in which CGRP activity was blocked acutely, permanent deletion of the α-CGRP gene does produce a significant increase in basal blood pressure. The reason for this discrepancy is currently under investigation.

Although a definitive role for CGRP has yet to be established, the weight of the evidence supports a role for this neuropeptide in the modulation of vasorelaxation in states of increased peripheral resistance or in an increase in blood flow to critical areas like the renal, coronary, and cerebral circulations. Under these conditions, it appears that activation of perivascular sensory nerves stimulates the release of neuropeptides that, in turn, regulates vascular tone, redistributes blood flow, and perhaps modulates systemic blood pressure. CGRP has also been implicated in other cardiovascular disease states such as congestive heart failure, myocardial infarction, ischemia/reperfusion injury, as well as other pathological conditions that produce significant alterations in cardiovascular functions *(1–7)*.

REFERENCES

1. Brain, S. D., William, T. J., Tippins, J. R., Morris, H. R., and MacIntyre, I. (1985) Calcitonin gene-related peptide is a potent vasodilator. *Nature* **313**, 54–56.
2. Wimalawansa, S. J. (1996) Calcitonin gene-related peptide and its receptors: molecular genetics, physiology, pathophysiology, and therapeutic potentials. *Endocr. Rev.* **17**, 533–585.
3. Breimer, L. H., MacIntyre, I., and Zaidi, M. (1988) Peptides from the calcitonin genes: molecular genetics, structure and function. *Biochem. J.* **255**, 377–390.

 4. Brown, M. J. and Morice, A. H. (1987) Clinical pharmacology of vasodilator peptides. *J. Cardiovasc. Pharmacol.* **10(12),** 582–590.
 5. Dockray, G. J. (1994) Physiology of enteric neuropeptides. In: *Physiology of the Gastrointestinal Tract* (Johnson, L. R., ed.), Raven, New York, p. 169.
 6. Gibson, S. J., Polak, J. M., Bloom, S. R., et al. (1984) Calcitonin gene-related peptide immuno-reactivity in the spinal cord of man and eight other species. *J. Neurosci.* **12,** 3101–3111.
 7. DiPette, D. J. and Wimalawansa, S. J. (1994) Cardiovascular actions of calcitonin gene-related peptide. In: *Calcium Regulating Hormones and Cardiovascular Function* (Crass, J. and Avioli, L. V., eds.), CRC, Ann Arbor, p. 239.
 8. Asimakis, G. K., DiPette, D. J., Conti, V. R., Holland, O. B., and Zwishenberger, J. B. (1987) Hemodynamic action of calcitonin gene-related peptide in the isolated rat heart. *Life Sci.* **41,** 597–603.
 9. DiPette, D. J., Schwarzenberger, K., Kerr, N., and Holland, O. B. (1989) Dose dependent systemic and regional hemodynamic effects of calcitonin gene-related peptide. *Am. J. Med. Sci.* **297,** 65–70.
10. Holzer, P. (1988) Local effector functions of capsaicin-sensitive sensory nerve endings: involvement of tackykinins, calcitonin gene-related peptide and other neuropeptides. *Neuroscience* **45,** 739–768.
11. Foord, S. M. and Marshall, F. H. (1999) RAMPS: accessory proteins for seven transmembrane domain receptors. *TIPS* **20,** 184–187.
12. Evans, B. N., Rosenblatt, M. I., Mnayer, L. O., Oliver, K. R., and Dickerson, I. M. (2000) CGRP-RCP, a novel protein required at CGRP and adrenomedullin receptors. *J. Biol. Chem.* **275,** 31,438–31,443.
13. Holzer, P. and Maggi, C. A. (1998) Dissociation of dorsal root ganglion neurons into afferent and efferent like neurons. *Neuroscience* **86,** 389–398.
14. Supowit, S. C., Hallman, D. M., Zhao, H., and DiPette, D. J. (1998) α_2-adrenoreceptor activation inhibits neuronal calcitonin gene-related peptide expression. *Brain Res.* **782,** 184–193.
15. Vasko, M. R., Campbell, W. B., and Waite, K. G. (1994) Prostaglandin E$_2$ enhances bradykinin stimulated release of neuropeptides from rat sensory neurons in culture. *J. Neurosci.* **14,** 4987–4997.
16. Supowit, S. C., Hallman, D. M., Zhao, H., and DiPette, D. J. (1995) Bradykinin regulates neuronal calcitonin gene-related peptide expression and release. *Hypertension* **26,** 564.
17. Kawasaki, H., Nuki, C., and Saito, A. (1990) Adrenergic modulation of calcitonin gene-related peptide (CGRP) containing nerve-mediated vasodilation in the rat mesenteric resistance vessel. *Brain Res.* **506,** 287–292.
18. Supowit, S. C., Christensen, M. D., Westlund, K. N., Hallman, D. M., and DiPette, D. J. (1995) Dexamethasone and activators of the protein kinase A and C signal transduction pathways regulate neuronal calcitonin gene-related peptide expression and release. *Brain Res.* **686,** 77–86.
19. Looi, S., Ekman, R., Lippton, J. C., and Keith, I. (1992) CGRP and somatostatin modulate chronic pulmonary hypertension. *Am. J. Physiol.* **263,** H681–H690.
20. Supowit, S. C., Guraraj, A., Ramana, C. V., Westlund, K. N., and DiPette, D. J. (1995) Enhanced neuronal expression of calcitonin gene-related peptide in mineralocorticoid-salt hypertension. *Hypertension* **25,** 1333–1338.
21. Supowit, S. C., Zhao, H., Hallman, D. M., and DiPette, D. J. (1997) Calcitonin gene-related peptide is a depressor of deoxycorticosterone-salt hypertension in the rat. *Hypertension* **29,** 945–950.
22. Supowit, C., Zhao, H., Hallman, D. M., and DiPette, D. J. (1998) Calcitonin gene-related peptide is a depressor in subtotal nephrectomy hypertension. *Hypertension* **31(2),** 391–396.
23. Gangula, P. R., Supowit, S. C., Wimalawansa, S. J., et al. (1997) Calcitonin gene-related peptide is a depressor in N^G-nitro-L-arginine methyl ester (L-NAME)-induced preeclampsia. *Hypertension* **29,** 248–253.
24. Deng, P. Y., Ye, F., Zhu, H. Q., Cai, W. J., Deng, H. W., and Li, Y.J. (2003) An increase in the synthesis and release of calcitonin gene-related peptide in two-kidney, one-clip hypertensive rats. *Regul. Pept.* **114,** 175–182.
25. Supowit, S. C., Zhao, H., and DiPette, D. J. (2001) Nerve growth factor enhances calcitonin gene-related peptide expression in the SHR. Hypertension **37,** 728–732.
26. Supowit, S. C., Watts, S. C., Zhao, H., Wang, D., and DiPette, D. J. (2000) Vascular reactivity to calcitonin gene-related peptide is enhanced in subtotal nephrectomy-salt hypertension. *Hypertension* **36,** 701.
27. Yallampalli, C., Dong, YU.-L., and Wimalawansa, S. J. (1996) Calcitonin gene-related peptide reverses the hypertension and significantly decreases the fetal mortality in preeclampsia rats induced by N^G-nitro-L-arginine methyl ester. *Hum. Reprod.* **11,** 895–899.
28. Keith, I. M. (2000) The role of endogenous lung peptides in regulation of the pulmonary circulation. *Physiol. Res.* **49,** 519–537.

29. Allen, K. M., Wharton, J., Polak, J. M., and Haworth, S. G. (1989) A study of nerves containing peptides in the pulmonary circulation of healthy infants and children of those with pulmonary hypertension. *Br. Heart J.* **62,** 353–360.
30. Uren, N. G., Ludman, P. F., Crake, T., and Oakley, C. M. (1992) Response of the pulmonary circulation to acetylcholine, calcitonin gene-related peptide, substance P, and oral nicardipine in patients with primary pulmonary hypertension. *J. Am. Coll. Cardiol.* **19,** 835–841.
31. Tjen-A-Looi, S., Kraiczi, H., Ekman, R., and Keith, I. M. (1998) Sensory CGRP depletion exacerbates hypoxia-induced pulmonary hypertension in rats. *Regul. Pept.* **74,** 1–10.
32. Bivalacqua, T. J., Hyman, A. L., Kadowitz, P. J., Paolocci, N., Kass, D. A., and Champion, H. C. (2002) Role of CGRP in chronic hypoxia-induced pulmonary hypertension in the mouse. Influence of gene transfer in vivo. *Regul. Pept.* **108,** 129–133.
33. Champion, H. C., Toyoda, K., Deistad, D. D., Hyman, A. L., and Kadowitz, P. J. (2000) In vivo gene transfer of prepro-calcitonin gene-related peptide to the lung attenuates chronic hypoxia-induced pulmonary hypertension in the mouse. *Circulation* **101,** 923–930.
34. Hoff, A. O., Thomas, P. M., Cote, G. J., Qiu, H., Bain, H., and Gagel, R. F. (1998) Generation of a calcitonin knockout mouse model. *Bone* **23,** S64.
35. Gangula, P. R., Zhao, H., Supowit, S. C., et al. (2000) Increased blood pressure in α-calcitonin gene-related peptide/calcitonin gene knockout mice. *Hypertension* **35,** 470–475.
36. Carlson, S. H. and Wyss, M. (2000) Long-term telemetric recording of arterial pressure and heart rate in mice fed basal and high NaCl diets. *Hypertension* **35,** E1–E5.
37. Zhao, H., Fink, G., DiPette, D. J., and Supowit, S. C. (2003) Telemetric recording of basal blood pressure and circadian rhythm in α-calcitonin gene-related peptide knockout mice. *Hypertension* **3,** 412.
38. Lu, J. T., Young-Jin, S., Lee, J., et al. (1999) Mice lacking α-calcitonin gene-related peptide exhibit normal cardiovascular regulation and neuromuscular development. *Mol. Cell Neurosci.* **14,** 99–120.
39. Oh-hashi, Y., Shindo, T., Kurihara, Y., et al. (2001) Elevated sympathetic nervous activity in mice deficient in α-CGRP. *Circ. Res.* **89,** 983–995.
40. Ma, H., Huang, R., Abela, G. S., et al. (2002) Coronary flow is decreased in the α-calcitonin gene-related peptide knockout mouse. *Hypertension* **40,** 384.
41. Yaoita, H., Sato, E., Kawaguchi, M., Saito, T., Maehara, K., and Maruyama, Y. (1994) Nonadrenergic noncholinergic nerves regulate basal coronary flow via release of capsaicin-sensitive neuropeptides in the rat heart. *Circ. Res.* **75,** 780–788.
42. Nishikimi, T., Mori, Y., Kobayashi, N., et al. (2002) Renoprotective effect of chronic adrenomedullin infusion in Dahl salt-sensitive rats. *Hypertension* **39,** 1077–1082.
43. Mori, Y., Nishikimi, T., Kobayashi, N., Ono, H., Kangawa, K., and Matsuoka, H. (2002) Long-term adrenomedullin infusion improves survival in malignant hypertensive rats. *Hypertension* **40,** 107–113.
44. Supowit, S. C., Rao, A. R., Bowers, M., et al. (2005) Calciton gene-related peptide protects against hypertension-induced heart and kidney damage. *Hypertension* **45,** 109–114.

10 The Renal Dopaminergic System, Hypertension, and Salt Sensitivity

Robin A. Felder, Robert M. Carey, and Pedro A. Jose

CONTENTS

1. INTRODUCTION

The kidney is the primary organ responsible for the long-term control of blood pressure by regulating sodium and chloride transport. Various renal autocrine/paracrine and endocrine mechanisms have evolved to increase or decrease sodium reabsorption in different segments of the nephron *(1,2)*.

Sodium chloride balance and blood pressure are the result of the interaction of many factors, such as the sympathetic nervous system and various interacting hormonal systems, such as the renin-angiotensin system and nitric oxide system. Short-term regulation of blood pressure by the kidney is mainly controlled by the autonomic nervous system using finely tuned, complex feed forward and feedback systems [reviewed elsewhere *(3)*]. Long-term regulation of blood pressure involves many of the same mechanisms involved with short-term blood pressure regulation, including the sympathetic nervous system *(4)* and the renin–angiotensin system *(4–9)*. However, for long-term regulation the blood volume involves slower cellular adaptive processes, such as upregulation and downregulation of cell surface receptors and their intracellular effectors *(10)* to increase or decrease sodium

From: *Contemporary Endocrinology: Hypertension and Hormone Mechanisms*
Edited by: R. M. Carey © Humana Press Inc., Totowa, NJ

reabsorption in the kidney. Because the kidney is such a key organ in the long-term regulation of blood pressure, many studies have focused on abnormal renal handling of sodium chloride in the pathogenesis of essential hypertension *(9,10)*, specifically, the increased sodium transport in the renal proximal tubule and medullary thick ascending limb *(11–13)*. Two principal pathways, the renin–angiotensin pathway *(7)* and the dopaminergic system *(14–26)*, are responsible for increasing or decreasing sodium reabsorption. These pathways may be antagonized or abetted by other systems, e.g., nitric oxide and endothelin.

2. RENAL DOPAMINE AND AUTOCRINE/PARACRINE FUNCTION

During the past decade dopamine has been shown to be an active modulator of sodium balance, by actions in the adrenal gland *(27,28)*, intestinal *(29–31)* and renal epithelia *(11,14–26,33–82)*, and sympathetic nervous system *(83)*. Although the dopaminergic system is active in various anatomic locations, the concentrations of dopamine found circulating in the blood (picomolar) are not high enough to activate the dopamine receptor because nanomolar concentrations are required for receptor activation. However, high nanomolar concentrations of dopamine can be generated locally by the conversion of L-DOPA found in the circulation to dopamine by L-aromatic amino acid decarboxlase found in dopamine-producing tissues (e.g., renal proximal tubule and jejunum). In the proximal tubule, dopamine does not become converted to norepinephrine (as in neurons) because renal tubules do not express dopamine β-hydroxylase. Dopamine produced intracellularly is then secreted into the tubular lumen, to a greater extent than in the peritubular areas, in which it acts as an autocrine/paracrine hormone to regulate sodium and chloride transport in the renal proximal tubule, thick ascending limb of Henle, and cortical collecting duct.

Long-term sodium (and chloride) balance during moderate sodium surfeit is regulated by locally generated dopamine, which acts on renal tubular and jejunal cells to decrease sodium transport. The dopaminergic renal control mechanism has a major impact on overall sodium balance because over 50% of incremental sodium excretion that occurs with increased sodium intake is regulated by dopamine receptors *(39,41,74,77,78,84)*. Renal hemodynamic mechanisms contribute to the increase in sodium excretion associated with protein loading *(171)*. However, the paracrine/autocrine dopaminergic regulation of sodium excretion during sodium surfeit is mediated by tubular but not by hemodynamic mechanisms *(42,74)*. Systemically administered dopaminergic drugs increase sodium excretion by both hemodynamic and tubular mechanisms. The clinical practice of systemically administering dopaminergic drugs during shock may not mimic the autocrine/paracrine function of dopamine because high doses of dopamine result in concentrations that can activate nondopaminergic receptors, such as the serotonin, α and β adrenergic receptors.

3. DOPAMINE RECEPTOR SUBTYPES

The two known families of dopamine receptors, the D_1-like and the D_2-like *(26,43–45,85,86)*, are structurally similar to all the G protein-coupled receptors in that they have seven-transmembrane domains with cytoplasmic carboxy terminal domains and a glycosylated extracellular amino terminal domain. The D_1-like receptor family consists of the D_1 and D_5 subtypes. Because the central D_1 and D_5 receptors have the same primary structure as the peripheral dopamine receptors (D_{1A} and D_{1B}, respectively in rodents) *(87)*, distinguishing "central" from "peripheral" dopamine receptors is no longer necessary. Despite similar affinities for dopamine, the distinct actions of the D_1 and D_5 receptors are a result of differential coupling to various intracellular G proteins associated with increases in intracellular enzymatic activity. For example, both the D_1 and D_5 couple to intracellular adenylyl cyclase to increase the conversion of ATP to cyclic adenosine monophosphate (cAMP) which in turn stimulates numerous intracellular events *(87)*. However, the D_1 receptor (in the presence of calcyon) but not the D_5 receptor activates phospholipase C leading to the generation of inositol phosphates and diacylglycerol.

The D_2-like dopamine receptor family consists of the D_2, D_3, and D_4 receptors, all which couple to the inhibitory G proteins $G\alpha_i$ and G_o. Unlike the D_1 receptors, the D_2-like receptors inhibit adenylyl cyclase and calcium channel activities, and modulate potassium channel activity *(45,88,89)*.

4. RENAL DOPAMINE RECEPTORS

The kidney is richly endowed with members of all the dopamine receptor subtypes. Prejunctional nerves are endowed with D_4 receptor *(88)*. Within the renal arterioles, the D_2, D_3, and D_4 receptors are located in the adventitia and the adventitia-media junction *(89)*, though the D_1, D_3, and D_5 receptors are expressed in the tunica media *(59,89)*. The expression of dopamine receptors in the endothelial cell layer in renal arterioles has not been described but the D_3 receptor is expressed in the endothelium of rat mesenteric arteries *(89)*. D_3 and D_4, but not D_1 and D_5, receptors are present in glomeruli *(57,59,89,90)*. The proximal tubule expresses D_1, D_5, D_3, and D_4 receptors *(54,57,59, 64,72,80,81,88)*. The medullary but not the cortical thick ascending limb of Henle expresses D_1, D_5, and D_3 receptors *(15,59,89,90)*. The collecting ducts (cortical and medullary) express D_1, D_5, D_3, and D_4 receptors *(57,59,75,89,90,92)*. The macula densa and juxtaglomerular cell express D_1 and D_3 receptors *(37,91,92)*. There may be species differences because the D_1 receptor is not expressed in human juxtaglomerular cells *(64)*.

Dopamine inhibits sodium transport at multiple sites along the nephron and acts on multiple transporters within each nephron segment such as the sodium hydrogen exchangers (NHE1 [SLC9A1], NHE3 [A3]), sodium phosphate cotransporter (Na/Pi [SLC34]), sodium bicarbonate exchanger (Na^+/HCO_3^- [SLC4]), chloride bicarbonate exchanger (Cl/HCO_3^- [SLC26A6]), and the active ATP-dependent sodium pump (Na^+/K^+-ATPase) *(15,16,18,33–36,40,48,51,52,55,66,67,70,71,93–114)*. The inhibitory effect of dopamine on sodium flux is highly influenced by the amount of intracellular sodium and calcium. Dopamine exerts its strongest effects in inhibiting Na^+/K^+-ATPase when intracellular sodium concentrations are greater than 20 mM and intracellular calcium concentrations are less than 120 nM *(95,101)*. There can be a substantial additive effect of incremental dopaminergic inhibition of sodium transport in each nephron segment.

5. RENAL SODIUM HANDLING AND DOPAMINE-MEDIATED HIGH BLOOD PRESSURE

Reduced renal sodium excretion is a central mechanism in the development and maintenance of essential hypertension. Subjects with elevated blood pressure have an inappropriate delay in responding to and excreting a salt load. D_1-like receptors are important in the regulation of basal blood pressure because blood pressure is increased when dopamine receptors are chronically blocked (saline-loaded Wistar rats and normotensive humans) (172,173). Some forms of hypertension can be the result of a decreased synthesis of dopamine, or a failure of proper D_1-like receptor signaling in the kidney. Interestingly, both human and rodent hypertension have similar defects in dopamine-regulated sodium excretion (12,13,26,42,45,47,86,115,116). In both rats and humans with genetic forms of hypertension, there is a well-documented failure of the normal inhibition by D_1-like receptors of the activities of NHE3, Na^+/HCO_3^-, Cl^-/HCO_3^-, and Na^+/K^+-ATPase (but not Na/Pi or NHE1) in the renal proximal tubule and thick ascending limb of Henle (14,48,51,55,65,66,98,102,105,107,114,117) that can lead to salt sensitivity (11–13,55).

Decreased renal synthesis of dopamine may also be involved in the pathogenesis of some forms of hypertension in some human subjects (47), and salt sensitivity in others (116,118–122). However, in other cases, renal dopamine production is normal or even increased, in either humans (47,123,124) or rodents (68,125,126). Furthermore, increasing renal dopamine production in the spontaneously hypertensive rat (SHR) does not enhance the ability of D_1-like agonists to inhibit renal cortical NHE3 activity or sodium excretion to the degree seen in Wistar–Kyoto (WKY) rats (42).

The principal dopaminergic defect in essential hypertension is a failure of D_1-like receptors to stimulate cAMP production in the renal proximal tubule and thick ascending limb of Henle (38,72) despite normal downstream effectors such as G protein subunits, adenylyl cyclase, phospholipase C, Na/K-ATPase, or NHE3 (14,26,37,38,42,46,48,51, 55,62,63,65,66,72,73,76,98,105,107,108,114,118,127–133). The impaired D_1-like receptor-mediated inhibition of epithelial sodium transport because of an uncoupling of the D_1-like receptor from its G protein/effector complex has been demonstrated in Dahl salt-sensitive rats, SHRs, and humans with essential hypertension, (14,26,37,38, 42,46,48,51,55,62,63,65,66,72,73,76,98,105,107,108,114,118,127–133). The uncoupling of the renal D_1-like receptor from its effector complex and second messenger (adenylyl cyclase) is receptor-specific because other adenylyl cyclase- linked receptors can operate normally (46,49,72,134,135). Additionally, the D_1-like receptor uncoupling is organ-selective because it is present in the kidney and small intestines (30), but not in the brain striatum (37). It is nephron-segment specific because it is observed in the renal proximal tubule and thick ascending limb of Henle (14,26,37,38,42,46,48,51,55,62,63,65,66,72, 73,76,98,105,107,108,114,118,127–133) but not in the cortical collecting duct (61). The activation of D_1-like receptors in cortical collecting ducts by the systemic administration of D_1-like drugs explains why these drugs are natriuretic in subjects with essential hypertension (58,136). This may not occur in rodent models of genetic hypertension (137–139).

6. GENETIC EVIDENCE FOR THE RENAL D1-LIKE RECEPTOR DEFECT IN HYPERTENSION

There is an evidence that the uncoupling of the D_1-like receptor in hypertension is genetic because it precedes the onset of hypertension in a variety of rodent models for genetically acquired hypertension (37,46,63,102,105,116). Furthermore, the hypertensive phenotype cosegregates with hypertension (genetically segregated—this term has a different meaning) in the SHR (62,140,141). There are polymorphisms in human D_5 receptor (142) and D_1 receptor (143). A polymorphism in the noncoding region of the

D_1 receptor has been associated with hypertension in one study *(143)*. There are no polymorphisms of the D_1 and D_5 receptors in SHRs but a renal D_5 receptor defect may still be present in genetic hypertension because D_5 receptor expression is decreased in the renal cortex of SHRs *(81)*.

7. ROLE OF G PROTEIN-COUPLED RECEPTOR KINASE TYPE 4

In humans with essential hypertension, the uncoupling of the D_1-like receptor from its G protein/effector complex has been shown to be a consequence of an activating variant in a member of the G protein-coupled receptor kinase (GRK) family of kinases that are responsible for G protein receptor inactivation following agonist stimulation. *(79,120,132,144–153)*. The complex of phosphorylated D_1 receptor, arrestin, and adaptor proteins undergo internalization, via clathrin-coated pits into an endosome in which the GPCR can be degraded by lysosomes or proteasomes, or dephosphorylated by phosphatases (e.g., GRK2A) *(28,33)* to be recycled back to the plasma membrane. Dephosphorylation can also occur directly at the plasma membrane *(154)*, and desensitization may be clathrin-independent *(133)*. Uncoupling of the D_1 like receptor in essential hypertension involves the D_1 receptor and not the D_5 receptor in hypertension [*(155,156)* and unpublished studies]. The D_1 receptor is hyper-serine-phosphorylated and not properly targeted to the cell surface membrane of the renal tubule cell, especially the proximal tubule *(72,134)*. Although an impaired protein phosphatase GRK2A function may play a role in the hyperphosphorylation of the renal D_1 receptor in the SHR *(29)*, the activity of the enzyme is actually increased in renal proximal tubule cells from hypertensive subjects (unpublished observations). However, the hyper-serine-phosphorylation of the D_1 receptor in the renal proximal tubule, in the absence of ligand occupation, is caused by increased GRK activity *(34)*. Indeed, decreasing GRK expression or activity in renal proximal tubule cells from hypertensive subjects normalizes the ability of D_1-like agonists to increase cAMP accumulation *(38)*.

There are seven GRKs, but in renal proximal tubules GRK4 is more important than other GRKs (e.g., GRK2) in the desensitization of D_1 receptors *(79)*. GRK4 activity is increased in renal proximal tubule cells from hypertensive humans, and the inhibition of GRK4 activity normalizes the ability of D_1-like receptors to increase cAMP production. In humans with essential hypertension, the constitutive desensitization of the D_1 receptor occurs as a result of a constitutively activated *GRK4* gene variant (*R65L*, *A142V*, and *A486V*) *(38)*. There is no difference in *GRK4* nucleotide sequence between WKY and SHRs. However, GRK4 activity is also increased in the kidneys of SHRs; chronic renal interstitial infusion of GRK4 antisense oligonucleotides blocks the increase in blood pressure that occurs with age in SHRs *(157)*. The D_1 receptor functional defect noted in renal proximal tubules and medullary thick ascending limb of Henle in hypertension is replicated by expression of *GRK4γ* gene variants in cell lines (CHO cells) and is rectified by the prevention of GRK4γ expression. In mice, overexpression of GRK4γ 142V impairs the natriuretic action of D_1 receptors and produces hypertension *(38)*. GRK4γ 142V transgenic mice have high blood pressure that is independent of sodium intake *(38)*. In contrast, GRK4γ 486V transgenic mice become hypertensive, after an increase in sodium intake *(78,158)*. The hypertensive phenotype in GRK4 transgenic mice is independent of transgene copy number and renal mRNA expression.

The *GRK4* locus, 4p16.3, is linked to hypertension *(159,160)*. We have reported that the *GRK4 486V* is associated with salt-sensitive hypertensive Italians, recapitulating the mouse transgenic study *(24)*. The latter study was recently corroborated by Speirs et al. in 168 unrelated Caucasians with essential hypertension *(161)*. In the Japanese, the presence of all three *GRK4* variants, *65L*, *142V*, and *486V*, predicts the salt-sensitive hypertensive phenotype with 94% accuracy *(162)*. The ability to excrete a sodium load in these hypertensive subjects is inversely related to the number of *GRK4* alleles with a high degree of correlation ($r^2 = 0.99$), indicating a gene dose effect. However, the presence of three *GRK4* variants impairs the natriuretic effect of a dopaminergic drug, even in normotensive subjects. Thus, salt sensitivity, *per se*, may be imparted by *GRK4* gene variants.

Six polymorphisms of *GRK4* have been reported (*GRK4 R65L*, *GRK4 A142V*, *GRK4 V247I*, *GRK4 A253T*, *GRK4 A486V*, and *GRK4 G562D*). The frequency of these polymorphisms varies according to ethnicity. A Japanese population was found to carry only the wild–type *GRK4 V247I*, *GRK4 A253T*, and *GRK4 G562D* (unpublished data). *GRK4 65L* and *142V* are more frequent among Ghanaians and African Americans than other ethnic groups studied (Chinese, Hispanics, Japanese, and Caucasians), whereas *GRK4 486V* is more frequent in Chinese and Japanese subjects [*(161–163)* and unpublished data]. Thirteen polymorphisms of eight genes in hypertensive Ghanaians (angiotensinogen, *AGT*; angiotensin-I-converting enzyme, *ACE*; angiotensin II receptor type 1, *AT$_1$R*; *GRK4*; nitric oxide synthases 1 and 3, *NOS1, NOS3*; and carbamyl phosphate synthase 1: *CPS1*, which affects NO production, and *CYP2C8*, the putative endothelium-derived hyperpolarizing factor synthase) were reported recently *(163)*. The best combination that was predictive of hypertension, not classified according to salt sensitivity, was *ACE* and *GRK4*, with an estimated prediction success of 70% *(163)*. Among Japanese, the best combination that was predictive of hypertension, not classified according to salt sensitivity, was *GRK4*, *ACE*, and *Cyp11B2*, with an estimated prediction success of 63% (unpublished data). We also found that the single best genetic model for low renin hypertension in Japanese included only *GRK4A142V* and *CYP11B2*, with an estimated prediction success of 84% [*(162)* and unpublished data]. These results show that underlying genetic models of salt sensitive, low renin, and possibly other subclasses of hypertension are different.

8. SUMMARY

The renal dopaminergic system is integral to the maintenance of normal long-term sodium homeostasis by primarily acting in the renal proximal tubule and thick ascending limb to decrease sodium transport. A reduction in sodium transport results in increased sodium excretion. A failure of proper functioning of the renal D$_1$-like receptor system results in a reduction in sodium excretion and an increase in blood pressure. Genetic polymorphisms in the G protein-coupled receptor kinase, *GRK4* causes a hyperphosphorylation of the D$_1$-like receptor resulting in its uncoupling from G protein/effector complex. Expression of *GRK4* variants in cell lines replicates the D$_1$ receptor defect noted in renal proximal tubules. Inhibition of *GRK4* function or expression normalizes D$_1$ receptor function in cell lines expressing *GRK4* gene variants and renal proximal tubule cells from humans with essential hypertension. Overexpression of *GRK4γ142V* variant in mice produces hypertension and impairs the natriuretic but not the acute vasodepressor effect of D_1 receptors. *GRK4γ 486V* imparts sodium sensitivity to mice that are otherwise normotensive. Moreover, selective renal inhibition of *GRK4* gene expression attenuates the increase in blood pressure in SHRs. These data fulfill the criteria recently proposed by Glazier et al. that are required to link genetic loci to the etiology of complex disease *(166)*. It is possible that *GRK4* inhibitors may lead to a novel treatment for salt sensitivity that would reduce the morbidity and mortality associated with this condition, even in normotensive subjects *(165–169)*.

ACKNOWLEDGMENT

This paper was supported in part by grants from the National Institutes of Health, DK39308, HL23081, DK52612, HL68686, HL074940, and HL65234.

REFERENCES

1. Zitnay, C. and Siragy, H. M. (1998) Action of angiotensin receptor subtypes on the renal tubules and vasculature: implications for volume homeostasis and atherosclerosis. *Miner Electrol. Metab.* **24(6),** 362–370.
2. Baum, M. A. and Harris, H. W. (1998) Recent insights into the coordinate regulation of body water and divalent mineral ion metabolism. *Am. J. Med. Sci.* **316(5),** 321–328. Review.
3. Ursino, M. and Magosso, E. (2003) Short-term autonomic control of cardiovascular function: a mini-review with the help of mathematical models. *J. Integr. Neurosci.* **2(2),** 219–247.
4. DiBona, G. F. (2002) Sympathetic nervous system and the kidney in hypertension. *Curr. Opin. Nephrol. Hypertens* **11,** 197–200.
5. Ferrario, C. M., Chappell, M. C., Tallant, E. A., Brosnihan K. B., and Diz, D. I. (1997) Counterregulatory actions of angiotensin-(1–7). *Hypertension* **30,** 535–541.
6. Fuchs, S., Frenzel, K., Xiao H. D., et al. (2004) Newly recognized physiologic and pathophysiologic actions of the angiotensin-converting enzyme. *Curr. Hypertens Rep.* **6,** 124–128.
7. Gurley, S. B., Le, T. H., and Coffman, T. M. (2002) Gene-targeting studies of the renin–angiotensin system: mechanisms of hypertension and cardiovascular disease. *Cold Spring Harb. Symp. Quant. Biol.* **67,** 451–457.
8. Lavoie, J. L. and Sigmund, C. D. (2003) Minireview: overview of the renin–angiotensin system—an endocrine and paracrine system. *Endocrinology* **144,** 2179–2183.
9. Navar, L. G., Harrison-Bernard, L. M., Nishiyama, A., and Kobori, H. (2002) Regulation of intrarenal angiotensin II in hypertension. *Hypertension* **39,** 316–322.
10. Hall, J. E., Brands, M. W., and Henegar, J. R. (1999) Angiotensin II and long-term arterial pressure regulation: the overriding dominance of the kidney. *J. Am. Soc. Nephrol.* **10(Suppl 12),** S258–S265.
11. Aviv, A., Hollenberg, N. K., and Weder, A. (2004) Urinary potassium excretion and sodium sensitivity in blacks. *Hypertension* **43,** 707–713.
12. Doris, P. A. (2000) Renal proximal tubule sodium transport and genetic mechanisms of essential hypertension. *J. Hypertens.* **18,** 509–519.
13. Ortiz, P. A. and Garvin, J. L. (2001) Intrarenal transport and vasoactive substances in hypertension. *Hypertension* **38,** 621–624.
14. Albrecht, F. E., Drago, J, Felder, R. A., et al. (1996) Role of the D_{1A} dopamine receptor in the pathogenesis of genetic hypertension. *J. Clin. Investig.* **97,** 2283–2288.
15. Aoki, Y., Albrecht, F. E., Bergman, K. R., and Jose, P. A. (1996) Stimulation of Na^+-K^+-2Cl- cotransport in rat medullary thick ascending limb by dopamine. *Am. J. Physiol.* **271,** R1561–R1567.
16. Aoki, Y., Aviles, D. H., and Jose, P. A. (2000) Biphasic effects of dopamine on [86]rubidium uptake in rat renal proximal tubules. *Clin. Exp. Hypertens.* **22,** 289–301.
17. Asghar, M., Hussain, T., and Lokhandwala, M. F. (2003) Overexpression of PKC-beta I and -delta contributes to higher PKC activity in the proximal tubules of old Fischer 344 rats. *Am. J. Physiol. Renal. Physiol.* **285,** F1100–F1107.
18. Asghar, M., Hussain, T., and Lokhandwala, M. F. (2001) Activation of dopamine D_1-like receptor causes phosphorylation of $alpha_1$-subunit of Na^+,K^+-ATPase in rat renal proximal tubules. *Eur. J. Pharmacol.* **411,** 61–66.

19. Asico, L. D., Ladines, C., Fuchs, S., et al. (1998) Disruption of the dopamine D3 receptor gene produces renin-dependent hypertension. *J. Clin. Investig.* **102,** 493–498.
20. Bacic, D., Kaissling, B., McLeroy, P., Zou, L., Baum, M., and Moe, O. W. (2003) Dopamine acutely decreases apical membrane Na/H exchanger NHE3 protein in mouse renal proximal tubule. *Kidney Int.* **64,** 2133–2141.
21. Baines, A. D. and Drangova, R. (1998) Does dopamine use several signal pathways to inhibit Na-Pi transport in OK cells? *J. Am. Soc. Nephrol.* **9,** 1604–1612.
22. Banday, A. A., Hussain, T., and Lokhandwala, M. F. (2004) Renal dopamine D1 receptor dysfunction is acquired and not inherited in obese Zucker rats. *Am. J. Physiol. Renal Physiol.* **287,** F109–F116.
23. Bek, M., Fischer, K. G., Greiber, S., Hupfer, C., Mundel, P., and Pavenstadt, H. (1999) Dopamine depolarizes podocytes via a D1-like receptor. *Nephrol. Dial. Transplant.* **14,** 581–587.
24. Bengra, C., Mifflin, T. E., Khripin, Y., et al. (2002) Genotyping essential hypertension SNPs using a homogenous PCR method with universal energy transfer primers. *Clin. Chem.* **48,** 2131–2140.
25. Bermak, J. C., Li, M., Bullock, C., and Zhou, Q. Y. (2001) Regulation of transport of the dopamine D1 receptor by a new membrane-associated ER protein. *Nat. Cell. Biol.* **3,** 492–498.
26. Carey, R. M. (2001) Theodore Cooper Lecture: Renal dopamine system: paracrine regulator of sodium homeostasis and blood pressure. *Hypertension* **38,** 297–302.
27. Aherne, A. M., Vaughan, C. J., Carey, R. M., and O'Connell, D. P. (1997) Localization of dopamine D1A receptor protein and messenger ribonucleic acid in rat adrenal cortex. *Endocrinology* **138,** 1282–1288.
28. Wu, K. D., Chen, Y. M., Chu, T. S., et al. (2002) Dopaminergic modulation of aldosterone secretions on changes of sodium intake in aldosterone-producing adenoma. *Am. J. Hypertens.* **15,** 609–614.
29. Lucas-Teixeira, V. A., Hussain, T., Serrao, P., Soares-da-Silva, P., and Lokhandwala, M. F. (2002) Intestinal dopaminergic activity in obese and lean Zucker rats: response to high salt intake. *Clin. Exp. Hypertens.* **24,** 383–396.
30. Lucas-Teixeira, V. A., Vieira-Coelho, M. A., Serrao, P., Pestana, M., and Soares-da-Silva, P. (2000) Salt intake and sensitivity of intestinal and renal Na$^+$–K$^+$-ATPase to inhibition by dopamine in spontaneous hypertensive and Wistar–Kyoto rats. *Clin. Exp. Hypertens.* **22,** 455–469.
31. Vieira-Coelho, M. A, Teixeira, V. A., Finkel, Y., Soares-Da-Silva, P., and Bertorello, A. M. (1998) Dopamine-dependent inhibition of jejunal Na$^+$–K$^+$-ATPase during high-salt diet in young but not in adult rats. *Am. J. Physiol.* **275,** G1317–G1323.
32. Brismar, H., Asghar, M., Carey, R. M., Greengard, P., and Aperia, A. (1998) Dopamine-induced recruitment of dopamine D1 receptors to the plasma membrane. *PNAS* **95,** 5573–5578.
33. Efendiev, R., Yudowski, G. A., Zwiller, J., et al. (2002) Relevance of dopamine signals anchoring dynamin-2 to the plasma membrane during Na$^+$,K$^+$-ATPase endocytosis. *J. Biol. Chem.* **277,** 44,108–44,114.
34. Felder, C. C., Albrecht, F. E., Campbell, T., Eisner, G. M., and Jose, P. A. (1993) cAMP-independent, G protein-linked inhibition of Na$^+$/H$^+$ exchange in renal brush border by D1 dopamine agonists. *Am. J. Physiol.* **264,** F1032–F1037.
35. Felder, C. C., Campbell, T., Albrecht, F., and Jose, P. A. (1990) Dopamine inhibits Na$^+$-H$^+$ exchanger activity in renal BBMV by stimulation of adenylate cyclase. *Am. J. Physiol.* **259,** F297–F303.
36. Felder, C. C., Jose, P. A., and Axelrod, J. (1989) The dopamine-1 agonist, SKF 82526, stimulates phospholipase-C activity independent of adenylate cyclase. *J. Pharmacol. Exp. Ther.* **248,** 171–175.
37. Felder, R. A., Kinoshita, S., Ohbu, K., et al. (1993) Organ specificity of the dopamine1 receptor/adenylyl cyclase coupling defect in spontaneously hypertensive rats. *Am. J. Physiol.* **264,** R726–R732.
38. Felder, R. A., Sanada, H., Xu, J., et al. (2002) G protein-coupled receptor kinase 4 gene variants in human essential hypertension. *Proc. Natl Acad. Sci. USA* **99,** 3872–3877.
39. Felder, R. A., Seikaly, M. G., Cody, P., Eisner, G. M., and Jose, P. A. (1990) Attenuated renal response to dopaminergic drugs in spontaneously hypertensive rats. *Hypertension* **15,** 560–569.
40. Grider, J., Kilpatrick, E., Ott, C., and Jackson, B. (1998) Effect of dopamine on NaCl transport in the medullary thick ascending limb of the rat. *Eur. J. Pharmacol.* **342,** 281–284.
41. Jose, P. A., Asico, L. D., Eisner, G. M., Pocchiari, F., Semeraro, C., and Felder, R. A. (1998) Effects of costimulation of dopamine D1- and D2-like receptors on renal function. *Am. J. Physiol.* **275,** R986–R994.
42. Jose, P. A., Eisner, G. M., Drago, J., Carey, R. M., and Felder, R. A. (1996) Dopamine receptor signaling defects in spontaneous hypertension. *Am. J. Hypertens.* **9,** 400–405.

43. Jose, P. A, Eisner, G. M., and Felder, R. A. (2003) Dopamine and the kidney: role in hypertension? *Curr. Opin. Nephrol. Hypertens.* **12,** 1189–1194.

44. Jose, P. A, Eisner, G. M., and Felder, R. A. (2002) Dopamine receptor-coupling defect in hypertension. *Curr. Hypertens. Rep.* **4,** 237–244.

45. Jose, P. A., Eisner, G. M., and Felder, R. A. (1998) Renal dopamine receptors in health and hypertension. *Pharmacol. Ther.* **80,** 149–182.

46. Kinoshita, S., Sidhu, A., and Felder, R. A. (1989) Defective dopamine-1 receptor adenylate cyclase coupling in the proximal convoluted tubule from the spontaneously hypertensive rat. *J. Clin. Investig.* **84,** 1849–1856.

47. Kuchel, O. G. and Kuchel, G. A. (1991) Peripheral dopamine in pathophysiology of hypertension: interaction with aging and lifestyle. *Hypertension* **18,** 709–721.

48. Kunimi, M., Seki, G., Hara, C., et al. (2000) Dopamine inhibits renal Na^+:HCO_3^- cotransporter in rabbits and normotensive rats but not in spontaneously hypertensive rats. *Kidney Int.* **57,** 534–543.

49. Ladines, C. A., Zeng, C., Asico, L. D., et al. (2001) Impaired renal D_1-like and D_2-like dopamine receptor interaction in the spontaneously hypertensive rat. *Am. J. Physiol. Regul. Integr. Comp. Physiol.* **281,** R1071–R1078.

50. Li, X. X, Bek, M., Asico, L. D, et al. (2001) Adrenergic and endothelin B receptor-dependent hypertension in dopamine receptor type-2 knockout mice. *Hypertension* **38,** 303–308.

51. Li, X. X., Albrecht, F. E., Xu, J., Robillard, J. E., Eisner, G. M., and Jose, P. A. (2001) D_1 dopamine receptor regulation of NHE3 during development in the spontaneously hypertensive rat. *Am. J. Physiol. Regul. Integr. Comp. Physiol.* **280,** R1650–R1656.

52. Meister, B., Fryckstedt, J., Schalling, M., et al. (1989) Dopamine- and cAMP-regulated phospho-protein (DARPP-32) and dopamine DA1 agonist-sensitive Na^+,K^+-ATPase in renal tubule cells. *Proc. Natl Acad. Sci. USA* **86,** 8068–8072.

53. Narkar, V. A., Hussain, T., Pedemonte, C., and Lokhandwala, M. F. (2001) Dopamine D_2 receptor activation causes mitogenesis via p44/42 mitogen-activated protein kinase in opossum kidney cells. *J. Am. Soc. Nephrol.* **12,** 1844–1852.

54. Nash, S. R., Godinot, N., and Caron, M. G. (1993) Cloning and characterization of the opossum kidney cell D1 dopamine receptor: expression of identical D1A and D1B dopamine receptor mRNAs in opossum kidney and brain. *Mol. Pharmacol.* **44,** 918–925.

55. Nishi, A., Eklof, A. C., Bertorello, A. M., and Aperia, A. (1993) Dopamine regulation of renal Na^+,K^+-ATPase activity is lacking in Dahl salt-sensitive rats. *Hypertension* **21,** 767–771.

56. Nowicki, S., Kruse, M. S., Brismar, H., and Aperia, A. (2000) Dopamine-induced translocation of protein kinase C isoforms visualized in renal epithelial cells. *Am. J. Physiol. Cell Physiol.* **279,** C1812–C1818.

57. O'Connell, D. P., Botkin, S. J., Ramos, S. I., et al. (1995) Localization of dopamine D1A receptor protein in rat kidneys. *Am. J. Physiol.* **268,** F1185–F1197.

58. O'Connell, D. P., Ragsdale, N. V., Boyd, D. G., Felder, R. A., and Carey, R. M. (1997) Differential human renal tubular responses to dopamine type 1 receptor stimulation are determined by blood pressure status. *Hypertension* **29,** 115–122.

59. O'Connell, D. P, Vaughan, C. J., Aherne, A. M., et al. (1998) Expression of the dopamine D3 receptor protein in the rat kidney. *Hypertension* **32,** 86–95.

60. Odlind, C., Reenila, I., Mannisto, P. T., Ekblom, J., and Hansell, P. (2001) The role of dopamine-metabolizing enzymes in the regulation of renal sodium excretion in the rat. *Pflugers Arch.* **442,** 505–510.

61. Ohbu, K. and Felder, R. A. (1993) Nephron specificity of dopamine receptor–adenylyl cyclase defect in spontaneous hypertension. *Am. J. Physiol.* **264,** F274–F279.

62. Ohbu, K., Hendley, E. D., Yamaguchi, I., and Felder, R. A. (1993) Renal dopamine-1 receptors in hypertensive inbred rat strains with and without hyperactivity. *Hypertension* **21,** 485–490.

63. Ohbu, K., Kaskel, F. J., Kinoshita, S., and Felder, R. A. (1995) Dopamine-1 receptors in the proximal convoluted tubule of Dahl rats: defective coupling to adenylate cyclase. *Am. J. Physiol.* **268,** R231–R235.

64. Ozono, R., O'Connell, D. P., Wang, Z. Q., et al. (1997) Localization of the dopamine D1 receptor protein in the human heart and kidney. *Hypertension* **30,** 725–729.

65. Pedrosa, R., Gomes, P., Zeng, C., Hopfer, U., Jose, P. A. and Soares-da-Silva, P. (2004) Dopamine D_3 receptor-mediated inhibition of the Na^+/H^+ exchanger in spontaneously hypertensive rat proximal tubular epithelial cells. *Br. J. Pharmacol.* **142,** 1343–1353.

66. Pedrosa, R., Jose, P. A., and Soares-Da-Silva, P. (2004) Defective D1-like receptor-mediated inhibition of Cl$^-$/HCO$_3^-$ exchanger in immortalized SHR proximal tubular epithelial cells. *Am. J. Physiol. Renal. Physiol.* **286**, F1120–F1126.

67. Perrichot, R., Garcia-Ocana, A., Couette, S., Comoy, E., Amiel, C., and Friedlander, G. (1995) Locally formed dopamine modulates renal Na-Pi co-transport through DA1 and DA2 receptors. *Biochem. J.* **312**, 433–437.

68. Pinho, M. J., Gomes, P., Serrao, M. P., Bonifacio, M. J., and Soares-da-Silva, P. (2003) Organ-specific overexpression of renal LAT2 and enhanced tubular L-DOPA uptake precede the onset of hypertension. *Hypertension* **42**, 613–618.

69. Pinho, M. J., Serrao, M. P., Gomes, P., Hopfer, U., Jose, P. A., and Soares-da-Silva, P. (2004) Overexpression of renal LAT1 and LAT2 and enhanced L-DOPA uptake in SHR immortalized renal proximal tubular cells. *Kidney Int.* **66**, 216–226.

70. Pinto-do-O, P. C., Chibalin, A. V., Katz, A. I., Soares-da-Silva, P., and Bertorello, A. M. (1997) Short-term vs. sustained inhibition of proximal tubule Na,K-ATPase activity by dopamine: cellular mechanisms. *Clin. Exp. Hypertens.* **19**, 73–86.

71. Saito, O., Ando, Y., Kusano, E., and Asano, Y. (2001) Functional characterization of basolateral and luminal dopamine receptors in rabbit CCD. *Am. J. Physiol. Renal. Physiol.* **281**, F114–F122.

72. Sanada, H., Jose, P. A., Hazen-Martin, D., et al. (1999) Dopamine-1 receptor coupling defect in renal proximal tubule cells in hypertension. *Hypertension* **33**, 1036–1042.

73. Sidhu, A., Vachvanichsanong, P., Jose, P. A., and Felder, R. A. (1992) Persistent defective coupling of dopamine-1 receptors to G proteins after solubilization from kidney proximal tubules of hypertensive rats. *J. Clin. Investig.* **89**, 789–793.

74. Siragy, H. M., Felder, R. A., Howell, N. L., Chevalier, R. L., Peach, M. J., and Carey, R. M. (1989) Evidence that intrarenal dopamine acts as a paracrine substance at the renal tubule. *Am. J. Physiol.* **257**, F469–F477.

75. Sun, D., Wilborn, T. W., and Schafer, J. A. (1998) Dopamine D4 receptor isoform mRNA and protein are expressed in the rat cortical collecting duct. *Am. J. Physiol.* **275**, F742–F751.

76. Uh, M., White, B. H., and Sidhu, A. (1998) Alteration of association of agonist-activated renal D1A dopamine receptors with G proteins in proximal tubules of the spontaneously hypertensive rat. *J. Hypertens.* **16**, 1307–1313.

77. Wang, Z. Q., Felder, R. A., and Carey, R. M. (1999) Selective inhibition of the renal dopamine subtype D1A receptor induces antinatriuresis in conscious rats. *Hypertension* **33**, 504–510.

78. Wang, Z. Q., Siragy, H. M., Felder, R. A., and Carey, R. M. (1997) Intrarenal dopamine production and distribution in the rat. Physiological control of sodium excretion. *Hypertension* **29**, 228–234.

79. Watanabe, H., Xu, J., Bengra, D., Jose, P. A., and Felder, R. A. (2002) Desensitization of renal D$_1$ dopamine receptors by G protein-coupled receptor. *Kidney Int.* **62**, 790–798.

80. Yamaguchi, I., Jose, P. A., Mouradian, M. M., et al. (1993) The expression of the dopamine D$_{1A}$ receptor gene in microdissected proximal convoluted tubules of rat kidney. *Am. J. Physiol.* **264**, F280–F285.

81. Zeng, C., Yang, Z., Wang, Z., et al. (2005) Interaction of AT$_1$ and D$_5$ dopamine receptors in renal proximal tubule cells. *Hypertension* **45(4)**, 804–810.

82. Chen, C. J. and Lokhandwala, M. F. (1992) An impairment of renal tubular DA-1 receptor function as the causative factor for diminished natriuresis to volume expansion in spontaneously hypertensive rats. *Clin. Exp. Hypertens. A* **14**, 615–628.

83. Hollon, T. R., Bek, M. J., Lachowicz, J. E., et al. (2002) Mice lacking D5 dopamine receptors have increased sympathetic tone and are hypertensive. *J. Neurosci.* **22**, 10,801–10,810.

84. Hansell, P. and Fasching, A. (1991) The effect of dopamine receptor blockade on natriuresis is dependent on the degree of hypervolemia. *Kidney Int.* **39**, 253–258.

85. Glickstein, S. B. and Schmauss, C. (2001) Dopamine receptor functions: lessons from knockout mice. *Pharmacol. Ther.* **91**, 63–83.

86. Hussain, T. and Lokhandwala, M. F. (1998) Renal dopamine receptor function in hypertension. *Hypertension* **32**, 187–197.

87. Sibley, D. R. (1999) New insights into dopaminergic receptor function using antisense and genetically altered animals. *Annu. Rev. Pharmacol. Toxicol.* **39**, 313–341.

88. Ricci, A., Marchal-Victorion, S., Bronzetti, E., Parini, A., Amenta, F., and Tayebati, S. K. (2002) Dopamine D4 receptor expression in rat kidney: evidence for pre- and postjunctional localization. *J. Histochem. Cytochem.* **50**, 1091–1096.

89. Amenta, F., Barili, P., Bronzetti, E., Felici, L., Mignini, F., and Ricci, A. (2000) Localization of dopamine receptor subtypes in systemic arteries. *Clin. Exp. Hypertens.* **22,** 277–288.

90. Zeng, C., Wang, D., Yang, Z., et al. (2004) Dopamine D1 receptor augmentation of D3 receptor action in rat aortic or mesenteric vascular smooth muscles. *Hypertension* **43,** 673–679.

91. Sanada, H., Yao, L., Jose, P. A., Carey, R. M., and Felder, R. A. (1997) Dopamine D3 receptors in rat juxtaglomerular cells. *Clin. Exp. Hypertens.* **19,** 93–105.

92. Yamaguchi, I., Yao, L., Sanada, H., et al. (1997) Dopamine D1A receptors and renin release in rat juxtaglomerular cells. *Hypertension* **29,** 962–968.

93. Bertorello, A. and Aperia, A. (1989) $Na^+–K^+$-ATPase is an effector protein for protein kinase C in renal proximal tubule cells. *Am. J. Physiol.* **256,** F370–F373.

94. Bertuccio, C. A., Cheng, S. X., Arrizurieta, E. E., Martin, R. S., and Ibarra, F. R. (2003) Mechanisms of $Na^+–K^+$-ATPase phosphorylation by PKC in the medullary thick ascending limb of Henle in the rat. *Pflugers Arch.* **447,** 87–96.

95. Budu, C. E., Efendiev, R., Cinelli, A. M., Bertorello, A. M., and Pedemonte, C. H. (2002) Hormonal-dependent recruitment of Na^+,K^+-ATPase to the plasmalemma is mediated by PKC beta and modulated by [Na^+]I. *Br. J. Pharmacol.* **137,** 1380–1386.

96. Cheng, S. X., Aizman, O., Nairn, A. C., Greengard, P., and Aperia, A. (1999) [Ca^{2+}]i determines the effects of protein kinases A and C on activity of rat renal Na^+,K^+-ATPase. *J. Physiol. (Lond)* **518(1),** 37–46.

97. Chibalin, A. V., Zierath, J. R., Katz, A. I., Berggren, P. O., and Bertorello, A. M. (1998) Phosphatidylinositol 3-kinase-mediated endocytosis of renal Na^+,K^+-ATPase alpha subunit in response to dopamine. *Mol. Biol. Cell* **9,** 1209–1220.

98. Debska-Slizien, A., Ho, P., Drangova, R., and Baines, A. D. (1994) Endogenous dopamine regulates phosphate reabsorption but not NaK-ATPase in spontaneously hypertensive rat kidneys. *J. Am. Soc. Nephrol.* **5,** 1125–1132.

99. de Toledo, F. G., Thompson, M. A., Bolliger, C., Tyce, G. M., and Dousa, T. P. (1999) γ-L-glutamyl-L-DOPA inhibits Na^+-phosphate cotransport across renal brush border membranes and increases renal excretion of phosphate. *Kidney Int.* **55,** 1832–1842.

100. Efendiev, R., Bertorello, A. M., and Pedemonte, C. H. (1999) PKC-beta and PKC-zeta mediate opposing effects on proximal tubule Na^+,K^+-ATPase activity. *FEBS Lett.* **456,** 45–48.

101. Efendiev, R., Bertorello, A. M., Zandomeni, R., Cinelli, A. R., and Pedemonte, C. H. (2002) Agonist-dependent regulation of renal Na^+,K^+-ATPase activity is modulated by intracellular sodium concentration. *J. Biol. Chem.* **277,** 11,489–11,496.

102. Gesek, F. A. and Schoolwerth, A. C. (1991) Hormone responses of proximal Na^+-H^+ exchanger in spontaneously hypertensive rats. *Am. J. Physiol.* **261,** F526–F536.

103. Glahn, R. P., Onsgard, M. J., Tyce, G. M., Chinnow, S. L., Knox, F. G., and Dousa, T. P. (1993) Autocrine/paracrine regulation of renal Na^+-phosphate cotransport by dopamine. *Am. J. Physiol.* **264,** F618–F622.

104. Gomes, P. and Soares-da-Silva, P. (2004) Dopamine acutely decreases type 3 Na^+/H^+ exchanger activity in renal OK cells through the activation of protein kinases A and C signalling cascades. *Eur. J. Pharmacol.* **488,** 51–59.

105. Horiuchi, A., Albrecht, F. E., Eisner, G. M., Jose, P. A., and Felder, R. A. (1992) Renal dopamine receptors and pre- and post-cAMP-mediated Na^+ transport defect in spontaneously hypertensive rats. *Am. J. Physiol.* **263,** F1105–F1111.

106. Hu, M. C., Fan, L., Crowder, L. A., Karim-Jimenez Z., Murer, H., and Moe, O. W. (2001) Dopamine acutely stimulates Na^+/H^+ exchanger (NHE3) endocytosis via clathrin-coated vesicles: dependence on protein kinase A-mediated NHE3 phosphorylation. *J. Biol. Chem.* **276,** 26,906–26,915.

107. Hussain, T. and Lokhandwala, M. F. (1996) Altered arachidonic acid metabolism contributes to the failure of dopamine to inhibit Na^+,K^+-ATPase in kidney of spontaneously hypertensive rats. *Clin. Exp. Hypertens.* **18,** 963–974.

108. Hussain, T. and Lokhandwala, M. F. (1996) Altered arachidonic acid metabolism contributes to the failure of dopamine to inhibit Na^+,K^+-ATPase in kidney of spontaneously hypertensive rats. *Clin. Exp. Hypertens.* **18,** 963–974.

109. Ibarra, F., Aperia, A., Svensson, L. B., Eklof, A. C., and Greengard, P. (1993) Bidirectional regulation of Na^+,K^+-ATPase activity by dopamine and an alpha-adrenergic agonist. *Proc. Natl Acad. Sci. USA* **90,** 21–24.

110. Khundmiri, S. J. and Lederer, E. (2002) PTH and DA regulate Na-K ATPase through divergent pathways. *Am. J. Physiol. Renal. Physiol.* **282,** F512–F522.
111. Li, X. X., Albrecht, F. E., Robillard, J. E., Eisner, G. M., and Jose, P. A. (2000) Gβ regulation of Na/H exchanger-3 activity in rat renal proximal tubules during development. *Am. J. Physiol. Regul. Integr. Comp. Physiol.* **78,** R931–R936.
112. Nowicki, S., Chen, S. L., Aizman, O., et al. (1997) 20-Hydroxyeicosa-tetraenoic acid (20 HETE) activates protein kinase C. Role in regulation of rat renal Na⁺,K⁺-ATPase. *J. Clin. Investig.* **99,** 1224–1230.
113. Wiederkehr, M. R., Di Sole, F., Collazo, R., et al. (2001) Characterization of acute inhibition of Na/H exchanger NHE-3 by dopamine in opossum kidney cells. *Kidney Int.* **59,** 197–209.
114. Xu, J., Li, X. X., Albrecht, F. E., Hopfer, U., Carey, R. M., and Jose, P. A. (2000) D₁ receptor, G$_s$α, and Na⁺/H⁺ exchanger interactions in the kidney in hypertension. *Hypertension* **36,** 395–399.
115. Contreras, F., Fouillioux, C., Bolivar, A., et al. (2002) Dopamine, hypertension and obesity. *J. Hum. Hypertens.* **16(Suppl 1),** S13–S17.
116. Lee, M. R. (1987) Dopamine, the kidney and essential hypertension. studies with gludopa. *Clin. Exp. Hypertens. A* **9,** 977–986.
117. Bianchi, G., Fox, U., Di Francesco, G. F., Giovanetti, A. M., and Pagetti, D. (1974) Blood pressure changes produced by kidney cross-transplantation between spontaneously hypertensive rats and normotensive rats. *Clin. Sci. Mol. Med.* **47,** 435–448.
118. Clark, B. A., Rosa, R. M., Epstein, F. H., Young, J. B., and Landsberg, L. (1992) Altered dopaminergic responses in hypertension. *Hypertension* **19,** 589–594.
119. Damasceno, A., Santos, A., Serrao, P., Caupers, P., Soares-da-Silva, P., and Polonia, J. (1995) Deficiency of renal dopaminergic-dependent natriuretic response to acute sodium load in black salt-sensitive subjects in contrast to salt-resistant subjects. *J. Hypertens.* **17,** 1995–2001.
120. Gill, J. R. Jr., Grossman, E., and Goldstein, D. S. (1991) High urinary dopa and low urinary dopamine-to-dopa ratio in salt-sensitive hypertension. *Hypertension* **18,** 614–621.
121. Gill, J. R. Jr., Gullner, H. G., Lake, C. R., Lakatua, D. J., and Lan, G. (1988) Plasma and urinary catecholamines in salt-sensitive idiopathic hypertension. *Hypertension* **11,** 312–319.
122. Sowers, J. R., Beck, F. W., and Eggena, P. (1984) Evidence for direct inhibitory effects of dopamine on zona glomerulosa secretion of 18-hydroxycorticosterone in rhesus monkeys. *Life Sci.* **34,** 2339–2346.
123. Saito, I., Itsuji, S., Takeshita, E., et al. (1994) Increased urinary dopamine excretion in young patients with essential hypertension. *Clin. Exp. Hypertens.* **16,** 29–39.
124. Saito, I., Takeshita, E., Saruta, T., Nagano, S., and Sekihara, T. (1986) Urinary dopamine excretion in normotensive subjects with or without family history of hypertension. *J. Hypertens.* **4,** 57–60.
125. Grossman, E., Hoffman, A., Tamrat, M., Armando, I., Keiser, H. R., and Goldstein, D. S. (1991) Endogenous dopa and dopamine responses to dietary salt loading in salt-sensitive rats. *J. Hypertens.* **9,** 259–263.
126. Racz, K., Kuchel, O., Buu, N. T., and Tenneson, S. (1996) Peripheral dopamine synthesis and metabolism in spontaneously hypertensive rats. *Circ. Res.* **57,** 889–897.
127. Chen, C., Beach, R. E., and Lokhandwala, M. F. (1993) Dopamine fails to inhibit renal tubular sodium pump in hypertensive rats. *Hypertension* **21,** 364–372.
128. Hussain, T. and Lokhandwala, M. F. (1997) Renal dopamine DA1 receptor coupling with G$_S$ and G$_{q/11}$ proteins in spontaneously hypertensive rats. *Am. J. Physiol.* **272,** F339–F346.
129. Sela, S., White, B. H., Uh, M., Kimura, K., Patel, S., and Sidhu, A. (1997) Dysfunctional D1A receptor-G protein coupling in proximal tubules of spontaneously hypertensive rats is not due to abnormal G proteins. *J. Hypertens.* **15,** 259–267.
130. Yao, L. P., Li, X. X., Yu, P. Y., Xu, J., Asico, L. D., and Jose, P. A. (1998) Dopamine D1 receptor and protein kinase C isoforms in spontaneously hypertensive rats. *Hypertension* **32,** 1049–1053.
131. Yu, P-Y., Asico, L. D., Eisner, G. M., Hopfer, U., Felder, R. A., and Jose, P. A. (2000) Renal protein phosphatase 2A activity and spontaneous hypertension in rats. *Hypertension* **36,** 1053–1058.
132. Yu, P. Y., Hopfer, U., Felder, R. A., and Jose, P. A. (2000) Increased serine-phosphorylation of the D₁ receptor in renal proximal tubule cells in hypertension. *Am. J. Hypertens.* **13,** 12A–13A.
133. Yu, P.-Y., Yang, Z. W., Jones, J. E., et al. (2004) D₁ dopamine receptor signaling involves caveolin-2 in HEK-293 cells. *Kidney Int.* **66,** 2167–2180.
134. Michel, M. C., Jager, S., Casto, R., et al. (1992) On the role of renal alpha-adrenergic receptors in spontaneously hypertensive rats. *Hypertension* **19,** 365–370.

135. Onsgard-Meyer, M. J., Berndt, T. J., Khraibi, A. A., and Knox, F. G. (1994) Phosphaturic effect of parathyroid hormone in the spontaneously hypertensive rat. *Am. J. Physiol.* **267,** R78–R83.
136. Murphy, M. B., Murray, C., and Shorten, G. D. (2001) Fenoldopam: a selective peripheral dopamine-receptor agonist for the treatment of severe hypertension. *N Engl. J. Med.* **345,** 1548–1557.
137. Chatziantoniou, C., Ruan, X., and Arendshorst, W. J. (1995) Defective G protein activation of the cAMP pathway in rat kidney during genetic hypertension. *Proc. Natl Acad. Sci. USA* **92,** 2924–2928.
138. de Vries, P. A., Navis, G., de Jong, P. E., de Zeeuw, D., and Kluppel, C. A. (1999) Impaired renal vascular response to a D_1-like receptor agonist but not to an ACE inhibitor in conscious spontaneously hypertensive rats. *J. Cardiovasc. Pharmacol.* **34,** 191–198.
139. Zeng, C., Wang, D., Asico, L. D., et al. (2004) Aberrant D1 and D3 dopamine receptor transregulation in hypertension. *Hypertension* **43(3),** 654–660.
140. Hendley, E. D. and Ohlsson, W. G. (1991) Two new inbred rat strains derived from SHR: WKHA, hyperactive, and WKHT, hypertensive, rats. *Am. J. Physiol.* **261,** H583–H589.
141. Hendley, E. D., Ohlsson, W. G., and Musty, R. E. (1992) Interstrain aggression in hypertensive and/or hyperactive rats: SHR, WKY, WKHA, WKHT. *Physiol. Behav.* **51,** 1041–1046.
142. Cravchik, A. and Gejman, P. V. (1999) Functional analysis of the human D5 dopamine receptor missense and nonsense variants: differences in dopamine binding affinities. *Pharmacogenetics* **9,** 199–206.
143. Sato, M., Soma, M., Nakayama, T., and Kanmatsue, K. (2000) Dopamine D1 receptor gene polymorphism is associated with essential hypertension. *Hypertension* **36,** 183–186.
144. Carman, C. V. and Benovic, J. L. (1998) G protein-coupled receptors: turn-ons and turn-offs. *Curr. Opin. Neurobiol.* **8,** 335–344.
145. Ferguson, S. S. (2001) Evolving concepts in G protein-coupled receptor endocytosis: the role in receptor desensitization and signaling. *Pharmacol. Rev.* **53,** 1–24.
146. Jackson, A., Iwasiow, R. M., Chaar, Z. Y., Nantel, M. F., and Tiberi, M. (2002) Homologous regulation of the heptahelical D1A receptor responsiveness: specific cytoplasmic tail regions mediate dopamine-induced phosphorylation, desensitization and endocytosis. *J. Neurochem.* **82,** 683–697.
147. Kim, O. J., Gardner, B. R., Williams, D. B., et al. (2004) The role of phosphorylation in D1 dopamine receptor desensitization: evidence for a novel mechanism of arrestin association. *J. Biol. Chem.* **279,** 7999–8010.
148. Kohout, T. A. and Lefkowitz, R. J. (2003) Regulation of G protein-coupled receptor kinases and arrestins during receptor desensitization. *Mol. Pharmacol.* **63,** 9–18.
149. Lamey, M., Thompson, M., Varghese, G., et al. (2002) Distinct residues in the carboxyl tail mediate agonist-induced desensitization and internalization of the human dopamine D1 receptor. *J. Biol. Chem.* **277,** 9415–9421.
150. Penn, R. B., Pronin, A. N., and Benovic, J. L. (2000) Regulation of G protein-coupled receptor kinases. *Trends Cardiovasc. Med.* **10,** 81–89.
151. Pitcher, J. A., Freedman, N. J., and Lefkowitz, R. J. (1998) G protein-coupled receptor kinases. *Annu. Rev. Biochem.* **67,** 653–692.
152. Pitcher, J. A., Tesmer, J. J., Freeman, J. L., Capel, W. D., Stone, W. C., and Lefkowitz, R. J. (1999) Feedback inhibition of G protein-coupled receptor kinase 2 (GRK2) activity by extracellular signal-regulated kinases. *J. Biol. Chem.* **274,** 34,531–34,534.
153. Tiberi, M., Nash, S. R., Bertrand, L., Lefkowitz, R. J., and Caron, M. G. (1996) Differential regulation of dopamine D1A receptor responsiveness by various G protein-coupled receptor kinases. *J. Biol. Chem.* **271,** 3771–3778.
154. Vickery, R. G. and von Zastrow, M. (1999) Distinct dynamin-dependent and -independent mechanisms target structurally homologous dopamine receptors to different endocytic membranes. *J. Cell. Biol.* **144,** 31–43.
155. Gardner, B., Liu, Z. F., Jiang, D., and Sibley, D. R. (2001) The role of phosphorylation/dephosphorylation in agonist-induced desensitization of D_1 dopamine receptor function: evidence for a novel pathway for receptor dephosphorylation. *Mol. Pharmacol.* **59,** 310–321.
156. Wang, X., Gildea, J., Bengra, C., et al. (2003) Human renal angiotensin type 1 receptor regulation by the D1 dopamine receptor. *Council for High Blood Pressure Research Abstracts.* American Heart Association, Washington, DC, p. 85.
157. Zeng, C., Luo, Y., Asico, L. D., et al. (2003) Perturbation of D1 dopamine and AT1 receptor interaction in spontaneously hypertensive rats. *Hypertension* **42,** 787–792.

158. Sanada, H., Yatabe, J., Yoneda, M., et al. (2002) In vivo targeting of the renal G protein-coupled receptor kinase type 4 (GRK4) with antisense oligonucleotides induces natriuresis in spontaneously hypertensive rats. *Circulation* **106(Suppl II),** II-234.

159. Wang, Z., Asico, L. D., Felder, R. A., Robillard, J. E., Jose, P. A. (2004) Human GRK4γ A142V variant produces hypertension in transgenic mice. *FASEB J.* **18,** A353.

160. Allayee, H., Dominguez, K. M., Aouizerat, B. E., et al. (2001) Genome scan for blood pressure in Dutch dyslipidemic families reveals linkage to a locus on chromosome 4p. *Hypertension* **38,** 773–778.

161. Casari, G., Barlassina, C., Cusi, D., et al. (1995) Association of the α-adducin locus with essential hypertension. *Hypertension* **25,** 320–326.

162. Speirs, H. J., Katyk, K., Kumar, N. N., Benjafield, A. V., Wang, W. Y., and Morris, B. J. (2004) Association of G protein-coupled receptor kinase 4 haplotypes, but not HSD3B1 or PTP1B polymorphisms, with essential hypertension. *J. Hypertens.* **22,** 931–936.

163. Williams, S. M., Addy, J. A., Phillips, J. A., III, et al. (2000) Combinations of variations in multiple genes are associated with hypertension. *Hypertension* **36,** 2–6.

164. Williams, S. M., Ritchie, M. D., Phillips, J. A., III, et al. (2004) Identification of multilocus genotypes that associate with high-risk and low-risk for hypertension. *Hum. Hered.* **57,** 28–38.

165. Glazier, A. M., Nadeau, J. H., and Aitman, T. J. (2002) Finding genes that underlie complex traits. *Science* **298,** 2345–2349.

166. de Wardener, H. E. and MacGregor, G. A. (2002) Harmful effects of dietary salt in addition to hypertension. *J. Hum. Hypertens.* **16,** 213–223.

167. He, J., Ogden, L. G., Vupputuri, S., Bazzano, L. A., Loria, C., and Whelton, P. K. (1999) Dietary sodium intake and subsequent risk of cardiovascular disease in overweight adults. *JAMA* **282,** 2027–2034.

168. Hu, G., Qiao, Q., and Tuomilehto, J. (2002) Nonhypertensive cardiac effects of a high salt diet. *Curr. Hypertens. Rep.* **4,** 13–17.

169. Tuomilehto, J., Jousilahti, P., Rastenyte, D., et al. (2001) Urinary sodium excretion and cardiovascular mortality in Finland: a prospective study. *Lancet* **357,** 848–851.

170. Weinberger, M. H., Fineberg, N. S., Fineberg, S. E., and Weinberger, M. (2001) Salt sensitivity, pulse pressure, and death in normal and hypertensive humans. *Hypertension* **37,** 429–432.

171. Luippold, G., Schneider, S., Stefanescu, A., Benohr, P., and Muhlbauer, B. (2001) Dopamine D2-like receptors and amino acid-induced glomerular hyperfiltration in humans. *Br. J. Clin. Pharmacol.* **51(5),** 415–421.

172. Shigetomi, S., Ueno, S., Tosaki, H., Kohno, H., Hashimoto, S., and Fukuchi, S. (1986) Increased activity of sympatho-adrenomedullary system and decreased renal dopamine receptor content after short-term and long-term sodium loading in rats. *Nippon Naibunpi Gakkai Zasshi* **62,** 776–783.

173. Haney, M., Ward, A.S., Foltin, R.W., and Fischman, M.W. (2001) Effects of ecopipam, a selective dopamine D1 antagonist, on smoked cocaine self-administration by humans. *Psychopharmacology (Berl)* **155,** 330–337.

III   METABOLIC DISORDERS AND HYPERTENSION

11 Insulin Resistance and Hypertension

James R. Sowers

CONTENTS

1. INTRODUCTION

The National Cholesterol Education Program Adult Treatment Panel III (NCEP ATP III) uses the term "metabolic syndrome" to describe a constellation of risk factors associated with insulin resistance, namely abdominal obesity, hypertension, dyslipidemia, and prothrombotic and proinflammatory states (1). These physiological abnormalities are produced through the interaction of genetic, hormonal, and lifestyle factors. Individuals with metabolic syndrome have a greatly heightened risk of developing diabetes, coronary heart disease, stroke, and renal disease, as well as increased all-cause and cardiovascular mortality rates. Hypertension, one of the most prevalent components of metabolic syndrome, contributes directly to many of these complications. The relationship between blood pressure and risk of cardiovascular disease (CVD) events is continuous, consistent, and independent; the higher the blood pressure, the greater the chance of myocardial infarction, heart failure, stroke, and renal disease. The CVD risk escalates further when other risk factors are present, as in patients with metabolic syndrome.

Data from the Third National Health and Nutrition Examination Survey (NHANES III; 1988–1994) suggest that 47 million US adults (23.7% of the population) have metabolic syndrome (2). Its prevalence increases with age, body mass index (BMI), sedentary

From: *Contemporary Endocrinology: Hypertension and Hormone Mechanisms*
Edited by: R. M. Carey © Humana Press Inc., Totowa, NJ

lifestyle, smoking, Mexican-American and Indian-American ethnicity, high carbohydrate intake, and postmenopausal status *(11,12)*. NHANES III data indicate that 44% of individuals aged 60–69 yr and 60% of men with a BMI ≥30 kg/m^2 have metabolic syndrome *(2)*. The current prevalence of metabolic syndrome is likely to be much higher than estimated in NHANES III, and is projected to increase further, with a parallel escalation in related health problems, as more and more individuals become severely or morbidly obese. Physicians are in a strategic position to improve the nation's health by early identification and management of individuals with metabolic syndrome, thereby blunting the impending epidemic of cardiovascular and end-organ insulin resistance should be a key initiative in rising to this challenge.

2. INSULIN RESISTANCE AND HYPERTENSION

Hypertension is frequently associated with decreased insulin sensitivity *(3)*; reduced insulin sensitivity has been observed in normotensive offspring of first-degree relatives of hypertensive patients, independent of obesity *(4)*. Insulin resistance also predates hypertension in normotensive persons. In a prospective investigation of CVD risk factors involving 840 normotensive persons, insulin sensitivity was inversely related to development of hypertension over a 5-yr period *(5)*. This observation has been confirmed in other large studies *(6)*.

There is accumulating data that insulin resistance is associated with abnormalities of the renin–angiotensin system *(3,7)*. For example, the level of insulin resistance in hypertensive persons is influenced by a relatively common polymorphism of the angiotensin-converting enzyme (ACE) gene, their being a significantly greater insulin resistance with the DD geno type *(8)*. Recent evidence suggests that tissue overexpression of the RAS leads to impaired insulin signaling, in part by increasing the generation of reactive oxygen species *(3,8)*. Further, abrogation of the RAS with ACE inhibitor and angiotensin receptor blocking agents has been shown to improve insulin sensitivity in animals and humans *(1,8,10)*.

3. DEFINITION AND DIAGNOSIS: WHAT IS THE METABOLIC SYNDROME?

Occurrence of three or more of the following prespecified risk factors is sufficient for a positive diagnosis: abdominal obesity (most common feature [Fig. 1D], hypertension, hypertriglyceridemia, low plasma high-density lipoprotein cholesterol, and elevated fasting plasma glucose) (*see* Table 1 for defining levels) *(1)*. Patients rarely present with all of the five factors.

Each determinant can be assessed easily in clinical practice; for example, measuring waist circumference (at the level of the iliac crest at the end of normal expiration) with a tape measure confirms abdominal obesity, and an oral glucose tolerance test is not needed. Because metabolic syndrome is typically asymptomatic, affected individuals will normally be identified at routine medical examinations or when presenting with other complaints. If metabolic syndrome is suspected at this consultation (e.g., because the patient is overweight and/or hypertensive), screening for other components of the syndrome is warranted.

Several other abnormalities cluster with metabolic syndrome (Table 2). These are probably related to insulin resistance/compensatory hyperinsulinemia, but are not

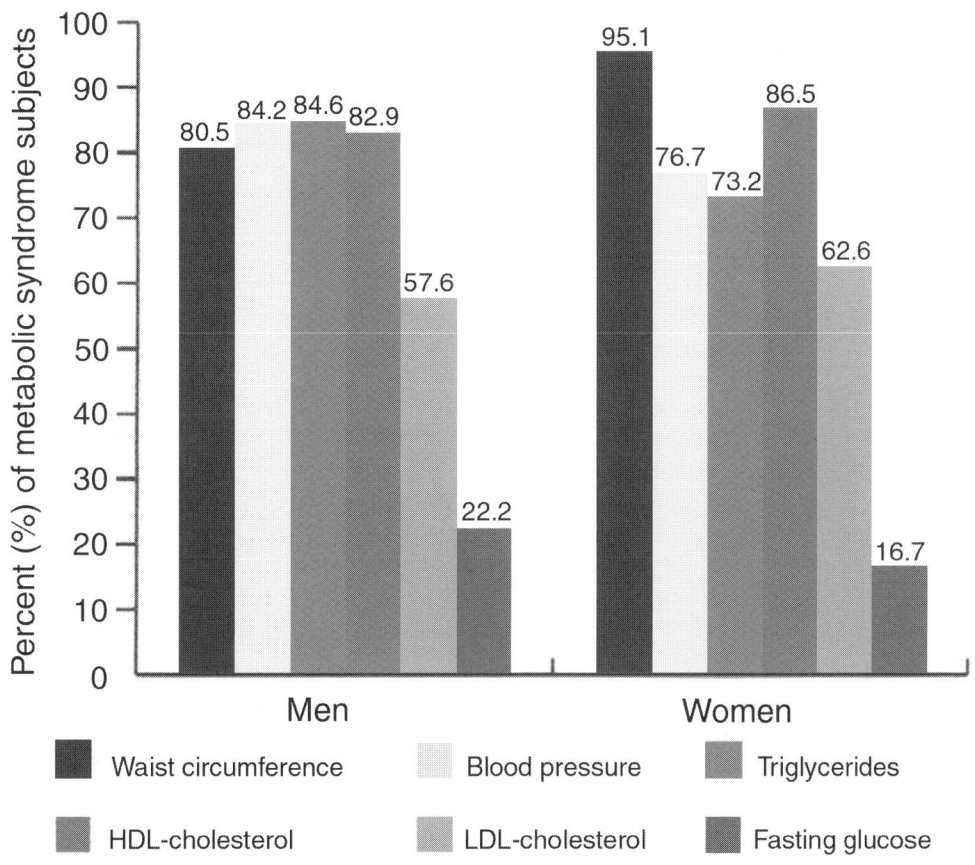

Fig. 1. Prevalence of selected risk factors among subjects with metabolic syndrome. From ref. *(15)*. (*See* color version of this figure on color plates.)

Table 1
Criteria for Identification of Metabolic Syndrome.
Metabolic Syndrome is Diagnosed When Three or More
of the Risk Determinants Listed in the Table are Present

Risk factor	Defining level
Abdominal obesity (waist circumference)	Men >102 cm (>40 in.) Women >88 cm (>35 in.)
Triglycerides	≥150 mg/dL (1.69 mmol/L)
High-density lipoprotein cholesterol	Men <40 mg/dL (1.03 mmol/L) Women <50 mg/dL (1.29 mmol/L)
Blood pressure	SBP ≥130 mmHg and/or DBP ≥85 mmHg
Fasting glucose	≥110 mg/dL (≥6.11 mmol/L)

SBP, systolic blood pressure; DBP, diastolic blood pressure. Adapted from ref. *(1)*.

Table 2
Abnormalittes Associated With Metabolic Syndrome

- Glucose intolerance
  - impaired fasting glucose
  - impaired glucose tolerance
  - type 2 diabetes mellitus
- Dyslipidemia
  - ↑ triglycerides
  - ↓ HDL-C
  - Small, dense LDL particles
  - ↑ postprandial lipemia
- Hemodynamic
  - ↑ sympathetic nervous system activity
  - ↑ renal sodium retention
  - ↑ blood pressure
- Microalbuminuria
- Hyperuricemima and gout
- ↑ oxidative stress
- ↑ renin-angiotensin-aldosterone system activity
- Chronic, low-grade inflammation
  - ↑ CRP
- Prothrombotic state
  - ↑ PAI-1
  - ↑ fibrinogen
  - ↑ von Willebrand factor levels
- Endothelial dysfunction
  - ↑ mononuclear cell adhesion
  - ↓ endothelium-dependent vasodilatation
- Polycstic ovary syndrome
- Non-alcoholic fatty liver disease
- Poor cardiorespiratory fitness

CRP, C-reactive protein; PAI-1, plasminogen activator inhibitor-1.

necessary for diagnosis. In other words, insulin resistance is not a disease *per se*; rather, it represents an increased risk of developing other abnormalities that further predispose to adverse clinical outcomes.

4. WHICH CLINICAL SEQUELA ARE ASSOCIATED WITH METABOLIC SYNDROME?

The next challenge for the physician is to appreciate and communicate to the patient the magnitude of the inherent risks of metabolic syndrome. Cardiovascular disease is the main adverse clinical outcome. This is not surprising given that coexistence of multiple CVD risk factors carries a greater susceptibility to cardiovascular morbidity and mortality than a disturbance in just one factor. The risk of a major cardiovascular event (myocardial infarction, sudden cardiac death, unstable angina, or stroke) is about twofold greater among individuals with metabolic syndrome than those without it *(13)*.

Metabolic syndrome also predisposes to type 2 diabetes mellitus. This is important from a CVD standpoint, because diabetes is regarded as a coronary risk equivalent *(1)*, meaning that the likelihood of a first major coronary event among patients with diabetes is as high as a recurrent event among individuals with established heart disease. Patients with diabetes and metabolic syndrome are thus at extremely high CVD risk. One report suggests that the incidence of cardiovascular events is five times higher among patients with diabetes and metabolic syndrome than among patients with diabetes alone *(14)*.

Individuals with metabolic syndrome are also susceptible to chronic renal disease, polycystic ovary syndrome, nonalcoholic fatty liver disease, cholesterol gallstones, asthma, sleep apnea, and some forms of cancer.

5. THE ROLE OF HYPERTENSION IN THE METABOLIC SYNDROME

Within the metabolic syndrome cluster, hypertension is defined as systolic blood pressure (SBP) ≥130 mmHg and diastolic blood pressure (DBP) ≥85 mmHg. It is present in 84.2% of men and 76.7% of women with metabolic syndrome (Fig. 1) *(15)*, and contributes directly to many adverse clinical outcomes. In its early stages, hypertension-related vascular and end-organ damage is often subclinical, manifesting itself only when a catastrophic cardiovascular event occurs (such as myocardial infarction or stroke). The development of microalbuminuria may serve as an early indicator of widespread vascular damage, being not only a pressure-dependent functional phenomenon in the glomerular vessels, but reflecting permanent atherosclerotic abnormalities throughout the entire vascular system.

Hypertension is also tightly associated with obesity. Obesity contributes to hypertension by activating the renin–angiotensin–aldosterone and sympathetic nervous systems. Chronic obesity also causes marked structural changes in the kidneys that eventually lead to a loss of nephron function and elevates arterial pressure further.

6. WHAT IS THE GOAL OF BLOOD PRESSURE MANAGEMENT?

The ultimate goal of antihypertensive therapy is to delay, prevent, or reverse blood pressure-related end-organ vascular damage. To achieve this most effectively, blood pressure should be reduced to target levels specified in the current guidelines. The current (seventh) report of the Joint National Committee on prevention, detection, evaluation, and treatment of high blood pressure (JNC7) recommends a goal of <140/90 mmHg in the general population *(16)*. However, a substantial proportion of patients with metabolic syndrome have diabetes or chronic kidney disease; JNC7 and the American Diabetes Association recommend a goal of <130/80 mmHg for such individuals *(16,17)*. Thus, the physician is challenged to be bold enough to adopt an intensive blood pressure management strategy to achieve and maintain goal blood pressure and protect the patient against future morbidity and mortality.

A survey utilizing the Framingham algorithm to evaluate coronary risk in NHANES III subjects with metabolic syndrome estimates that the controlling blood pressure to normal levels (120–129/80–84 mmHg) would prevent 28.1% of coronary events in men and 12.5% of events in women *(15)*. Control to optimal levels (<120/80 mmHg) was expected to prevent 28.2% of coronary events in men and 45.2% of events in women. However, clinical end point data are needed to confirm these figures.

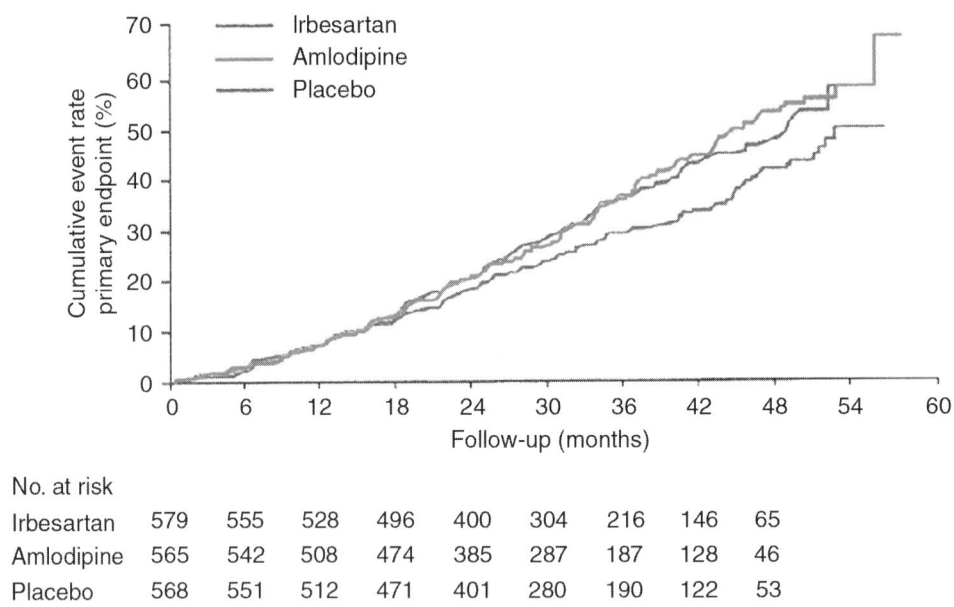

No. at risk

Irbesartan	579	555	528	496	400	304	216	146	65
Amlodipine	565	542	508	474	385	287	187	128	46
Placebo	568	551	512	471	401	280	190	122	53

Fig. 2. Algorithm for the treatment of hypertension. (*See* color version of this figure on color plates.)

Metabolic syndrome patients with hypertension should be managed according to current guidelines, which comprise lifestyle modifications and pharmacological therapy (Fig. 2) *(16)*.

7. REDUCING BLOOD PRESSURE THROUGH LIFESTYLE CHANGES

Therapeutic lifestyle changes focusing on weight reduction, exercise, and healthy eating (restricted sodium intake, the dietary approaches to stop hypertension [DASH] eating plan, and moderate alcohol consumption) is the foundation of hypertension management in persons with metabolic syndrome (Table 3) *(16)*. Individuals should also be counseled to stop smoking to reduce their overall CVD risk. A realistic weight loss target is 10% of initial weight over 6 mo. Losing 22 lbs (10 kg) reduces SSP by 5–20 mmHg in a large proportion of overweight individuals *(16)*.

Lifestyle interventions also prevent the development of diabetes, an important consideration in patients with metabolic syndrome. A program comprising weight loss and physical activity reduced the onset of diabetes by almost 60% vs placebo—and was significantly more effective than metformin—in prediabetic individuals with elevated fasting and postload plasma glucose levels *(18)*. Lifestyle modifications also reduce the overall CVD risk by improving other disturbances characteristic of metabolic syndrome, including dyslipidemia, insulin resistance, plasma glucose, and serum levels of C-reactive protein and plasminogen activator inhibitor-1 *(19)*.

Motivating patients to maintain lifestyle changes as a means of long-term blood pressure control presents another challenge to the physician. For example, many patients find it difficult to adhere to weight-reduction programs, or regain the lost weight after discharge from clinical care. Continued observation and encouragement with combined lifestyle interventions and antihypertensive therapy can help patients attain their blood

Table 3
Lifestyle Modifications to Prevent and Manage Hypertension

Modification	Recommendation	Approximate SSP reduction (range)
Weight reduction	Achieve and maintain normal body weight (BMI: 18.5–24.9 kg/m²) e.g.. – decrease portion sizes for meals, snacks – reduce portion sizes or frequency of consumption of high-calorie beverages – reduce energy intake by 500 kcal/d	5–20 mmHg/10 kg
Adopt DASH eating plan	Consume a diet rich in fruits, vegetables, and low-fat dairy products with a reduced content of saturated and total fat	8–14 mmHg
Dietary sodium reduction	Reduce dietary sodium intake to ≤100 mmol/d (2.4 g sodium or 6 g sodium chloride) NB. a high sodium intake is especially deleterious in overweight individuals	2–8 mmHg
Physical activity	Engage in regular aerobic physical activities that raise the heart rate, such as brisk walking (≥30 min/d, most days of the week)	4–9 mmHg
Moderation of alcohol	Limit consumption to ≤2 drinks (e.g., 24 oz beer, 10 oz wine, or 3 oz 80-proof whiskey) per day in most men and to ≤1 drink per day in women and lighter-weight persons	2–4 mmHg

BMI, body mass index; DASH, dietary approaches to stop hypertension. From ref. (16).

181

pressure goal, making them more likely to adhere to the lifestyle changes through positive reinforcement.

8. USE OF ANTIHYPERTENSIVE DRUGS

Once a decision has been made to adopt a pharmacological approach to hypertension management, the challenge is to select the most appropriate drug. According to JNC7, thiazide diuretics, β-blockers, ACE inhibitors, angiotensin receptor blockers (ARBs), and calcium channel blockers are suitable for reducing blood pressure and preventing hypertensive complications in patients with metabolic syndrome (16). Antihypertensive drug selection should be tailored to the individual, taking into account the metabolic syndrome determinants present and any comorbid conditions, such as renal disease, that are compelling indications for specific agents.

8.1. Thiazide Diuretics

Thiazide diuretics are widely regarded as the cornerstone of antihypertensive drug therapy. JNC7 recommends initial therapy with a thiazide diuretic in patients with uncomplicated hypertension, either alone or combined with drugs from other classes. At high doses, however, diuretics may cause untoward metabolic disturbances (e.g., hypokalemia, hyperuricemia, impaired glucose control, and increased insulin resistance), which are of concern in metabolic syndrome patients. Combining a low dose of diuretic with another antihypertensive agent provides additive blood pressure– lowering efficacy and minimizes drug-related, dose-dependent side effects. Diuretic-induced potassium depletion can be offset by coadministering an ARB or ACE inhibitor.

8.2. β-Blockers

β-Blockers can have adverse effects on insulin sensitivity in patients with diabetes or obesity, and have been shown to predispose to weight gain and the onset of type 2 diabetes in some population studies. These potentially adverse effects need to be balanced against the proven benefits of beta-blockers in reducing cardiovascular risk. β-Blockers are especially useful in patients with ischemic heart disease.

8.3. Calcium Channel Blockers

Because calcium channel blockers have neutral effects on lipid and glucose metabolism, they are appropriate for patients with metabolic syndrome. Clinical outcome trials, such as the hypertension optimal treatment (HOT) trial (20) and the antihypertensive and lipid-lowering treatment to prevent heart attack trial (ALLHAT) (21) showed that calcium channel blockers are safe and effective in controlling blood pressure and reducing CVD events in patients with diabetes. Side effects associated with vasodilatation, such as flushing, headache, and ankle edema, can be troublesome.

8.4. ACE Inhibitors

Several large clinical trials, including the heart outcomes prevention evaluation (HOPE) study (22,23), demonstrated that ACE inhibitors have cardioprotective and renoprotective properties beyond their effect on blood pressure. These benefits extend to patients with diabetes (23). ACE inhibitors also appear to delay the onset of diabetes (22). The most common adverse effect of ACE inhibitors is a chronic dry cough.

8.5. Angiotensin Receptor Blockers

Renoprotection data from clinical trials, such as the irbesartan diabetic nephropathy trial (Fig. 3), indicate that ARBs slow the progression of renal disease in patients with type 2 diabetes *(24–27)*. Other outcome trials indicate that ARBs also delay the onset of diabetes and prevent cardiovascular events *(28,29)*. The incidence of adverse effects with ARBs appears to be lower than with other currently available antihypertensive agents.

8.6. Combination Therapy

Clinical trials consistently show that most patients require two or more antihypertensive agents to reach blood pressure goal. Most national and international hypertension management guidelines recognize the need for multidrug therapy *(16,17,30)*, and some recommend first-line treatment with a combination of two drugs in certain patients. For example, JNC7 recommends considering initial treatment with two drugs if blood pressure is >20/10 mmHg above goal *(16)*, and the International Society on Hypertension in Blacks recommends combination therapy if blood pressure is ≥15/10 mmHg above goal *(30)*. The combination should include a diuretic in almost all cases *(16)*.

Using fixed-dose combinations containing two antihypertensive agents eases the process of blood pressure control. Selecting efficacious, well-tolerated, once daily combinations allows goal blood pressure to be achieved quickly in a broad range of patients, and may encourage patient compliance by reducing pill burden. Such formulations are also cost effective.

8.7. Microalbuminuria and Antihypertensive Medication

Microalbuminuria (urinary albumin excretion 30–300 mg/d) clusters with metabolic syndrome, the prevalence being significantly higher among those with than without metabolic syndrome (12.3% vs 4.7%; $p = 0.004$) *(31)*. In many patients, microalbuminuria is attributable to diabetic nephropathy.

The presence of microalbuminuria demands attention because it is associated with a 50% increase in cardiovascular risk in the general population *(32)*, suggesting that it reflects more widespread vascular damage. Of the individual metabolic syndrome components, microalbuminuria confers the strongest risk of cardiovascular death *(33)*.

Rigorous blood pressure control is paramount to prevent the development and progression of microalbuminuria. Guidelines typically recommend a target of <130/80 mmHg in patients with renal disease, using a regimen that includes an ARB or ACE inhibitor (i.e., antihypertensive agents with proven renoprotective properties) *(16,17,30)*.

9. CONCLUSIONS

With the expected explosion in prevalence of metabolic syndrome, as the number of obese and overweight individuals increases, the consequences of ignoring it are clear: a dramatic increase in cardiovascular morbidity and mortality, and an increase in diabetes and its complications. The downstream costs of these healthcare problems will be substantial. Early intervention will reap future rewards for the physician, the patient, and the healthcare provider.

Hypertension is a highly prevalent component of metabolic syndrome that dramatically heightens the risk of stroke and accelerates the progression of atherosclerosis and renal

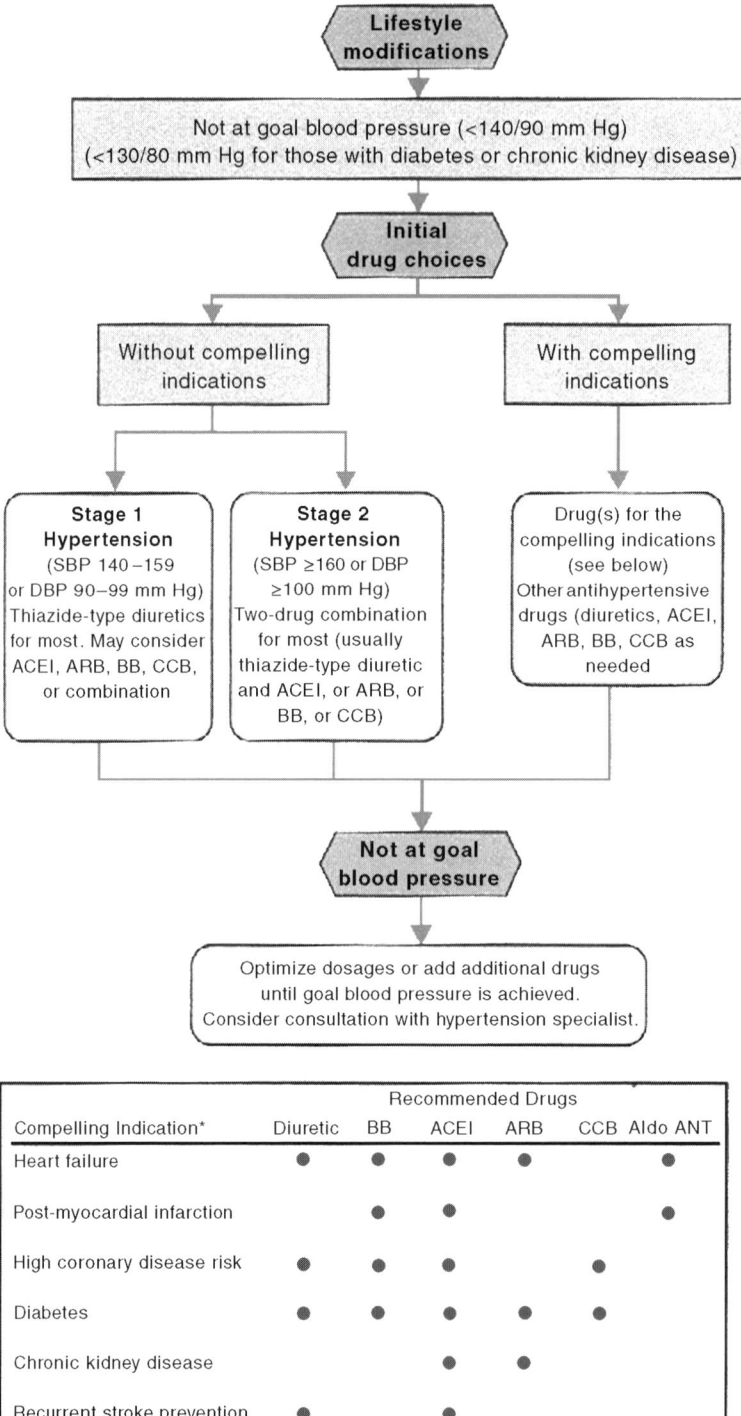

Fig. 3. Cumulative proportions of patients with the primary composite end point (doubling of baseline serum creatinine, development of end-stage renal disease, or death from any cause) in 1715 patients with nephropathy due to type 2 diabetes treated with irbesartan 300 mg, amlodipine 10 mg, or placebo in the Irbesartan Diabetic Nephropathy Trial. (*See* color version of this figure on color plates.)

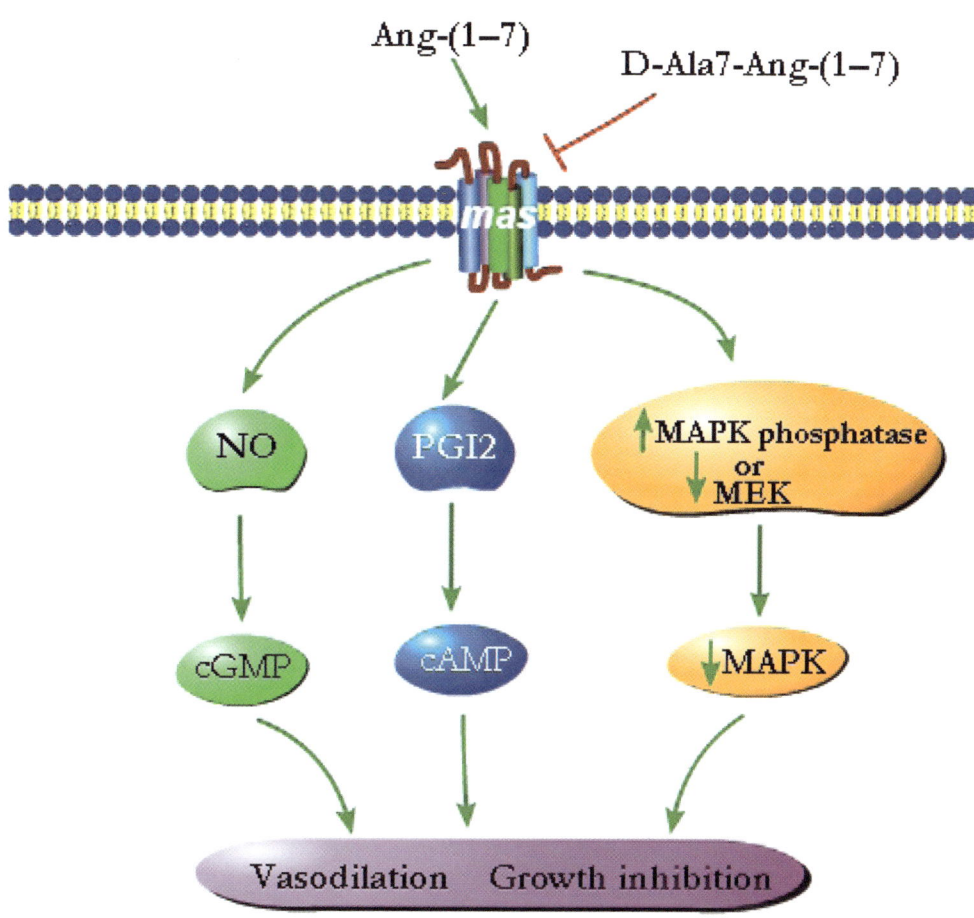

Color Plate 3. Chapter 3, Fig. 4. The major signal transduction pathways for Ang-(1–7). Ang-(1–7) activates the G protein-coupled *mas* receptor to increase the production of nitric oxide (NO) and prostacyclin (PGI_2) to increase cGMP and cAMP, respectively. Ang-(1–7) also reduces the mitogen-activated protein kinases (MAPKs) by either increasing MAPK phosphatases or reducing the MAPK kinase MEK. The increase in cAMP and cGMP and the decrease in MAPK activity cause vasodilation and inhibit cell growth. (*See* discussion on p. 52.)

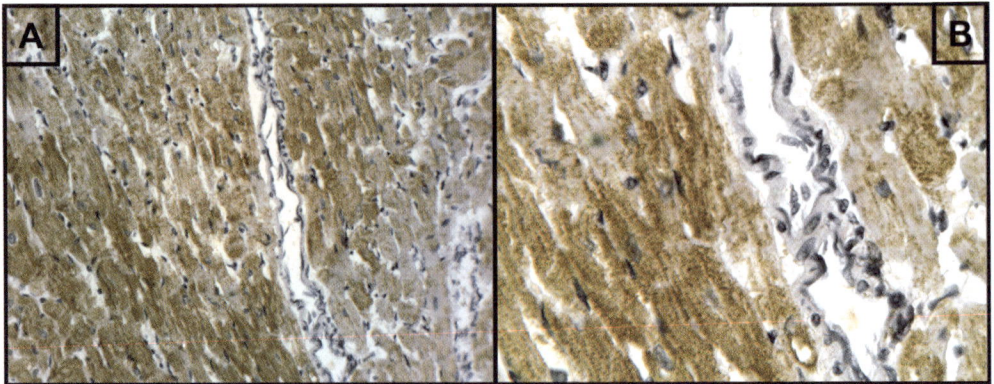

Color Plate 1. Chapter 3, Fig. 2. Expression of Ang-(1–7)-like cardiac immunoreactivity in the rat. Ang-(1–7) staining was restricted to ventricular myocytes whereas it appeared as a granular reaction product throughout the cytoplasm (Panel **A**). The absence of Ang-(1–7) staining in endothelial and vascular smooth muscle cells of coronary vessels is best illustrated in the higher power magnification of Panel **B**. (*See* discussion on p. 46.)

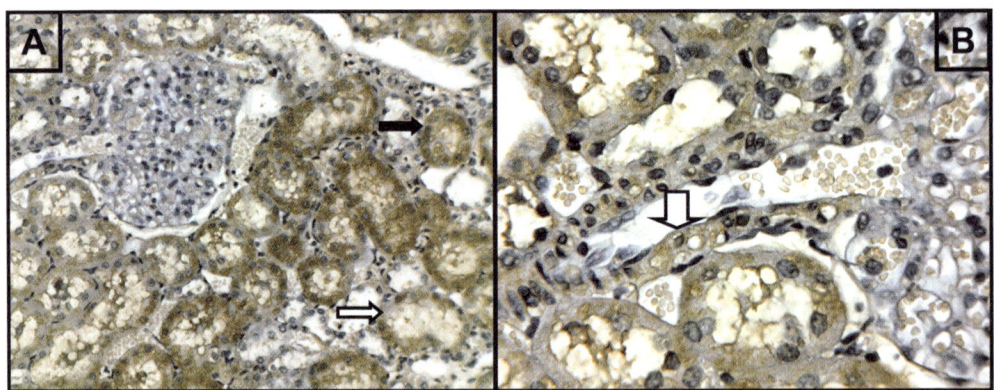

Color Plate 2. Chapter 3, Fig. 3. Characteristics of Ang-(1–7)-like immunoreactivity in rat kidney. The most intense staining for Ang-(1–7) was in the thick-walled epithelial cells of the proximal-convoluted tubule (filled arrow in Panel **A**). A less intense staining for the peptide was observed in the thin-walled epithelial cells of collecting ducts (open arrow of Panel **A**). At both low (Panel A) and high (Panel **B**) power magnifications, there is essentially no staining for Ang-(1–7) in the glomerulus. Panel B also illustrates modest staining in the afferent arteriole (arrowhead in Panel B). (*See* discussion on p. 47.)

20. Hansson, L., Zanchetti, A., Carruthers, S. G., et al. (1998) Effects of intensive blood pressure lowering and low-dose aspirin in patients with hypertension: principal results of the hypertension optimal treatment (HOT) randomised trial. *Lancet* **351(9118)**, 1755–1762.

21. The ALLHAT Officers and Coordinators for the ALLHAT Collaborative Research Group. (2002) Major outcomes in high-risk hypertensive patients randomized to angiotensin-converting enzyme inhibitor or calcium channel blocker vs diuretic. The antihypertensive and lipid-lowering treatment to prevent heart attack trial (ALLHAT). *JAMA* **288(23)**, 2981–2997.

22. The Heart Outcomes Prevention Evaluation Study Investigators. (2002) Effects of an angiotensin-converting-enzyme inhibitor, ramipril, on cardiovascular events in high-risk patients. *N Engl. J. Med.* **342(3)**, 145–153.

23. Heart Outcomes Prevention Evaluation Study Investigators. (2000) Effects of ramipril on cardiovascular and microvascular outcomes in people with *Diabetes mellitus*: results of the HOPE study and MICRO-HOPE substudy. *Lancet* **355(9200)**, 253–259.

24. Lewis, E. J., Hunsicker, L. G., Clarke, W. R., et al. (2001) Renoprotective effect of the angiotensin-receptor antagonist irbesartan in patients with nephropathy due to type 2 diabetes. *N Engl. J. Med.* **345(12)**, 851–860.

25. Brenner, B. M., Cooper, M. E., de Zeeuw, D., et al. (2001) Effects of losartan on renal and cardiovascular outcomes in patients with type 2 diabetes and nephropathy. *N Engl. J. Med.* **345(12)**, 861–869.

26. Parving, H. H., Lehnert, H., Brochner-Mortensen, J., et al. (2001) The effect of irbesartan on the development of diabetic nephropathy in patients with type 2 diabetes. *N Engl. J. Med.* **345(12)**, 870–878.

27. Viberti, G. and Wheeldon, N. M. (2002) Microalbuminuria reduction with valsartan in patients with type 2 *Diabetes mellitus*: a blood pressure-independent effect. Circulation **106(6)**, 672–678.

28. Dahlöf, B., Devereux, R. B., Kjeldsen, S. E., et al. (2002) Cardiovascular morbidity and mortality in the Losartan intervention for endpoint reduction in hypertension study (LIFE): a randomised trial against atenolol. *Lancet* **359(9311)**, 995–1003.

29. Pfeffer, M. A., Swedberg, K., Granger, C. B., et al. (2003) Effects of candesartan on mortality and morbidity in patients with chronic heart failure: the CHARM- Overall Programme. *Lancet* **362(9386)**, 759–766.

30. Douglas, J. G., Bakris, G. L., Epstein, M., et al. (2003) Management of high blood pressure in African Americans: consensus statement of the Hypertension in African Americans Working Group of the International Society on Hypertension in Blacks. *Arch. Intern. Med.* **163(5)**, 525–541.

31. Chen, J., Muntner, P., Hamm, L. L., et al. (2004) The metabolic syndrome and chronic kidney disease in U.S. adults. *Ann. Intern. Med.* **140(3)**, 167–174.

32. Hillege, H. L., Fidler, V., Diercks, G. F., et al. (2002) Urinary albumin excretion predicts cardiovascular and noncardiovascular mortality in general population. *Circulation* **106(14)**, 1777–1782.

33. Isomaa, B., Almgren, P., Tuomi, T., et al. (2001) Cardiovascular morbidity and mortality associated with the metabolic syndrome. *Diab. Care* **24(4)**, 683–689.

disease, yet is easily treated. By emphasizing the importance of a healthy lifestyle and making informed choices in drug selection, physicians can rise to the challenge of achieving goal blood pressure in all their metabolic syndrome patients. Reducing blood pressure to goal should translate into immense public health benefits by preventing future morbidity and mortality.

REFERENCES

1. Expert Panel on Detection, Evaluation, and Treatment of High Blood Cholesterol in Adults. (2001) Executive summary of the Third Report of the National Cholesterol Education Program (NCEP) Expert Panel on detection, evaluation, and treatment of high blood cholesterol in adults (Adult Treatment Panel III). *JAMA* **285(19),** 2486–2497.
2. Ford, E. S., Giles, W. H., and Dietz, W. H. (2002) Prevalence of the metabolic syndrome among US adults: findings from the Third National Health and Nutrition Examination Survey. *JAMA* **287(3),** 356–359.
3. Sowers, J. R. (2004) Insulin resistance and hypertension. *Am. J. Physiol. Heart Circ. Physiol.* **286,** H1597–H1602.
4. Balletshofer, B. M., Rittig, K., Enderle, M. D., et al. (2000) Endothelial dysfunction is detectable in young normotensive first-degree relatives of subjects with type 2 diabetes in association with insulin resistance. *Circulation* **101,** 1780–1784.
5. Goff, D. C. Jr., Zaccaro, D. J., Haffner, S. M., et al. (2003) Insulin sensitivity and the risk of incident hypertension: insights from the insulin resistance atherosclerosis study. *Diab. Care* **26,** 805–809.
6. Ferrannini, E. (2003) Analysis of data on insulin resistance from the European group for the study of insulin resistance: focus on obesity and hypertension. *Endocrinol. Pract.* **9,** 43–49.
7. McFarlane, S., Kumar, A., and Sowers, J. R. (2003) Mechanisms by which angiotensin-converting enzyme inhibitors prevent diabetes and cardiovascular disease. *Am. J. Cardiol.* **91(Suppl),** 30H–37H.
8. Perticone, F., Ceravolo, R., Iacopino, S., et al. (2001) Relationship between angiotensin-converting enzyme gene polymorphism and insulin resistance in never-treated hypertensive patients. *J. Clin. Endocrinol. Metab.* **86,** 172–178.
9. Blendea, M. C., Jacobs, D., Stump, C. S., et al. (2005) Abrogation of oxidative stress improves insulin sensitivity in the Ren2 Rat model of tissue angiotensin II overexpression. *Am. J. Physiol. Endocrinol. Metab.* **288(2),** E353–E359.
10. Sowers, J. R. and Stump, C. S. (2004) Insights into the biology of diabetic vascular disease: What's new? *Am. J. Hypertens.* **17(11 Suppl),** S2–S6.
11. Park, Y. W., Zhu, S., Palaniappan, L., et al. (2003) The metabolic syndrome: prevalence and associated risk factor findings in the US population from the third national health and nutrition examination survey, 1988–1994. *Arch. Intern. Med.* **163(4),** 427–436.
12. Resnick, H. E. (2002) Metabolic syndrome in American Indians. *Diab. Care* **25(7),** 1246–1247.
13. Ninomiya, J. K., L'Italien, G., Criqui, M. H., et al. (2004) Association of the metabolic syndrome with history of myocardial infarction and stroke in the Third National Health and Nutrition Examination Survey. *Circulation* **109(1),** 42–46.
14. Bonora, E., Targher, G., Formentini, G., et al. (2004) The metabolic syndrome is an independent predictor or cardiovascular disease in type 2 diabetic subjects. Prospective data from the verona diabetes complications study. *Diabet. Med.* **21(1),** 52–58.
15. Wong, N. D., Pio, J. R., Franklin, S. S., et al. (2003) Preventing coronary events by optimal control of blood pressure and lipids in patients with the metabolic syndrome. *Am. J. Cardiol.* **91(12),** 1421–1426.
16. Chobanian, A. V., Bakris, G. L., Black, H. R., et al. (2003) Seventh report of the Joint National Committee on prevention, detection, evaluation, and treatment of high blood pressure. *Hypertension* **42(6),** 1206–1252.
17. American Diabetes Association. (2004) Hypertension management in adults with diabetes. *Diab. Care* **27(Suppl 1),** S65–S67.
18. Knowler, W. C., Barrett-Connor, E., Fowler, S. E., et al. (2002) Reduction in the incidence of type 2 diabetes with lifestyle intervention or metformin. *N Engl. J. Med.* **346(6),** 393–403.
19. Grundy, S. M., Brewer, H. B. Jr, Cleeman, J. I., et al. (2004) Definition of metabolic syndrome: report of the National Heart, Lung, and Blood Institute/American Heart Association conference on scientific issues related to definition. *Circulation* **109(3),** 433–438.

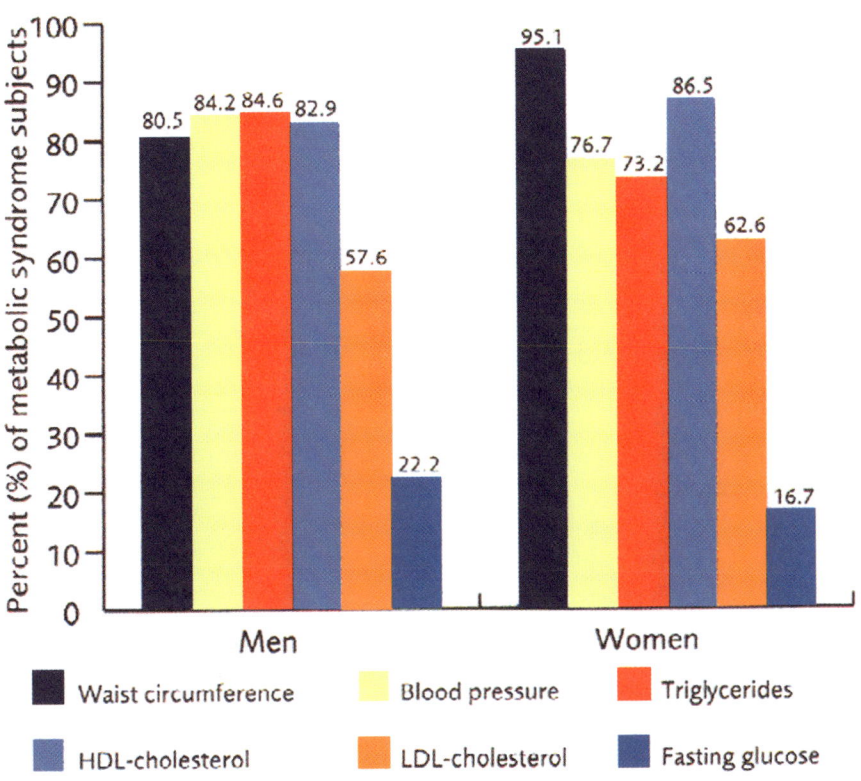

Color Plate 4. Chapter 11, Fig. 1. Prevalence of selected risk factors among subjects with metabolic syndrome. From ref. *(15)*. (*See* discussion on p. 179.)

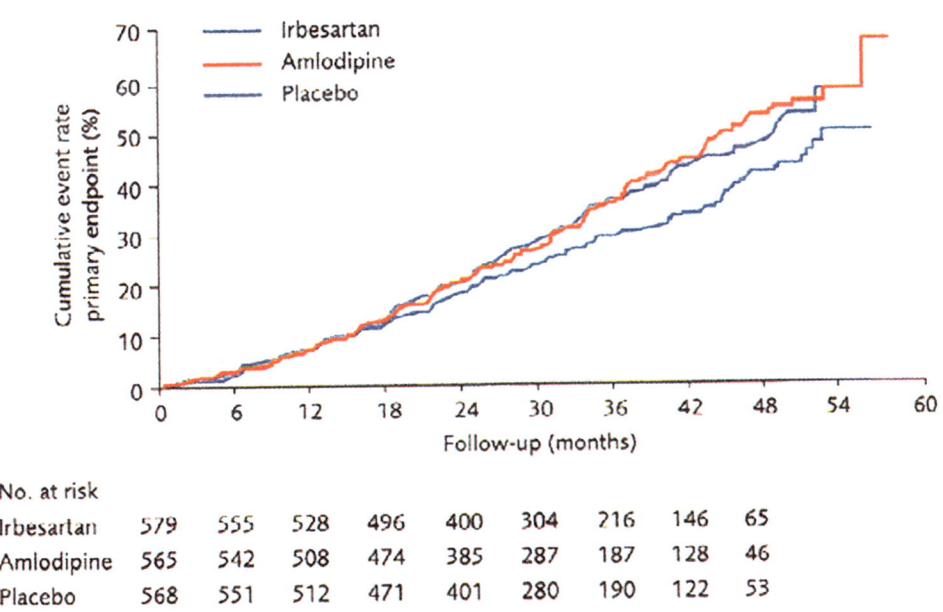

No. at risk									
Irbesartan	579	555	528	496	400	304	216	146	65
Amlodipine	565	542	508	474	385	287	187	128	46
Placebo	568	551	512	471	401	280	190	122	53

Color Plate 5. Chapter 11, Fig. 2. Algorithm for the treatment of hypertension. (*See* discussion on p. 180.)

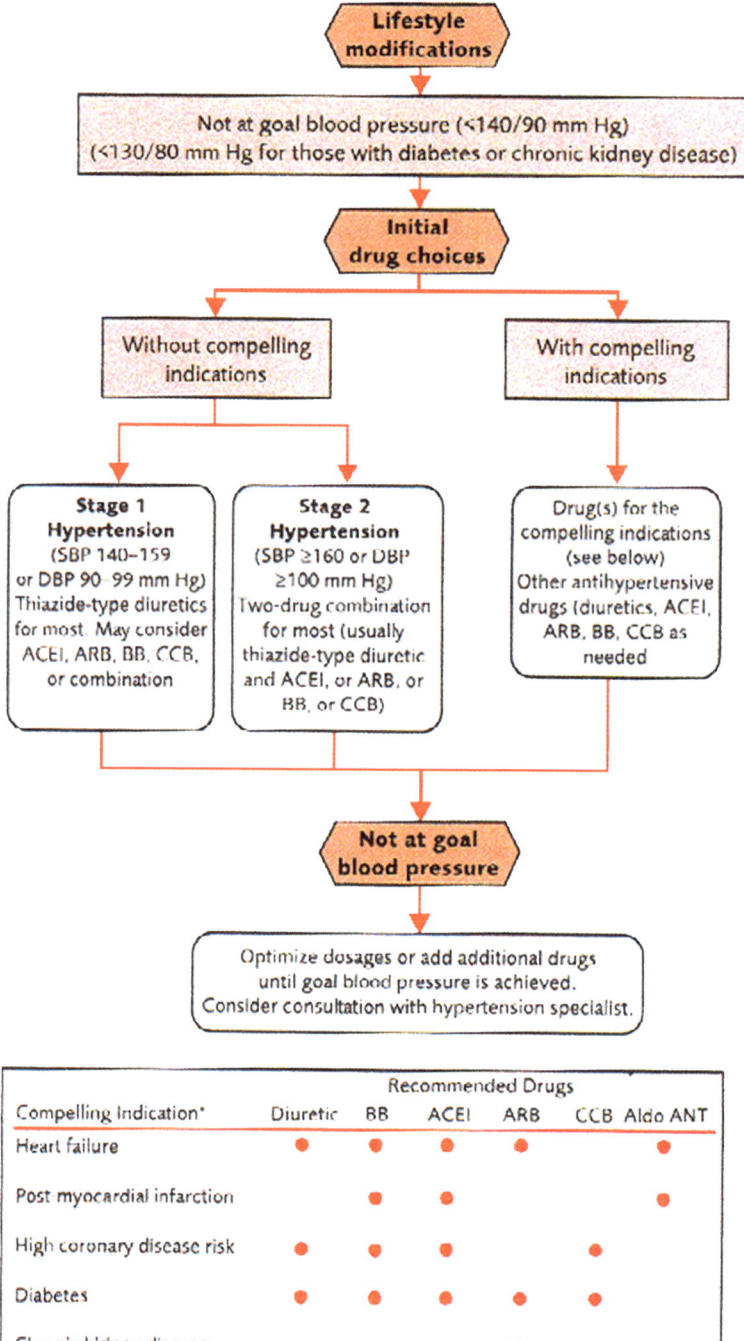

Color Plate 6. Chapter 11, Fig. 3. Cumulative proportions of patients with the primary composite end point (doubling of baseline serum creatinine, development of end-stage renal disease, or death from any cause) in 1715 patients with nephropathy due to type 2 diabetes treated with irbesartan 300 mg, amlodipine 10 mg, or placebo in the Irbesartan Diabetic Nephropathy Trial. (*See* discussion on p. 183.)

12 Fatty Acids, Cell Signaling, and Cardiovascular Risk

Brent M. Egan

CONTENTS

1. FATTY ACIDS AND CARDIOVASCULAR RISK: CLINICAL EPIDEMIOLOGY

Abdominal obesity is linked to increased non-esterified fatty acid (NEFA) concentrations and turnover that are resistant to suppression by insulin *(1,2)*. Similarly, physical activity and maximal oxygen consumption, a marker of physical fitness, are inversely associated with plasma NEFA concentrations measured as the area under-the-curve during a standard 2-h oral glucose tolerance test *(3)*. Familial combined hyperlipidemia, a relatively common autosomal dominant trait, is associated with high plasma NEFAs as well as greater and more prolonged elevation of NEFAs following a fat load *(4)*. Obesity, sedentary lifestyles, and familial combined hyperlipidemia are associated with high blood pressure, abnormal glucose and lipid metabolism, and more cardiovascular events including sudden death *(5–7)*.

NEFAs may be a common denominator linking diverse entities such as central obesity, physical inactivity, and familial combined hyperlipidemia to elevated blood pressures and greater cardiovascular risk. In the Paris Prospective Study, e.g., elevated fasting NEFA concentrations were independently predictive of the development of hypertension and sudden death *(8,9)*. In the same study, hypertensive men had higher fasting NEFA concentrations than normotensive men with the greatest differences evident in leaner than more obese subjects *(10)*. Moreover, in 50-yr-old Swedish men, higher serum levels

From: *Contemporary Endocrinology: Hypertension and Hormone Mechanisms*
Edited by: R. M. Carey © Humana Press Inc., Totowa, NJ

of saturated fatty acids and oleic acid were independently predictive of left ventricular hypertrophy assessed at age 70 *(11)*. Collectively, these data suggest that abnormalities of NEFA metabolism characterized by relatively high plasma concentrations that do not suppress normally in response to insulin may participate in increasing metabolic and hemodynamic risk factors for cardiovascular disease and events. Clinical physiologial evidence supporting the notion that abnormalities of NEFAs contribute to metabolic and hemodynamic risk will now be examined (Fig. 1).

2. FATTY ACIDS AND CARDIOVASCULAR RISK: CLINICAL PHYSIOLOGY

In this section, we will focus on the (patho)physiological actions of insulin at several key targets in cardiovascular risk and disease. The next section will examine potential signaling mechanisms underlying the physiological observations.

2.1. Fatty Acid and Glucose Metabolism

NEFAs may promote impaired fasting glucose and diabetes mellitus by one or more mechanisms. Potential processes include reducing hepatic insulin uptake *(12)*, increasing hepatic glugoneogenesis *(13)*, impairing pancreatic β-cell responses to glucose-stimulated insulin secretion *(14)*, inducing apoptosis of pancreatic islet cells *(15)*, and decreasing both oxidative and nonoxidative glucose metabolism in skeletal muscle *(16,17)*.

2.2. Fatty Acids and Lipid Metabolism

NEFAs may also promote a complex dyslipidemia characterized by increased VLDL-triglyceride rich particles, reduced levels of HDL-cholesterol, and an increased number of small dense LDL-cholesterol particles. Potential mechanisms by which NEFAs may contribute to these complex disturbance of lipid metabolism include increasing hepatic apoprotein B production and VLDL synthesis, with an increase in the number of VLDL-triglyceride rich particles *(4)*. HDL-cholesterol concentrations fall in part as cholesterol is transferred from HDL to VLDL by the activity of cholesterol–ester transfer protein (CETP). As triglycerides are hydrolyzed from the greater number of VLDL-particles by endothelial lipoprotein lipase, large numbers of small, dense LDL particles are produced *(18)*.

2.3. Fatty Acids and Endothelial Function

High-fat meals impair flow-mediated dilation, a marker of endothelial function *(19)*. Endothelial function is also impaired in patients with insulin resistance including abdominal obesity and diabetes mellitus *(20)*. The adverse effects of high-fat meals, central obesity, and diabetes on endothelial function may be mediated by NEFAs. NEFAs, especially cis-unsaturated fatty acids, produce a concentration dependent inhibition of Ca^{2+}-calmodulin dependent nitric oxide synthase activity in endothelial cells *(21,22)*. Moreover, short-term elevations of plasma NEFAs produced by simultaneous infusion of intralipid, a source of triglycerides, and heparin, which activates endothelial lipoprotein lipase, also reduce endothelial cell nitric oxide production and impair responses to endothelium-dependent vasodilators such as metacholine and acetylcholine *(23)*. In addition to suppressing endothelial nitric oxide synthase activity, NEFAs also enhance

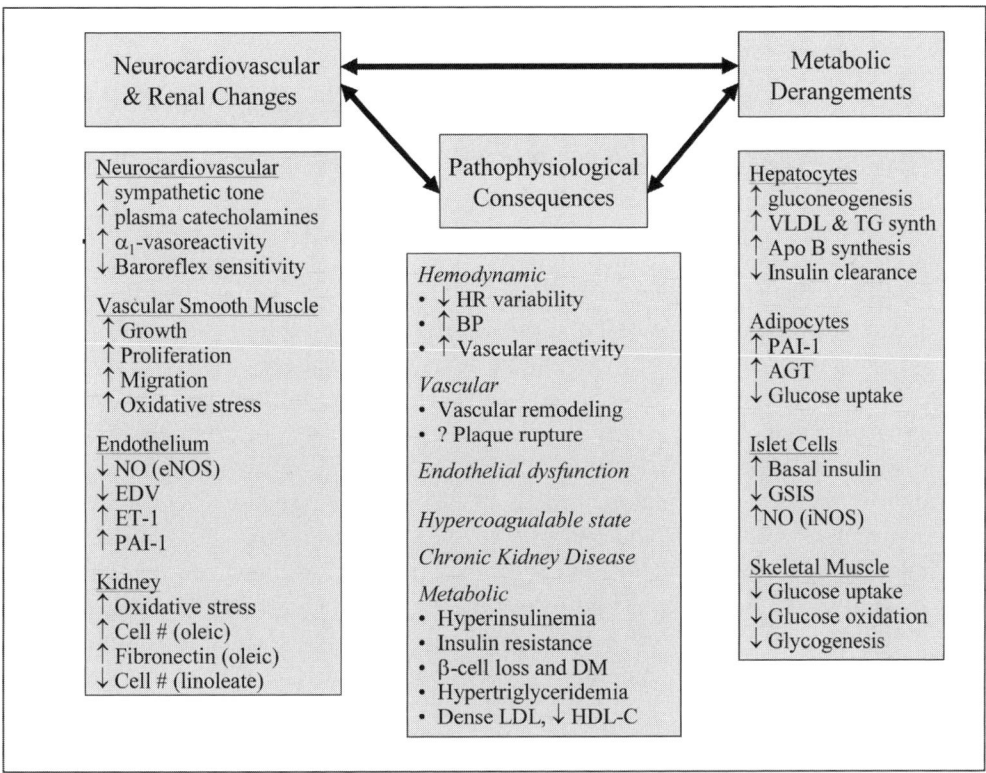

Fig. 1. Selected target organ system and cellular effects of NEFAs are shown at key sites mediating hemodynamic, cardiovascular, renal, and metabolic effects of fatty acids. The pathophysiological consequences reflect an interplay of the neurocardiovascular, renal, and metabolic derangements. The interactions between these factors are bidirectional and reinforcing, which help explain the high incidence of cardiovascular and renal disease and long-term worsening of metabolic disturbances in metabolic syndrome patients. For example, impairment of nitric oxide synthase can impair renal pressure natriuresis, raise in blood pressure, and worsen insulin resistance, whereas hypertension, dyslipidemia, and hyperglycemia exacerbate endothelial dysfunction. See text for further discussion and references.

endothelin and plasminogen activator inhibitor-1 (PAI-1) production in cultured endothelial cells *(24,25)*.

2.4. Fatty Acids and Vascular Reactivity

Obese patients have increased vascular α-adrenergic reactivity and tone *(26,27)*. In part, this appears to reflect increased sympathetic nerve activity and structural vascular changes. Moreover, increasing NEFA concentrations locally in the dorsal hand veins of healthy, normotensive volunteers induces a two- to threefold increase in the vasoconstrictor sensitivity to phenylephrine, a selective α_1-agonist but not to clonidine, a partial α_2-agonist *(28,29)*. When NEFA concentrations are raised systemically with a co-infusion of intralipid and heparin, the pressor sensitivity to phenylephrine is enhanced in lean normotensive volunteers, obese hypertensive subjects, and in patients with chronic kidney disease *(30,31)*. The enhanced vasoconstrictor responses to phenylephrine in human dorsal hand veins were blocked by pretreatment with indomethacin *(32)*. These data suggest that fatty acids induced the production of cyclo-oxygenase products, which augmented vascular α_1-adrenergic reactivity.

2.5. Fatty Acids and Autonomic Function

When plasma NEFA concentrations are elevated over the course of 4 h with infusion of intralipid and heparin, blood pressure, and heart rate are elevated at 2 h and rise further by 4 h in human volunteers (33). With the infusion of intralipid and heparin, plasma epinephrine and norepinephrine concentrations increase, and the ratio of low frequency to high frequency bands on power spectral analysis of heart rate variability also increases (34). The data from power spectral analysis of heart rate variability suggest that NEFAs increase the preponderance of sympathetic to parasympathetic control of heart rate, which is a characteristic of obese patients (35). These data further suggest that NEFAs can activate the sympathetic nervous system and inhibit parasympathetic function.

In response to short-term elevation of NEFAs produced by co-infusion of intralipid and heparin, the sympathomimetic effects of NEFAs predominate (33). More specifically, the pressor response to the elevation of NEFAs is associated with an increase of catecholamines, heart rate, and the ratio of sympathetic to parasympathetic control of heart rate variability (34). However, a short-term elevation of blood pressure typically activates carotid and other arterial baroreceptors, which suppress plasma catecholamines, reduce heart rate, and decrease sympathetic to parasympathetic control of the heart (36).

2.6. Abdominal Obesity, Fatty Acids, and Neurogenic Hypertension

As noted previously, NEFAs have been linked epidemiologically to hypertension and its genesis. NEFAs have several actions that could contribute to hypertension and help explain the link between the obesity epidemic and increasing prevalence of hypertension (37). Hypertensive patients are more likely to be overweight and obese than normotensive individuals. Moreover, when matched for body mass index, hypertensives are more likely to have a centralized fat pattern and a greater amount of visceral to subcutaneous abdominal fat than normotensives (38). Even within the normotensive range, abdominally obese subjects have higher blood pressures than individuals with gluteofemoral obesity, and these blood pressure differences are related to insulin resistance (39).

Subjects with abdominal obesity are not only resistant to insulin-mediated glucose disposal, but they are also resistant to insulin's NEFA lowering actions (1,2,40). Moreover, resistance to insulin's effects on fatty acids during a euglycemic clamp coincides with higher plasma NEFAs over 24 h and with a higher plasma NEFA nadir following a mixed meal (40–42). The NEFA abnormality in obese hypertensives is especially prominent. NEFAs were suppressed in upper body obese normotensives by roughly 50% and turnover by approximately one-third when plasma insulin was raised just 5 µU/mL (2). Abdominally obese hypertensives did not suppress NEFA concentration and turnover by 50% even when plasma insulin was raised ~100 µU/mL (32). NEFA concentration and turnover during the clamp correlated directly with blood pressure measured at the screening visit in these volunteers. The correlations persisted when lean normotensives were excluded and after controlling for hyperinsulinemia and insulin-mediated glucose disposal. The finding of a direct and independent relationship between NEFAs and blood pressure was confirmed in a larger group of volunteers undergoing a 15-min insulin tolerance test (1). In a subsequent study, the angiotensin-converting enzyme inhibitor enalapril significantly improved the action of insulin to suppress plasma NEFAs during a euglycemic clamp *(43)*. The blood pressure reduction during enalapril treatment in obese hypertensive patients correlated with the improvement in insulin's capacity to suppress plasma NEFAs.

Another condition associated with hypertension and insulin resistance is familial combined hyperlipidemia *(44)*. Patients with familial combined hyperlipidemia have plasma NEFAs of ~1.5±0.5 m*M* (SD) after a high-fat test meal *(4)*. These are close to the NEFA levels that caused vasoconstriction and a pressor response in minipigs *(45)*. Moreover, hypertriglyceridemic family members of proband cases with familial combined hyperlipidemia have a tendency to higher fasting insulin and NEFAs as well as higher systolic blood pressure than family members having normal triglycerides *(4)*. Patients with familial combined hyperlipidemia comprise ~1–2% of the general population but ~12% of hypertensive patients, i.e., familial dyslipidemic hypertension *(44)*. The findings that patients with familial combined hyperlipidemia have elevated plasma NEFAs *(4)* and are more likely to be hypertensive *(44)*, that their affected family members have a tendency to increased NEFAs and blood pressure *(4)*, and that elevating NEFAs raises blood pressure *(45)* suggest that NEFAs may link this genetic disorder and hypertension. This link is consonant with the data from the Paris Prospective Study that plasma NEFAs were positively and independently related to a new onset hypertension *(8)*.

The link between visceral obesity and elevated blood pressures remains unknown *(38,39)*. As noted, NEFAs have effects on multiple targets that participate in blood pressure regulation including a reduced endothelial cell nitric oxide synthase activity and endothelium-dependent vasodilation *(21,23)*, increased endothelial cell endothelin production *(24)*, enhanced vascular tone and reactivity *(28,30)*, vascular and renal structural remodeling *(46,47)*, impaired baroreflex sensitivity *(48)*, augmented oxidative stress *(49)*, and elevated sympathetic to parasympathetic tone *(34)*. The effects on impaired nitric oxide production could potentially reset renal pressure natriuresis to a higher level *(50)*, which is fundamentally important in sustaining high blood pressure.

Although the mechanisms by which NEFAs may change autonomic control are unknown, the visceral fat mass is active with rapid lipolysis and re-esterification of triglycerides *(2)*. Thus, abdominally obese individuals would have increased portal delivery of NEFAs to the liver. In rats, increasing the delivery of oleic acid into the hepatic portal circulation elicits a neurogenically mediated pressor response *(51)*. In fact, obesity-induced hypertension in rats, rabbits, and dogs has a strong neurogenic component, and several studies on obese hypertensive humans identified evidence for neurogenic hypertension *(26,52–54)*. These observations are consistent with studies demonstrating that acute elevations of NEFAs in humans raise plasma catecholamines and increases the ratio sympathetic to parasympathetic control of the heart *(34)*.

2.7. Fatty Acids and Oxidative Stress

Oxidative stress is implicated in the pathogenesis of hypertension, and short-term elevations of NEFAs increase oxidative stress in humans *(49,55)*. F2-isoprostanes are produced mainly as a result of nonenymatic interactions of reactive oxygen species (ROS) with arachidonic acid. The F2-isoprostanes are stable biomarkers of oxidative stress, and measurements of these lipid biomarkers have facilitated clinical studies of oxidative stress. When plasma NEFA concentrations are increased in human volunteers by co-infusion of intralipid and heparin, plasma and urine F2-isoprostanes are elevated by 2 h and remain elevated at 4 h of the infusion *(49)*. Of note, F2-isoprostanes increase significantly more in African Americans than Caucasians, despite identical infusion rates of intralipid and heparin *(56)*. The implications of this observation for the higher rates of hypertension, stroke, and end-stage renal disease in African Americans than Caucasians merits further investigation.

Clinical studies in humans are limited by difficulties in elucidating the cellular signaling mechanisms by which NEFAs exert (patho)physiological effects. This limitation can be partially addressed by animal experiments and in vitro studies of cells and tissues to assess the specific effects of individual NEFAs. In the next section, signal transduction mechanisms by which NEFAs may mediate pathophysiological actions will be examined.

3. FATTY ACIDS AND CELL SIGNALING

3.1. Overview

NEFAs have many cellular actions which could impact cardiovascular pathobiology. Although this review focuses principally on the cardiovascular system, NEFAs also have cellular actions implicated in cancer *(57–59)*. Because obese patients are not only at a greater risk for cardiovascular disease but also for cancers of the colon, breast, uterus, and prostate *(60–62)*, NEFAs may be one of the factors contributing to these seemingly disparate observations.

Among the cellular actions of NEFAs are included effects on membrane fluidity and ion transport, e.g., Na^+/K^+-ATPase, Na^+ and K^+ channels, and Ca^{2+} currents *(63)*. The effects of these ion channels on cell function are protean. As examples of potential biological relevance, the capacity of selected cis-unsaturated NEFAs including oleic acid to blunt basal and stimulated release of growth hormone from pituitary cells and nitric oxide from endothelial cells is mediated by inhibitory effects on Ca^{2+} signaling *(22,64)*. Growth hormone and endothelial function are altered in obesity and may reflect in disordered part NEFA metabolism.

NEFAs enhanced α_1-adrenoceptor-mediated vascular reactivity through a cyclo-oxygenase sensitive mechanism *(32)*. In cultured vascular smooth muscle cells (VSMCs), oleic and linoleic acids induced a rise of 6-keto-$PGF_{1\alpha}$, a stable metabolite of prostacyclin *(65)*. Although prostacyclin is a vasodilator, a precursor, endoperoxide (PGH_2) is an agonist at the thromboxane A2 receptor, which promotes vascular smooth muscle contraction and growth. In these experiments, the mechanism underlying the rise of eicosanoids appeared to be a protein kinase C (PKC)-independent activation of phospholipase A_2 (PLA_2). Similarly, cis-unsaturated fatty acids including oleic acid facilitated neurotransmission in the hippocampus by a PLA_2 signaling pathway *(66)*.

In Raji cells, oleic acid induced cell proliferation *(67)*. In these cells, oleic and arachidonic acids independently affected the expression of genes for cytokines, transcription factors and proteins for cell cycle, defense and repair as well as apoptosis, DNA synthesis, cell adhesion, cytoskeleton, and hormone receptors. The greatest effects of the fatty acids occurred on the genes coding for signal transduction proteins. Although the mechanisms by which NEFAs affect transcription are not fully known, some genes appear to have an oleate response element in the promoter region *(68)*. NEFAs activate peroxisome proliferators-activated receptors and NF-κB, which function as nuclear transcriptional regulators *(24,69)*. NEFAs also induce a PKC-dependent increase in mitogen activated/extracellular-regulated protein kinase (MEK) *(70)*, which have downstream effects on nuclear transcription *(71)*.

Cis-unsaturated NEFAs, including oleic and linoleic acids, can directly activate the typical and atypical isoforms of PKC by a diacylglycerol (DAG)-independent mechanism *(72,73)*. Selected NEFAs bind to the regulatory domain of PKC at a site separate from that of DAG. NEFAs, in general, appear to be full agonists for the Ca^{2+}-independent and atypical PKC isoforms and partial agonists for the Ca^{2+}-independent isoforms *(74)*. The EC_{50} for activation of PKC for selective isoforms is within the range of estimated intracellular concentrations, which raises the possibility that cis-unsaturated NEFAs are biologically relevant regulators of cell signaling processes.

3.2. Fatty Acids and Signaling in Selected Target Cells

3.2.1. PANCREATIC CELLS

In cultured pancreatic β-cells, oleic acid increases basal insulin secretion but inhibits glucose-stimulated insulin release *(14)*. Oleic acid regulated the expression of 45 genes that participate in metabolism, cell growth, signal transduction, transcription, and protein processing. The radical scavenger N-acetylcysteine essentially blocked the effects of oleic acid on cell growth and differentiation but did not affect the other activities. In another study, cis-unsaturated but not saturated NEFAs-induced phosphorylation of NDP kinase and the β subunit of heterotrimeric G proteins, which are implicated in insulin secretion *(75)*. The capacity of NEFAs to induce apoptosis of the pancreatic β-cells was mediated by increased expression of inducible nitric oxide synthase and *de novo* ceramide production *(15)*. These experiments may elucidate the observation at the cellular level that some diabetic patients have enhanced basal insulin release but impaired insulin responses to glucose *(14,76)*. The cellular actions of NEFAs may also account for some of the progressive loss of β-cell function over time in most diabetic patients *(15,77)*.

3.2.2. ENDOTHELIAL CELLS

As noted, cis-unsaturated NEFAs suppress Ca^{2+}-calmodulin dependent nitric oxide synthase activity in endothelial cells under basal and stimulated conditions *(22)*. The diminution in nitric oxide synthase activity is associated with reduced Ca^{2+} signaling and with enhanced production of superoxide. Unsaturated NEFAs also enhance PAI-1 production by endothelial cells. The effects of unsaturated fatty acids including oleic, linoleic, and linolenic acids on endothelial PAI-1 production appear to be mediated by activation of PPARα and/or PPARγ *(25)*. Oleic acid also stimulates endothelin-1 expression in cultured endothelial cells. The latter effects of oleic acid are mediated by activation of PKC, especially the Ca^{2+}-dependent isoforms α and βII, and NF-κB *(24)*. Collectively, these studies implicate elevations of unsaturated NEFAs in the endothelial dysfunction that accompanies many insulin resistant states, which include patients with abdominal obesity, diabetes mellitus, familial combined hyperlipidemia, and the metabolic syndrome.

3.2.3. VASCULAR SMOOTH MUSCLE CELLS

Activation of PKC by cis-unsaturated fatty acids, in turn, stimulates NADPH oxidase *(78)* and induces the respiratory burst in leukocytes *(79,80)*, mesangial cells *(81)*, and VSMCs *(82)*. ROS in VSMCs activate a range of processes that are linked to vascular remodeling and cardiovascular events. In VSMCs, for example, ROS are associated with the activation of ERKs, transcription factors, PLA$_2$, and matrix metalloproteinases, with increases in IGF-1 and reduction in IGF binding proteins, and with increases in DNA synthesis. When oleic acid is combined with angiotensin II, a synergistic increase in VSMC ROS production and proliferation occur *(70)*.

3.2.4. PROXIMAL RENAL TUBULAR CELLS

Patients with proteinuria have an increase in tubulointerstitial matrix proteins including fibronectin. Fatty acids are rarely "free" in extracellular fluid but rather combined to albumin. When proximal tubular cells in culture are treated with oleic acid bound to albumin, a PKC-dependent increase in fibronectin production occurs, whereas linoleate bound albumin was inhibitory and cytotoxic *(47)*. Stearate and palmitate neither stimulated fibronectin production nor were cytotoxic. These data provide one potential link by which obesity and diabetes may lead to progressive renal disease by increasing delivery of albumin-bound oleate and linoleate to the proximal renal tubule.

4. FATTY ACIDS, PKC, AND ROS: POTENTIAL RELEVANCE TO HYPERTENSION AND VASCULAR DISEASE

Activation of PKC is involved in regulation of vascular tone *(83)* and VSMC growth *(84)* and may contribute to impaired endothelial function *(85)*, decreased microvessel formation *(86)* and metabolic aspects of the risk factor cluster *(87)*. The ζ isoform of PKC is of interest, because it is nutritionally regulated *(88)*, elevated in insulin-resistant patients with diabetes mellitus independently of hyperglycemia *(89)*, fully activated by selected cis-unsaturated NEFAs including oleic acid *(90)*, and linked to mitogenic responses *(91,92)*.

Glutathione, a key component of the cellular antioxidant defense mechanism, inhibits activation of PKC *(93)*. Diets deficient in antioxidants could lower the amount of reduced glutathione to attenuate PKC activity. The typical Western diet, which is high in fat and sugar but low in antioxidants, creates an imbalance whereby oxidant stressors, e.g., NEFAs, are increased relative to antioxidant mechanisms, e.g., vitamins C and E, and flavonoids. Thus, factors activating PKC would tend to predominate over those that oppose activation.

The notion that a decrease in antioxidant defenses contributes to hypertension is supported by an experiment in normotensive, Sprague–Dawley rats *(94)*. Addition of the glutathione synthase inhibitor, buthionine sulfoximine to drinking water for 2 wk, reduced tissue glutathione ~70%, decreased urinary nitrate excretion, a marker for nitric oxide, by over 60% and increased systolic blood pressure ~75 mmHg. Addition of vitamins C and E attenuated the rise of blood pressure by ~50% and corrected the defect in urinary nitrate excretion without significantly altering tissue glutathione content.

In addition to adverse effects on VSMCs as noted earlier, ROS can impair endothelial function *(19,95)*. Moreover, matrix metalloproteinases are present in significant amounts in the shoulder regions of human atherosclerotic plaque *(96)*. This is the region of plaque that is prone to rupture and initiate cardiovascular events *(97)*. ROS activate matrix metalloproteinases by destabilizing the sulfhydryl bonds, which maintain the inactive state *(98)*.

ROS play a critical role in mitogenic signaling in VSMCs mediated by angiotensin and oleic acid, separately and in combination *(99,100)*. A number of in vitro and in vivo studies indicate an important role for angiotensin II in cardiac and vascular remodeling. Angiotensin II increases ROS via an NADH/NADPH oxidase-dependent mechanism *(99,101)*. p22phox, a cytochrome-*b*-like protein, participates in the transfer of oxygen in the genesis of ROS *(99)*. These upstream signaling events lead to the subsequent activation of p38 MAP kinase and early response genes *(101,102)*. Angiotensin II and oleic acid induce a synergistic mitogenic response in VSMCs associated with a synergistic effect on ROS *(70)*. These studies demonstrate that ROS play an important role in the mitogenic signaling response of VSMCs.

The NADH/NADPH-mediated generation of ROS also participate in the hypertensive response to angiotensin II. Hypertension in rats induced by a long-term infusion of angiotensin leads to a doubling of vascular superoxide production *(101,103)*. The aortic rings of the angiotensin-induced hypertension in rats also generate more superoxide ex vivo than aortic rings from control animals. Pretreatment of the aortic rings with diphenyleniodinium, a selective inhibitor of NADH/NADPH oxidase reverses the excess superoxide production in the aortic ring studies. The blood pressure of hypertensive rats receiving angiotensin declined an impressive 60 mmHg with liposomal delivery of superoxide dismutase *(103)*. Vascular superoxide rapidly associates with nitric oxide and produces the *peroxynitrite*, which is not a vasodilator *(104)*. Although more stable than superoxide, peroxynitrite is also a reactive molecule that interacts with the tyrosine residues of proteins to produce 3-nitrotyrosine.

4.1. ROS May Contribute to Insulin Resistance

Adipocytes exposed to H_2O_2 in vitro manifest impaired lipid synthesis, glycogen synthetase activity, and glucose uptake in response to insulin *(105)*. Type II diabetics show an inverse relationship between measures of oxidant stress and insulin action *(106,107)*. Antioxidant therapy with vitamin E was associated with improved glucose metabolism in some studies of diabetics *(108)*. Collectively, the studies implicate oxidant stress in the metabolic components of insulin resistance observed in subjects with the risk factor cluster.

If ROS participate in cardiovascular risk and disease, then benefits of antioxidants should be evident among high-risk subjects, e.g., those in the heart outcomes prevention evaluation (HOPE) study *(109)*. In this study, vitamin E had no significant benefit, whereas the ACE inhibitor ramipril reduced risk. However, vitamin E in a wide range of concentrations of the racemic mixture as well as specific enantiomers had no effect on ROS produced by VSMCs stimulated with oleic acid and angiotensin II (unpublished observations). Consequently, vitamin E, which is lipophilic, may not block some important signaling events, many of which occur in the cytosol, in the genesis of vascular disease in humans.

In contrast to specific antioxidant supplements, natural foods contain several antioxidants and bioflavonoids that collectively could affect a wide range of signal transduction processes involved in the initiation and progression of vascular disease. Several reports indicate that foods high in antioxidants are associated with a reduction in cardiovascular disease, whereas trials of specific antioxidants are less consistent *(100–113)*. Thus, negative studies with a single antioxidant supplement are insufficient evidence to conclude that reactive oxygen intermediates and oxidative stress are not involved in the pathogenesis of cardiovascular risk and disease. As a general principal, rationale and effective antioxidant therapy requires an understanding of the molecular pathways mediating a disease process and the specific antioxidants that can interrupt that pathway. The antioxidant(s) must then be delivered in adequate concentrations and for a sufficient time to the microenvironment(s) in which the relevant biomolecular processes occur.

The DASH combination diet, which is high in fruits, vegetables, and low-fat dairy products, lowered systolic blood pressure by 11.4 mmHg in hypertensives but only 3.5 mmHg in normotensives (114). The high fruits and vegetables diet lowered systolic pressure by 7.2 mmHg in hypertensives but only 0.8 mmHg in normotensives. Thus, much of the benefit of DASH in hypertensives reflected greater intake of fruits and vegetables, which are high in antioxidants, K^+, Mg^{2+}, and fiber. The trial of hypertension prevention found that diets supplemented with K^+, Ca^{2+}, and Mg^{2+} had minimal effects on blood pressure (115). Thus, most of the blood pressure reduction with fruits and vegetables may reflect effects of antioxidants in fruits and vegetables.

The effects of DASH compared to a usual (low-antioxidant) diet for 4 wk each in random sequence on plasma total antioxidant capacity and blood pressure were studied in 12 obese hypertensives and 12 lean, demographically matched, normotensives (116). Although adherence with the DASH eating plan was ~50% in these free-living subjects, the DASH raised antioxidant levels in obese but not in lean volunteers and eliminated the difference between the two groups observed at baseline. Blood pressure fell with DASH in obese subjects ~8/6 mmHg, $p < 0.01$, but did not change in lean controls. The magnitude of the decline in blood pressure in obese hypertensives on DASH was inversely related to the increase in antioxidant capacity.

5. LIMITATIONS OF THE NEFA AND CARDIOVASCULAR DISEASE LINK

This literature reviewed implicates cis-unsaturated fatty acids in the pathophysiology of cardiovascular risk and disease. However, oleic acid has beneficial effects in vitro under selected conditions, so that not all cellular effects of this fatty acid are deleterious. Perhaps of greater relevance, diets high in mono- and poly-unsaturated, e.g., the Mediterranean Diet, are linked to lower rates of cardiovascular disease (117,118). It is, therefore, important to distinguish among the fatty acid content of diets, circulating fatty acids, and membrane fatty acid composition. The fatty acid content and composition of the diet are not closely related to circulating fatty acid levels (118). In contrast, the lipid content of cholesterol esters and phospholipids is strongly related to diet (118,119). Patients with obesity and insulin resistance tend to have high levels of circulating NEFAs (1,2,40–42). Diets with a high sugar content can induce fatty acid synthesis, including oleic acid, by the liver and adipose tissue (120–123).

This review has focused principally on the signaling effects of "free" cis-unsaturated fatty acids at membrane, cytosolic, and nuclear signaling targets. Many signaling actions may not be directly linked in time to circulating plasma NEFA concentrations. Moreover, linoleic and especially arachidonic acids, unlike oleic acid, have numerous metabolites that have diverse signaling effects in virtually every cell type (124,125). Saturated and trans-unsaturated fatty acids can also have deleterious effects, which were not examined in this work (126,127).

6. CONCLUSIONS

Although fatty acids are critical in energy metabolism, these lipids do not sit quietly in adipose stores or circulating in plasma waiting for the next fast. NEFAs are physiologically important regulators of cell function in key target organs including the pituitary, pancreas, liver, and vascular endothelium as well as cardiac, skeletal, and vascular smooth muscles. Disordered NEFA metabolism is implicated in multiple pathophysiological conditions including hypertension, diabetes, and dyslipidemia as well as the oxidative stress, endothelial dysfunction, altered vascular reactivity, hypercoagulable state, vascular remodeling, and related complications. At the cellular level, NEFAs can affect multiple important signaling targets including cation transport, PKC, PLA_2, cyclic AMP, protein kinase A, mitogen-activated protein kinase, and NF-κB to mention just a few. Cis-unsaturated NEFAs also activate peroxisome proliferators-activated receptors and modulate the transcription of numerous genes coding for proteins involved in cell metabolism, growth, proliferation, differentiation, and death.

This review has focused on NEFAs and cardiovascular risk. NEFAs are also implicated as tumor promoters. Obesity is associated with a significant increase for cardiovascular events and several cancers including breast, uterus, kidney, prostate, colon, and esophagus. A better understanding of NEFAs in health and disease is providing a foundation for refining and designing interventions to better manage the array of health problems associated with obesity and insulin resistance. That challenge is complicated by the fact that NEFAs exert important effects on key target cells through diverse signaling pathways. Moreover, some NEFAs, e.g., linoleic and arachidonic acid have multiple metabolites that are important in signal transduction with diverse effects in virtually every known tissue. Thus, inhibiting single pathways, though beneficial, may have limited effects. The data suggest that interventions to normalize NEFA metabolism might have more generalized benefits. In this regard, lifestyle changes including weight loss and exercise and pharmacological therapies such as angiotensin-converting enzyme inhibitors *(43,128)* and thiazolidinediones *(128,129)* may exert a range of beneficial effects in part through the capacity to improve NEFA metabolism.

ACKNOWLEDGMENTS

This work was supported in part by HL04290, HL58794, and P60-MD00267 (EXPORT) from the National Heart Lung and Blood Institute.

REFERENCES

1. Egan, B. M., Hennes, M. M. I., O'Shaughnessy, I. M., Stepniakowski, K. T., Kissebah, A. H., and Goodfriend, T. L. (1996) Obesity hypertension is more closely related to impairment of insulin's fatty acid than glucose lowering action. *Hypertension* **27(2),** 723–728.
2. Jensen, M. D., Haymond, M. W., Rizza, R. A., Cryer, P. E., and Miles, J. M. (1989) Influence of body fat distribution on free fatty acid metabolism in obesity. *J. Clin. Investig.* **83,** 1168–1173.
3. Franks, P. W., Wong, M.-Y., Luan, J., Mitchell, J., Hennings, S., and Wareham, N. J. (2002) Non-esterified fatty acid levels and physical inactivity: the relative importance of low habitual energy expenditure and cardio-respiratory fitness. *Br. J. Nutr.* **88,** 307–313.
4. Cabezas, M. C., deBruin, T. W. A., deValk, H. W., Shoulders, C. C., Jansen, H., and Erkelens, D. W. (1993) Impaired fatty acid metabolism in familial combined hyperlipidemia: a mechanism associating hepatic apolipoprotein B overproduction and insulin resistance. *J. Clin. Investig.* **92,** 160–168.

5. Quillot, D., Fluckiger, L., Zannad, F., Drouin, P., and Ziegler, O. (2001) Impaired autonomic control of heart rate and blood pressure in obesity: the role of age and of insulin resistance. *Clin. Auton. Res.* **11,** 79–86.

6. Martinson, B. C., O'Connor, P. J., and Pronk, N. P. (2001) Physical inactivity and short-term all-cause mortality in adults with chronic disease. *Arch. Intern. Med.* **161,** 1173–1180.

7. Carr, M. C. and Brunzell, J. D. (2004) Abdominal obesity and dyslipidemia in the metabolic syndrome: importance of type 2 diabetes and familial combined hyperlipidemia in coronary artery disease risk. *J. Clin. Endo. Metab.* **89,** 2601–2607.

8. Fagot-Campagna, A., Balkau, B., Simon, D., et al. (1998) High free fatty acid concentration: an independent risk factor for hypertension in the Paris prospective study. *Internat J. Epidemiol.* **27,** 808–813.

9. Jouven, X., Charles, M. A., Desnos, M., and Ducimetiere, P. (2001) Circulating nonesterified fatty acid level as a predictive risk factor for sudden death in the population. *Circulation* **104,** 756–761.

10. Filipovsky, J., Ducimetière, P., Eschwège, E., Richard, J. L., Rosselin, G., and Claude, J. R. (1996) The relationship of blood pressure with glucose, insulin , heart rate, free fatty acids and plasma cortisol levels according to the degree of obesity. *J. Hypertens.* **14,** 229–235.

11. Sundström, J., Lind, L., Bessby, B., Andrén, B., Aro, A., and Lithel, H. O. (2001) Dyslipidemia and an unfavorable fatty acid profile predict left ventricular hypertrophy 20 years later. *Circulation* **103,** 836–841.

12. Strömblad, G. and Björntorp, P. (1986) Reduced hepatic insulin clearance in rats with dietary-induced obesity. *Metabolism* **35,** 323–327.

13. Ferrannini, E., Barrett, E. J., and Bevilacqua, S. (1983) Effect of fatty acids on glucose production and utilization in man. *J. Clin. Investig.* **72,** 1737–1747.

14. Wang, X., De Leo, D., Guo, W., et al. (2004) Gene and protein kinase expression profiling of reactive oxygen species-associated lipotoxicity in the pancreatic β-cell line MIN6. *Diabetes* **53,** 129–140.

15. Shimabukuro, M., Zhou, Y.-T., and Unger, R. H. (1998) Fatty acid-induced β cell apoptosis: A link between obesity and diabetes. *Proc. Natl Acad. Sci.* **95,** 2498–2502.

16. Randle, P. J., Garland, P. B., Hales, C. N., and Newsholme, E. A. (1963) The glucose fatty-acid cycle: its role in insulin sensitivity and the metabolic disturbances of diabetes mellitus. *Lancet* **1,** 785–789.

17. Boden, G., Chen, X., Ruiz, J., White, J. V., and Rossetti, L. (1994) Mechanisms of fatty acid-induced inhibition of glucose uptake. *J. Clin. Investig.* **93,** 2438–2446.

18. Krauss, R. M. (2004) Lipids and lipoproteins in patients with type 2 diabetes. *Diab. Care* **27,** 1496–1504.

19. Tasi, W. C., Li, Y. H., Lin, C. C., Chao, T. H., and Chen, J. H. (2004) Effects of oxidative stress on endothelial function after a high-fat meal. *Clin. Sci.* **106,** 315–319.

20. Hamdy, O., Ledbury, S., Jullooly, C., et al. (2003) Lifestyle modification improves endothelial function in obese subjects with the insulin resistance syndrome. *Diab. Care* **26,** 2119–2125.

21. Davda, R. K., Stepniakowski, K. T., Lu, G., Ullian, M. E., Goodfriend, T. L., and Egan, B. M. (1995) Oleic acid inhibits endothelial cell nitric oxide synthase by a PKC-independent mechanism. *Hypertension* **26,** 764–770.

22. Esenabhalu, V. E., Schaeffer, G., and Graier, W. F. (2003) Free fatty acid overload attenuates Ca^{2+} signaling and NO production in endothelial cells. *Antioxid. Redox. Signal* **5,** 147–153.

23. Steinberg, H. O., Tarshoby, M., Monestel, R., et al. (1997) Elevated circulating free fatty acid levels impair endothelium-dependent vasodilation. *J. Clin. Investig.* **100,** 1230–1239.

24. Park, J.-Y., Kim, Y. M., Son, H. S., et al. (2003) Oleic acid induces endothelin-1 expression through activation of protein kinase C and NF-κB. *Biochem. Biophys. Res. Commun.* **303,** 891–895.

25. Ye, P., Hu, X., and Zhao, Y. (2002) The increase in plasminogen activator inhibitor type-1 expression by stimulation of activators for peroxisome proliferators-activated receptors in human endothelial cells. *Chin. Med. Sci. J.* **17,** 112–116.

26. Egan, B., Panis, R., Hinderliter, A., Schork, N., and Julius, S. (1987) Mechanism of increased α-adrenergic vasoconstriction in human essential hypertension. *J. Clin. Investig.* **80,** 812–817.

27. Egan, B. M., Schork, N. J., and Weder, A. B. (1989) Regional hemodynamic abnormalities in overweight men: focus on alpha-adrenergic vascular responses. *Am. J. Hypertens.* **2,** 428–434.

28. Stepniakowski, K. T., Goodfriend, T. L., and Egan, B. M. (1995) Fatty acids enhance vascular α-adrenergic sensitivity. *Hypertension* **25(2),** 774–778.

29. Stepniakowski, K. T., Sallee, R. F., Goodfriend, T. L., Zhang, Z., and Egan, B. M. (1996) Fatty acids enhance neurovascular reflex responses by effects on α1-adrenoceptors. *Am. J. Physiol.* **270,** R1240–R1346.

30. Haastrup, A., Stepniakowski, K. T., Goodfriend, T. L., and Egan, B. M. (1998) Lipids enhance α1-adrenergic receptor mediator pressor reactivity. *Hypertension* **32,** 693–698.

31. Gadegbeku, C. A., Shrayyef, M. Z., LaPorte, F. B., and Egan, B. M. (2004) Lipids enhance alpha1-adrenoceptor pressor sensitivity in patients with chronic kidney disease. *Am. J. Kid. Dis.* **44,** 446–454.

32. Stepniakowski, K. T., Lu, G., Davda, R. K., and Egan, B. M. (1997) Fatty acids enhance endothelium-dependent dilation in hand veins by a cyclo-oxygenase dependent mechanism. *Hypertension* **30,** 1634–1639.

33. Stojiljkovic, M. P., Zhang, D., Lopes, H. F., Lee, C. G., Goodfriend, T. L., and Egan, B. M. (2001) Hemodynamic effects of lipids in humans. *Am. J. Physiol.* **R280,** 1674–1679.

34. Palisso, G., Manzella, D., Rizzo, M. R., et al. (2000) Elevated plasma fatty acid concentrations stimulate the cardiac autonomic nervous system in healthy subjects. *Clin. Nutr.* **72,** 723–730.

35. Andersson, B., Wikstrand, J., Ljung, T., Bjork, S., Wennmalm, A., and Bjorntorp, P. (1998) Urinary albumin excretion and heart rate variability in obese women. *Int. J. Obes. Relat. Metab. Disord.* **22,** 399–405.

36. Egan, B., Fitzpatrick, M. A., and Julius, S. (1987) The heart and the regulation of renin. *Circulation* **75(Suppl 5),** S103–S107.

37. Fields, L. E., Burt, V. L., Cutler, J. A., Hugher, J., Roccella, E. J., and Sorlie, P. (2004) The burden of adult hypertension in the United States 1999 to 2000: a rising tide. *Hypertension* **44,** 398–404.

38. Stern, M. and Haffner, S. (1986) Body fat distribution and hyperinsulinemia as risk factors for diabetes and cardiovascular disease. *Arteriosclerosis* **6,** 123–129.

39. Peiris, A., Sothmann, M., Hoffmann, R., et al. (1989) Adiposity, fat distribution and cardiovascular risk. *Ann. Int. Med.* **110,** 867–872.

40. Chen, Y.-D. I., Golay, A., Swislocki, A. L. M., and Reaven, G. M. (1987) Resistance to insulin suppression of plasma free fatty acid concentrations and insulin stimulation of glucose uptake in noninsulin-dependent diabetes mellitus. *J. Clin. Endocrinol. Metab.* **64,** 17–21.

41. Roust, L. R. and Jensen, M. D. (1993) Postprandial free fatty acid kinetics are abnormal in upper body obesity. *Diabetes* **42,** 1567–1573.

42. Reaven, G. M., Hollenbeck, C., Jeng, C. Y., Wu, M. S., and Chen, Y. D. I. (1988) Measurement of plasma glucose, free fatty acids, lactate, and insulin for 24 hours in patients with NIDDM. *Diabetes* **37,** 1020–1024.

43. Hennes, M. M., O'Shaugnessy, I. M., Kelly, T. M., Labelle, P., Egan, B. M., and Kissebah, A. H. (1996) Insulin resistant lipolysis in abdominally obese hypertensives: role of the renin–angiotensin system. *Hypertension* **28,** 120–126.

44. Williams, R. R., Hunt, S. C., Hopkins, P. N., et al. (1988) Familial dylipidemic hypertension: evidence from 58 Utah families for a syndrome present in ~12% of patients with essential hypertension. *JAMA* **259,** 3579–3586.

45. Bülow, J., Madsen, J., and Hojgaard, L. (1990) Reversibility of the effects on local circulation of high lipid concentrations in blood. *Scand. J. Clin. Lab. Investig.* **50,** 291–296.

46. Lu, G., Morinelli, T. A., Meier, K. A., Rosenzweig, S. A., and Egan, B. M. (1996) Oleic acid-induced mitogenic signaling in vascular smooth muscle cells a role for protein kinase C. *Circ. Res.* **79,** 611–618.

47. Arici, M., Brown, J., Williams, M., Harris, K. P. G., Walls, J., and Brunskill, N. J. (2002) Fatty acids carried on albumin modulate proximal tubular cell fibronectin production: a role for protein kinase C. *Nephrol. Dial. Trnasplant.* **17,** 1751–1757.

48. Gadegbeku, C. A., Dhandayuthapani, A., Sadler, Z. E., and Egan, B. M. (2002) Raising lipids acutely reduces baroreflex sensitivity. *Am. J. Hypertens.* **15,** 479–485.

49. Stojiljkovic, M. P., Lopes, H. F., Zhang, D., Morrow, J. D., Goodfriend, T. L., and Egan, B. M. (2002) Raising fatty acids increases plasma and urine F2-isoprostanes in humans. *J. Hypertens.* **20,** 1–7.

50. Granger, J. P., Alexander, B. T., Llinas, M. T., Bennett, W. A., and Khalil, R. A. (2001) Pathophysiology of hypertension during preeclampsia linking placental ischemia with endothelial dysfunction. *Hypertension* **38(2),** 718–722.

51. Grekin, R. J., Dumont, C. J., Vollmer, A. P., Watts, S. W., and Webb, R. C. (1997) Mechanisms in the pressor effects of hepatic portal venous fatty acid infusion. *Am. J. Physiol.* **273,** R324–R330.

52. Rocchini, A. P., Moorehead, C. P., DeRemer, S., and Blondi, D. (1989) Pathogenesis of weight related changes of blood pressure in dogs. *Hypertension* **13,** 922–928.

53. Hall, J. E., Brands, M. W., Dixon, W. N., and Smith, M. J. Jr. (1993) Obesity-induced hypertension: renal function and systemic hemodynamics. *Hypertension* **22,** 292–299.

54. Sowers, J. R., Nyby, M., Stern, N., et al. (1982) Blood pressure and hormone changes associated with weight reduction in the obese. *Hypertension* **4,** 686–691.

55. Lauresen, J. B., Rajagopalan, S., Galis, Z., Tarpey, M., Freeman, B. A., and Harrison, D. G. (1997) Role of superoxide in angiotensin II-induced but not catecholamine-induced hypertension. *Circulation* **95,** 588–593.

56. Lopes, H. F., Morrow, J. D., Stojiljkovic, M. P., Goodfriend, T. L., and Egan, B. M. (2003) Acute hyperlipidemia increases oxidative stress more in African Americans than in Caucasian Americans. *Am. J. Hypertens.* **16,** 331–336.

57. Hardy, S., Langelier, Y., and Prentki, M. (2000) Oleate activates phophatidylinositol 3-kinase and promotes proliferation and reduces apoptosis of MDA-MS-231 breast cancer cells, whereas palmitate has opposite effects. *Cancer Res.* **61,** 6353–6358.

58. Palmantier, R., George, M. D., Akiyama, S. K., Wolber, F. M., Olden, K., and Roberts, J. D. (2001) Cis-unsaturated fatty acids stimulate beta1 integrin-mediated adhesion of human breast carcinoma cells to type IV collagen by activating protein kinase C-epsilon and -mu. *Cancer Res.* **61,** 2445–2452.

59. Yoshida, M., Okamura, S., Kodaki, T., Mori, M., and Yamashita, S. (1998) Enhanced levels of oleate-dependent and Arf-dependent phospholipase D isoforms in experimental colon cancer. *Oncol. Res.* **10,** 399–406.

60. Garfinkel, L. (1985) Overweight and cancer. *Ann. Int. Med.* **103(6),** 1034–1036.

61. Bianchini, F., Kaaks, R., and Vainio, H. (2002) Overweight, obesity, and cancer risk. *Lancet Oncol.* **3,** 545–574.

62. Jun, R. T. (1997) Obesity as a disease. *Br. Med. Bull.* **53,** 307–321.

63. Ordway, R. W., Singer, J. J., and Walsh, J. V. (1991) Direct regulation of ion channels by fatty acids. *Trends Neurosci.* **14,** 96–100.

64. Perez, F. R., Casabiell, X., Camina, J. P., Zugaza, J. L., and Casaneuva, F. F. (1997) Cis-unsaturated free fatty acids block growth hormone and prolactin secretion in thyrotropin-releasing hormone-stimulated GH3 cells by perturbing the function of plasma membrane integral proteins. *Endocrinology* **138,** 264–272.

65. Haastrup, A., Gadegbeku, C. A., Zhang, D., et al. (2001) Intralipid stimulates the production of 6-keto-PGF$_{1\alpha}$ in human dorsal hand veins. *Hypertension* **38,** 858–861.

66. Nomura, T., Nishizaki, T., Enomoto, T., and Itoh, H. (2001) A long-lasting facilitation of hippocampal neurotransmission via a phspholipase A2 signaling pathway. *Life Sci.* **68,** 2885–2891.

67. Verlengia, R., Gorjao, R., Kanunfre, C. C., et al. (2003) Genes regulated by arachidonic and oleic acids in Raji cells. *Lipids* **38,** 1157–1165.

68. Rottensteiner, H., Palmier, L., Hartig, A., et al. (2002) The peroxisomal transporter gene ANT2 is regulated by a deviant oleate response element (ORE): characterization of the signal for fatty acid induction. *Biochem. J.* **365(1),** 109–117.

69. Jump, D. B. (2004) Fatty acid regulation of gene transcription. *Crit. Rev. Clin. Lab. Sci.* **41,** 41–78.

70. Lu, G., Meier, K. E., Jaffa, A. A., Rosenzweig, S. A., and Egan, B. M. (1998) Oleic acid and angiotensin induce a synergistic mitogenic response. *Hypertension* **31,** 978–985.

71. Engelman, J. A., Chu, C., Lin, A., et al. (1998) Caveolin-meidated regulatoin of signaling along the P42/44 MAP kinase cascade in vivo: a role for the caveolin-scaffolding domain. *FEBS Lett.* **428,** 205–211.

72. Touny, S. E., Khan, W., and Hannun, Y. (1990) Regulation of platelet protein kinase C by oleic acid. *J. Biol. Chem.* **265,** 16,437–16,443.

73. Khan, W. A., Blobe, G., Halpern, A., et al. (1993) Selective regulation of protein kinase C isozymes by oleic acid in human platelets. *J. Biol. Chem.* **268,** 5063–5068.

74. Egan, B. M., Lu, G., and Greene, E. L. (1999) Vascular effects of non-esterified fatty acids: implications for the cardiovascular risk factor cluster. *Prostagl. Leukotr. Essen. Fatty Acids* **60,** 411–420.

75. Kowluru, A. (2004) Differential regulation by fatty acids of protein histidine phosphorylation in rat pancreatic islets. *Mol. Cell. Biochem.* **266,** 175–182.

76. Garcia-Webb, P., Bonser, A. M., Pelham, J., and Whiting, D. (1982) Basal insulin secretion increases with the onset of non-insulin dependent diabetes. *Pathology* **14,** 323–325.

77. Haupt, E., Haupt, A., Herrmann, R., Benecke-Timp, A., Vogel, H., and Walter, C. (1999) The KID study V: the natural history of type 2 diabetes in younger patients still practicing a profession. Heterogeneity of basal and reactive C-peptide levels in relation to BMI, duration of disease, age and HbA1. *Exp. Clin. Endo. Diab.* **107,** 236–243.

78. Cox, J. A., Jeng, A. Y., Sharkey, N. A., Blumberg, P. M., and Tauber, A. I. (1985) Activation of the human neutrophil nicotinamide adenine dinucleotide phosphate (NADPH)-oxidase by protein kinase C. *J. Clin. Investig.* **76,** 1932–1938.

79. Myers, M. A., McPhail, L. C., and Snyderman, R. (1985) Redistribution of protein kinase C activity in human monocytes: correlation with activation of the respiratory burst. *J. Immunol.* **135,** 3411–3416.

80. McPhail, L. C., Clayton, C. C., and Snyderman, R. (1984) A potential second messenger role for unsaturated fatty acids: activation of Ca^{2+}-dependent protein kinase. *Science* **224,** 622–625.

81. Fiorani, M., Cantoni, O., Tasinato, A., Boscoboinik, D., and Azzi, A. (1995) Hydrogen peroxide and fetal bovine serum-induced DNA synthesis in vascular smooth muscle cells: positive and negative regulation by protein kinase C isoforms. *Biochim. Biophys. Acta* **1269,** 98–104.

82. Lu, G., Greene, E. L., Toshi, J. I., and Egan, B. M. (1998) Reactive oxygen species are critical in the oleic acid-mediated mitogenic signaling pathway in vascular smooth muscle cells. *Hypertension* **32,** 1003–1010.

83. Osol, G., Laher, I., and Cipolla, M. (1991) Protein kinase C modulates basal myogenic tone in resistance arteries from the cerebral circulation. *Circ. Res.* **68,** 359–367.

84. Dzau, V. J. and Gibbons, G. H. (1991) Endothelium and growth factors in vascular remodeling in hypertension. *Hypertension* **18(Suppl),** III115–III121.

85. Morrison, K. J. and Pollock, D. (1990) Impairment of relaxation to acetylcholine and nitric oxide by a phorbol ester in rat isolated aorta. *Br. J. Pharmacol.* **101,** 432–436.

86. Doctrow, S. R. and Folkman, J. (1987) Protein kinase C activators suppress stimulation of capillary endothelial cell growth by angiogenic endothelial mitogens. *J. Cell. Biol.* **104,** 679–687.

87. Heydrick, S. J., Ruderman, N. B., Kurowski, T. G., et al. (1991) Enhanced stimulation of diacylglycerol and lipid synthesis by insulin in denervated muscle: altered PKC activity and possible link to insulin resistance. *Diabetes* **40,** 1707–1711.

88. Nair, S. C., Toshkov, I. A., Yaktine, A. L., Barnett, T. D., Chaney, W. G., and Birt, D. F. (1994) Dietary energy restriction-induced modulation of protein kinase ζ isozyme in the hamster pancreas. *Mol. Carcinol.* **14,** 10–15.

89. Considine, R. V., Nyce, M. R., Allen, L. E., et al. (1995) Protein kinase C ζ is increased in the liver of humans and rats with non-insulin-dependent diabetes mellitus. An alteration not due to hyperglycemia. *J. Clin. Investig.* **95,** 2938–2944.

90. Nakanishi, H. and Exton, J. H. (1992) Purification and characterization of the ζ isoform of protein kinase C from bovine kidney. *J. Biol. Chem.* **267,** 16,347–16,354.

91. Liao, D.-F., Monia, B., Dean, N., and Berk, B. C. (1997) Protein kinase C-ζ mediates angiotensin II activation of ERK-1 and -2 in vascular smooth muscle cells. *J. Biol. Chem.* **272,** 6146–6150.

92. Berra, E., Dioa-Meco, M. T., Dominguez, I., et al. (1993) Protein kinase C ζ is critical for mitogenic signal transduction. *Cell* **74,** 555–563.

93. Ward, N. E., Pierce, D. S., Chung, S. E., Gravitt, K. R., and O'Brian, C. A. (1998) Irreversible inactivation of protein kinase C by glutathione. *J. Biol. Chem.* **273,** 12,558–12,566.

94. Nosratola, D., Vaziri, D., Wang, X. Q., Oveisi, F., and Rad, B. (2000) Induction of oxidative stress by glutathione depletion causes severe hypertension in normal rats. *Hypertension* **36,** 142–146.

95. Gumusel, B., Tel, B. C., Demirdamar, R., and Sahin-Erdemli, I. (1996) Reactive oxygen species-induced impairment of endothelium-dependent relaxation in rat aortic rings: protection by L-arginine. *Eur. J. Pharmacol.* **306,** 107–112.

96. Galis, Z. S., Sukhova, G., Lark, M. W., and Libby, P. (1994) Increased expression of matrix metalloproteinases and matrix degrading activity in vulnerable regions of human atherosclerotic plaques. *J. Clin. Investig.* **94,** 2493–2503.

97. Rajagopalan, S., Meng, X. P., Ramasamy, S., Harrison, D. G., and Galis, Z. S. (1996) Reactive oxygen species produced by macrophage-derived foam cells regulate the activity of vascular matrix metalloproteinases in vitro. Implications for atherosclerotic plaque stability. *J. Clin. Investig.* **98,** 2572–2579.

98. Rajagopalan, S., Meng, X. P., Ramasamy, S., et al. (1996) Reactive oxygen species produced by macrophage-derived foam cells regulate the activity of matrix metalloproteinases. *J. Clin. Investig.* **98,** 2572–2579.

99. Ushio-Fukai, M., Zafari, A. M., Fukui, T., Ishizaka, N., and Griendling, K. K. (1996) $p22^{phox}$ is a critical component of the superoxide-generating NADH/NADPH oxidase system and regulates angiotensin II-induced hypertrophy in vascular smooth muscle cells. *J. Biol. Chem.* **271,** 23,317–23,321.

100. Puri, P. L., Avantaggiati, M. L., Burgio, V. L., et al. (1995) Reactive oxygen intermediates mediate angiotensin II-induced c-jun/c-fos heterodimer DNA binding activity and proliferative hypertrophic responses in myogenic cells. *J. Biol. Chem.* **270,** 22,129–22,134.

101. Rajagopalan, S., Kurz, S., Munzel, T., et al. (1996) Angiotensin II-mediated hypertension in the rat increases vascular superoxide production via membrane NADH/NADPH oxidase activation. *J. Clin. Investig.* **97,** 1916–1923.

102. Ushio-Fukai, M., Alexander, R. W., Akers, M., and Griendling, K. K. (1998) p38 mitogen-activated protein kinase is a critical component of the redox-sensitive signaling pathways activated by angiotensin II. *J. Biol. Chem.* **273,** 15,022–15,029.

103. Liao, D. F., Monia, B., Dean, N., and Berk, B. C. (1997) Protein kinase C-zeta mediates angiotensin II activation of ERK1/2 in vascular smooth muscle cells. *J. Biol. Chem.* **272,** 6146–6150.

104. Ferdinandy, P. and Schulz, R. (2003) Nitric oxide, superoxide, and peroxynitrite in myocardial ischaemia-reperfusion injury and preconditioning. *Br. J. Pharmacol.* **138,** 532–543.

105. Rudich, A., Kozlovsky, N., Patashnik, R., and Bashan, N. (1997) Oxidant stress reduces insulin responsiveness in 3T3-L1 adipocytes. *Am. J. Physiol.* **272,** E935–E940.

106. Paolisso, G., D'Amopre, A., Volpe, C., et al. (1994) Evidence for a relationship between oxidative stress and insulin action in non-insulin-dependent (type II) diabetic patients. *Metabol. Clin. Exp.* **43,** 1426–1429.

107. Sano, T., Umeda, F., Hashimoto, T., Nawata, H., and Utsumi, H. (1998) Oxidative stress measurement by in vivo electron spin resonance spectroscopy in rats with streptozotocin-induced diabetes. *Diabetologia* **41,** 1355–1360.

108. Jain, S. K., McVie, R., Jaramillo, J. J., Palmer, M., and Smith, T. (1996) Effect of modest vitamin E supplementation on blood glycated hemoglobin and triglyceride levels and red cell indices in type 1 diabetic patients. *J. Am. Coll. Nutr.* **15,** 458–461.

109. Yusuf, S., Dagenais, G., Pogue, J., Bosch, J., and Sleight, P. (2000) Vitamin E supplementation and cardiovascular events in high-risk patients. The heart outcomes prevention evaluation study. *N. Engl. J. Med.* **342,** 154–160.

110. Keli, S. O., Hertog, M. G. L., Feskens, E. J. M., and Kromhout, D. (1996) Dietary flavonoids, antioxidant vitamins and incidence of stroke. *Arch. Intern. Med.* **154,** 637–642.

111. Geleijnse, J. M., Launer, L. J., Hofman, A., Pols, H. A. P., and Witteman, J. C. M. Tea flavonoids may protect against atherosclerosis. The Rotterdam study. *Arch. Intern. Med.* **159,** 2170–2174.

112. Joshipura, K. J., Ascherio, A., Manson, J. E., et al. (1999) Fruit and vegetable intake in relation to risk of ischemic stroke. *JAMA* **282,** 1233–1239.

113. Ascherio, A., Rimm, E. B., Hernan, M. A., et al. (1999) Relation of consumption of vitamin E, vitamin C, and carotenoids to risk for stroke among men in the United States. *Ann. Int. Med.* **130,** 963–970.

114. Appel, L. J., Moore, T. J., Obarzanek, E., et al. (1997) A clinical trial of the effects of dietary patterns on blood pressure. *N. Engl. J. Med.* **336,** 1117–1124.

115. Whelton, P. K., Kumanyika, S. K., Cook, N. R., et al. (1997) Efficacy of nonpharmacologic interventions in adults with high-normal blood pressure: results from phase 1 of the trials of hypertension prevention. Trials of hypertension prevention collaborative group. *Am. J. Clin. Nutr.* **65(2 Suppl),** 652S–660S.

116. Lopes, H. F., Martin, K. L., Nashar, K., Morrow, J. D., Goodfriend, T. L., and Egan, B. M. (2003) Effects of the DASH diet on blood pressure, antioxidant capacity and acute lipid-induced oxidative stress. *Hypertension* **41,** 422–430.

117. Massora, M., Carluccio, M. A., and Caterina, R. D. (1999) Direct vascular antiatherogenic effects of oleic acid: a clue to the cardioprotective effects of the Mediterranean diet. *Cardiologia* **44,** 507–513.

118. de Lorgeril, M., Salen, P., Martin, J. L., Monjaud, I., Boucher, P., and Mamelle, N. (1998) Mediterranean dietary pattern in a randomized trial: prolonged survival and possible reduced cancer rate. *Arch. Int. Med.* **158,** 1181–1187.

119. Raatz, S. K., Bibus, D., Thomas, W., and Kris-Ehterton, P. (2001) Total fat intake modifies plasma fatty acid composition in humans. *J. Nutr.* **131,** 231–234.

120. Chajes, V., Elmstahl, S., Martinez-Garcia, C., Van Kappel, A. L., Bianchini, F., Kaaks, R., and Riboli, E. (2001) Comparison of fatty acid profile in plasma phospholipids in women from Granada (southern Spain) and Malmo (southern Sweden). *Int. J. Vit. Nutr. Res.* **71,** 237–242.

121. Hudgins, L. C., Hellerstein, M., Seidman, C., Neese, R., Diakun, J., and Hirsch, J. (1996) Human fatty acid synthesis is stimulated by a eucaloric low fat, high carbohydrate diet. *J. Clin. Investig.* **97,** 2081–2091.

122. Cahscione, C., Elwyn, D. H., Davila, M., Gil, K. M., Askanazi, J., and Kinney, J. M. (1987) Effect of carbohydrate intake on *de novo* lipogenesis in human adipose tissue. *Am. J. Physiol.* **253(6),** E664–E669.

123. Nakamura, M. T. and Nara, T. Y. (2004) Structure, function, and dietary regulation of delta6, delta5, and delta9 desaturases. *Ann. Rev. Nutr.* **24,** 345–376.

124. Rao, G. N., Alexander, R. W., and Runge, M. S. (1995) Linoleic acid and its metabolites, hydroperoxyoctadecadeienoic acids, stimulate c-fos, c-jun, c-myc mRNA expression, mitrogen-activated protein kinase activation and growth in rat aortic smooth muscle cells. *J. Clin. Investig.* **96,** 842–847.

125. Nie, D. and Honn, K. V. (2004) Eicosanoid regulation of angiogenesis in tumors. *Sem. Thromb. Hemo.* **30,** 119–125.

126. Hunnicutt, J. W., Hardy, R. W., Williford, J., and McDonald, J. M. (1994) Saturated fatty acid-induced insulin resistance in rat adipocytes. *Diabetes* **43,** 540–545.

127. Kummerow, F. A., Zhou, Q., Mahfouz, M. M., Smiricky, M. R., Grieshop, C. M., and Schaeffer, D. J. (2004) Trans fatty acids in hydrogenated fat inhibited the synthesis of polyunsaturated fatty acids in the phospholipids of arterial cells. *Life Sci.* **74,** 2707–2723.

128. Yamauchi, S., Takeishi, Y., Minamihaba, O., et al. (2003) Angiotensin converting enzyme inhibition improves cardiac fatty acid metabolism in patients with congestive heart failure. *Nucl. Med. Commun.* **24,** 901–906.

129. Natali, A., Baldeweg, S., Toschi, E., et al. (2004) Vascular effects of improving metabolic control with metformin or rosiglitazone in type 2 diabetes. *Diab. Care* **27,** 1349–1357.

13 Goal-Oriented Hypertension Management in Diabetic and Nondiabetic Patients

Gregory M. Singer, John F. Setaro, and Henry R. Black

CONTENTS

INTRODUCTION
HYPERTENSION GUIDELINES (1972–2005)
LESSONS FROM CLINICAL TRIALS ABOUT OPTIMAL
    PHARMACOLOGICAL TREATMENT FOR THE DIABETIC HYPERTENSIVE
GOAL-ORIENTED MANAGEMENT
CONCLUSIONS
REFERENCES

1. INTRODUCTION

Despite increasing evidence favoring intensive therapy of high blood pressure (BP) *(1–5)*, lower treatment goals have yet to be realized in clinical practice. This chapter will explore the evolution of practice guidelines, with a focus on trial findings that demonstrate benefits of vigorous BP management, especially in the diabetic population. We will review pharmacologic strategies derived from clinical trials, with an emphasis on optimal treatment for hypertensives with and without diabetes.

In the 1940s, hypertension was identified as a modifiable risk factor in preventing cardiovascular (CV) and renal complications. Despite better understanding of the benefits of BP reduction with treatment and with goals evolving downward since the 1970s, clinician acceptance and incorporation of these goals into practice have lagged. "Physician inertia" *(6)* is a powerful force, and arises from concerns that intensive therapy may increase costs and side effects. For example, despite clear advantages of BP reduction, it has been hypothesized that overtreatment may precipitate myocardial infarction (MI) in patients with coronary heart disease (CHD; the "J"-curve phenomenon), or strokes in those with cerebrovascular disease.

The Veterans Affairs (VA) trials in the 1960s and 1970s unambiguously showed that treating hypertensives with diastolic blood pressure (DBP) ≥ 105 mmHg reduced

From: *Contemporary Endocrinology: Hypertension and Hormone Mechanisms*
Edited by: R. M. Carey © Humana Press Inc., Totowa, NJ

cerebrovascular and CV events, but optimal treatment goals remained uncertain. The Hypertension Detection and Follow-Up Program (HDFP) was the first large randomized trial that examined this issue (1972–1979). HDFP illustrated the benefits of intensive therapy, even with DBP 90–104 mmHg. Later trials, including Hypertension Optimal Treatment (HOT) Study, United Kingdom Prospective Diabetes Study (UKPDS) trial in diabetics, and African–American Study of Kidney Disease (AASK) in subjects with renal insufficiency, have addressed this issue.

By 2005, clinical trials had not only revealed benefit, but also indicated no harm from intensive therapy. Guideline committees reinforced BP targets <140/90 mmHg for most hypertensives, and espoused even more stringent criteria for high-risk patients, especially diabetics. Newer, stricter goals in turn have challenged clinicians in their efforts to optimize BP lowering through the use of currently available medications. This chapter will survey contemporary trial data suggesting that attaining goal, rather than specific drug choice, is the highest priority. We will review how goal-oriented management can be successful, and we will discuss whether currently available therapy is adequate for reaching ambitious new goals, especially in diabetic hypertensives. With greater focus on multiple drug regimens, we can approach these goals as we wait for new and better therapies.

2. HYPERTENSION GUIDELINES (1972–2005)

Since the first VA trials, treatment of hypertension has been linked to better outcomes for stroke and CV disease. Goals, as well as the tools to reach those goals, have evolved simultaneously with greater appreciation of the advantages of lower BP. Before the introduction of thiazide diuretics in 1957, only hypertensives with life threatening levels of BP were the candidates for treatment. Sympathectomy or poorly tolerated and toxic drugs (ganglionic blockers, peripheral adrenergic blockers, and vasodilators) were too risky to use in any other patients. The VA trials employed a fixed dose combination of a thiazide diuretic, a peripheral sympathetic blocker, and a vasodilator. These studies demonstrated the efficacy and tolerability of these newer antihypertensive therapies and enlarged the number of patients who could be treated safely (7,8). With the development of more effective and better-tolerated medications (Table 1), safe drugs could now be offered to hypertensive patients with lesser elevations of BP and who were at lower risk of complications. The risk/benefit ratio had become much more favorable (9).

2.1. JNC I (1976)

Based on results from Task Force I of the National High Blood Pressure Education Program (10), the National Heart, Lung, and Blood Institute (NHLBI; then called the National Heart Institute), commissioned the first Joint National Committee on the detection, evaluation, and treatment of high blood pressure (JNC I) to set criteria for hypertension evaluation and management. Initial goals were conservative by modern standards, advocating treatment for DBP > 105 mmHg, individualized intervention for DBP from 90 to 104 mmHg, and observation alone for those with a systolic blood pressure (SBP) > 160 mmHg (11). JNC I based recommendations on DBP alone, because the benefit of treating SBP was not yet proven even though the risk of elevated SBP had been convincingly demonstrated. Kannel et al. in the Framingham Heart Study had even

Table 1
Development of Antihypertensive Agents From 1940 to the Present

1940s	Thiocyanates
	Ganglion blocking agents
	Catecholamine depletors
1950s	Vasodilators
	Peripheral sympathetic inhibitors
	Monoamine oxidase inhibitors
	Diuretics
1960s	Central α2-agonists
	β-Blockers
	Nondihydropyridine calcium channel blockers (NDHPCCBs)
1970s	Peripheral α_1 adrenergic blockers
	α–β-Blockers
	Angiotensin converting enzyme inhibitors (ACE-I)
1980s	Dihydropyridine calcium channel blockers (DHPCCBs)
1990s	Angiotensin II receptor antagonists (ARBs)

Adapted from ref. *(9)*.

shown in 1971 that SBP was a *better* determinant of risk than DBP, especially in elderly people *(12)*. The goal of treatment for DBP was <90 mmHg with no goal suggested for SBP. JNC I recognized that the available compounds harbored potential adverse effects, and permitted relaxation of goal, if adverse effects served as an obstacle to treatment. For DBP = 90–104 mmHg, the Committee endorsed individualized therapy to be shaped by the presence of additional risk factors such as SBP, target organ damage, family history of complications, elevated cholesterol, and diabetes.

2.2. JNC II (1980)

Influenced by HDFP, the next committee (JNC II) noted reduced all-cause mortality and CV disease when "mild" hypertension (DBP: 90–104 mmHg) was treated, and therefore recommended initiating therapy for those patients. JNC II identified stroke protection, heart failure (HF) prevention, and the arrest of hypertension progression from mild to severe as advantages proven in both VA and HDFP studies. HDFP also showed a 20.3% mortality reduction and a significant reduction in cardiac events *(13)*. JNC II supported a DBP goal of <90 mmHg, but asserted that "a reasonable further goal is the lowest diastolic pressure consistent with safety and tolerance" *(14)*. The Committee recognized the risk of isolated systolic hypertension (ISH), then defined as SBP ≥ 160 with DBP ≤90 mmHg. Cautious treatment was advised for elderly patients, although no data yet supported therapy for elevated DBP or ISH in this group. The stated goal for elderly persons was 140–160 mmHg systolic, with diastolic <90 mmHg.

2.3. JNC III (1984)

JNC III echoed these recommendations and again declared that the lowest, safely tolerated DBP should be the goal, implying additional benefit from lowering BP to an unspecified lower goal when target organ damage, diabetes or major cardiac risk factors were present. Special populations, such as diabetics and elderly patients, were singled out as particularly vulnerable to sequela of inadequately treated hypertension. Improved outcomes were already recognized in elderly patients treated for ISH (SBP 160–219 mmHg) in the Systolic Hypertension in the Elderly Program Pilot Study (SHEP-PS), a feasibility trial completed in 1984 *(15)*. JNC III reclassified ISH, however no treatment was required unless SBP was consistently >160 mmHg. In aged subjects, treatment goal of SBP 140–160 mmHg was recommended, however the committee suggested further reduction to <140 mmHg, if tolerated and accomplished without side effects *(16)*.

2.4. JNC IV (1988)

The fourth JNC report redefined the criteria for the diagnosis of hypertension, incorporating SBP as well as treatment goals of <140/90 mmHg *(17)*. The Working Group on Hypertension in Diabetes further underscored the vulnerability of patients with both diagnoses, and cited ideal BP below 140/90 mmHg as tolerated, yet did not formally recommend a lower goal for these patients *(18)*.

2.5. JNC V (1993)

JNC V created a significant paradigm shift in the evaluation and treatment of hypertension. As part of a major reclassification of hypertension, JNC V called "Stage I" what was previously termed mild hypertension (DBP: 90–104 mmHg). These patients were candidates for pharmacologic treatment after a reasonable trial of lifestyle modification. Hypertension was now defined as ≥140 mmHg SBP and/or ≥90 DBP. More than 50 million Americans were hypertensive using this new definition. Most experts agreed that a BP of <120/80 mmHg reflected the lowest risk group, with 120–140/ 80–90 mmHg an intermediate risk population. But there was no proof of the treatment benefit in those with intermediate risk, and no specific recommendations were made *(19)*. JNC V highlighted the downward trend in stroke, CHD, and all-cause mortality from 1972 to 1990 per findings of the National Center for Health Statistics; a development strongly linked to heightened awareness and treatment of hypertension.

Emerging trial data allowed JNC V to recommend treatment in two important groups, those with ISH and aged persons with elevated DBP. In both, treatment superiority had previously not been proven before JNC V and some experts doubted the safety of pharmacotherapy. The Systolic Hypertension in the Elderly (SHEP) main trial in 1991 provided JNC V with an evidence-based management rationale. SHEP, with entry criteria of SBP ≥160 mmHg and DBP <90 mmHg, achieved a 32% risk reduction for all CV morbidity and mortality with active treatment (thiazide-like diuretic with a β-blocker if needed) vs placebo. SHEP goals mandated SBP reduction by 20 mmHg, if 160–179 mmHg at entry; or below 160 mmHg, if ≥180 mmHg at entry *(20)*. JNC V adopted these goals. Although treating Stage 2 and above ISH (SBP ≥160 mmHg) was now firmly evidence-based, no data existed then or even now regarding Stage 1 ISH (SBP = 140–159 mmHg and DBP <90 mmHg).

Studies examining therapy for aged persons with increased DBP (who typically have high SBP as well) were incorporated into JNC V. The Medical Research Council (MRC) trial in the elderly and the first Swedish Trial on Old Patients with Hypertension

(STOP-Hypertension-1) both documented unequivocal risk reduction with treatment for aged persons and validated earlier recommendations to treat these hypertensives *(21,22)*.

By the time of JNC V, clinical trial data were still lacking regarding the value of intensive therapy in diabetics. Yet diabetes was understood to confer significantly increased CV risk, and JNC V advised that higher risk patients (such as diabetics) be treated to the goal of <130/85 mmHg. This was the first time that diabetics were assigned a lower therapeutic target *(19)*.

2.6. WHO/ISH 1993

Concurrently, 1993 World Health Organization/International Society of Hypertension (WHO/ISH) recommendations mirrored JNC V guidelines, advocating treatment of "mild" hypertension (DBP = 90–105 mmHg and/or SBP = 140–180 mmHg), a term they kept and still in use, as well as ISH (SBP ≥140 mmHg and DBP < 90 mmHg). Diabetes was acknowledged as a frequent co-morbid condition in hypertensives, and intensive BP management was credited with delaying the deterioration of renal function and reducing the progression of microalbuminuria. Despite advocating a desirable BP of 120–130/80 mmHg in younger patients, <140/90 mmHg in aged diabetic hypertensives, and SBP <140 mmHg in patients with ISH, the 1993 WHO/ISH paper did not stratify targets as the JNC V did for diabetic hypertensives or those with increased CV risk *(23)*.

2.7. WHO/ISH 1996

The next WHO/ISH guidelines continued to use the terms "mild," "moderate," and "severe hypertension" and categorized hypertensives by "grades" rather than stages as did JNC V. CV risk assessment and evaluation of target organ damage, however, were integrated into the treatment decision process, and more intensive goals for diabetic hypertensives of <130/85 mmHg were promoted as in JNC V *(24)*.

2.8. JNC VI (1997)

JNC VI had considerably more clinical trial data favoring the long-term value of treating hypertension on which to base its recommendations. Yet in contrast, data from the US National Health and Nutrition Examination Survey (NHANES) parts III-1 and III-2 (1988–1994) pointed to the alarming situation that the improving trend for continued reduction of stroke and CHD rates in the United States had stopped, co-incident with a decline in awareness, treatment, and control of high BP. This problem became the key feature of JNC VI, rather than the usual attention to the initial drug therapy recommendations. In addition, JNC VI focused on stratifying hypertensives by risk and suggested starting drug treatment at different levels depending on the risk strata of individual patients. Diabetes was accepted as an independent risk for CV disease, and directly placed patients into the highest risk group (C), with recommendations for immediate initiation of drug therapy for SBP >130 mmHg or DBP >85 mmHg. This document emphasized therapeutic titration to BP goal, and recommended that patients who were not at goal on two medications be referred to a hypertension specialist, the first time that the special expertise of these individuals was recognized *(25)*.

The recommendation to treat high-risk patients more aggressively was not strictly "evidence-based" since the trials that supported a more aggressive approach in diabetics, as an example of high-risk hypertensives, were not completed when JNC VI was written. They came soon thereafter. The first was the United Kingdom Prospective Diabetes Study (UKPDS 38), which demonstrated a 30% mortality benefit when diabetic subjects were treated to a "tight" BP goal (<150/85 mmHg) vs "less-tight" control (≤180/105 mmHg). The tight control group had 10/5 mmHg additional BP lowering (144/82 mmHg compared to 154/87 mmHg in the less-tight control group) without additional adverse reactions. In this trial, tight control of glycemia was not as effective at reducing events as was tight control of BP (26).

The second study supporting aggressive treatment in diabetic hypertensives was the HOT study. These investigators examined the goals of treatment to evaluate the "J"-curve phenomenon and determine whether intensive therapy was harmful. Using the same pharmacologic regimens, HOT randomized volunteers to three DBP goals (<80 mmHg vs <85 mmHg vs <90 mmHg). Unfortunately, HOT was not designed to compare SBP goals as well. The overall trial failed to show the advantage of more intensive therapy, but also did not show additional risk in those with a lower treatment goal ("J"-curve). Diabetics ($n = 1501$) was the only subgroup looked at where the intensive therapy was beneficial. Diabetics treated to DBP <80 mmHg had 51% fewer CV events vs diabetics treated to DBP <90 mmHg. In the overall cohort, the CV risk was optimally reduced at a mean-treated BP of 138/82 mm Hg (1). These data were not provided for the diabetic subgroup.

2.9. WHO/ISH 1999

UKPDS and HOT findings were integrated into 1999 WHO/ISH guidelines. As in JNC VI, diabetes was adopted as a valid criterion for considering a hypertension to be high risk (27). Because UKPDS and HOT conclusions were not yet available when JNC VI was being prepared, the more stringent target of <130/85 mmHg for diabetics was not yet strictly "evidence-based." With completion of these trials and publication of similar recommendation by the 1999 WHO/ISH, the foresight of JNC VI was validated. In 2001, the American Diabetes Association (ADA) reduced the goal still further to a new and lower target of <130/80 mmHg for diabetic hypertensives (28).

2.10. JNC 7 (2003)

The latest US guidelines appear in the seventh JNC statement. JNC 7 significantly revised the classification of hypertension. Previously "high-normal" or normal BP (120–139/80–89 mmHg) was now recategorized as "prehypertension" (Table 2). This reclassification underscored the continuum of escalating risk for men and women as BP rises from clearly normal levels (<120/80 mmHg) to definitely hypertensive values (>140/90 mmHg). The new classification system recommended in JNC 7 was strongly influenced by a meta-analysis of more than 1 million volunteers in observational studies showing that CV risk begins at 115/75 mmHg and doubles with each increment of 20/10 mmHg (29), JNC 7 continued the approach of JNC VI, focusing on attaining goal BP, but updated the goals in parallel with other guideline committees and newer data. Although no new trials yet supported the lower goal of <130/80 mmHg for diabetics, JNC 7 choose to also recommend this target (30) (Table 3). JNC 7 further emphasized the importance of titrating to BP goal, and cited all classes of antihypertensives that were acceptable for initial therapy were fundamentally equivalent.

Table 2
Comparison of Classifications of BP of JNC VI and JNC 7

JNC VI[a]	Systolic (mmHg)		Diastolic (mmHg)	JNC 7[b]
Optimal	<120	and	<80	Normal
	120–139	or	80–89	Prehypertension
Normal	<130	and	<85	
High normal	130–139	or	85–89	
Stage 1 hypertension	140–159	or	90–99	Stage 1 hypertension
Stage 2 hypertension	160–179	or	100–109	Stage 2 hypertension
Stage 3 hypertension	≥180	or	≥110	

[a]JNC VI: The sixth report of the Joint National Committee on the detection, evaluation, and treatment of high BP.

[b]JNC 7: The seventh report of the Joint National Committee on the detection, evaluation, and treatment of high BP.

Table 3
Comparison of Hypertension Goals of JNC VI and JNC 7

	<140/90 mmHg	<130/85 mmHg	<130/80 mmHg	<125/75 mmHg
Uncomplicated	a,b			
Diabetes		a	b	
Chronic kidney disease		a	b	
Proteinuria in excess of 1 g/24 h			b	a

[a]JNC VI: The sixth report of the Joint National Committee on the detection, evaluation, and treatment of high BP.

[b]JNC 7: The seventh report of the Joint National Committee on the detection, evaluation, and treatment of high BP.

3. LESSONS FROM CLINICAL TRIALS ABOUT OPTIMAL PHARMACOLOGICAL TREATMENT FOR THE DIABETIC HYPERTENSIVE

The choice of specific drug regimens for hypertension and for diabetic hypertensives has evolved along with the JNC recommendations. At the time of JNC I, only 28 drugs were available. In 2005, there are more than 125 agents and over 50 fixed-dose combinations, yet the ideal choice remains controversial. Until JNC VI introduced the idea of starting with two drugs in combination for some patients, all panels advised starting therapy with a single drug class. JNC I and all subsequent committees recommended diuretics as initial therapy. JNC III added β-blockers and JNC IV added angiotensin-converting enzyme inhibitors (ACE-I) and calcium channel blockers (CCBs) although no long-term trials had yet documented that these agents were equivalent or superior to diuretics or β-blockers for prevention of unfavorable outcomes. JNC V declared diuretics and β-blockers as "preferred" classes of drugs, but allowed another form of initial therapy in specific clinical situations.

JNC VI formalized this concept in which certain agents could be given for "specific indications," such as peripheral α_1 blockers for hypertensive men with prostatism, through which a co-morbid condition could be addressed with the same agent. JNC VI also recommended choosing certain compounds if a "compelling indication" were present. These compelling indications emerged from large trials assessing the conditions related to hypertension, such as diabetes or heart failure, treated with drugs that are also used to treat hypertension (ACE-I for heart failure or after an MI, for example) by which favorable CV outcomes had been demonstrated. In those conditions, initial therapy other than diuretic or β-blocker was permitted. JNC 7 expanded this group of drugs and conditions in light of trials reported between 1996 and 2003 (Table 4).

Of particular interest are several studies illustrating superior outcomes with inhibition of the renin–angiotensin–aldosterone system in patients who have type 2 diabetes mellitus. These trials led to both ACE-I and angiotensin receptor blockers (ARBs) being recommended as initial therapy in patients with diabetic nephropathy.

A fundamental debate in BP management centers on the question of ideal strategy when the initial choice fails to attain goal BP: should additional agents be added (stepped-care) or should the first agent be stopped in favor of another class of agents (sequential monotherapy)? JNC V allowed both approaches but JNC VI strongly favored stepped-care unless there was no therapeutic response or intolerable side effects with the first choice. Advocates of sequential monotherapy reasoned that BP can be successfully controlled if an agent with a specific mechanism of action is matched with a patient whose hypertension arises from dysregulation of that specific BP control mechanism. But this concept has two basic flaws. First, Page and many others have pointed out that hypertension is a mosaic and that many systems (renal volume regulation, sympathetic nervous system, the renin–angiotensin–aldosterone system, kinins, and other naturally occurring vasodilators to name a few) are implicated in hypertension. It is rare for only a single abnormality to be present (31,32). Second, all antihypertensive drugs are likely to lower BP by more than one mechanism. For example, diuretics reduce plasma volume but are also direct vasodilators, and ACE-I suppress the renin–angiotensin–aldosterone system but also slow the degradation of kinins and thereby stimulating vasodilation. ARBs block the AT_1 receptor but may also work through the effects of unopposed AT_2 receptor stimulation. Stepped-care exploits the antihypertensive activity of multiple drugs, with less focus on mechanisms of action and greater emphasis on goal achievement.

Before 1996, no published data addressed the treatment of hypertensive type 2 diabetics, and only the captopril trial by Lewis et al. in 1993 evaluated treatment for type 1 diabetics (33). Since that time, insight on management of diabetic hypertensive patients proceeds from two sources: trials enrolling diabetic hypertensives, and subgroup analyses of larger studies of which a proportion of subjects had diabetes.

The first trial in diabetics with hypertension was UKPDS 38. This protocol examined BP and glycemic control by examining 1148 diabetic hypertensives, randomizing them to either what was called "tight" or "less-tight" BP control. Investigators tracked both micro- and macrovascular complications of diabetes, as well as CV and all-cause mortality. Subjects were followed for a mean of 8.4 yr and multiple drugs were required in most of the tight BP control group and many of the less-tight BP control group. In the tight vs less-tight BP control groups, diabetic complications were 24% fewer

Table 4
Comparison of Drug Class Recommendations for High-Risk
Conditions with Compelling Indications by JNC VI and JNC 7

	Diuretic	β-Blocker	ACE Inhibitor	ARB	CCB	Aldosterone antagonist
Heart failure	a,b	b	a,b	b		b
Post-MI		a,b	a,b			b
High coronary disease risk	b	b	b		b	
Diabetes	b	b	a,b	b	b	
Chronic kidney disease			b	b		
Recurrent stroke prevention	b		b			
Isolate systolic hypertension	a,b				a	

[a]JNC VI: The sixth report of the Joint National Committee on the detection, evaluation, and treatment of high BP.
[b]JNC 7: The seventh report of the Joint National Committee on the detection, evaluation, and treatment of high BP.

($p = 0.0046$), diabetes-related deaths 32% fewer ($p = 0.019$), strokes 44% fewer ($p < 0.013$), and MI 21% fewer (p = nonsignificant). Tight blood glucose control was associated with only a 12% reduction in diabetic complications, underscoring the importance of BP regulation in diabetics, though optimization of both BP and glucose are clearly essential (34).

The UKPDS trial also addressed this issue of whether one specific drug class is more effective at reducing events. In 758 type 2 diabetics, approximately half received the β-blocker atenolol and half the ACE-I, captopril. Outcomes were similar with no evidence of superiority for the ACE-I, the result that experts most would not have predicted (35).

Most insights concerning the higher risk and greater benefit for treatment in diabetic hypertensives come from subgroup analyses of large BP trials. SHEP showed that in the 583 diabetics vs 4149 nondiabetic subjects, the absolute risk reduction for cardiovascular disease (CVD) events was 101/1000 in diabetics compared to 51/1000 in nondiabetics with active treatment compared to placebo, over the 5 yr of the study (36). Of the 1501 diabetics among 18,790 HOT volunteers, a 51% reduction in CV mortality was demonstrated in the group randomized to the lowest DBP goal (<80 mmHg). No other subgroup had benefit, though none showed harm from aggressive therapy. A variety of drugs were used in these trials. UKPDS used ACE-I and beta blockers; SHEP used diuretics and a β-blocker or centrally acting agent, if needed; and HOT used CCBs, beta blockers, ACE-I, and diuretics (1,20,34).

Several small and underpowered studies such as the Appropriate Blood Pressure Control in Diabetes ABCD trial and the Fosinopril vs Amlodipine Cardiovascular Events Randomized Trial (FACET) focused on specific classes of drugs and levels of BP control, but these results are difficult to interpret. Recent larger trials have helped to clarify the issues. In the heart outcomes protection evaluation (HOPE) study, ACE-I were proven effective in diabetics: there was a 22% relative risk reduction in CV events for the 3577 diabetic patients of the 9297 enrolled. This trial of high risk and not necessarily hypertensive individuals, compared the ACE-I ramipril to placebo. Although investigators claim that small differences in BP between study groups do not account for the beneficial effects of ACE-I, many observers believe that BP reduction explains much of the positive results, so that the advantage of active therapy was not a special property of ACE-I beyond their ability to lower BP (37). The Comparison of Amlodipine vs Enalapril to Limit Occurrences of Thrombosis (CAMELOT) study, evaluating a three arm protocol of enalapril vs amlodipine vs placebo in 1991 normotensive patients with CAD, showed cardioprotective effects in treated patients after 2 yr. Patients randomized to amlodipine had a 5/3 mmHg reduction from a baseline BP of 129/77 mmHg, similar to the 5/2 mmHg reduction achieved with enalapril, yet only the amlodipine group experienced a 31% reduction in CV events. This suggested that ACE-I do not have protective effects beyond BP reduction as suggested by the HOPE study (38).

Two studies published in 2001 examined the efficacy of ARBs in diabetics with nephropathy and further examined specific benefits of drugs vs the degree of BP control achieved. The Irbesartan Type II Diabetic Nephropathy Trial (IDNT) (irbesartan), and the Reduction of End Points in Non-Insulin Dependent Diabetes Mellitus with Angiotensin II [AII] Antagonist Losartan (RENAAL) Trial (losartan), demonstrated specific renal protective benefits of AII blockade in delaying the progression of renal dysfunction to end stage renal disease (ESRD). In both studies, there was equally good BP control in the ARB treatment arm vs the non-ARB treatment arm. Both sets of investigators concluded that the 20–30% risk reduction in renal endpoints was attributable to the inherent properties of ARBs rather than degree of BP control achieved (39,40).

Three other trials with large diabetic cohorts have been completed. The Controlled Onset Verapamil Investigation of Cardiac Endpoints (CONVINCE) trial enrolled 3239 diabetics among 16,602 volunteers. Subjects were randomized to controlled-onset extended release CCB (verapamil) vs β-blocker (atenolol) or a diuretic (hydrochlorothiazide). Likewise International Verapamil–Trandolapril Study (INVEST) compared hypertension treatment randomized to the CCB verapamil plus ACE-I vs the β-blocker atenolol plus ACE-I in a large subgroup of diabetics (6400 of 22,576). Neither study showed superiority of any agent in mortality, nonfatal MI, or stroke outcomes (2,41).

The Antihypertensive and Lipid-Lowering Treatment to Prevent Heart Attack (ALLHAT) study represents the largest diabetic subgroup analysis in any clinical hypertension trial. There were 13,101 diabetics, an additional 1399 volunteers with impaired fasting glucose (IFG), and 17,012 normoglycemic (NG) patients. ALLHAT randomized subjects to three different first-line agents: diuretics, CCBs, or ACE-I. A fourth group received a peripheral α-adrenergic blocker, doxazosin, as initial therapy but that arm of the trial was stopped early. ALLHAT tested whether first-line antihypertensive therapy beginning with a CCB (amlodipine) or ACE-I (lisinopril) was superior to the thiazide-like diuretic, chlorthalidone (4).

Results from ALLHAT showed no evidence of superiority in patients initially treated with the newer agents in any of the three glycemic subgroups or in the overall trial. As expected, the event rate for nonfatal MI and fatal CHD was higher in diabetics compared to those with impaired fasting glucose or normoglycemia, but this finding was observed equally in all treatment arms. Likewise, there was no significant difference in rates of stroke or combined CVD in diabetic participants among treatment arms. There was a 3–4 mg/dL increase in fasting glucose levels among normoglycemics at 4 yr in patients assigned to the chlorthalidone group vs amlodipine or lisinopril, with a consequent 3% increased incidence of fasting glucose levels >126 mg/dL, the definition of diabetes. However, no significant increase in fasting glucose was noted in patients previously classified as diabetic *(42)*. There were differences, however, in the incidence of new diabetes in the volunteers randomized to each class of drugs. Only 8.1% of those randomized to lisinopril developed new diabetes compared to 9.8% receiving amlopidine and 11.6% receiving chlorthalidone *(4)*. The significance of these findings is unclear because the diabetic subgroup of ALLHAT that started therapy with chlorthalidone did as well or better than those randomized to begin treatment with the other drugs. There was nothing in ALLHAT to confirm the expected special benefit of ACE-I for diabetics, for any outcome including HF or renal disease. The early reduction in SBP in subjects who began with chlorthalidone compared to other agents best explains the overall study results.

Observations common to all three large studies (CONVINCE, INVEST, and ALLHAT) relate to quality of BP control. Over 3–5 yr, reduction to goal (<140 for SBP and <90 mmHg for DBP) was achieved in 60% of participants, irrespective of initial agent. The great majority required multiple drugs to attain goal. DBP objective was achieved in >90% of volunteers, whereas only 60–65% reached SBP goal. We have coined the term, the "60–90 rule" to characterize this phenomenon. These findings reinforce JNC VI and JNC 7 guidelines that favor combination therapy and stepped-care approach to management. ALLHAT and CONVINCE did not mandate a lower goal for diabetics as recommended by the guidelines, however INVEST sought a BP goal for diabetics <130/85 mmHg *(3)*. INVEST also showed that fewer participants developed new diabetes in the ACE-I/CCB combination group compared to the β-blocker/ACE-I group *(41)*.

The above trials furnished the main rationale for the JNC 7 recommendation advocating thiazide or thiazide-like diuretics for first-line therapy for most hypertensives; for initiating combination therapy for diabetics with ≥150 mmHg SBP and/or ≥90 mmHg DBP; and for a goal in diabetic hypertensives of <130/80 mmHg. For diabetic hypertensives, JNC 7 stated that combination regimens are usually required, and that ACE-I or ARB should be included, especially in diabetics with nephropathy. Achieving goal was emphasized as previously, but what was not addressed was how difficult it may be to attain such stringent goals.

Compared to national surveys, in which only 27–31% of hypertensives were at goal, these clinical trials used a forced-titration algorithm and demonstrated superior BP control rates. CONVINCE and ALLHAT reached goal in >60% of participants, regardless of initial agent (except for the discontinued doxazosin arm), and showed that multiple agents were usually necessary to accomplish these control rates. ALLHAT enrolled over 42,000 participants from primary care practices, but treatment changes were protocol-driven and implemented by study coordinators *(4)*. Compared with the general patient population, volunteers may have experienced better BP control because they agreed to the study after being selected by investigators to participate. They were more likely to attend study visits and adhere to medical therapy, and less likely to be lost to followup. Trained clinical staffs focused on outcomes and side effect issues, and may have devoted more energy to goal achievement in study subjects when compared to patients seen in other settings where reaching goal is not as much of a priority. Such differences may explain much of the disparity in target goal success rates in trails vs practice *(43)*.

4. GOAL-ORIENTED MANAGEMENT

Although considerable evidence now strongly validates the intensive recommendations of JNC 7, it remains to be seen if these goals can be achieved in clinical practice. Favorable outcomes from clinical trials are compelling, yet methods must be devised to translate trial conclusions into practice if physicians are to improve the disappointing rates of BP control in the United States and throughout the world. Though a dichotomized goal (above or below a prespecified target) is clearly artificial and not physiologic, we believe it is easier in a busy practice to implement a goal that provides a specific number, than it would be to encourage vigorous treatment without offering a target to shoot for. This approach will also make it easier to assess performance and sets a clear basis for comparison of the quality of management between different healthcare providers and different healthcare delivery systems.

The choice of an appropriate goal is also a key issue. A goal that cannot be reached is too severe and thus unachievable, but a goal that is too easily reached will not optimize outcomes in high-risk subjects. Results from CONVINCE and ALLHAT have shown that excellent control rates are available in clinical trials in which study coordinators maintain fidelity to protocols that demand forced titration or the addition of a new drug or drugs, if goal BP is not reached.

Although the Hypertension Service at Rush University manages patients via individual physician encounters and has doctors with different practice styles, we believed that a University hospital-based Hypertension Specialty Clinic could equal BP control rates seen in clinical trials. Alternatively, if excellent BP control rates could not be acquired in a clinic staffed by knowledgeable specialists such as the Rush Clinic, then the outlook would indeed be poor for good BP control in other settings.

In our study of 437 consecutive patients seen at Rush, we judged our performance against (1) the Health Employer Data Information Set (HEDIS) 2000 measures, (2) JNC VI, and (3) the more stringent goals of the ADA and National Kidney Foundation (NKF) for diabetic patients. Most patients were referred by physicians because of difficult-to-manage or resistant hypertension. Using "goal-oriented management," our four physicians aimed at satisfying current guideline criteria for BP control. Similar to forced-titration algorithms in clinical trials, "goal-oriented management" requires stepping up therapy until goal is achieved. No specific drug treatment algorithm was mandated and our physicians were free to choose any lifestyle or drug combination they wished. The American Society of Hypertension has certified three of our physicians as clinical specialists; two are certified by the ABIM in Nephrology, one in Endocrinology and one in Clinical Pharmacology. A dedicated Hypertension Fellow assists us.

Results from this study parallel evidence from large clinical trials. Similar to CONVINCE and ALLHAT, 59% of patients achieved the SBP goal <140 mmHg and DBP goal <90 mmHg, with 86% having DBP <90 mmHg. As in HOT and CONVINCE, in which 30% and 32% of participants received monotherapy at 3 yr respectively, over two-thirds of patients required two or more medications *(44)*. In diabetics, 52% achieved a BP <140/90 mmHg, the HEDIS criteria, but only 22% of diabetics reached the JNC VI target of <130/85 mmHg, and a dismal 15% got to the ADA, NKF, and JNC 7 target of <130/80 mmHg (45).

A similar study was published by a group of specialists from Spain who examined 4049 difficult-to-control subjects in 47 hospital-based hypertension clinics. Using similar methods, overall goal BP (<140/90 mmHg) in uncomplicated hypertensives was reached in 42% of patients, with DBP goal reached in 70% and SBP goal in 47%. However, only 36.7% of diabetics were <140 mmHg for SBP and also <90 mmHg for DBP. Similar to our results, only 13.2% were <130/85 mmHg and fewer (10.5%) were <130/80 mmHg (46).

Further studies have analyzed guideline adherence and goal achievement in the managed care setting, in which many hypertensive patients are treated. A retrospective analysis of 502 patients in three primary care clinics operated by a commercial Managed Care Organization (MCO) looked at target achievement based on HEDIS and JNC VI guideline criteria for uncomplicated hypertensives and diabetics. Subjects had full health insurance including prescription coverage. Goal of ≤140/90 mmHg was attained by 74% of patients, with 46% of the 148 diabetics being <130/85 mmHg (47).

A study in 792 randomly selected adults covered by commercial health insurance, seen in the offices of 32 different physicians, showed a 55% prevalence rate of hypertension with a 43% control rate based on contemporary HEDIS and JNC standards (SBP <140 mmHg and DBP <90 mmHg). The 126 diabetics were difficult to control with only 45% at the HEDIS 3.0 and JNC V standard of <140/90 mmHg and 15% at the JNC VI target of <130/85 mmHg (48).

Although results of these analyses are disappointing, control rates in other setting are often worse. In a VA study of 800 patients (one-third of whom were diabetic), hypertensive patients with diabetes were actually less intensively treated than other hypertensives. The intensity of therapy was judged by the frequency of regimen modification during visits by which the BP above target was recorded. Because this analysis was done in VA clinics, the cost of medication and access to care were not barriers to clinicians' prescribing behavior. Physician inertia again may have been a factor. Similar lack of BP control was seen as in the above studies (45–47), with no clearly identified reason for the lack of clinician intensity in this higher risk group (49).

We doubt that specific algorithms can be applied in the general practice settings or that such recommendations are appropriate. The pathophysiology of hypertension in individual patients varies widely, and some will certainly respond better to certain agents or combinations of agents than others. Access, cultural, language, and economic factors will introduce further variation. It is critically important to allow physicians to choose the regimen they view as best for each patient. Contrary to recent critics, JNC 7 and other contemporary guidelines grant considerable flexibility to clinicians in allowing for choices based on judgment about how an individual patient will respond, what other diseases or risk factors are present, and what economic factors exist. Whereas a forced-titration algorithm specifies which drug to add when a patient is not at goal and is appropriate for a clinical trial, a goal-oriented algorithm advocates vigorous drug titration using available and well-tolerated agents regardless of initial drug therapy or life-style modification approach.

We are not at all certain about what element of our practice or other specialty practices is responsible for our relative success. We are staffed by hypertension specialists which should improve our results, but we see more difficult-to-manage patients, increasing our challenge. The clinical experience of the specialists, however, may allow them to add necessary medications or increase doses to attain goal with less hesitation regarding adverse effects. Mandating a particular regimen is unlikely to work, but a goal-oriented approach can be successful in achieving outcomes resembling those of clinical trials.

Although goal-oriented management is effective in an outpatient-specialist setting, adaptation to general practice may present a challenge. Less-experienced physicians may hesitate to titrate drug regimens vigorously, or may be excessively concerned that lowering BP too far or too fast will cause side effects. ALLHAT and the newly completed VALUE study suggest that these concerns are overstated and that intensive treatment in high-risk hypertensives can save many more lives. VALUE showed fewer endpoints with early intensive BP reduction, the amlodipine (CCB) group achieving 4.0/2.1 mmHg greater difference in BP reduction after 1 mo compared to the valsartan (ARB) group. The groups averaged 13.9/7.2 mmHg (amlodipine) and 11.3/5.3 mmHg (valsartan) reduction in the first 6 mo: however, the differences in BP reduction were less (1.5/1.3 mmHg) after 1 yr. The 63% excess strokes in the valsartan group occurred in the first 6 mo, and 76% within the first year, perhaps reflecting benefit of early intensive BP reduction *(5)*.

Because excellent results can be achieved in practice settings such as ALLHAT, CONVINCE, INVEST, and VALUE, it is possible that similar results are achievable in primary care setting using a team approach. One suggestion is that a team can be composed of one primary care physician, two nonphysician practitioners (physician associates, physician assistants, or nurse practitioners), three members of the nursing staff (nurses or medical assistants), and an administrative coordinator *(50)*. By applying a goal-oriented approach in a team setting, a physician promotes intensive follow up of BP control with frequent visits with nonphysician staff. Motivated by a goal-oriented philosophy and guided by preset interim adjustments, patients may achieve goal earlier and maintain goal longer. Medication complications, adverse reactions, or lack of efficacy will prompt follow up with the physician, but nonphysicians manage the majority of visits.

In a study of 1407 diabetics in a British hospital-based clinic, patients were randomized to a specialist nurse-led hypertension clinic vs usual care with their diabetologist. In the hypertension clinic arm, patients identified as uncontrolled (BP ≥140/≥80 mmHg initially received life-style modification education with an individualized action plan, and if persistently uncontrolled, were begun on medication. At regular follow-up visits every 4–6 wk, the clinician reinforced life-style modification, reviewed medication tolerance, and titrated according to a stepped-care preset protocol. Patients needing more medications were discussed with physicians, who initiated additional therapy. This strategy contrasted with the usual care arm that included biannual visits to a diabetologist, who made written suggestions to the primary doctor. The same titration algorithm used in the nurse-specialist clinics was available to the general practitioners, who had ultimate autonomy about whether to initiate or change treatment.

Nurse-led specialty clinics effectively improved rates of goal achievement when their skills were added to routine diabetes care. Although there was only a modest improvement from 31% to 37% controlled, mortality benefit was statistically significant (odds ratio 0.55 [95% CI 0.32–0.92], $p = 0.02$). BP goals for diabetic hypertensives were higher than currently recommended, and mean visit frequency was only twice per year during the 1.5 yr follow up period in the nurse specialist arm for hypertension *(51)*.

Despite less stringent targets and few follow-up visits, when diabetic patients received specific attention to multiple-risk factors, they experienced great benefits. Further studies are indicated to examine this clinical strategy, with more energetic titration and frequent follow up, aimed at more stringent targets. Although it must be pointed out that the results seen in the Rush University Hypertension Clinic were achieved by physicians without benefit of other health-care providers.

5. CONCLUSIONS

As reflected in the evolution of guideline recommendations, tighter BP control yields significant morbidity and mortality benefit, especially in higher risk diabetic hypertensives. The question of whether reducing BP to more strict targets improves outcomes for diabetic hypertensives remains to be answered, and we must be cautious until the proof is in hand. We may be surprised. For example, the African American Study of Kidney Disease (AASK) failed to prove that lower goal BP (mean arterial pressure, MAP <92 mmHg or approximately <125/75 mmHg, which was achieved), led to better clinical outcomes in more than 1100 African Americans with renal insufficiency due to reasons other than diabetic nephropathy (52). But otherwise the current data consistently show that intensive antihypertensive therapy benefits high-risk individuals, and that combination therapy will likely be required to realize goals. However, until the Avoiding Cardiovascular Events Through Combination Therapy in Patients Living with Systolic Hypertension (ACCOMPLISH) trial is completed in 5–7 yr, we will not have the necessary evidence to help us select the optimal combination of currently available drugs (53).

But we need to act while waiting for definitive answers. Intensive therapy using goal-oriented management can bring a large percentage of hypertensive patients to goal, many more than we are at goal now. Although diabetic hypertensives are more difficult to control, it is also clear that they receive greater benefit if goal is vigorously pursued and reached. The inclusion of specific drugs is less important as we strive for increasingly lower levels of BP, because the overwhelming majority of patients, especially diabetics, will require multiple drug regimens to reach goal. Although inhibitors of the renin–angiotensin–aldosterone system may provide additional benefit beyond BP, the insightful clinician will use all modalities, including life style modifications, and focus more on arriving at goal rather than on any specific way to get there. As the prevalence and incidence of diabetes rises, and dialysis units are increasingly populated by patients with diabetic nephropathy and hypertension, the potential for reducing morbidity, delaying mortality, and lowering the cost of the care of diabetics is now an urgent national priority (54).

REFERENCES

1. Hansson, L., Zanchetti, A., Carruthers, S. G., et al. (1998) Effects of intensive BP lowering and low-dose aspirin in patients with hypertension: principal results of the hypertension optimal treatment (HOT) randomized trial. *Lancet* **351,** 1755–1762.
2. Black, H. R., Elliott, W. J., Grandits, G., et al. (2003) CONVINCE research group. Principal results of the controlled onset verapamil investigation of CV end points (CONVINCE) trial. *JAMA* **289,** 2073–2082.
3. Pepine, C. J., Handberg, E. M., Cooper-DeHoff, R. M., et al. (2003) INVEST investigators. A calcium antagonist vs a noncalcium antagonist hypertension treatment strategy for patients with coronary artery disease. The international verapamil-trandolapril study (INVEST): a randomized controlled trial. *JAMA* **290,** 2805–2816.

 4. The ALLHAT Officers and Coordinators for the ALLHAT Collaborative Group (2002) Major outcomes in high-risk hypertensive patients randomized to angiotensin converting enzyme inhibitor or calcium channel blocker vs diuretic. The antihypertensive and lipid-lowering treatment to prevent heart attack trial (ALLHAT). *JAMA* **288**, 1981–1997.
 5. Julius, S., Kjeldsen, S. E., Weber, M., et al. (2004) Zanchetti a for the VALUE trial group. Outcomes in hypertensive patients a high CV risk treated with regimens based on valsartan or amlodipine: the VALUE randomized trial. *Lancet* **363**, 2022–2031.
 6. Phillips, L. S., Branch, W. T. Jr., Cook, C. B., et al. (2001) Clinical inertia. *Ann. Intern. Med.* **135**, 825–834.
 7. Veterans Administration Cooperative Study Group on Antihypertensive Agents (1970) Effects of treatment on morbidity in hypertension. II. Results in patients with diastolic BP averaging 90 through 114 mmHg. *JAMA* **213**, 1143–1152.
 8. Veterans Administration Cooperative Study Group on Antihypertensive Agents (1967) Effects of treatment on morbidity in hypertension. Results in patients with diastolic BP averaging 115 through 129 mmHg. *JAMA* **202**, 1028–1034.
 9. Moser, M. (1997) Evolution of the treatment of hypertension from the 1940s to JNC V. *Am. J. Hypertens.* **10(3)**, 2S–8S.
10. National High BP Education Program (1973) Report to the hypertension information and education advisory committee. Task Force I Data Base. Recommendations for a national high BP program database for effective antihypertensive therapy. DHEW Publication No. (NIH) 75-593, September 1.
11. Report of the Joint National Committee on Detection (1977) Evaluation and treatment of high BP (JNC I). *JAMA* **237**, 255–261.
12. Kannel, W. B., Gordon, T., and Schwartz, M. J. (1971) Systolic versus diastolic BP and risk of coronary heart disease. The Framingham study. *Am. J. Cardiol.* **27**, 335–346.
13. Hypertension Detection and Follow-up Program Cooperative Group (1979) Five-year findings of the hypertension detection and follow-up program (HDFP). Reduction in mortality of persons with high BP, including mild hypertension. *JAMA* **242**, 2562–2571.
14. The 1980 report of the Joint National Committee on Detection, Evaluation, and Treatment of High BP (1980) *Arch. Intern. Med.* **140**, 1280–1285.
15. Hulley, S. B., Furberg, C. D., Gurland, B., et al. (1985) Systolic hypertension in the elderly program (SHEP): antihypertensive efficacy of chlorthalidone. *Am. J. Cardiol.* **56**, 913–920.
16. The 1984 report of the Joint National Committee on Detection, Evaluation, and Treatment of High BP (1984) *Arch. Intern. Med.* **144**, 1045–1057.
17. Report of the Joint National Committee on Detection, Evaluation and Treatment of High BP (JNC IV) (1988) *Arch. Intern. Med.* **148**, 1023–1038.
18. Working Group on Hypertension in Diabetes (1987) Statement on hypertension in diabetes mellitus: final report. *Arch. Intern. Med.* **147**, 830–842.
19. Report of the Joint National Committee on Detection, Evaluation and Treatment of High BP (JNC V) (1993) *Arch. Intern. Med.* **153**, 154–183.
20. Systolic Hypertension in the Elderly Program Cooperative Research Group (1991) Prevention of stroke by antihypertensive drug treatment in older persons with isolated systolic hypertension. Final results of the systolic hypertension in the elderly program (SHEP). *JAMA* **265**, 3255–3264.
21. MRC Working Party (1992) Medical research council trial of treatment of hypertension in older adults: principal results. *BMJ* **304**, 405–412.
22. Dahlöf, B., Lindholm, L. H., Hansson, L., et al. (1991) Morbidity and mortality in the Swedish trial in old patients with hypertension (STOP-Hypertension). *Lancet* **338**, 1281–1285.
23. 1993 Guidelines for the Management of Mild Hypertension (1993) Memorandum from a World Health Organization/International Society of Hypertension Meeting. Guidelines Subcommittee of the WHO/ISH Mild Hypertension Liaison Committee. *Hypertension* **22**, 392–403.
24. Chalmers J. and Zanchetti A. (1996) The 1996 report of a World Health Organization Expert Committee on hypertension control. *J. Hypertens.* **14**, 929–933.
25. Joint National Committee on Prevention, Detection, and Treatment of High BP (1997) The sixth report of the Joint National Committee on prevention, detection, and treatment of high BP (JNC VI). *Arch. Intern. Med.* **157**, 2413–2446.
26. Laasko, M. (1999) Benefits of strict glucose and BP control in type 2 diabetes: lessons from the UK prospective diabetes study. *Circulation* **99**, 461–462.
27. 1999 World Health Organization–International Society of Hypertension Guidelines for the Management of Hypertension (1999) Guidelines Subcommittee. *J. Hypertens.* **17**, 151–183.

28. American Diabetes Association: Clinical Practice Recommendations (2001) *Diabetes Care* **24,** S33–S43.

29. Lewington, S., Clarke, R., Qizilbash, N., Peto, R., and Collins, R. (2002) Age-specific relevance of usual BP to vascular mortality: a meta-analysis of individual data for one million adults in 61 prospective studies. *Lancet* **360,** 1903–1913.

30. Chobanian, A. V., Bakris, G. L., Black, H. R., et al. (2003) The seventh report of the Joint National Committee on the prevention, detection, evaluation, and treatment of high BP. *JAMA* **289,** 2560–2572.

31. Page, I. H. (1949) Pathogenesis of arterial hypertension. *JAMA* **140,** 451–458.

32. Khosla, M. C., Page, I. H., and Bumpus, F. M. (1979) Interrelations between various BP regulatory systems and the mosaic theory of hypertension. *Biochem. Pharmacol.* **28,** 2867–2882.

33. Lewis, E. J., Hunsicker, L. G., Bain, R. P., and Rohde R. D., for the Collaborative Study Group. (1993) The effect of angiotensin-converting-enzyme inhibition on diabetic nephropathy. *NEJM* **329,** 1456–1462.

34. UK Prospective Diabetes Study Group (1998) Tight BP control and risk of macrovascular and microvascular complications in type 2 diabetes: UKPDS 38. *BMJ* **317,** 703–713.

35. UK Prospective Diabetes Study Group (1998) Efficacy of atenolol and captopril in reducing macrovascular and microvascular complications in type 2 diabetes: UKPDS 39. *BMJ* **317,** 713–720.

36. Curb, J. D., Pressel, S. L., Cutler, J. A., et al. (1996) Effect of diuretic-based antihypertensive treatment on CV disease risk in older diabetic patients with isolated systolic hypertension. Systolic hypertension in the elderly program cooperative research group. *JAMA* **276,** 1886–1892.

37. Yusuf, S., Sleight, P., Pogue, J., Bosch, J., Davies, R., and Dagenais, G. (2000) Effects of an angiotensin-converting-enzyme inhibitor, ramipril, on CV events in high-risk patients. The heart outcomes prevention evaluation study investigators. *NEJM* **342,** 145–153.

38. Nissen, S. E., Tuzcu, E. M., Libby, P., et al. (2004) Effect of antihypertensive agents on cardiovascular events in patients with coronary disease and normal blood pressure The CAMELOT study: a randomized controlled trial. *JAMA* **292,** 2217–2226.

39. Lewis, E. J., Hunsicker, L. G., Clarke, W. R., et al. (2001) Renoprotective effect of the angiotensin receptor antagonist irbesartan in patients with nephropathy due to type 2 diabetes. *NEJM* **345,** 851–860.

40. Brenner, B. M., Cooper, M. E., de Zeeuw, D., et al. (2001) For the reduction of end points in non-insulin-dependent diabetes mellitus with the angiotensin II antagonist losartan (RENAAL) study investigators. Effects of losartan on renal and CV outcomes in patients with type 2 diabetes and nephropathy. *NEJM* **345,** 861–869.

41. Bakris, G. L., Gaxiola, E., Messerli, F. H., et al. (2004) Clinical outcomes in the diabetes cohort of the international verapamil SR-trandolapril study. *Hypertension* **44,** 1–6.

42. Whelton, P. K., Barzilay, J., Cushman, W. C., et al. (2005) Clinical outcomes in ALLHAT antihypertensives trial participants with Type 2 diabetes, impaired fasting glucose, and normoglycemia. *Arch. Intern. Med.* **165(12),** 1401–1409.

43. LaCroix, A. Z. Ott, S. M. Ichikawa, L., Scholes, D., and Barlow, W. E. (2000) Low-dose hydrochlorothiazide and preservation of bone mineral density in older adults. A randomized, double-blind, placebo-controlled trial. *Ann. Intern. Med.* **133,** 516–526.

44. Singer, G. M., Izhar, M., and Black, H. R. (2002) Goal-oriented management of hypertension: translating clinical trial results into practice. *Hypertension* **40,** 464–469.

45. Singer, G. M., Izhar, M., and Black, H. R. (2004) Guidelines of hypertension: are quality assurance measures on target? *Hypertension* **43,** 198–202.

46. Banegas, J. R., Segura, J., Ruilope, L. M., et al. (2004) BP control and physician management of hypertension in hospital hypertension units in Spain. *Hypertension* **43,** 1338–1344.

47. Romain, T. M., Patel, R. T., Heaberlin, A. M., and Zarowitz, B. J. (2003) Assessment of factors influencing BP control in a managed care population. *Pharmacotherapy* **23,** 1060–1070.

48. Elliott, W. J., Toth, S. J., Stemer, A., and Cadwalader, J. H., for the Ispat Inland/United Steelworkers of America Health Care Network. (1999) Detection, treatment, and control of adult hypertension in northwest Indiana. *Am. J. Hypertens.* **12,** 830–834.

49. Berlowitz, D., Ash, A., Hickey, E., Glickman, M., Friedman, R., and Kader, B. (2003) Hypertension management in patients with diabetes: the need for more aggressive therapy. *Diabetes Care* **26,** 355–359.

50. Bodenheimer, T. (2003) Innovations in primary care in the United States. *BMJ* **326,** 796–799.

51. New, J., Mason, J., Freemantle, N., et al. (2003) Treat and control hypertension and hyperlipidemia in diabetes (SPLINT) a randomized controlled trial. *Diabetes Care* **26,** 2250–2255.

52. Wright, J. T., Agodoa, L., Contreras, G., et al. (2002) Successful BP control in the African American study of kidney disease and hypertension. *Arch. Intern. Med.* **162,** 1636–1643.
53. Jamerson, K. A. (2003) The first hypertension trial comparing the effects of two fixed-dose combination therapy regimens on CV events: avoiding CV events through combination therapy in patients living with systolic hypertension (ACCOMPLISH). *J. Clin. Hypertens.* **5(4 Suppl 3),** 29–35.
54. Elliott, W. J., Weir, D. R., and Black, H. R. (2000) Cost-effectiveness of the lower treatment goal (of JNC VI) for diabetic hypertensive patients. *Arch. Intern. Med.* **160,** 1277–1283.

IV ENDOTHELIAL HORMONES AND AUTOCOIDS IN HYPERTENSION

14 Nitric Oxide and Hypertension

David L. Mattson and Allen W. Cowley Jr.

CONTENTS

1. INTRODUCTION

Nitric oxide (NO) is a paracrine/autocrine factor that is important in the physiological regulation of numerous biological processes including neurotransmission, cardiovascular control, cell growth, apoptosis, and inflammation *(1–3)*. Numerous mammalian tissues and organs express NO synthase (NOS) and are therefore capable of producing NO under different physiological and pathophysiological conditions *(1,2,3)*. The role of NO in the control of renal function has been extensively studied. Works to date indicate that NO participates in the control of renal and glomerular hemodynamics, the tubulo-glomerular feedback response, the release of renin and sympathetic transmitters, tubular ion transport, and renal water and sodium excretion *(2,4,5)*. The focus of this chapter is on the role of NO in the control of renal water and sodium excretion. Because renal excretion of sodium and water is a primary determinant of extracellular fluid volume and arterial blood pressure *(6)*, this report emphasizes the importance of NO in the long-term control of arterial blood pressure.

2. SYNTHESIS OF NO IN THE KIDNEY

NO is synthesized from L-arginine by NOS that catalyzes the oxidation of one of the terminal guanidine nitrogen atoms of L-arginine resulting in NO and L-citrulline. This enzymatic reaction requires molecular oxygen and nicotinamide adenine dinucleotide phosphate (NADPH). Cofactors include calmodulin, tetrahydrobiopterin, flavin adenine dinucleotide (FAD), and flavin mononucleotide (FMN) *(2,7)*. The redox form of NO, nitric oxide (NO$^{\bullet}$), is preferentially generated by the oxidation of L-arginine, which is

From: *Contemporary Endocrinology: Hypertension and Hormone Mechanisms*
Edited by: R. M. Carey © Humana Press Inc., Totowa, NJ

catalyzed by NOS. NO can be interconverted among different redox forms such as NO•, nitroxyl anion (NO⁻), and nitrosonium cation (NO⁺) *(3)*. The generation and conversion of NO among these redox forms are influenced by a variety of factors including the different NOS isoforms, substrate depletion, and overall tissue redox status *(8,9)*. Different redox forms of NO can target different molecules in cells of different tissues and may lead to a wide variety and complexity of reactions. The measurement of the different redox forms of NO within biological tissue and differentiation of the effects of these redox forms is difficult. Currently, our understanding of the biological function of NO is based on the concept of the nitrogen monoxide complex, referred to in the literature as NO, as the biologically active molecule.

2.1. NOS Isoforms in the Kidney

Although reports have indicated that NO can be transported in blood by binding to hemoglobin in red blood cells or other plasma carrier protein and molecules *(3)*, the role and physiological regulation of NO as a circulating hormone is not clear. As a result, it is generally accepted that it is the endogenously produced NO in the kidney that determines its renal actions. There is now a considerable evidence demonstrating that NO produced in the kidney influences renal tubular and vascular function in a paracrine or autocrine manner. The kidney expresses the mRNA, protein and enzymatic activity of neuronal (nNOS, NOS I, and NOS 1), inducible (iNOS, NOS II, and NOS 2) and endothelial NOS (eNOS, NOS III, and NOS 3). The enzymatic activity of nNOS and eNOS is dependent on intracellular Ca^{2+}/calmodulin levels. Moreover, although nNOS and eNOS are both considered to be "constitutively expressed" enzymes, the expression of these enzymes can be regulated by different physiological stimuli including hypoxia, ischemia, and shear stress *(1,2,3,10,11)*. The other major NOS isoform, known as inducible NOS, was originally named based on its transcriptional induction in macrophage cells by a number of cytokines or immunologic stimuli. The activity of iNOS is believed to be Ca^{2+}/calmodulin independent, though a calmodulin consensus sequence is present in this isoform and recent studies indicate that iNOS is twice as active in the presence of Ca^{2+} as its absence *(12)*. Moreover, as described below, this enzyme is expressed in different cell types of the kidney under normal physiological conditions, so it may therefore be more appropriate to consider iNOS as a constitutively expressed molecule in the same manner as nNOS and eNOS.

A number of techniques have been used to localize the protein or mRNA of the different NOS isoforms within different tubular and/or vascular segments of the kidney. Immunohistochemical studies have demonstrated the presence of large amounts of nNOS protein in the macula densa *(13,14)*. *In situ* hybridization and RT-PCR of microdissected renal vessels and tubules have shown nNOS mRNA in the macula densa, inner and outer medullary collecting duct, glomerulus, arcuate artery, and in renal nerves in perivascular connective tissue *(13,15–18)*. Further RT-PCR studies have detected eNOS mRNA in the glomeruli, arcuate arteries, interlobular arteries, and afferent arteriole *(19,20)*, and eNOS protein has been identified in the endothelium of pre- and post-glomerular vessels by immunohistochemical techniques *(13)*. The mRNA encoding iNOS has been found in arcuate and interlobular arteries, glomeruli, proximal tubules, thick ascending limbs, and collecting ducts by *in situ* hybridization and RT-PCR of microdissected segments

(18,19,21,22). Although these types of studies localized different NOS isoforms within the renal vascular and tubular structures, experiments of this type do not permit the quantification of NOS enzymatic activity or NO levels in the individual structures.

2.2. NO Concentration and NOS Enzymatic Activity in the Renal Cortex and Medulla

Work in our laboratory has focused on the role of NO in the regulation of renal sodium excretion and in the long-term control of arterial blood pressure. We utilized a series of techniques to quantify NOS protein and enzymatic activity in kidney tissue and NO concentration in the renal interstitial space. By using these quantitative analyses, a unique feature of the distribution of intrarenal NO and NOS activity along cortical–medullary axis has been revealed. Early experimental results indicated that the renal medulla of dogs *(23)* and rats *(24,25)* had a greater capacity to produce NO than the renal cortex. As shown in Fig. 1, measurements of total NOS enzymatic activity in tissue homogenates of the renal cortex, outer medulla, and inner medulla have demonstrated that NOS enzymatic activity is as much as 25 times greater in the inner medulla than in the renal cortex *(18)*. This observation has been confirmed at the level of NOS protein. By immunoblotting, relatively large amounts of immunoreactive eNOS, nNOS, and iNOS proteins are detected in whole tissue homogenates of the renal inner medulla whereas none of the NOS isoforms were detectable using this technique in renal cortical homogenates *(26)*. On a whole tissue basis, the renal medulla is enriched in NO synthetic capacity.

To examine the segmental distribution of NOS enzymatic activity in the kidney, an analysis of NOS activity in isolated renal tubular and vascular segments of the rat kidney was performed *(18,19)*. As illustrated in Fig. 2, the inner medullary collecting duct was found to have the greatest NOS activity in the segments examined, the vasa recta and glomeruli possessed moderate NOS activity, which was significantly lower than in IMCD, but significantly higher than in the other renal structures. The other renal structures studied, including proximal tubules, thick ascending limb, and cortical collecting duct, exhibited minimal NOS enzymatic activity. The tubular and vascular structures of the renal medulla thus possess a greater potential to produce NO than other portions of the kidney *(18,19)*. These types of data, however, still do not permit the quantification of NO in vivo.

To assess the potential importance of the increased NOS protein and enzymatic activity in the renal medulla on NO production, further studies were performed to measure the concentration of NO in different kidney regions in anesthetized rats using an in vivo microdialysis system perfused with oxygenated hemoglobin (OxyHb) to trap NO. Results of these experiments have demonstrated that NO concentration is markedly elevated in the renal medulla compared to the renal cortex of anesthetized rats (Fig. 1; *[27,28]*). These results indicate that NOS in the renal medulla is a major source of intrarenal tissue NO and raise the possibility that the NO gradient between the renal medulla and cortex and the bulk flow in ascending tubules and vasa recta may lead to the movement of NO from the renal medulla to the cortex. This view is supported by the observations that blockade of the NOS activity selectively in the renal medulla by medullary interstitial infusion of L-NAME significantly decreases NO concentrations in both the renal cortex and medulla, changes that could not be explained by recirculating L-NAME *(28)*.

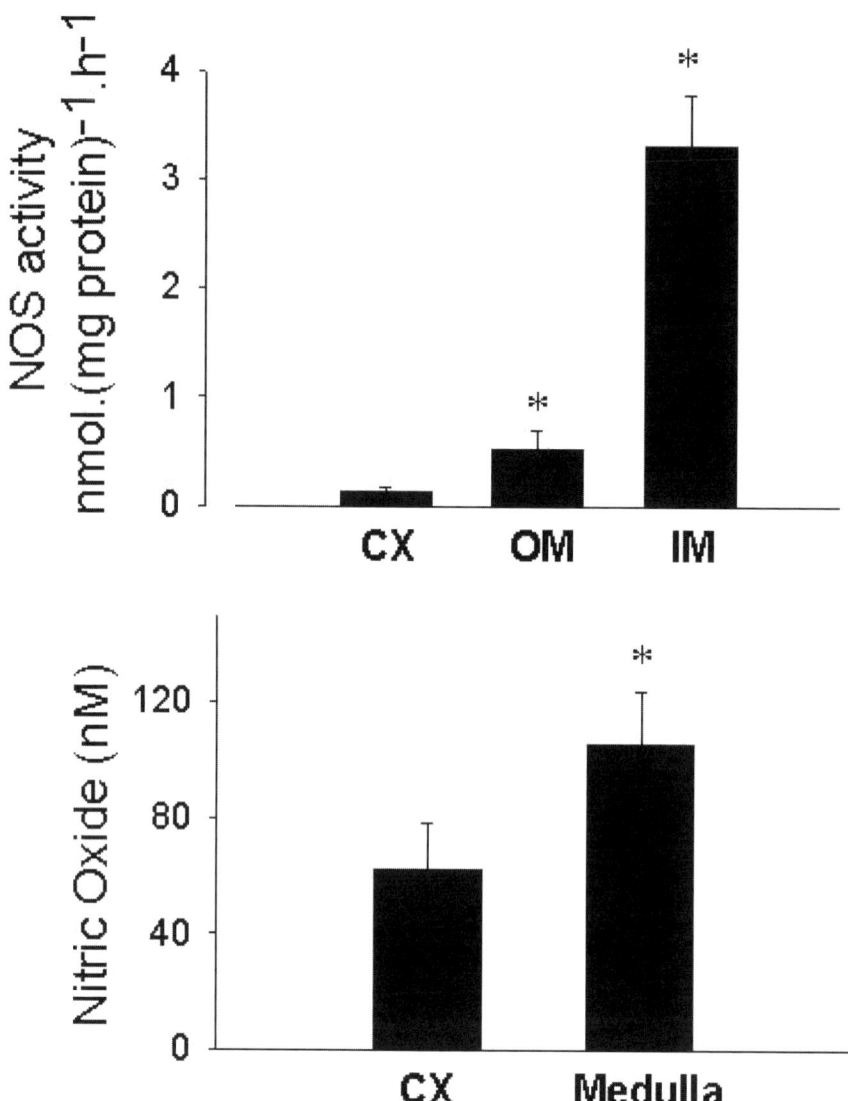

Fig. 1. *Top:* Nitric oxide synthase enzymatic activity measured in protein homogenates of renal cortex (CX), outer medulla (OM), and inner medulla (IM). Asterisk (*) indicates significantly different ($p < 0.05$) from CX. Data regraphed from the original manuscript *(18)*. *Bottom:* Nitric oxide concentration in the renal cortical and medullary interstitial space of Sprague–Dawley rats. Data regraphed from the original manuscript *(27)*.

2.3. Autocrine and Paracrine Actions of NO in the Kidney

Recently, a number of studies have been performed to assess the autocrine/paracrine nature of NO in the kidney by utilizing fluorescent microscopy techniques in thin microtissue strips of renal outer medullary tissue *(29–31)*. Studies were performed to examine the role of AngII to increase NO in the vasa recta, the blood vessels of the renal medulla. Previous studies demonstrated that the vasoconstrictor actions of AngII in the renal medullary circulation are blunted by an increase in NO release *(28)*. The studies

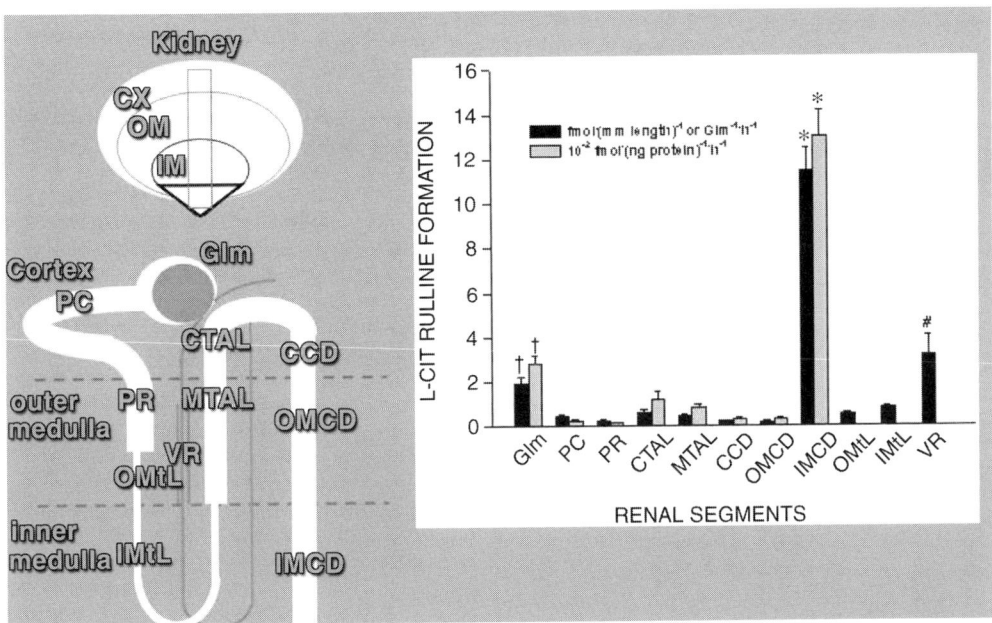

Fig. 2. Localization of NOS enzymatic activity in microdissected renal tubular and vascular segments obtained from the renal cortex (CX), outer medulla (OM) or inner medulla (IM) of the Sprague–Dawley rat. The filled bars represent total NOS activity normalized to segment length; the shaded bars represent NOS activity normalized to protein content. The result for each segment was obtained from 6 to 8 separate assays from 3 to 4 rats. Segments examined include glomeruli (Glm); pars convoluta (PC); pars recta (PR); cortical (CTAL) and medullary thick ascending limb (MTAL); cortical (CCD), outer medullary (OMCD), and inner medullary collecting duct (IMCD); the outer medullary (OMtL) and inner medullary thin loop of Henle (IMtL); and the vasa recta (VR). Asterisk (*) indicates significant difference ($p < 0.05$) compared to all other segments; † indicates significant difference ($p < 0.05$) compared to all segments except VR; # indicates significant difference ($p < 0.05$) compared to all segments except Glm. Data replotted from the original manuscript (18).

in the microtissue strips demonstrated that AngII increases intracellular NO ($[NO]_i$) in pericytes of the vasa recta only when these blood vessels are surrounded by renal tubular segments, mostly medullary thick ascending limbs of the loop of Henle (mTAL). In the absence of the adjacent mTAL, neither the vascular endothelium nor the pericytes of the vasa recta can directly increase NO production in response to AngII. Despite their inability to increase NO following AngII stimulation, AngII does increase intracellular calcium concentration in the pericytes of the descending vasa recta as part of its constrictor action on these vessels. This experimental evidence, therefore, indicates that the constrictor response to AngII in vasa recta is buffered by NO, which diffuses from the tubular elements surrounding the vasa recta within the outer medulla. These studies provide direct evidence, at the level of individual renal tubules and blood vessels, that NO can serve a paracrine function; an event that has been termed "tubulo-vascular cross talk." In a broader sense, these studies indicate that NO can diffuse from cell type to cell type and could affect a number of different functions in the kidney. These complex interactions remain to be fully explored and understood regarding the role of NO in the integrated function of the kidney.

3. ROLE OF NO IN THE REGULATION
OF RENAL SODIUM EXCRETION

The role of NO in the control of renal sodium excretion has been extensively studied. It is generally agreed that NO is important in the control of renal sodium excretion under physiological condition and is also critical in the chronic adaptation to a high-salt intake *(2,5)*. Given a wide range of its effects on renal hemodynamic and tubular function, NO likely regulates sodium excretion through a number of different mechanisms.

3.1. Actions of NO on Glomerular Filtration Rate

A constancy of glomerular filtration rate (GFR) is important to prevent extreme changes in renal excretion. Increases in GFR would result in a significant increase in urine flow and solute excretion if tubular reabsorption remains constant, and reductions in GFR would lead to a decrease in excretion rate. Under normal physiological conditions, GFR autoregulation and glomerulotubular balance mechanisms prevent large changes in renal excretion of water and solute in the face of changes in renal perfusion pressure or renal vasoconstrictors. The maintenance of GFR plays an important role in the control of renal sodium and water excretion.

There is strong evidence to support the idea that NO favors an increase in GFR and hence facilitates sodium and water excretion *(1,9)*. First, NO dilates renal afferent arterioles and increases glomerular perfusion and filtration. Numerous studies have been performed to define the role of NO in the control of glomerular perfusion and filtration. Micropuncture studies revealed that NOS inhibition increased renal vascular resistance and decreased renal blood flow and GFR *(32,33)*. Studies in the isolated perfused rat juxtamedullary microvascular preparation have demonstrated that NO primarily alters afferent vascular tone and modulates the autoregulatory response of the preglomerular vasculature to an elevation of perfusion pressure *(34)*. Studies using in vitro isolated microperfused rabbit arterioles also indicated that locally generated NO controls both afferent and efferent arteriolar resistance *(35)*. Based on these studies, it appears that endogenous NO in the kidney increases GFR.

NO also has been shown to modulate the tubuloglomerular feedback (TGF) response and in this manner also participates in the control of GFR. Studies have demonstrated that nNOS is abundant at the juxtaglomerular apparatus and that NOS in macula densa cells is activated by tubular solute reabsorption to release NO. Afferent arteriolar tone is thus reduced by NO that reduces the strength of the TGF response *(14,36,37)*. The attenuation of TGF by NO would promote glomerular filtration and increase water and sodium delivery into the tubules.

There is also evidence that NO can influence the glomerular capillary ultrafiltration coeffecient (K_f). Blockade of NOS leads to a reduction of K_f as well as an increase in renal vascular resistance *(32,33)*. It has been reported that glomerular mesangial cells express NOS, primarily iNOS. Furthermore, NO relaxes glomerular mesangial cells studied in vitro *(38)*, and blockade of endogenous NO production inhibits AngII-induced mesangial cell contraction *(39)*. In conclusion, these studies indicated that endogenously produced NO moderates mesangial cell contraction, thereby increasing K_f and GFR and the delivery of sodium into the tubules.

3.2. Direct Effects of NO on Tubular Reabsorption

The pressure natriuresis–diuresis response is depressed in anesthetized dogs following administration of the NOS inhibitor, L-NAME *(40)*. This effect was observed independent of changes in whole-kidney hemodynamics, suggesting that an alteration in medullary blood flow or direct tubular effects may be an important mechanism of NO action on sodium and water excretion *(40)*. Studies in the isolated perfused rat kidney have demonstrated that NOS inhibition produced a reduction in fractional sodium reabsorption, probably owing to specific tubular effects *(41)*. Recent studies using isolated perfused tubule preparations or cultured tubular cells support these functional data. It has been demonstrated that endogenous NO inhibits sodium reabsorption in proximal tubules, TAL and collecting ducts *(4,42–48)*. The effects of NO on sodium reabsorption are associated with its direct inhibitory action on Na^+/H^+ exchange, Na^+/K^+-ATPase and/or amiloride-sensitive Na^+ channels in these tubular segments *(4)*. Moreover, in mTAL cells transfected with iNOS, the expression of NOS inhibits Na^+/K^+-ATPase activity *(49)*. Based on these results, it appears that the direct inhibitory effects of NO on different tubules are important in the control of sodium excretion.

There is a recent evidence that oxidative stress within the kidney that is associated with hypertension and diabetes can alter the bioavailability and actions of NO. The physiological consequences of elevating superoxide $(O_2^{\bullet-})$ levels in the renal outer medulla have been shown to be mediated in part through the reduction of NO *(50)*. An interaction between NO and $O_2^{\bullet-}$ was found to regulate NaCl transport in the thick ascending loop of Henle. *(43,51)*. Because excess sodium (or glucose) transport in the mTAL increases $O_2^{\bullet-}$ production *(52)*, it appears that the associated reductions in the bioavailability of NO would increase the activity of the Na^+/H^+ exchanger and produce greater $O_2^{\bullet-}$. These events could also reduce the overall medullary bioavailability of NO and thereby reduce medullary blood flow. We have proposed this positive feedback cycle as a contributing factor to the chronic progressive injury that is seen in hypertension and diabetes *(52)*.

3.3. Influence of NO on Renal Medullary Hemodynamics

A large body of work has been performed to test the hypothesis that the renal medulla is an important site of the action of NO in the control of sodium and water homeostasis *(6,24,26,28,29,53,54)*. As discussed earlier, NOS protein expression, NOS enzymatic activity, and interstitial NO concentration are much greater in the renal medulla than in the renal cortex *(18,27,29)*. Acute infusion directly into the renal medullary interstitial space of the NOS inhibitor N^G-nitro-L-arginine methyl ester (L-NAME) selectively reduced renal medullary blood flow, renal interstitial hydrostatic pressure and sodium excretion, suggesting a tonic regulatory action of NO on medullary blood flow and sodium excretion *(53)*. Furthermore, selective stimulation of NO in the renal medullary interstitial space of anesthetized rats resulted in an increase in medullary blood flow with an accompanying natriuresis and diuresis *(55)*. In anesthetized dogs, Salom et al. demonstrated that nonpressor doses of the NOS inhibitor, L-NAME depresses the pressure–natriuretic response independent of changes in whole-kidney hemodynamics, suggesting that medullary vascular reaction or tubular effects may be an important mechanism of the NO action on sodium and water excretion *(56)*. These data strongly indicate that NO in the renal medulla also plays an important role in the long-term regulation of sodium and water excretion.

4. ROLE OF NO IN THE LONG-TERM CONTROL
OF ARTERIAL PRESSURE

It is widely accepted that NO is an important endogenous antihypertensive factor that plays a significant role in the control of fluid and electrolyte homeostasis and the regulation of arterial blood pressure. A dysfunction of NOS in many tissues has been observed in genetically hypertensive rats such as the Dahl salt-sensitive (Dahl SS) rat *(57,58)*. In addition, genetic deletion of eNOS has been proven to lead to hypertension in mice *(59,60)*. Despite substantial data demonstrating the importance of NO in the development of hypertension; however, the mechanisms of the NO-mediated antihypertensive effects remain a subject of debate. Because NO appears critical in the regulation of sodium excretion, many studies have explored the renal mechanism of hypertension induced by NO inhibition and/or a deficiency in NO under various physiological and pathophysiological conditions.

4.1. Hypertension Induced by Chronic Inhibition of NO Synthesis

Long-term administration of NOS inhibitors by oral or intravenous administration has been demonstrated to result in sustained hypertension in different species such as mice, rats, rabbits, and dogs *(2,5,6,15)*. Common characteristics of this hypertension model are systemic hypertension, renal vasoconstriction, a reduction in glomerular K_f, and sodium retention *(32,33,38,61)*. In addition to the renal effects, which lead to retention of sodium and water, the increase in arterial blood pressure is also associated with systemic vasoconstriction owing to the blockade of the tonic vasodilating effect of NO. In addition, there is evidence that increases in renin release and activation of the renin–angiotensin II system also contribute to the development of hypertension during chronic systemic inhibition of the NOS activity *(62)*. Although chronic oral or intravenous administration of NOS inhibitors produce hypertension, it is unclear whether the observed hypertension was primarily a result of generalized systemic vasoconstriction, an effect of NO reduction in brain, or a primary consequence of reduced renal excretory function.

4.2. Importance of Medullary NO Production in the Long-Term Control
of Medullary Blood Flow and Arterial Pressure

The first evidence that basal NO production in the renal medulla plays an important role in determining the long-term level of arterial blood pressure arose from observations made in our laboratory that indicated the chronic intravenous administration of the NOS inhibitor L-NAME led to a selective decrease in blood flow in the renal medulla, the retention of sodium, and the development of hypertension in conscious rats *(63)*. It was unclear, however, whether the medullary NO production *per se* played an important role in the long-term regulation of renal medullary blood flow, sodium excretion, and arterial pressure. Further studies were then performed in which L-NAME was infused chronically into the renal medullary interstitium of Sprague–Dawley rats for 5 d *(64)*. As shown in Fig. 3, the renal medullary interstitial infusion of L-NAME resulted in a sustained reduction of renal medullary blood flow (~30%) with no measurable changes of cortical flow. The selective reduction of medullary perfusion was associated with the retention of sodium, and the development of hypertension *(64)*. These experiments demonstrated that selective blockade of NO production in the renal medulla could reduce medullary blood flow and produce hypertension in normal animals. It had been

Chronic Renal Interstitial
L-NAME Infusion

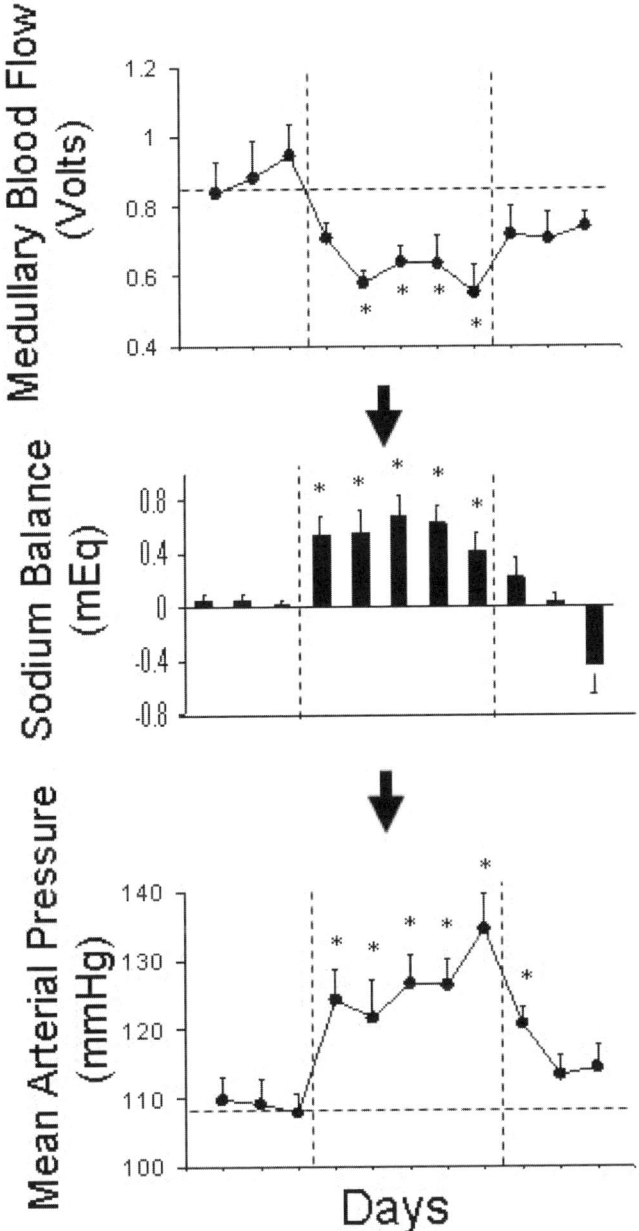

Fig. 3. Chronic influence of renal medullary interstitial infusion of the nitric oxide synthase inhibitor N^G-nitro-L-arginine methyl ester (L-NAME, 8.6 mg/kg/d) on renal medullary blood flow (top), daily sodium balance (middle), and mean arterial blood pressure (bottom) in conscious Sprague–Dawley rats. Vertical hashed marks indicate the L-NAME infusion period. Asterisk (*) indicates significance from control ($p < 0.05$). Data replotted from the original manuscript (64).

previously assumed that hypertension resulting from systemically administered L-NAME was probably related to a reduction of total renal blood flow and an overall increase in systemic vascular resistance related to vascular and central nervous system NOS inhibition. Although these effects are undoubtedly important, the present studies with both systemic and renal medullary delivery of L-NAME demonstrated that the production of NO specifically within the medulla is of primary importance in the long-term regulation of medullary perfusion and sodium homeostasis, and that a reduction of NOS activity in the renal medulla alone could produce chronic hypertension.

The potential mechanisms by which NOS inhibition or deficiency can produce hypertension are summarized in Fig. 4. Reduction of the NO levels within the whole kidney may decrease GFR through the enhancement of renal vascular constriction, enhancement of the TGF response and/or reduction of the glomerular ultrafiltration coefficient, thereby decreasing filtered load. In addition, a reduction of renal NO levels leads to a decrease in renal medullary blood flow and increased activity of tubular Na^+/H^+ exchange, Na^+/K^+-ATPase and amiloride-sensitive Na^+ channels. Collectively, these effects would lead to an increase in tubular sodium reabsorption that would blunt pressure natriuresis and diuresis and result in sodium retention and hypertension.

4.3. Interaction Between Vasoconstrictors and NO

Numerous studies have been performed to test the interaction of NO and different vasoconstrictors in animal experiments (65–68). Zou and Cowley demonstrated that NO concentration in the renal cortex and medulla of rats increased in response to intravenous infusion of subpressor doses of vasoconstrictors such as AngII (28). Studies by Deng et al. demonstrated that intravenous infusion of AngII increased renal excretion of the stable NO metabolites, nitrite, and nitrate (66). Siragy and Carey further defined the role of the subtypes of AngII receptors in mediating stimulation of AngII to NO production in the renal cortex and suggested that the AT_2 subtype mediates AngII-stimulated NO production (69).

The functional significance of increased renal NO production induced by AngII has been further addressed in anesthetized rat experiments. Infusion of a subpressor dose of AngII (5 ng/kg/min) did not alter renal medullary blood flow under baseline conditions. This dose of AngII reduced medullary blood flow by 23% without altering renal cortical blood flow, however, when a subpressor dose of L-NAME was infused into the renal medullary interstitial space. These experiments indicated that NO is increased in the renal medulla in response to small elevations of circulating AngII in order to buffer the vasoconstrictor effects of this peptide (28). Further experiments were performed in chronically instrumented rats; intravenous infusion of AngII at a subpressor dose (3 ng/ng/min) did not affect arterial blood pressure. A threshold dose of L-NAME was determined (75 µg/kg/h), which did not produce significant acute or chronic changes in medullary blood flow and mean arterial blood pressure when administered alone. In rats pretreated with this dose of L-NAME, the intravenous infusion of AngII resulted in a 30% reduction of medullary blood flow and a 30 mmHg rise of mean arterial blood pressure (70). These results indicate that even moderate reductions of renal medullary NOS activity sensitize the medullary circulation to the vasoconstrictor actions of AngII, whereby even small physiological plasma elevation of this peptide can result in chronic reduction of medullary blood flow and lead to hypertension (70).

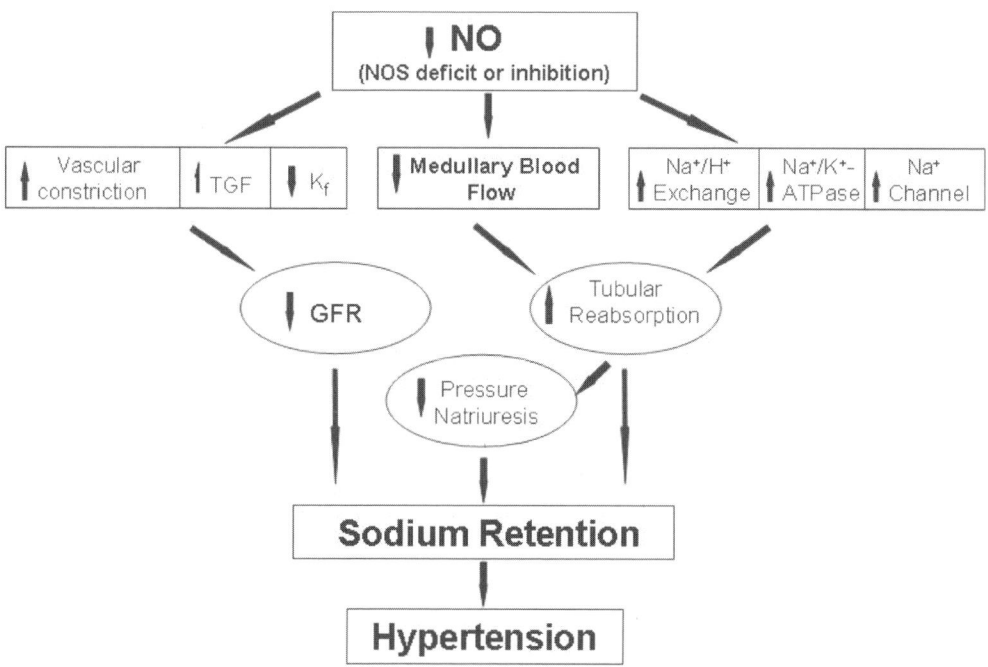

Fig. 4. Schematic diagram summarizing proposed mechanisms promoting hypertension during conditions in which NO is reduced in the kidney.

Similar results were observed during the administration of norepinephrine (NE). Experiments have indicated that NE can induce NO release through the α2-receptors *(71,72)*. Studies examined the in vivo effects of NE on the renal medullary circulation. Following an intravenous infusion of a subpressor dose of norepinephrine (0.1 μg/kg/min), medullary [NO] increased 43% *(72)*. This response was inhibited with a selective α2-adrenergic inhibitor *(72)*. As was observed in the AngII studies, when medullary NOS activity was blunted by medullary infusion with a low dose of L-NAME, the NE-induced rise of tissue NO was abolished and a reduction of both MBF and tissue PO_2 of nearly 30% was observed *(72)*. Experiments were then performed in conscious rats and demonstrated that chronic intravenous infusion of NE (0.1 μg/kg/min) did not alter mean arterial pressure greater than 5 mmHg when infused for 5–7 d to normal Sprague–Dawley rats. The infusion of NE in addition to the non-hypertensive dose of L-NAME, however, led to a sustained elevation of arterial blood pressure *(73)*. These results, along with similar experiments performed during the infusion of AVP *(74)* demonstrated the importance of the NO to counter the prohypertensive actions of different vasoconstrictor agents.

4.4. Salt-Sensitive Hypertension and Inhibition of NOS

There is a considerable evidence indicating that NO contributes to an adaptive increase in sodium excretion in response to high-salt intake. An impaired L-arginine–NO system would be predicted to increase the sensitivity of arterial blood pressure not only to vasoconstrictor agents but also to elevated sodium intake. It has been reported that NO production increases in rats in response to chronic salt loading *(57,75)*. An increase in NO production may be because of the upregulation of mRNA or protein and/or activation of enzyme activity. Maintenance of Sprague–Dawley rats on a high-salt diet for 3 wk led to a significant increase in eNOS, nNOS, and iNOS immunoreactive proteins in the renal inner medulla, but not in the renal cortex and aorta. These observations suggest that increased levels of NOS in the renal medulla may reflect a chronic adaptation to increased salt intake *(26)*. This, however, has not been a consistent finding among laboratories. Ni and Vaziri observed a decrease in medullary protein expression of nNOS and iNOS following 3 wk of an 8% sodium diet *(76)*, whereas other groups have observed no change in mRNA expression of any of the NOS isoforms in the renal medulla *(16,45)*.

To define the functional significance of salt-induced adaptive increases in renal NO, Tolins and Shultz determined the hypertensive effect of a high-salt diet in normotensive rats in which NOS activity was blunted. They demonstrated that administration of L-NAME in a dose that did not alter arterial blood pressure in normotensive Sprague–Dawley rats on low salt diet, significantly elevated arterial blood pressure in rats receiving a high-salt diet *(77)*. Likewise, low doses of L-NAME have also been found to increase the sensitivity of arterial blood pressure to high-salt intake in rats *(26)* and dogs *(2,78)*. Taken together, these results indicate that the L-arginine–NO system participates in the physiologic adaptation to increased dietary salt intake although the precise role of NOS in the renal medulla in this process remains to be clarified. Nevertheless, these adaptive changes in endogenous NO production appear to play a critical role in sodium and blood pressure homeostasis.

4.5. Hypertension Induced by NOS Deficit in the Dahl SS Rat

The Dahl salt-sensitive (Dahl SS) rat has a reduced capacity to generate NO in the renal medulla. The mRNA and immunoreactive protein for each of the NOS isoforms is reduced in the outer medulla of Dahl SS rats compared to normotensive Brown Norway (BN) control rats (Fig. 5; *[29,79,80]*). Consistent with these observations, total NOS enzyme activity was found to be nearly one-third less in the outer medulla of SS rats than in normotensive salt-resistant BN rats *(79)*. Of greatest importance, though, is the observation that the baseline concentration of NO in the renal medullary interstitial space is significantly lower in the Dahl SS compared to BN rats *(79)*. Moreover, it was observed that the increase in NO in the renal medulla in response to AngII infusion was blunted in the Dahl SS rat, indicating a diminished capacity to release NO following in vivo stimulation *(79)*. These observations indicate that the vasculature and tubules of the kidney of the Dahl SS rat may be overly sensitive to small elevations of circulating vaso-constrictor agents (e.g., AngII, vasopressin, and norepinephrine) because of the lack of an NO counter–regulatory system.

A series of studies were performed to determine whether Dahl SS rats respond similarly to normal rats in which NOS activity in the renal medulla was blunted by selective delivery of L-NAME to the medullary interstitium. Chronic intravenous infusion of AngII (3.0 ng/kg/min) did not induce an increase of arterial blood pressure in normotensive BN rats maintained on a low NaCl (0.4%) diet *(79)*. In marked contrast, intravenous infusion of the identical dose of AngII led to a sustained hypertension in Dahl SS rats, which were also maintained on the low salt diet. Interestingly, a low dose of AngII significantly reduced MBF in SS rats, but not in BN rats *(79)*. These studies demonstrate

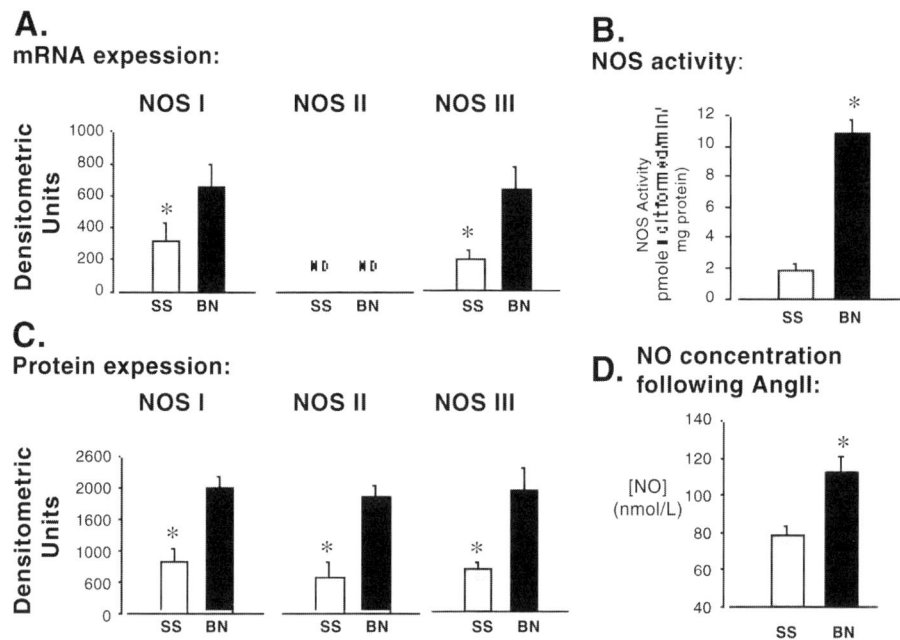

Fig. 5. Summary of studies demonstrating the reduced capacity of the Dahl SS rat to generate NO within the outer medulla when compared to the Brown Norway (BN) rats. Panel **A** shows the significantly reduced mRNA expression (determined by Northern blot) of the two detectable NOS isoforms in SS rats compared to the BN rats *(80)*. NOS activity in the outer medulla of SS rats is also significantly decreased as depicted in Panel **B** *(79)*. Panel **C** summarizes the results of the Western blot analysis of protein expression of the three NOS isoforms in which all three isoforms were significantly lower in the SS rat compared to BN rat *(79)*. Panel **D** illustrates the changes in NO in the renal medulla following an intravenous infusion of angiotensin II (AngII) in the BN and the SS rat. Asterisk (*) designates a significant difference between the SS and BN in panels A–C and in Panel D, indicates a significant difference from the pre-Ang II control.

that the ability of the BN rats to buffer AngII induced reductions of medullary blood flow is dependent on the release of medullary interstitial NO because of Dahl SS rats that failed to increase medullary NO in response to AngII exhibited a significant reduction of blood flow *(79)*. Similar results to those observed with infusion of AngII were observed when AVP was infused continuously to Dahl SS rats *(80)*. Together, these results indicate that a deficit in the ability of the outer medullary tissue of Dahl SS rats to produce NO in response to AngII or AVP results in a chronic elevation of arterial pressure in the Dahl SS rat with elevations of pressor agents that normally do not produce hypertension.

4.6. NO Regulation and L-Arginine Uptake in Renal Medulla

The studies outlined above indicate that a deficit in NO synthetic ability in the renal medulla may be important in the development of hypertension. The deficit in NO production could be related to NOS enzyme as described above *(79)*, or this effect could be mediated by other alterations in the NO synthetic pathway. Related to this possibility, it has been demonstrated that supplementation of L-arginine (L-Arg), the substrate for NOS, is capable of preventing salt-induced hypertension in Dahl SS rats when administered by oral or intravenous routes *(81–84)*. Experiments in anesthetized rats demonstrated that the pressure–natriuretic response and the transmission of perfusion pressure into the renal interstitium were normalized by L-Arg treatment *(83,84)*. These observations led us to hypothesize that the major antihypertensive actions of L-Arg in Dahl SS rats could be mediated through actions of this NO precursor in the renal medulla. A dose of L-Arg (300 µg/kg/min) was then infused into the renal medullary interstitial space of Dahl SS to determine the effects of selective administration of L-Arg administration on salt-induced hypertension *(54,85)*. Remarkably, as dietary salt content was increased from 0.4 to 4.0% NaCl, mean arterial pressure remained nearly unchanged for a week in Dahl SS rats receiving the medullary infusion of L-Arg (Fig. 6). In contrast, in Dahl SS rats receiving the saline vehicle infusion, mean arterial pressure increased over 40 mmHg during the same time period. The same dose of L-Arg that prevented salt-induced hypertension in SS rats when administered into the renal medullary interstitial space failed to blunt the development of hypertension when infused intravenously. Moreover, it was found that SS rats receiving the high-salt diet exhibited a significant reduction of MBF, which was prevented by chronic medullary interstitial delivery of L-Arg *(54)*. These data, as summarized in Fig. 6, indicated that the prevention of salt-sensitivity in SS rats was due specifically to the action of L-Arg on the renal medullary function and that SS rats may have a deficit of medullary substrate availability that could account in part for the observed reduction in NO production in this region of the kidney. Taken together, these studies in the Dahl SS rat indicate that an impairment of NO synthetic capacity in the renal medulla is important in the development of hypertension in response to both small elevations of circulating vasoconstrictor compounds, such as AngII, and in response to a high-salt diet.

5. SUMMARY AND CONCLUSIONS

The data summarized in this chapter demonstrate that NOS is widely expressed along the renal vasculature and nephron, with the three major NOS isoforms present in a number of different tubular and vascular segments. Current evidence indicates that NO serves as a paracrine and autocrine agent within the kidney. Under physiological conditions, NO is important in the regulation of renal vascular resistance, the glomerular ultrafiltration coefficient and the sensitivity of the tubuloglomerular feedback response. The overall effects of NO favor an increase GFR. In addition, NO directly affects renal tubular sodium handling that leads to decreased tubular sodium reabsorption. Under physiological condition, NO serves as an intrarenal natriuretic factor and plays an important role in the long-term control of arterial blood pressure.

Biochemical studies demonstrated that NOS mRNA, immunoreactive protein, and enzymatic activity are enriched in the renal medulla relative to the renal cortex. This enrichment of NOS synthetic activity in this portion of the kidney is associated with elevated interstitial levels of NO. Moreover, studies in anesthetized rats demonstrated that selective stimulation or inhibition of NO in the renal medullary interstitial space is associated with a preferential alteration in blood flow in the medulla and corresponding changes in sodium excretion and urine flow rate. Further experiments demonstrated

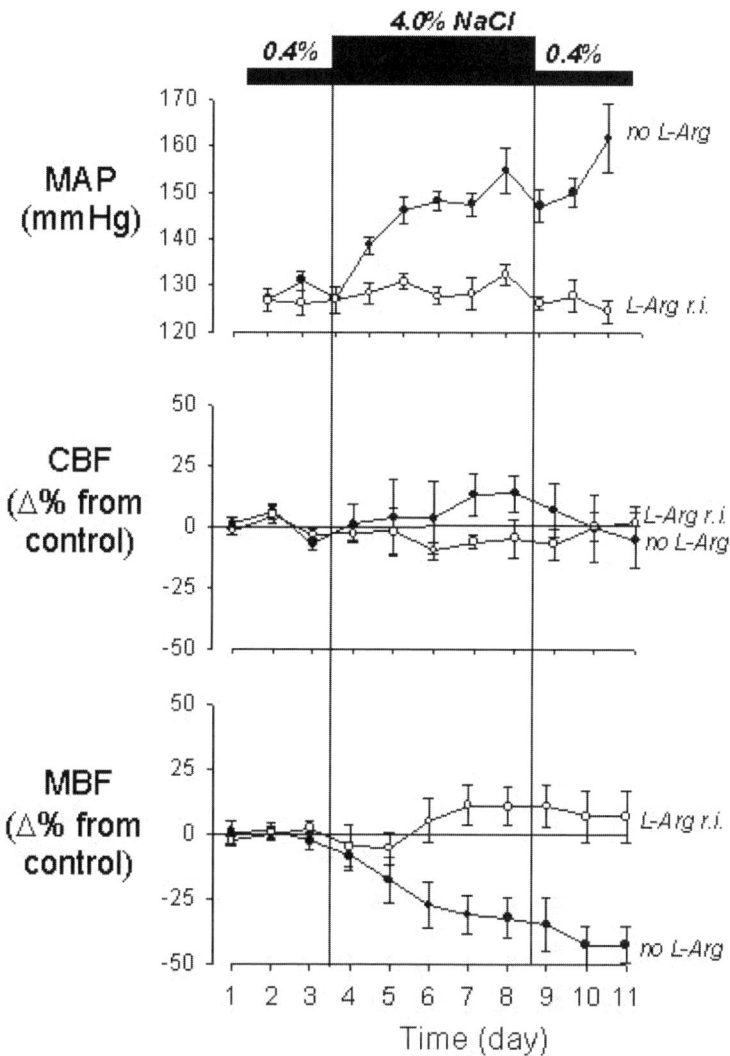

Fig. 6. Effects of renal medullary interstitial infusion of L-Arginine (L-Arg; 300 μg/kg/min) in Dahl SS rats on high-salt diet-induced changes in mean arterial pressure (MAP), cortical blood flow (CBF), and medullary blood flow (MBF). SS rats infused with L-Arg r.i. are indicated by the open circle. SS rats not infused with L-Arg but undergoing the same change in diet are indicated by the closed circle. These data are regraphed from the original manuscript *(54)*.

that chronic inhibition of NO in the renal medulla of conscious rats led to a sustained reduction in medullary blood flow, the retention of sodium, and the development of hypertension. An additional set of experiments in conscious rats demonstrated that the use of nonpressor doses of NOS inhibitors could attenuate the ability of the renal medulla to increase NO in response to vasoconstrictor agents that was associated with a sustained elevation in arterial blood pressure. Finally, it was demonstrated that a genetic model of hypertension, the Dahl SS rat, has a reduction in NO synthetic capacity on the renal medulla. Functional studies demonstrated that this deficit leads to a hypertensive response of these rats to small doses of exogenous vasoconstrictors. Moreover, supplementation of NOS substrate to increase the NO synthetic capacity of the medulla of the Dahl SS rat prevents the hypertension that occurs when these animals are placed on a high-salt diet. The production of NO in the kidney, particularly in the renal medulla, is therefore of extreme importance in the regulation of extracellular fluid homeostasis and arterial blood pressure regulation.

ACKNOWLEDGMENTS

The work from our laboratories most frequently cited in this report was supported by National Heart, Lung and Blood Institute Grant HL-29587.

REFERENCES

1. Gross, S. S. and Wolin, M. S. (1995) Nitric oxide: pathophysiological mechanism. *Ann. Rev. Physiol.* **57**, 737–769.
2. Kone, B. C. and Baylis, C. (1997) Biosynthesis and homeostatic roles of nitric oxide in the normal kidney. *Am. J. Physiol.* **272**, F561–F578.
3. Stamler, J. S., Singel, D. J., and Loscalzo, J. (1992) Biochemistry of nitric oxide and its redox-activated forms. *Science* **258**, 1898–1902.
4. Ortiz, P. A. and Garvin, J. L. (2002) Role of nitric oxide in the regulation of nephron transport. *Am. J. Physiol.* **282**, F777–F784.
5. Schnackenberg, C., Patel, A. R., Kirchner, K. A., and Granger, J. P. (1997) Nitric oxide, the kidney and hypertension. *Clin. Exp. Pharmacol. Physiol.* **24**, 600–606.
6. Cowley, A. W. Jr. (1997) Role of the renal medulla in volume and arterial pressure regulation. *Am. J. Physiol.* **273**, R1–R15.
7. Bredt, D. S. and Snyder, S. H. (1994) Nitric oxide: a physiologic messenger molecule. *Ann. Rev. Biochem.* **63**, 175–195.
8. Fukuto, J. M., Wallace, G. C., Hszieh, R., and Chaudhuri, G. (1992) Chemical oxidation of N-hydroxyguanidine compounds. Release of nitric oxide, nitroxyl and possible relationship to the mechanism of biological nitric oxide generation. *Biochem. Pharmacol.* **43**, 607–613.
9. Mayer, B., John, M., Heinzel, B., et al. (1991) Brain nitric oxide synthesis is a biopterin- and flavin-containing multi-functional oxido-reductase. *FEBS Lett.* **288**, 187–191.
10. Forstermann, U. and Kleinert, H. (1995) Nitric oxide synthase: expression and expressional control of the three isoforms. *Naunyn Schmiedbergs Arch. Pharmacol.* **352**, 351–364.
11. Harrison, D. G., Sayegh, H., Ohara,Y., Inoue, N., and Venema, R. C. (1996) Regulation of expression of the endothelial cell nitric oxide synthase. *Clin. Exp. Pharmacol. Physiol.* **23**, 251–255.
12. Venema, R. C., Sayegh, H. S., Kent, J. D., and Harrison, D. G. (1996) Identification, characterization, and comparison of the calmodulin binding domains of the endothelial and inducible nitric oxide synthases. *J. Biol. Chem.* **271**, 6435–6440.
13. Bachman, S., Bosse, H. M., and Mundel, P. (1995) Topography of nitric oxide synthesis by localizing constitutive NO synthases in mammalian kidney. *Am. J. Physiol.* **268**, F885–F898.
14. Wilcox, C. S., Welch, W. J., Murad, F., et al. (1992) Nitric oxide synthase in macula densa regulates glomerular capillary pressure. *Proc. Natl Acad. Sci. USA* **89**, 11,993–11,997.
15. Bachmann, S. and Mundel, P. (1994) Nitric oxide in the kidney: synthesis, localization, and function. *Am. J. Kid. Dis.* **24**, 112–129.
16. Singh, I., Grams, M., Wang, W. H., et al. (1996) Coordinate regulation of renal expression of nitric oxide synthase, rennin, and angiotensinogen mRNA by dietary salt. *Am. J. Physiol.* **270**, F1027–F1037.
17. Terada, Y., Tomita, K., Nonoguchi, H., and Marumo, F. (1992) Polymerase chain reaction localization of constitutive nitric oxide synthase and soluble guanylate cyclase messenger RNAs in microdissected rat nephron segments. *J. Clin. Investig.* **90**, 659–665.
18. Wu, F., Park, F., Cowley, A. W. Jr., and Mattson, D. L. (1999) Nitric oxide synthase activity in microdissected segments of the Sprague Dawley rat kidney. *Am. J. Physiol.* **276**, F874–F881.

19. Mattson, D. L. and Wu, F. (2000) Nitric oxide synthase activity and isoforms in the rat renal vasculature. *Hypertension* **35**, 337–341.
20. Ujiie, K., Yuen, J., Hogarth, L., Danziger, R., and Starr, R. A. (1994) Localization and regulation of endothelial NO synthase mRNA expression in rat kidney. *Am. J. Physiol.* **267**, F296–F302.
21. Ahn, K. Y., Mohaupt, M. G., Madsen, K. M., and Kone, B. C. (1994) *In situ* hybridization localization of mRNA encoding inducuble nitric oxide synthase in rat kidney. *Am. J. Physiol.* **267**, F748–F757.
22. Mohaupt, M. G., Elzie, J. L., Ahn, K. Y., et al. (1994) Differential expression and induction of mRNAs encoding two inducible nitric oxide synthases in rat kidney. *Kidney Int.* **46**, 653–665.
23. Biondi, M. L. and Romero, J. C. (1990) Nitric oxide-mediated reactions stimulate cyclic GMP levels in the dog kidney. *J. Vasc. Med. Biol.* **2**, 294–298.
24. Mattson, D. L. (2003) Importance of the renal medullary circulation in the control of sodium excretion and blood pressure. *Am. J. Physiol.* **284**, R13–R27.
25. Moridani, B. A. and Kline, R. L. (1996) Effect of endogenous L-arginine on the measurement of nitric oxide synthase activity in the rat kidney. *Can. J. Physiol. Pharmacol.* **74**, 1210–1214.
26. Mattson, D. L. and Higgins, D. (1996) Influence of dietary sodium intake on renal medullary nitric oxide synthesis. *Hypertension* **27**, 688–692.
27. Zou, A.-P. and Cowley, A. W. Jr. (1997) Nitric oxide in renal cortex and medulla: an in vivo microdialysis study. *Hypertension* **29**, 194–198.
28. Zou, A. P., Wu, F., and Cowley, A. W. Jr. (1998) Protective effect of angiotensin II-induced increase in nitric oxide in the renal medullary circulation. *Hypertension* **31**, 271–276.
29. Cowley, A. W. Jr., Mori, T., Mattson, D. L., and Zou, A.-P. (2003) Role of renal NO production in the regulation of medullary blood flow. *Am. J. Physiol.* **284**, R1335–R1369.
30. Dickhout, J. G., Mori, T., and Cowley, A. W. Jr. (2002) Tubulovascular nitric oxide crosstalk: buffering of angiotensin II-induced vasoconstriction. *Circ. Res.* **91**, 487–493.
31. Mori, T., Dickhout, J. G., and Cowley, A. W. Jr. (2002) Vasopressin increases intracellular nitric oxide concentration via Ca^{2+} signaling in inner medullary collecting duct. *Hypertension* **39**, 465–469.
32. Deng, A. Y. and Baylis, C. (1993) Locally produced EDRF controls preglomerular resistance and ultrafiltration coefficient. *Am. J. Physiol.* **264**, F212–F215.
33. Zatz, R. and de Nucci, G. (1991) Effects of acute nitric oxide inhibition on rat glomerular microcirculation. *Am. J. Physiol.* **261**, F360–F362.
34. Imig, J. D. and Roman, R. J. (1992) Nitric oxide modulates vascular tone in preglomerular arterioles. *Hypertension* **19**, 770–774.
35. Ito, S., Airma, S., Ren, Y. L., Juncos, L. A., and Carretero, O. A. (1993) Endothelium-derived relaxing factor/nitric oxide modulates angiotensin II action in the isolated microperfused rabbit afferent arterioles but not efferent arteriole. *J. Clin. Investig.* **91**, 2012–2019.
36. Welch, W. J. and Wilcox, C. S. (1997) Macula densa arginine delivery and uptake in the rat regulate glomerular capillary pressure. Effect of salt intake. *J. Clin. Investig.* **100**, 2235–2242.
37. Welch, W. J. and Wilcox, C. S. (1997) Role of nitric oxide in tubuloglomerular feedback: effect of dietary salt. *Clin. Exp. Pharmacol. Physiol.* **24**, 582–586.
38. Raij, L. and Baylis, C. (1995) Glomerular action of nitric oxide. *Kidney Int.* **48**, 20–32.
39. Shultz, P. J., Schorer, A. E., and Raij, L. (1990) Effects of endothelium-derived relaxing factor and nitric oxide on rat mesangial cells. *Am. J. Physiol.* **258**, F162–F167.
40. Romero, J. C., Lahera, V., Salom, M. G., and Biondi, M. L. (1992) Role of the endothelium-dependent relaxing factor nitric oxide on renal function. *J. Am. Soc. Nephrol.* **2**, 1371–1387.
41. Radermacher, J., Klanke, B., Schurek, H. J., Stolte, H. F., and Frolich, J. C. (1992) Importance of EDRF/NO for glomerular and tubular function: Studies in the isolated perfused rat kidney. *Kidney Int.* **41**, 1549–1559.
42. Mckee, M., Scavone, C., Nathanson, J. A. (1994) Nitric oxide, cGMP, and hormone regulation of active sodium transport. *Proc. Natl Acad. Sci. USA* **91**, 12,056–12,060.
43. Ortiz, P. A. and Garvin, J. L. (2002) Interaction of O_2^- and NO in the thick ascending limb. *Hypertension* **39**, 591–596.
44. Plato, C. F., Stoos, B. A., Wang, D., and Garvin, J. L. (1999) Endogenous nitric oxide inhibits chloride transport in the thick ascending limb. *Am. J. Physiol.* **276**, F159–F163.
45. Roczniak, A., Zimpelmann, J., and Burns, K. D. (1998) Effect of dietary salt on neuronal nitric oxide synthase in the inner medullary collecting duct. *Am. J. Physiol.* **275**, F46–F54.

46. Stoos, B. A., Garcia, N. H., and Garvin, J. L. (1995) Nitric oxide inhibits sodium reabsorption in the isolated perfused cortical collecting duct. *J. Am. Soc. Nephrol.* **6,** 89–94.
47. Roczniak, A. and Burns, K. D. (1996) Nitric oxide stimulates guanylate cyclase and regulates sodium transport in rabbit proximal tubule. *Am. J. Physiol.* **270,** F106–F115.
48. Ortiz, P. A. and Garvin, J. L. (2000) NO inhibits NaCl absorption by rat thick ascending limb through activation of cGMP stimulated phosphodicsterase. *Hypertension* **37,** 467–471.
49. Kone, B. C. and Higham, S. (1999) Nitric oxide inhibits transcription of the Na^+-K^+-ATPase alpha1-subunit gene in an MTAL cell line. *Am. J. Physiol.* **276,** F614–F621.
50. Mori, T. and Cowley, A. W. Jr. (2003) Angiotensin II–NAD(P)H oxidase-stimulated superoxide modifies tubulovascular nitric oxide cross-talk in renal outer medulla. *Hypertension* **42,** 588–593.
51. Ortiz, P. A. and Garvin, J. L. (2002) Superoxide stimulates NaCl absorption by the thick ascending limb. *Am. J. Physiol.* **283,** F957–F962.
52. Mori, T. and Cowley, A. W. Jr. (2004) Renal oxidative stress in medullary thick ascending limbs produced by elevated NaCl and glucose. *Hypertension* **43,** 341–346.
53. Mattson, D. L., Roman, R. J., and Cowley, A. W. Jr. (1992) Role of nitric oxide in renal papillary blood flow and sodium excretion. *Hypertension* **19,** 766–769.
54. Miyata, N. and Cowley, A. W. Jr. (1999) Renal intramedullary infusion of L-arginine prevents reduction of medullary blood flow and hypertension in Dahl salt-sensitive rats. *Hypertension* **33,** 446–450.
55. Mattson, D. L. and Cowley, A. W. Jr. (1993) Kinin actions on renal papillary blood flow and sodium excretion. *Hypertension* **21,** 961–965.
56. Salom, M. G., Lahera, V., Miranda-Guardiola, F., and Romero, J. C. (1992) Blockade of pressure natriuresis induced by inhibition of renal synthesis of nitric oxide in dogs. *Am. J. Physiol.* **262,** F718–F722.
57. Hayakawa, H. and Raij, L. (1998) Nitric oxide synthase activity and renal injury in genetic hypertension. *Hypertension* **31,** 266–270.
58. Ikeda, Y., Saito, K., Kim, J. I., and Yokoyama, M. (1995) Nitric oxide synthase isoform activities in kidney of Dahl salt-sensitive rats. *Hypertension* **26,** 1030–1034.
59. Huang, P. L., Huang, Z., Mashimo, H., et al. (1995) Hypertension in mice lacking the gene for endothelial nitric oxide synthase. *Nature* **377,** 239–242.
60. Shesely, E. G., Maeda, N., Kim, H. S., et al. (1996) Elevated blood pressures in mice lacking endothelial nitric oxide synthase. *Proc. Natl Acad. Sci. USA* **93,** 13,176–13,181.
61. Baylis, C., Mitruka, B., and Deng, A. (1992) Chronic blockade of nitric oxide synthesis in the rat produces systemic hypertension and glomerular damage. *J. Clin. Investig.* **90,** 278–281.
62. Pollock, D. M., Polakowski, J. S., Divish, B. J., and Opgenorth, T. J. (1993) Angiotensin blockade reverses hypertension during long-term nitric oxide synthase inhibition. *Hypertension* **21,** 660–666.
63. Nakanishi, K., Mattson, D. L., and Cowley, A. W. Jr. (1995) Role of renal medullary blood flow in the development of L-NAME hypertension in rats. *Am. J. Physiol.* **268,** R317–R323.
64. Mattson, D. L., Lu, S., Nakanishi, K., Papanek, P. E., and Cowley, A. W. Jr. (1994) Effect of chronic renal medullary nitric oxide inhibition on blood pressure. *Am. J. Physiol.* **266,** H1918–H1926.
65. Baylis, C., Harvey, J., and Engels, K. (1994) Acute nitric oxide blockade amplifies the renal vaso-constrictor actions of angiotensin II. *J. Am. Soc. Nephrol.* **5,** 211–214.
66. Deng, X., Welch, W. J., and Wilcox, C. S. (1993) Role of nitric oxide in short term and prolonged effects of angiotensin II on renal hemodynamics. *Hypertension* **27,** 1173–1179.
67. Du, Z. Y., Dusting, G. J., and Woodman, O. L. (1992) Inhibition of nitric oxide synthase specifically enhances adrenergic vasoconstriction in rabbits. *Clin. Exp. Pharmacol. Physiol.* **19,** 523–530.
68. Parekh, N., Dobrowolski, L., Zou, A.-P., and Steinhausen, M. (1996) Nitric oxide modulates angiotensin II- and norepinephrine-dependent vasoconstriction in rat kidney. *Am. J. Physiol.* **270,** R630–R635.
69. Siragy, H. M. and Carey, R. M. (1997) The subtype 2 (AT_2) angiotensin receptor mediates renal production of nitric oxide in conscious rats. *J. Clin. Investig.* **100,** 264–269.
70. Szentivanyi, M. Jr., Maeda, C. Y., and Cowley, A. W. Jr. (1999) Local renal medullary L-NAME enhances the effect of long-term angiotensin II treatment. *Hypertension* **33,** 440–445.
71. Ikenaga, H., Fallet, R. W., and Carmines, P. K. (1996) Basal nitric oxide production curtails arteriolar vasoconstrictor responses to ANG II in rat kidney. *Am. J. Physiol.* **271,** F365–F373.
72. Zou, A.-P. and Cowley, A. W. Jr. (2000) Alpha-2 adrenergic receptor-mediated increase in NO production buffers renal medullary vasoconstriction. *Am. J. Physiol.* **279,** R769–R777.

73. Szentivanyi, M. Jr., Zou, A. P., Maeda, C. Y., Mattson, D. L., and Cowley, A. W. Jr. (2000) Increase in renal medullary nitric oxide synthase activity protects from norepinephrine-induced hypertension. *Hypertension* **35,** 418–423.
74. Szentivanyi, M. Jr., Park, F., Maeda, C. Y., and Cowley, A. W. Jr. (2000) Nitric oxide in the renal medulla protects from vasopressin-induced hypertension. *Hypertension* **35,** 740–745.
75. Shultz, P. J. and Tolins, J. P. (1993) Adaptation to increased dietary salt intake in the rat. Role of endogenous nitric oxide. *J. Clin. Invest.* **91,** 642–650.
76. Ni, Z. and Vaziri, N. D. (2000) Effect of salt loading on nitric oxide xynthase expression in normotensive rats. *Am. J. Hypertension* **14,** 155–163.
77. Tolins J. P. and Shultz P. J. (1994) Endogenous nitric oxide synthesis determines sensitivity to the pressor effect of salt. *Kidney Int.* **46,** 230–236.
78. Yamada, S. S., Sassaki, A. L., Fujihara, C. K., et al. (1996) Effect of salt intake and inhibitor dose on arterial hypertension and renal injury induced by chronic nitric oxide blockade. *Hypertension* **27,** 1165–1172.
79. Szentivanyi, M. Jr., Zou, A.-P., Mattson, D. L., et al. (2001) Renal medullary nitric oxide deficit of Dahl S rats enhances hypertensive actions of angiotensin II. *Am. J. Physiol.* **283,** R266–R272.
80. Yuan, B. and Cowley, A. W. Jr. (2001) Evidence that reduced renal medullary nitric oxide synthase activity of Dahl S rats enables small elevations of arginine vasopressin to produce sustained hypertension. *Hypertension* **37,** 524–528.
81. Chen, P. Y. and Sanders, P. W. (1993) Role of nitric oxide synthase in salt-sensitive hypertension in Dahl/Rapp rats. *Hypertension* **22,** 812–818.
82. Hu, L. and Manning, R. D. Jr. (1995) Role of nitric oxide in regulation of long-term pressure–natriuresis relationship in Dahl rats. *Am. J. Physiol.* **268,** H2375–H2383.
83. Patel, A. R., Granger, J. P., and Kirchner, K. A. (1994) L-arginine improves transmission of perfusion pressure to the renal interstitium in Dahl salt-sensitive rats. *Am. J. Physiol.* **266,** R1730–R1735.
84. Patel, A. R., Layne, S., Watts, D., and Kirchner, K. A. (1993) L-arginine administration normalizes pressure natriuresis in hypertensive Dahl rats. *Hypertension* **22,** 863–869.
85. Miyata, N., Zou, A. P., Mattson, D. L., and Cowley, A. W. Jr. (1998) Renal medullary interstitial infusion of L-arginine prevents hypertension in Dahl salt-sensitive rats. *Am. J. Physiol.* **275,** R1667–R1673.

15 Role of Endothelin-1 in Hypertension

Ernesto L. Schiffrin

CONTENTS

1. INTRODUCTION

It has been recognized for many years that the endothelium produces vasoconstrictor agents. In 1985, Hickey et al. showed the presence of a vasoconstrictor peptide secreted by endothelial cells *(1)*. Three years later, Yanagisawa et al. isolated and cloned the 21 amino-acid peptide endothelin (ET) *(2)*. It has since become evident that not one but several ETs are produced by many organs, subserving various functions. Of the different ETs, ET-1 is the peptide that appears to be the more important ET produced by vascular cells. Secreted by endothelial cells abluminally toward underlying smooth muscle cells, it acts in a paracrine or autocrine manner *(3)*.

Endothelin-converting enzyme (ECE) occurs as two different species (ECE-1 and ECE-2). ECE-2 is present on smooth muscle cells and converts big ET-1 to ET-1 at this level in the proximity of ET receptors on smooth muscle cells, from which ET-1 may be protected from degradation. ECE-1 occurs in four isoforms (ECE-1a–1d) encoded by one gene. There are four alternative promoters that result in the production of the four isoforms *(4)*. These isoforms differ only by their N-terminal amino-acid end, which is responsible for their cellular localization. ECE-1b is an intracellular enzyme *(5)*. The three remaining isoforms have their catalytic domain oriented toward the outside of the cell. It has been proposed that ECE-1b may heterodimerize with the other ECE-1 isoforms and regulates extracellular ECE-1 activity *(6)*. In addition, there are non-ECE ET-generating enzymes (chymase and neutral endopeptidase) *(5)*.

Effects of ET-1 are mediated through ET_A and ET_B receptors. ET_B receptors localized on endothelial cells induce vasodilation through the production of nitric oxide (NO) and cyclooxygenase-derived prostacyclin. ET_A and ET_B receptors localized on vascular smooth muscle cells participate in the vasoconstrictor, proliferative and hypertrophic

From: *Contemporary Endocrinology: Hypertension and Hormone Mechanisms*
Edited by: R. M. Carey © Humana Press Inc., Totowa, NJ

effects of ET-1. In arteries, ET_A receptors are predominant, whereas in veins and in the pulmonary circulation, vasoconstrictor ET_B may predominate over ET_A receptors. Interestingly, there are few endothelial vasodilator ET_B receptors in the coronary circulation, and accordingly, ET-1 is predominantly a coronary vasoconstrictor. Because of this bifunctional action, it is still unclear whether ET is a vasoconstrictor or a vasodilator under physiological conditions.

Inactivation of the ET-1 or the ET_A receptor gene in mice induces a slightly raised blood pressure as a result of craniofacial developmental abnormalities that affect ventilation [7,8]. Associated with this are large conduit artery abnormalities that demonstrate the role of the ET-1/ET_A axis in development of the aorta. ET-3 on the other hand is a neuropeptide with a critical role in neural crest cell migration, and mutations or gene inactivation of ET_B receptors, for which ET-3 is the preferred ligand, induce pigmentary abnormalities and aganglionic megacolon [9]. Indeed, in many cases of hereditary Hirschprung's disease, characterized by aganglionic megacolon, mutations in the ET_B receptor have been noted. Interestingly, heterozygous mice for inactivation of the ET_B receptor present slightly increased blood pressure, suggesting that ET_B receptors are predominantly vasodilator, even if there are also vasoconstrictor ET_B receptors.

2. VASCULAR EFFECTS OF ET-1

ET-1 generation is modulated by shear stress that downregulates its release by endothelial cells [10]. NO production, stimulated by shear stress, is an important inhibitor of ET-1 release [11], and may thus be a mediator of this effect. Hypoxia, epinephrine, thrombin, Ang II, vasopressin, cytokines, insulin, and growth factors such as TGF-β1 stimulate endothelial release of ET-1. Leptin has also been shown to upregulate ET-1 production by endothelial cells [12], which could explain in part increases of ET-1 in obesity. This may represent a mechanism that relates obesity to frequently associated cardiovascular conditions including hypertension and atherosclerosis, or that contributes to the evolution of the metabolic syndrome toward type 2 diabetes. Peroxisome proliferator-activated receptors (PPARs) are nuclear factors involved in adipocyte differentiation and insulin sensitivity that have been recently shown to exhibit potent anti-inflammatory and antigrowth properties [13–15]. Both PPARα and γ have been shown in vivo, to inhibit the enhanced expression of preproET-1 mRNA and prevent the progression of hypertension in DOCA-salt rats [16], in which the ET system is activated [17]. This effect of fibrates (PPARα activators) and thiazolidinediones (glitazones, PPARγ activators) was accompanied by decreased vascular ET-1 expression.

In deoxycorticosterone acetate (DOCA)-salt rats, associated with an increased vascular ET-1 production [17] "enhanced" vascular superoxide generation by reduced nicotinamide adenine dinucleotide phosphate (NADPH) oxidase has been demonstrated, which may contribute to decreased bioavailability of NO, and accordingly, induce endothelial dysfunction [16].

2.1. Long-Term Effects of ET-1 on Blood Vessels in Experimental Hypertension

ET-1 participates in the remodeling of large and small arteries found in hypertension [18]. In some models of experimental hypertension, particularly those that are salt-induced, such as DOCA-salt hypertension or in Dahl salt-sensitive rats, as well as in severe hypertension, there is typically hypertrophic remodeling of resistance arteries with increased cross-sectional area rather than the eutrophic remodeling without true vascular hypertrophy more often found in essential hypertension and in spontaneously hypertensive rats (SHR) *(18)*. This hypertrophic remodeling appears to be the signature of an effect of ET-1 *(19,20)*, in contrast to the effects of endogenous Ang II, which is associated with eutrophic remodeling *(21)*. Collagen deposition participates in the remodeling occurring in hypertension. EGF receptor transactivation appears to play an important role in the vascular fibrotic component of remodeling *(22)*. In transgenic mice harboring the luciferase gene under the control of the collagen I-α2 chain promoter, ET-1 induced a rapid phosphorylation of the mitogen-activated protein kinase (MAPK) and activation of the collagen I gene in aorta, effect that was blocked by an EGF receptor phosphorylation inhibitor, and by a blocker of MAPK. The EGF receptor inhibitor also reduced vasoconstrictor effects in vitro and pressor responses in vivo to ET-1.

We recently created a genetically engineered mouse that transgenically expresses human preproET-1 limited to the endothelium (by use of the endothelium-specific promoter Tie-2) *(23)*. This induced a phenotype that, in the absence of significant blood pressure elevation, was associated with small artery hypertrophic remodeling and endothelial dysfunction, in support of our previous proposal that ET-1 induced vascular hypertrophy directly and independently of blood pressure elevation *(19,20)*. Interestingly, NADPH oxidase activity was enhanced, indicating increased generation of superoxide anion that could contribute to the decreased endothelium-dependent relaxation through reduced NO bioavailability.

Bakker et al. have investigated in organoid culture some of the mechanisms involved in the remodeling induced by ET-1 in small arteries *(24)*. Three-day activation with ET-1 induced vasoconstriction and eutrophic remodeling, which could be enhanced by an antibody directed to β_3-integrin. Inward eutrophic remodeling was shown to be a response to sustained contraction, which may involve collagen reorganization through β_3-integrins. The same group showed that stimulation with ET-1 induced significant increase in c-fos mRNA, which could not be blocked by inhibitors of tyrosine kinases, MAP kinases, or conventional protein kinase C, but was inhibited by staurosporine and the calcium chelator BAPTA, suggesting a role for intracellular calcium *(25)*. Thus, ET-1 induced increased expression of c-fos independent of MAP kinase via a calcium-dependent mechanism in the absence of wall stress.

ET_B receptors have been suggested to play a pro-apoptotic role *(26)*, whereas ET_A receptors mediate cell growth and apoptosis through NFκB activation *(27)*. However, the overall effect of ET-1 appears to be a survival and anti-apoptotic action and is associated with attenuation of the caspase-3 pathway activation *(28)*.

Reactive oxygen species (ROS), which are involved in the pathophysiology of hypertension and in vascular damage, are potent inducers of ET-1 synthesis in endothelial cells *(29)*. In addition, as already mentioned in relation to endothelial dysfunction, ET-1 is able to activate NADPH oxidase in smooth muscle cells and in blood vessels *(20)*. Its mitogenic effects may be in part mediated via an increase in the production of ROS *(30)*, as already mentioned. In aldosterone-infused rats exposed to a normal salt diet, systolic blood pressure, plasma ET, systemic oxidative stress, and vascular NADPH activity increased in association with small artery hypertrophic remodeling. Laser confocal microscopy showed increased collagen, fibronectin, and intercellular adhesion molecule (ICAM-1) content in the vessel wall of aldosterone-infused rats. ET_A receptor antagonism decreased oxidative stress, normalized the hypertrophic remodeling, decreased collagen and fibronectin deposition, and reduced ICAM-1 abundance in the vascular wall of aldosterone-infused rats, whereas hydralazine lowered blood pressure and reduced NADPH activity in aorta but did not affect the other vascular changes. ET blockade thus exerts beneficial effects on vascular remodeling, fibrosis, oxidative stress, and adhesion molecule expression in aldosterone-induced hypertension *(31)*. In salt-loaded stroke-prone SHR (SHR-SP) rats, whose hypertension has an ET-1 component, administration of antioxidants such as the superoxide dismutase mimetic Tempol decreased the media to lumen ratio of mesenteric arteries *(32)*. However, whereas in mice NADPH oxidase appears to be of major importance in mediation of ROS generation induced by ET-1 *(23,33)*, in rats and in human smooth muscle cells ET-1 appears to induce superoxide anion formation also through activation of other mechanisms, including xanthine oxidase and mitochondrial sources of free radicals *(34)*. It is known that ET-1 influences mitochondrial function and ROS formation in cultured cardiomyocytes *(35)*. Interestingly, superoxide anion from different sources including mitochondrial ROS modulates ET-1 production *(35,36)*. Ang II-induced redox-sensitive ERK signaling plays a role in ET-1 gene expression in rat aortic smooth muscle cells *(37)* and ET-1 synthesis depends on intracellular ROS generation in human VSMCs *(38)*. Increased ET-1 could in turn stimulate mitochondrial-derived ROS production. Although Ang II activates p38MAPK, JNK, and ERK5 primarily through NAD(P)H oxidase-generated ROS *(34)*, ET-1 stimulates these kinases via redox-sensitive processes that involve mitochondrial-derived ROS. Thus, redox-dependent activation of MAPKs by Ang II and ET-1 occurs through distinct ROS-generating systems that contribute to the differential signaling in vascular smooth muscle cells by these agents.

ET-1 stimulates cell migration and VEGF production *(39,40)*, which could imply its involvement in angiogenesis. ET-1 antagonists block angiogenesis and tumor progression *(41)*. However, ET_A/ET_B antagonism has improved survival after myocardial infarction, which may relate to improved perfusion resulting from triggering of an angiogenic response *(42)*. In a model of hindlimb ischemia the ET system is activated and ET antagonists increase neovascularization *(43)*. Capillary density in the left ventricular myocardium is decreased in DOCA-salt rats *(44)*. This rarefaction may be prevented by use of an ET_A receptor blocker, which suggests that ET-1 has detrimental effects on the microcirculation, whereas ET_A receptor blockers favor angiogenesis. The role of ET-1 in angiogenesis post-ischemia or on tumor growth remains therefore undefined. A recent study examined the role of ET-1 in the development of coronary vasa vasorum in experimental hypercholesterolemia in pigs using microscopic-computed tomography *(45)*. Vasa vasorum density was higher in the hypercholesterolemic group associated with increased VEGF expression in the coronary arterial wall. These changes were abrogated by an ET_A receptor antagonist, supporting an involvement of ET in vasa vasorum neovascularization in early coronary atherosclerosis.

2.2. ET-1 and Renal and Cardiac Target Organ Damage in Experimental Hypertension

ET-1 plays a role in renal and cardiac target organ damage in hypertension. ET-1 production is enhanced under conditions of salt loading, and via renal ET_B receptor activation, inhibits sodium re-absorption *(46)*. Ang II infusion combined with high salt increases renal ET-1 *(47)*. In Ang II-infused mice, the dual ET_A/ET_B receptor blocker bosentan partially prevented the activation of the procollagen gene *(48)*. However, Rothermund et al. studied transgenic rats overexpressing the *ren2* gene (TGR(mRen2)27) that have renin-dependent hypertension (Ren2) and were treated between 10 and 30 wk of age with the selective ET_A receptor antagonist darusentan or the ET_A/ET_B receptor antagonist LU420627 *(49)*. The elevated blood pressure and mortality of Ren2 was not affected by either ET receptor antagonist. Proteinuria and glomerulosclerosis, tubulo-interstitial damage, and renal osteopontin mRNA expression were reduced by an angiotensin receptor blocker but were unchanged in ET receptor blocker-treated Ren2-rats, indicating that ET-1 is not involved in the renal damage and mortality in primary renin-dependent hypertension. On the other hand, in salt-loaded SHR-SP, increases in renal ET-1 were associated with increases in transforming growth factor (TGF)-β1, basic fibroblast growth factor (bFGF), procollagen I expression and matrix metallo-proteinase (MMP)-2 activity, which in turn were normalized by a selective ET_A antagonist. This indicates that ET-1 plays a role in renal fibrosis through growth factors and induction of inflammation *(50)*.

In the heart, ET_A blockade prevented enhanced TGF-β1 expression and collagen deposition in DOCA-salt rats *(51)*. ET_A receptors modulated the expression of inflammatory mediators such as NFκB and adhesion molecules, and the activation of the anti-apoptotic molecule X inhibitor of apoptosis peptide (xIAP) *(52)*. Thus, regulation of the inflammatory process may affect mechanisms that play a role in cardiac remodeling such as apoptosis and cell hypertrophy. Inhibition of NFκB has indeed prevented anti-apoptotic and hypertrophic actions of ET-1 *(53)*. NFκB is redox sensitive and is activated by NADPH oxidase-derived superoxide anion *(54)*. ET-1-dependent cardiac hypertrophy is induced by the activation of NADPH oxidase and MAPK *(55)*. Combined ET_A/ET_B prevented target organ damage in Ang II-infused rats through decreased activation of NFκB and downregulation of ICAM-1, vascular cellular adhesion molecule (VCAM)-1, and tissue factor, underlining the pro-inflammatory effects of ET-1 that occur partly interacting with the renin–angiotensin–aldosterone system (RAAS) *(56)*. However, it should be noted that there is an evidence that ET-1 and the RAAS act in parallel rather than in series, as suggested by recent work *(49,57,58)*. Indeed, in the TGR(mRen2)27, a primary form of renin-dependent hypertension, bosentan was ineffective in lowering blood pressure *(56)* as also reported with an ET_A selective blocker in other studies *(58)*. Among components of the RAAS, aldosterone may contribute to both cardiac and vascular damage mediated by ET-1, similarly to effects already described for the mineralocorticoid DOCA. Indeed, we recently showed that ET_A antagonism prevents vascular remodeling and cardiac and vascular fibrosis in aldosterone-infused rats *(31,59,60)*.

3. THE ET SYSTEM IN ESSENTIAL HYPERTENSION

Immunoreactive ET plasma levels, which reflect poorly ET-1 tissue production, are not elevated in essential hypertension *(61)*, except in African Americans, in whom the circulating ET is elevated in hypertensive subjects *(62)*. Hirai et al. *(63)* recently studied immunoreactive ET in plasma in 1492 subjects and showed by multiple stepwise regression analysis that age, creatinine, and smoking were significantly correlated to plasma ET. No relation was demonstrated between plasma ET and BP, suggesting that high ET is not related to hypertension, but to subclinical renal dysfunction and smoking. However, vascular levels of immunoreactive ET are increased in patients with moderate-to-severe hypertension (Stage 2 of the JNC 7 classification), compared with normotensive subjects or patients with mildly elevated blood pressure (Stage 1) *(64)*. Studies in hypertensive humans have shown that ET_A receptor antagonists cause a greater degree of vasodilatation in forearm vessels of essential hypertensive patients compared with normotensive subjects *(65)*, which may suggest a predominant role of ET_A receptors in the regulation of vascular tone by endogenous ET-1. The ET_A antagonist BQ-123 improved impaired vasodilation in hypertensive patients. On the other hand, the ET_B antagonist BQ-788 induced vasoconstriction on forearm resistance arteries in normotensive subjects *(66,67)*. This suggests that ET_B receptors may play a vasodilator role in normotensive subjects. BQ-788 had a vasodilator action on the forearm circulation of hypertensive subjects *(66)*, indicating that a vasoconstrictor effect of ET_B receptors could be found in hypertensive but not in normotensive individuals. Black American patients appear to have increased numbers of smooth muscle vasoconstrictor ET_B receptors *(68,69)*, which may underlie the ET-dependency that has been suggested in these subjects. In a recently published study, forearm blood flow responses to BQ-123 in normotensives was similar in white and black subjects, whereas in hypertensive patients the vasodilator effect of ET_A receptor blockade was significantly higher in blacks than in whites *(70)*. ET-1 induced a significant vasoconstriction without differences between white and black patients. Together, this data suggested that in hypertensive blacks there is increased ET_A-dependent tone that participates in vasoconstriction and contributes to blood pressure elevation. Human subjects infused with stepwise increasing intravenous doses of Ang II exhibited decreased renal plasma flow and glomerular filtration rate, and increased blood pressure and renal vascular resistance, which were unaffected by co-administration of the selective ET_A-receptor antagonist BQ-123 *(71)*, which suggests as indicated earlier *(55)* that the pressor responses to Ang II cannot be attributed to the action of ET-1.

ET-1 potentiates the action of vasoconstrictors such as phenylephrine or serotonin at low concentrations (10^{-11} mol/L) *(72)*. This mechanism has been demonstrated to be enhanced in hypertensive patients *(73)* and is affected by a polymorphism (*EDN1 K198N*) located in the coding region of the prepro-ET-1 gene *(74)*. This phenomenon could contribute to increased vascular tone in hypertensive patients.

Cardiac hypertrophy and fibrosis have been attributed to the effects of mineralocorticoids and ET-1 in experimental studies *(51,52)*. Recent studies in human hypertension using the analysis of the ultrasonic backscatter signal that arises from tissue heterogeneity within the myocardium and describes myocardial texture have allowed investigation of relations between myocardial fibrosis and circulating aldosterone and immunoreactive ET in human hypertension *(75)*. In patients with essential hypertension, primary aldosteronism, or renovascular hypertension, myocardial-integrated backscatter correlated with plasma aldosterone and immunoreactive ET, suggesting that aldosterone and ET-1 may induce myocardial fibrosis in human hypertension.

3.1. ET Antagonists in Essential Hypertension

Because ET_B receptors are both vasoconstrictor and vasodilator, and additionally at least in the mouse have a natriuretic effect, there has been ongoing controversy on whether selective ET_A or combined ET_A/ET_B receptor blockers would be more efficacious therapeutically in cardiovascular diseases including hypertension. However, there are no clinical trials available comparing an ET_A antagonist to a combined ET_A/ET_B blocker.

The combined ET_A/ET_B antagonist bosentan (500 mg to 2000 mg/d for 4 wk) given to patients with mild-to-moderate essential hypertension lowered blood pressure by 5.7 mmHg, comparable to the reduction observed with the ACE inhibitor enalapril (20 mg/d) *(76)*. More recently, the selective ET_A antagonist darusentan was shown to reduce systolic blood pressure by 6.0 (at 10 mg/d for 6 wk) to 11.3 mmHg (at 100 mg/d) *(77)*. Elevation of liver enzymes, a side effect sometimes found with bosentan, was not encountered with darusentan. Although these results have been promising, whether ET receptor antagonists will become part of the therapeutic armamentarium in essential hypertension and associated target organ damage remains unclear, and none of these agents are currently being developed for this indication. Recently, however, trials have been started for treatment of resistant hypertension using ET_A selective endothelin antagonists such as darusentan. Some initial promising preliminary results have been reported, but we will have to wait for definitive larger trials to determine whether indeed resistant, severe or uncontrolled hypertension becomes an indication for the use of ET antagonists.

3.2. ET Antagonists in Heart Failure, Renal Failure, and Diabetes Mellitus

Although initial studies of heart failure demonstrated beneficial effects of ET blockade both acutely *(78)* and with bosentan over 14 d with improved systemic and pulmonary hemodynamics *(79)*, recent studies such as ENABLE demonstrated increased risk of worsening heart failure in patients treated with bosentan *(80)*. On the other hand, ET_A selective antagonists (darusentan) increased cardiac index after 3 wk of treatment in the HEAT study, although pulmonary capillary wedge pressure, pulmonary arterial pressure, pulmonary vascular resistance, and right atrial pressure remained unchanged. However, systemic vascular resistance decreased significantly. High dosage of darusentan induced adverse events, but were associated in some cases with early aggravation of heart failure and even death. Thus, in a large patient population selective ET_A receptor blockade for 3 wk improved some indices of heart failure, but long-term studies are still needed to conclude whether ET_A blockade is beneficial in congestive heart failure *(81)*. Other recent studies such as RITZ-4 and 5 with the intravenous ET_A/ET_B antagonist tezosentan in acute heart failure do not seem to support much evidence of efficacy of ET blockers in acute left ventricular dysfunction *(82)*. On the other hand, and on the basis of clinical trials *(83)*, bosentan was approved for the treatment of primary pulmonary hypertension, which is currently the only approved indication of ET receptor antagonists. New studies suggest as well the use potential use for this indication of ET_A selective blockers.

Selective ET_A antagonists have prevented the progression of diabetic nephropathy in rat models *(84)*. In an acute, randomized, placebo-controlled, double-blind, four-way crossover study, the selective ET_A (BQ-123) and ET_B (BQ-788) receptor antagonists were given alone and in combination to patients with chronic renal failure *(85)*. The ET$_A$ receptor blocker lowered blood pressure and induced renoprotective effects in the chronic renal failure patients. Because the ET$_B$ receptor has renal vasodilatory action, combined ET$_A$/ET$_B$ receptor blockade did not confer these renal benefits, although it did lower blood pressure.

Hyperinsulinemic insulin-resistant individuals have relatively elevated circulating levels of immunoreactive ET, suggesting that ET-1 plays a role in endothelial dysfunction and vascular damage found in these conditions *(86)*. In patients with type 2 diabetes, ET$_A$ receptor blockade restored impaired vasodilatation *(87)*. In nondiabetic obese and in type 2 diabetic subjects, arterial administration of BQ-123 produced significant vasodilatation *(83)*. ET$_A$ blockade did not affect basal NO flux, which suggests the presence of increased ET constrictor tone in these subjects. Stimulated NO flux increased in response to ET$_A$ blockade in obese and type 2 diabetic subjects. Thus, ET contributes to endothelial dysfunction and the regulation of vascular tone in obesity and type 2 diabetes *(88)*.

On the basis of the experimental and clinical data reported above, a clinical trial has recently been initiated in diabetic nephropathy using an ET$_A$ selective receptor blocker. The results of this study, when available, will allow further conclusions on the potential of inhibition of the endothelin system to stop progression of this critical complication of diabetes mellitus.

3.3. Genetics of the ET System

A polymorphism (*EDN1 K198N*) located in the coding region of the prepro-ET-1 gene *(89)* has been associated with increased vascular reactivity, and as already mentioned, could contribute to increased vascular tone in hypertensive patients *(74)*. This polymorphism has also been associated with blood pressure levels in overweight individuals *(88)*. A polymorphism of ECE-1b (*ECE1 C-388A*) in the 5′-regulatory region of the ECE-1b gene (338 bp upstream from the translation start site), resulting in a binding site for the transcription factor E2F-2 was recently described in two cohorts of hypertensive patients. This C-to-A substitution is associated with increased promoter activity, as demonstrated in promoter–reporter gene experiments *(90)*. In a group of untreated hypertensive German women, the A allele of this polymorphism had a codominant effect on daytime and night time systolic and diastolic BP *(90)*. In another cohort from the Étude du Vieillissement Artériel (EVA) study, an epidemiological study in France, this finding was in part confirmed in 1198 subjects (698 women) *(91)*. The association of BP and the polymorphism was found in women but not in men. Females homozygous for the A allele had significantly higher systolic, diastolic, and mean BP levels, which suggest a recessive effect of this variant in this French population. The A allele may raise expression of ECE-1b, resulting in increased production of ET-1, which remains to be proven. The *EDN1 K198N* polymorphism of the preproET-1 gene was not associated with BP values in either men or women in this study, but interacted with the *ECE1 C-338A* variant to influence systolic and mean BP levels in women *(91)*. Although the *EDN1* variant did not correlate with BP, the effect of the *ECE1 C-338A* variant on BP occurred only in homozygous *EDN1* KK women. The reason why the ECE-1b effect was observed only in females remains undetermined but could be related to interactions between sex hormones and the ET system. Stimulation of the ET system by androgens might explain the lack of effect in males.

4. CONCLUSIONS

ET-1 has pro-inflammatory, hypertrophic, and pro-fibrotic properties on the heart, kidney, and blood vessels. Beneficial actions of ET receptor antagonists could contribute to prevent hypertensive, atherosclerotic, and diabetic complications. ET blockade may present important blood pressure-independent effects on cardiovascular growth, inflammation, and fibrosis, which may contribute to its therapeutic potential in hypertension and other cardiovascular disorders, including chronic renal failure and diabetes. We must now wait for the results of ongoing trials of ET_A receptor blockers in resistant or uncontrolled essential hypertension and in diabetic nephropathy to find out whether the promise of therapeutic effectiveness of ET blockade in human disease is realized.

ACKNOWLEDGMENTS

This work was supported by a grant 37917 and a group grant to the Multidisciplinary Research Group on Hypertension, both from the Canadian Institutes of Health Research.

REFERENCES

1. Hickey, K. A., Rubanyi, G., Paul, R. J., and Highsmith, R. F. (1985) Characterization of a coronary vasoconstrictor produced by cultured endothelial cells. *Am. J. Physiol.* **248,** C550–C556.
2. Yanagisawa, M., Kurihara, H., Kimura, S., et al. (1988) A novel potent vasoconstrictor peptide produced by vascular endothelial cells. *Nature* **332,** 411–415.
3. Wagner, O. F., Christ, G., Wojta, J., et al. (1992) Polar secretion of endothelin-1 by cultured endothelial cells. *J. Biol. Chem.* **267,** 16,066–16,068.
4. Valdenaire, O., Lepailleur-Enouf, D., Egidy, G., et al. (1999) A fourth isoform of endothelin-converting enzyme (ECE-1) is generated from an additional promoter molecular cloning and characterization. *Eur. J. Biochem.* **264,** 341–349.
5. D'Orléans-Juste, P., Plante, M., Honoré, J. C., Carrier, E., and Labonté, J. (2003) Synthesis and degradation of endothelin-1. *Can J. Physiol. Pharmacol.* **81,** 503–510.
6. Muller, L., Barret, A., Etienne, E., et al. (2003) Heterodimerization of endothelin-converting enzyme-1 isoforms regulates the subcellular distribution of this metalloprotease. *J. Biol. Chem.* **278,** 545–555.
7. Kurihara, Y., Kurihara, H., Suzuki, H., et al. (1994) Elevated blood pressure and craniofacial abnormalities in mice deficient in endothelin-1. *Nature* **368,** 703–710.
8. Clouthier, D. E., Hosoda, K., Richardson, J. A., et al. (1998) Cranial and cardiac neural crest defects in endothelin-A receptor-deficient mice. *Development* **125,** 813–824.
9. Hosoda, K., Hammer, R. E., Richardson, J. A., et al. (1994) Targeted and natural (piebald-lethal) mutations of endothelin-B receptor gene produce megacolon associated with spotted coat color in mice. *Cell* **79,** 1267–1276.
10. Malek, A. and Izumo, S. (1992) Physiological fluid shear stress causes downregulation of endothelin-1 mRNA in bovine aortic endothelium. *Am. J. Physiol.* **263,** C389–C396.
11. Boulanger, C. and Luscher, T. F. (1990) Release of endothelin from the porcine aorta: inhibition by endothelium-derived nitric oxide. *J. Clin. Investig.* **85,** 587–590.
12. Quehenberger, P., Exner, M., Sunder-Plassmann, R., et al. (2002) Leptin induces endothelin-1 in endothelial cells in vitro. *Circ. Res.* **90,** 711–718.
13. Diep, Q. N., El Mabrouk, M., Cohn, J. S., et al. (2002) Structure, endothelial function, cell growth, and inflammation in blood vessels of angiotensin II-infused rats. Role of peroxisome proliferator-activated receptor-γ. *Circulation* **105,** 2296–2302.
14. Diep, Q. N., Amiri, F., Touyz, R. M., Cohn, J. S., Endemann, D., and Schiffrin, E. L. (2002) PPARα activator effects on Ang II-induced vascular oxidative stress and inflammation. *Hypertension* **40,** 866–871.
15. Schiffrin, E. L., Amiri, F., Benkirane, K., Iglarz, M., and Diep, Q. N. (2003) Peroxisome proliferators-activated receptors: vascular and cardiac effects in hypertension. *Hypertension* **42,** 664–668.
16. Iglarz, M., Touyz, R. M., Amiri, F., Lavoie, M.-F., Diep, Q. N., and Schiffrin, E. L. (2003) Effect of peroxisome proliferator-activated receptor-α and -γ activators on vascular remodeling in endothelin-dependent hypertension. *Arterioscl. Thromb. Vasc. Biol.* **23,** 45–51.

17. Larivière, R., Thibault, G., and Schiffrin, E. L. (1993) Increased endothelin-1 content in blood vessels of deoxycorticosterone acetate-salt hypertensive but not in spontaneously hypertensive rats. *Hypertension* **21,** 294–300.

18. Intengan, H. D. and Schiffrin, E. L. (2000) Structure and mechanical properties of resistance arteries in hypertension: role of adhesion molecules and extracellular matrix determinants. *Hypertension* **36,** 312–318.

19. Li, J. S., Larivière, R., and Schiffrin, E. L. (1994) Effect of a nonselective endothelin antagonist on vascular remodeling in deoxycorticosterone acetate-salt hypertensive rats. Evidence for a role of endothelin in vascular hypertrophy. *Hypertension* **24,** 183–188.

20. Schiffrin, E. L. (1995) Endothelin: potential role in hypertension and vascular hypertrophy. *Hypertension* **25,** 1135–1143.

21. Li, J. S., Knafo, L., Turgeon, A., Garcia, R., and Schiffrin, E. L. (1996) Effect of endothelin antagonism on blood pressure and vascular structure in renovascular hypertensive rats. *Am. J. Physiol. Heart Circ. Physiol.* **40,** H88–H93.

22. Flamant, M., Tharaux, P. L., Placier, S., et al. (2002) Epidermal growth factor receptor transactivation mediates the tonic and fibrogenic effects of endothelin in the aortic wall of transgenic mice. *FASEB J.* **16,** 254–272.

23. Amiri, F., Virdis, A., Neves, M. F., et al. (2004) Endothelium-restricted overexpression of human endothelin-1 causes vascular remodelling and endothelial dysfunction. *Circulation* **110,** 2233–2240.

24. Bakker, E. N. T. P., Buus, C. L., VanBavel, E., et al. (2004) Activation of resistance arteries with endothelin-1: from vasoconstriction to functional adaptation and remodeling. *J. Vasc. Res.* **41,** 174–182.

25. Buus, C. L., Kristensen, H. B., Bakker, E. N. T. P., et al. (2004) Force-independent expression of c-fos mRNA by endothelin-1 in rat intact small mesenteric arteries. *Acta Physiol. Scand.* **181,** 1–11.

26. Shichiri, M., Kato, H., Marumo, F., and Hirata, Y. (1997) Endothelin-1 as an autocrine/paracrine apoptosis survival factor for endothelial cells. *Hypertension* **30,** 1198–1203.

27. Mangelus, M., Galron, R., Naor, Z., and Sokolovsky, M. (2001) Involvement of nuclear factor-kappaB in endothelin-A-receptor-induced proliferation and inhibition of apoptosis. *Cell Mol. Neurobiol.* **21,** 657–674.

28. Diep, Q. N., Intengan, H. D., and Schiffrin, E. L. (2000) Endothelin-1 attenuates omega3 fatty acid-induced apoptosis by inhibition of caspase 3. *Hypertension* **35,** 287–291.

29. Kahler, J., Mendel, S., Weckmuller, J., et al. (2000) Oxidative stress increases synthesis of big endothelin-1 by activation of the endothelin-1 promoter. *J. Mol. Cell. Cardiol.* **32,** 1429–1437.

30. Wedgwood, S., Dettman, R. W., and Black, S. M. (2001) ET-1 stimulates pulmonary arterial smooth muscle cell proliferation via induction of reactive oxygen species. *Am. J. Physiol.* **281,** L1058–L1067.

31. Pu, Q., Neves, M. F., Virdis, A., Touyz, R. M., and Schiffrin, E. L. (2003) Endothelin antagonism on aldosterone-induced oxidative stress and vascular remodeling. *Hypertension* **42,** 49–55.

32. Park, J. B., Touyz, R. M., Chen, X., and Schiffrin, E. L. (2002) Chronic treatment with a superoxide dismutase mimetic prevents vascular remodeling and progression of hypertension in salt-loaded stroke-prone spontaneously hypertensive rats. *Am. J. Hypertens.* **15,** 78–84.

33. Li, L. X., Fink, G. D., Watts, S. W., et al. (2003) Endothelin-1 increases vascular superoxide via endothelinA-NADPH oxidase pathway in low-renin hypertension. *Circulation* **107,** 1053–1058.

34. Touyz, R. M., Yao, G., Viel, E., Amiri, F., and Schiffrin, E. L. (2004) Angiotensin II and endothelin-1 regulate MAP kinases through different redox-dependent mechanisms in human vascular smooth muscle cells. *J. Hypertens.* **22,** 1141–1149.

35. Yuhki, K. I., Miyauchi, T., Kakinuma, Y., et al. (2001) Endothelin-1 production is enhanced by rotenone, a mitochondrial complex I inhibitor, in cultured rat cardiomyocytes. *J. Cardiovasc. Pharm.* **38,** 850–858.

36. Lopez-Ongil, S., Saura, M., Zaragoza, C., et al. (2002) Hydrogen peroxide regulation of bovine endothelin-converting enzyme-1. *Free Radic. Biol. Med.* **32,** 406–413.

37. Hong, H. J., Chan, P., Liu, J. C., et al. (2004) Angiotensin II induces endothelin-1 gene expression via extracellular signal-regulated kinase pathway in rat aortic smooth muscle cells. *Cardiovasc. Res.* **61,** 159–168.

38. Kahler, J., Ewert, A., Weckmuller, J., et al. (2001) Oxidative stress increases endothelin-1 synthesis in human coronary artery smooth muscle cells. *J. Cardiovasc. Pharm.* **38,** 49–57.

39. Noiri, E., Hu, Y., Bahou, W. F., Keese, C. R., Giaever, I., and Goligorsky, M. S. (1997) Permissive role of nitric oxide in endothelin-induced migration of endothelial cells. *J. Biol. Chem.* **272,** 1747–1752.

40. Matsuura, A., Yamochi, W., Hirata, K., Kawashima, S., and Yokoyama, M. (1998) Stimulatory interaction between vascular endothelial growth factor and endothelin-1 on each gene expression. *Hypertension* **32,** 89–95.
41. Kopetz, E. S., Nelson, J. B., and Carducci, M. A. (2002) Endothelin-1 as a target for therapeutic intervention in prostate cancer. *Investig. New Drugs* **20,** 173–182.
42. Mulder, P., Richard, V., Derumeaux, G., et al. (1997) Role of endogenous endothelin in chronic heart failure: effect of long-term treatment with an endothelin antagonist on survival, hemodynamics, and cardiac remodeling. *Circulation* **96,** 1976–1982.
43. Iglarz, M., Silvestre, J. S., Duriez, M., Henrion, D., and Levy, B. I. (2001) Chronic blockade of endothelin receptors improves ischemia-induced angiogenesis in rat hindlimbs through activation of vascular endothelial growth factor-NO pathway. *Arterioscler. Thromb. Vasc. Biol.* **21,** 1598–1603.
44. Larouche, I. and Schiffrin, E. L. (1999) Cardiac microvasculature in DOCA-salt hypertensive rats: effect of endothelin ET(A) receptor antagonism. *Hypertension* **34,** 795–801.
45. Herrmann, J., Best, P. J., Ritman, E. L., et al. (2002) Chronic endothelin receptor antagonism prevents coronary vasa vasorum neovascularization in experimental hypercholesterolemia. *J. Am. Coll. Cardiol.* **39,** 1555–1561.
46. Plato, C. F., Pollock, D. M., and Garvin, J. L. (2000) Endothelin inhibits thick ascending limb chloride flux via ET(B) receptor-mediated NO release. *Am. J. Physiol.* **279,** F326–F333.
47. Sasser, J. M., Pollock, J. S., and Pollock, D. M. (2002) Renal endothelin in chronic angiotensin II hypertension. *Am. J. Physiol.* **283,** R243–R248.
48. Fakhouri, F., Placier, S., Ardaillou, R., Dussaule, J. C., and Chatziantoniou, C. (2001) Angiotensin II activates collagen type I gene in the renal cortex and aorta of transgenic mice through interaction with endothelin and TGF-beta. *J. Am. Soc. Nephrol.* **12,** 2701–2710.
49. Rothermund, L., Kossmehl, P., Neumayer, H.-H., Paul, M., and Kreutz, R. (2003) Renal damage is not improved by blockade of endothelin receptors in primary renin-dependent hypertension. *J. Hypertens.* **21,** 2389–2397.
50. Tostes, R. C., Touyz, R. M., He, G., Ammarguellat, F., and Schiffrin, E. L. (2002) Endothelin A receptor blockade decreases expression of growth factors and collagen and improves matrix metalloproteinase-2 activity in kidneys from stroke-prone spontaneously hypertensive rats. *J. Cardiovasc. Pharmacol.* **39,** 892–900.
51. Ammarguellat, F., Larouche, I. I., and Schiffrin, E. L. (2001) Myocardial fibrosis in DOCA-salt hypertensive rats: effect of endothelin ET(A) receptor antagonism. *Circulation* **103,** 319–324.
52. Ammarguellat, F. Z., Gannon, P. O., Amiri, F., and Schiffrin, E. L. (2002) Fibrosis, matrix metalloproteinases, and inflammation in the heart of DOCA-salt hypertensive rats: role of ET(A) receptors. *Hypertension* **39,** 679–684.
53. Hirotani, S., Otsu, K., Nishida, K., et al. (2002) Involvement of nuclear factor-kappaB and apoptosis signal-regulating kinase 1 in G protein-coupled receptor agonist-induced cardiomyocyte hypertrophy. *Circulation* **105,** 509–515.
54. Wei, Z., Costa, K., Al-Mehdi, A. B., Dodia, C., Muzykantov, V., and Fisher, A. B. (1999) Simulated ischemia in flow-adapted endothelial cells leads to generation of reactive oxygen species and cell signaling. *Circ. Res.* **85,** 682–689.
55. Tanaka, K., Honda, M., and Takabatake, T. (2001) Redox regulation of MAPK pathways and cardiac hypertrophy in adult rat cardiac myocyte. *J. Am. Coll. Cardiol.* **37,** 676–685.
56. Muller, D. N., Mervaala, E. M., Schmidt, F., et al. (2000) Effect of bosentan on NF-kappaB, inflammation, and tissue factor in angiotensin II-induced end-organ damage. *Hypertension* **36,** 282–290.
57. Schiffrin, E. L. (2003) The angiotensin–endothelin relationship: does it play a role in cardiovascular and renal pathophysiology? Editorial Commentary. *J. Hypertens.* **21,** 2245–2247.
58. Rossi, G. P., Sacchetto, A., Rizzoni, D., et al. (2000) Blockade of angiotensin II type 1 receptor and not of endothelin receptor prevents hypertension and cardiovascular disease in transgenic (mREN2)27 rats via adrenocortical steroid-independent mechanisms. *Arterioscler. Thromb. Vasc. Biol.* **20,** 949–956.
59. Park, J. B. and Schiffrin, E. L. (2002) Cardiac and vascular fibrosis and hypertrophy in aldosterone-infused rats: role of endothelin-1. *Am. J. Hypertens.* **15,** 164–169.
60. Park, J. B. and Schiffrin, E. L. (2001) ET(A) receptor antagonist prevents blood pressure elevation and vascular remodeling in aldosterone-infused rats. *Hypertension* **37,** 1444–1449.
61. Schiffrin, E. L. (1999) Role of endothelin-1 in hypertension. *Hypertension* **34(2),** 876–881.

62. Ergul, S., Parish, D. C., Puett, D., et al. (1996) Racial differences in plasma endothelin-1 concentrations in individuals with essential hypertension. *Hypertension* **28,** 652–655.

63. Hirai, Y., Adachi, H., Fujiura, Y., Hiratsuka, A., Enomoto, M., and Imaizumi, T. (2004) Plasma endothelin-1 level is related to renal function and smoking status but not to blood pressure: an epidemiological study. *J. Hypertens.* **22,** 713–718.

64. Schiffrin, E. L., Deng, L. Y., Sventek, P., and Day, R. (1997) Enhanced expression of endothelin-1 gene in resistance arteries in severe human essential hypertension. *J. Hypertens.* **15,** 57–63.

65. Cardillo, C., Kilcoyne, C. M., Waclawiw, M., Cannon, R. O. 3rd, and Panza, J. A. (1999) Role of endothelin in the increased vascular tone of patients with essential hypertension. *Hypertension* **33,** 753–758.

66. Cardillo, C., Campia, U., Kilcoyne, C. M., Bryant, M. B., and Panza, J. A. (2002) Improved endothelium-dependent vasodilation after blockade of endothelin receptors in patients with essential hypertension. *Circulation* **105,** 452–456.

67. Verhaar, M. C., Strachan, F. E., Newby, D. E., et al. (1998) Endothelin-A receptor antagonist-mediated vasodilatation is attenuated by inhibition of nitric oxide synthesis and by endothelin-B receptor blockade. *Circulation* **97,** 752–756.

68. Ergul, A., Tackett, R. L., and Puett, D. (1999) Distribution of endothelin receptors in saphenous veins of African Americans: implications of racial differences. *J. Cardiovasc. Pharmacol.* **34,** 327–332.

69. Grubbs, A. L., Anstadt, M. P., and Ergul, A. (2002) Saphenous vein endothelin system expression and activity in African American patients. *Arterioscler. Thromb. Vasc. Biol.* **22,** 1122–1127.

70. Campia, U., Cardillo, C., and Panza, J. A. (2004) Ethnic differences in the vasoconstrictor activity of endogenous endothelin-1 in hypertensive patients. *Circulation* **109,** 3191–3195.

71. Bayerle-Eder, M., Langenberger, H., Pleiner, J., et al. (2002) Endothelin ET_A receptor-subtype specific antagonism does not mitigate the acute systemic or renal effects of exogenous angiotensin II in humans. *Eur. J. Clin. Investig.* **32,** 230–235.

72. Yang, Z. H., Richard, V., von Segesser, L., et al. (1990) Threshold concentrations of endothelin-1 potentiate contractions to norepinephrine and serotonin in human arteries. A new mechanism of vasospasm? *Circulation* **2,** 188–195.

73. Haynes, W. G., Hand, M. F., Johnstone, H. A., Padfield, P. L., and Webb, D. J. (1994) Direct and sympathetically mediated venoconstriction in essential hypertension. Enhanced responses to endothelin-1. *J. Clin. Investig.* **94,** 1359–1364.

74. Iglarz, M., Benessiano, J., Philip, I., et al. (2002) Preproendothelin-1 gene polymorphism is related to a change in vascular reactivity in the human mammary artery in vitro. *Hypertension* **39,** 209–213.

75. Kozàkovà, M., Buralli, S., Palombo, C., et al. (2003) Myocardial ultrasonic backscatter in hypertension—relation to aldosterone and endothelin. *Hypertension* **41,** 230–236.

76. Krum, H., Viskoper, R. J., Lacourcière, Y., Budde, M., and Charlon, V. (1998) The effect of an endothelin-receptor antagonist, bosentan, on blood pressure in patients with essential hypertension. Bosentan hypertension investigators. *N. Engl. J. Med.* **338,** 784–790.

77. Nakov, R., Pfarr, E., and Eberle, S. (2002) Darusentan: an effective endothelin A receptor antagonist for treatment of hypertension. *Am. J. Hypertens.* **15,** 583–589.

78. Kiowski, W., Sütsch, G., Hunziker, P., et al. (1995) Evidence for endothelin-1-mediated vasoconstriction in severe chronic heart failure. *Lancet* **346,** 732–736.

79. Sutsch, G., Kiowski, W., Yan, X. W., et al. (1998) Short-term oral endothelin-receptor antagonist therapy in conventionally treated patients with symptomatic severe chronic heart failure. *Circulation* **98,** 2262–2268.

80. Kalra, P., Moon, J., and Coats, A. (2002) Do results of the ENABLE (endothelin antagonist bosentan for lowering cardiac events in heart failure) study spell the end for non-selective endothelin antagonism in heart failure? *Int. J. Cardiol.* **85,** 195.

81. Lüscher, T. F., Enseleit, F., Pacher, R., et al. (2002) Hemodynamic and neurohumoral effects of selective endothelin A (ET_A) receptor blockade in chronic heart failure—the heart failure ET_A receptor blockade trial (HEAT). *Circulation* **106,** 2666–2672.

82. Rich, S. and McLaughlin, V. V. (2003) Endothelin receptor blockers in cardiovascular disease. *Circulation* **108,** 2184–2190.

83. Rubin, L. J., Badesch, D. B., Barst, R. J., et al. (2002) Bosentan therapy for pulmonary arterial hypertension. *N. Engl. J. Med.* **346,** 896–903.

84. Sugimoto, K., Tsuruoka, S., and Fujimura, A. (2002) Renal protective effect of YM598, a selective endothelin ET(A) receptor antagonist, against diabetic nephropathy in OLETF rats. *Eur. J. Pharmacol.* **450,** 183.
85. Goddard, J., Johnston, N. R., Hand, M. F., et al. (2004) Endothelin-A receptor antagonism reduces blood pressure and increases renal blood flow in hypertensive patients with chronic renal failure—a comparison of selective and combined endothelin receptor blockade. *Circulation* **109,** 1186–1193.
86. Morise, T., Takeuchi, Y., Kawano, M., Koni, I., and Takeda, R. (1995) Increased plasma levels of immunoreactive endothelin and von Willebrand factor in NIDDM patients. *Diabetes Care* **18,** 87–89
87. Cardillo, C., Campia, U., Bryant, M. B., and Panza, J. A. (2002) Increased activity of endogenous endothelin in patients with type II diabetes mellitus. *Circulation,* **106,** 1783–1787.
88. Mather, K. J., Mirzamohammadi, B., Lteif, A., et al. (2002) Endothelin contributes to basal vascular tone and endothelial dysfunction in human obesity and type 2 diabetes. *Diabetes* **51,** 3517–3523.
89. Tiret, L., Poirier, O., Hallet, V., et al. (1999) The Lys198Asn polymorphism in the endothelin-1 gene is associated with blood pressure in overweight people. *Hypertension* **33,** 1169–1174.
90. Funke-Kaiser, H., Reichenberger, F., Köpke, K., et al. (2003) Differential binding of transcription factor E2F-2 to the endothelin-converting enzyme-1b promoter affects blood pressure regulation. *Hum. Mol. Genet.* **12,** 423–433.
91. Funalot, B., Courbon, D., Brousseau, T., et al. (2004) Genes encoding endothelin-converting enzyme-1 and endothelin-1 interact to influence blood pressure in women: the EVA study. *J. Hypertens.* **22,** 739–743.

16

The Kallikrein–Kinin System and Hypertension

Julie Chao and Lee Chao

Contents

1. TISSUE KALLIKREIN–KININ SYSTEM COMPONENTS

Tissue (glandular or renal) kallikrein (E.C. 3.4.21.35) belongs to a subgroup of serine proteinases and processes low molecular weight kininogen substrate to release vasoactive kinin peptides *(1)*. The well-recognized function of tissue kallikrein is mediated by lysyl-bradykinin (Lys-BK or kallidin) and bradykinin (BK), which consist of 10 and 9 amino-acid peptides, respectively. Kinins are then degraded by enzymes such as kininases I and II and neutral endopeptidase (NEP) to produce a number of kinin metabolites or inactive fragments. Intact kinins bind to kinin B2 receptors, whereas kinin metabolites, such as Des–Arg^9–BK or Des–Arg^{10}–Lys-BK, bind to kinin B1 receptors. The physiological functions of the KKS are mediated by the constitutively expressed B2 receptor. Unlike the B2 receptor, the B1 receptor is expressed at low levels in the heart, vasculature, and kidney and is induced by trauma or inflammation *(2)*. The binding of kinins to their respective receptors activates second messengers such as NO, cGMP, prostacyclin, and cAMP, which trigger a broad spectrum of biological effects including vasodilation, smooth muscle contraction and relaxation, inflammation, and pain *(3,4)*. Figure 1 shows the inter-relationship of the tissue kallikrein–kinin system components.

The KKS can be regulated at different steps through system-specific inhibitors, kininases and antagonists, as well as through a kininase shared with the renin–angiotensin system (RAS). Expression of the tissue kallikrein gene is regulated by a number of hormones *(5,6)*. The activity and metabolism of kallikrein are modulated post-translationally by

From: *Contemporary Endocrinology: Hypertension and Hormone Mechanisms*
Edited by: R. M. Carey © Humana Press Inc., Totowa, NJ

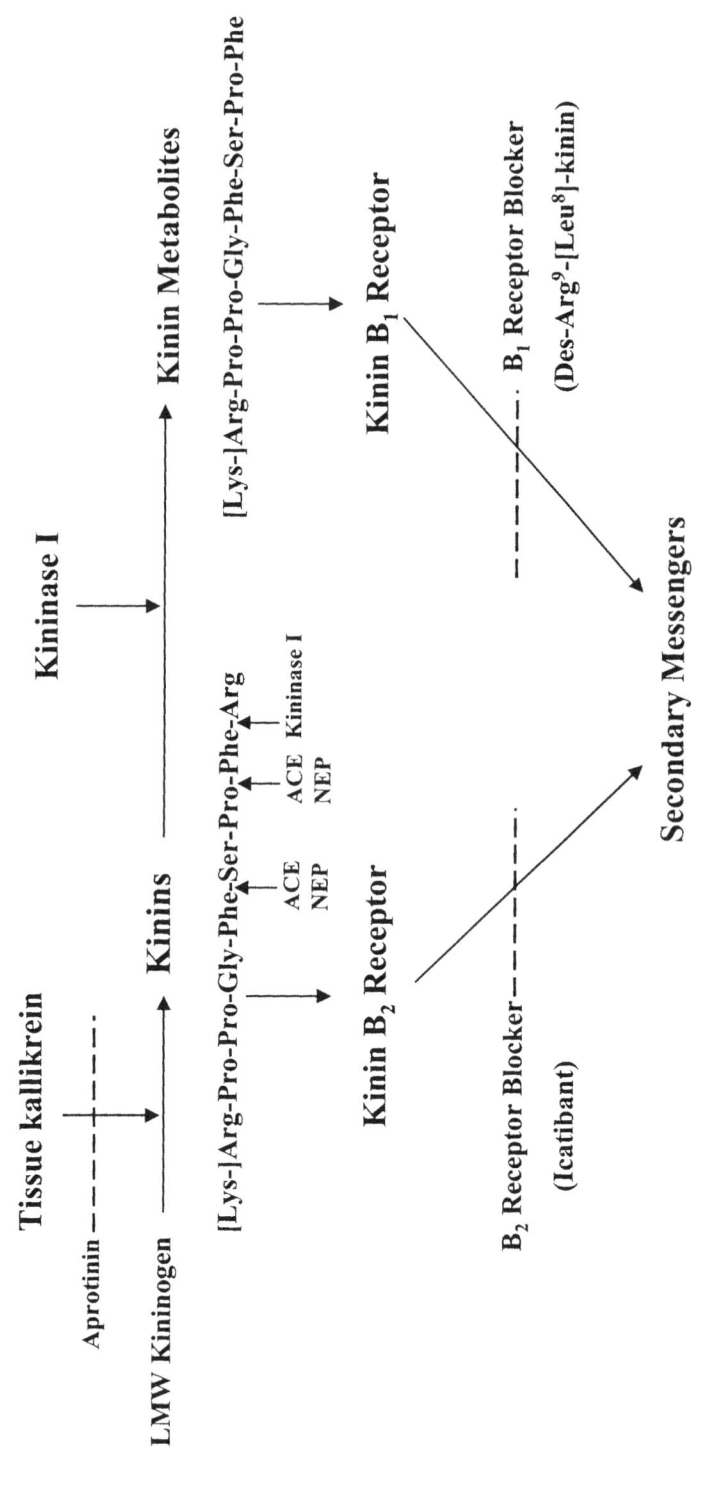

Fig. 1. The interrelationship of the tissue kallikrein–kinin sysyem components.

kallistatin, an endogenous and specific tissue kallikrein-binding protein and inhibitor *(7–9)*. Kallistatin is a potent vasodilator, which induces blood pressure reduction in anesthesized rats and vasorelaxation in isolated aortic rings independent of its kallikrein inhibitory activity *(10)*. The KKS can be blocked by tissue kallikrein inhibitors (kallistatin or aprotinin), icatibant (Hoe 140, a specific B2 receptor antagonist) or Des–Arg^9–[Leu^8] BK (a specific B1 receptor antagonist) *(1,3)*. The KKS and RAS are linked by angiotensin-converting enzyme (ACE), a dipeptidase, which is the same enzyme as kininase II. ACE has dual functions: it not only converts angiotensin I to vasoconstrictor peptide angiotensin II (Ang II), but also degrades kinin to release a dipeptide fragment, Phe–Arg, from the carboxyl end of the kinin peptide, rendering kinin inactive. Therefore, the beneficial effects of ACE inhibition in hypertension, cardiovascular, and renal diseases may also be attributed to kinin accumulation, as icatibant can partially abolish these effects *(11–13)*. Hypertension could result from either an excess of vasoconstrictor substances or a deficiency in vasodilator substances. Manipulation of the vasodilator KKS by a continuous supply of tissue kallikrein through gene transfer or protein infusion could potentially counter-balance the vasopressor effect of the RAS in blood pressure homeostasis and cardiovascular complications.

2. TISSUE KALLIKREIN IN HYPERTENSION

Tissue kallikrein was first discovered as a hypotensive substance in 1909 by Abelous and Bardier as they showed that intravenous injection of human urine into the anesthetized dog causes a transient reduction of blood pressure *(14)*. This hypotensive substance was later isolated and identified as an enzyme, which was called kallikrein, a Greek synonym for pancreas *(15,16)*. Although pancreas has been shown to be the major site of human tissue kallikrein synthesis *(17)*, urinary kallikrein mainly originates from the kidney *(18)*. Tissue kallikrein is widely expressed in tissues relevant to cardiovascular and renal function including heart, kidney, brain, and blood vessels. Reduced renal (urinary) kallikrein levels in the patients of essential hypertension were documented in 1934 *(19)*. Four decades later, this important finding was verified by a series of studies showing abnormally low kallikrein excretion in patients with essential hypertension and renovascular hypertension and in hypertensive animal models *(20–22)*. Furthermore, long-term studies indicated that urinary kallikrein excretion was familiarly aggregated, markedly reduced in African-American compared to caucasian children, and inversely related to blood pressure in these normotensive populations *(23)*. An association between reduced excretion of kallikrein and human hypertension has also been reported both in Caucasian and African-American individuals *(23–25)*. The influence of both race and dietary sodium intake on kallikrein excretion in hypertensive patients is greater compared to normotensive individuals. Moreover, a study using highly informative family pedigrees in Utah indicated that a dominant gene expressed as renal or urinary kallikrein may be associated with a reduced risk of hypertension *(26)*. These findings suggest a protective role of tissue kallikrein in the development of high blood pressure in human populations.

Reduced urinary kallikrein excretion has also been described in a number of genetically hypertensive rat models such as spontaneously hypertensive rats (SHR), New Zealand rats, Fawn-Hooded rats, and Dahl-SS hypertensive rats *(27–31)*. Restriction fragment length polymorphisms (RFLPs) have been mapped in the rat tissue kallikrein gene between SHR and normotensive Wistar–Kyoto (WKY) rats *(32)*, and a tissue kallikrein RFLP has been shown to cosegregate with high blood pressure in the F2 offspring of SHR and normotensive Brown Norway crosses *(33)*. These findings suggest a close linkage between the kallikrein gene locus and the hypertensive phenotype in SHR. Kinin appears to play a role in blood pressure regulation in SHR fed a salt-deficient diet, because the administration of a kinin receptor antagonist caused an increase in blood pressure *(34)*. Furthermore, kininogen-deficient (Brown Norway–Katholiek) rats, which cannot generate kinin, are susceptible to the development of salt-induced hypertension *(35)*. In humans and rats, low dietary sodium intake, high potassium intake, or sodium-retaining steroids all increased kallikrein excretion, whereas spirolactone decreases it *(36,37)*. Since urinary kallikrein originates in the kidney, increased urinary kallikrein levels would suggest increased synthesis in the kidney. High potassium diet in SHR resulted in upregulation of renal kallikrein and kinin B2 receptor expression, which was accompanied by blood pressure reduction *(38)*.

2.1. Genetic Linkage of Human Tissue Kallikrein Gene Polymorphism

Essential hypertension is commonly recognized as a complex disorder with a significant degree of genetic and environmental components *(39)*. A high dietary salt intake has been suggested to be one of the most important environmental risk factors for hypertension *(40–42)*. However, the blood pressure responses to salt intake or depletion vary dramatically in humans *(43)*. Stratification of salt sensitivity in the general population is a major problem for the application of dietary sodium restriction as a nonpharmacological therapy for essential hypertension. Therefore, it is important to identify individuals with gene(s) and their allelic variants that confer an increased risk to develop hypertension under a high-salt diet. In this regard, we have identified 14 polymorphic alleles in the proximal promoter region of the human tissue kallikrein gene *(KLK1) (44)*. This region contains a poly-guanine length polymorphism coupled with multiple substitution polymorphisms that constitute at least ten differential haplotypes in the –121 to –131 nucleotides from the transcription initiation site. Promoter activity assays with a reporter gene indicated that this polymorphic site regulates the expression of the kallikrein gene. The high variability of the promoter and its proximity to the tissue kallikrein gene render it suitable for investigating the correlation between this polymorphism and blood pressure regulation.

In response to dietary restriction, individuals with a lower kallikrein excretion under habitual high-salt diet showed a higher mean blood pressure reduction than the groups with a higher kallikrein excretion. Furthermore, the blood pressure response to dietary sodium was significantly correlated with the kallikrein promoter genotype. These findings indicate that this kallikrein promoter polymorphism may directly participate in the regulation of kallikrein gene expression and the blood pressure regulation in response to dietary sodium restriction in human populations. Moreover, a recent study reported that the systemic and renal KKS act in tandem to modulate the response to salt intake *(45)*. The systemic KKS is activated during high salt intake and counterbalances increased vascular response to pressors. With sodium restriction, the renal system is activated and counter-balances the increased sodium-retaining state induced by activation of the RAS. With hypertension, these modulating effects are diminished or lost, indicating a role of the KKS and RAS in the development on maintenance of hypertension.

Low urinary kallikrein excretion has been associated with hypertension and renal disease *(20,21,23)*. Because urinary kallikrein originates in the kidney, reduced kallikrein excretion would suggest impaired renal function. To identify the source of differential kallikrein excretion, we evaluated the linkage of the human tissue kallikrein gene promoter alleles with end-stage renal disease (ESRD) in African-Americans. The results show that the kallikrein gene promoter is uniquely polymorphic and the alleles of the kallikrein gene promoter are associated with hypertension and/or hypertension-associated ESRD *(46)*.

2.2. Hypotension in Transgenic Mice Expressing Human Tissue Kallikrein or Kinin B2 Receptor

Although epidemiological and genetic linkage analyses implicate a protective role of tissue kallikrein in the development of hypertension, molecular evidence documenting a direct link between kallikrein gene expression, and alteration of blood pressure is lacking. This is because of the difficulty in eliciting and maintaining high levels of either kinin or kallikrein in experimental animals. Gene transfer technology provides a novel approach to study the role of the KKS in blood pressure regulation. In order to evaluate the physiological role of the KKS, we have established transgenic mouse lines expressing KKS components. Transgenic mice expressing human tissue kallikrein were permanently hypotensive throughout their lifetime compared to their control littermates *(47–49)*. Similarly, transgenic rats expressing human tissue kallikrein are also hypotensive *(50)*. Administration of aprotinin or icatibant to the transgenic mice raised their blood pressures to normal levels *(47,48)*. These results indicate that the expression of functional human tissue kallikrein can permanently alter the blood pressure setting in the transgenic animals and that the effect is mediated by the kinin B2 receptor. This conclusion is reinforced by a study showing that transgenic mice expressing human kinin B2 receptor are hypotensive when compared to their control littermates *(51)*.

3. ENDOGENOUS KKS IN BLOOD PRESSURE HOMEOSTASIS AND CARDIOVASCULAR FUNCTION

Gene knockout is a powerful approach used to study the physiological role of a gene by analyzing the phenotype in an animal model deficient in the encoded gene product. Kinin B2 receptor-deficient mice had a significantly higher systemic blood pressure when maintained on a high-salt diet, compared to knockout mice on a normal sodium diet *(52)*. However, there was no difference in blood pressure in normal mice fed either a normal or a high-sodium diet. These findings indicate that kinin and the B2 receptor contribute to the prevention of salt-sensitive hypertension, possibly by maintaining renal blood flow under conditions of high salt intake. Another study showed that mice lacking the B2 receptor have elevated systolic blood pressure *(53)*. In addition, systemic blood pressure in B2 heterozygous mice was initially shown to be similar to that of control mice, but gradually increased to hypertensive levels at the age of 6 mo *(54)*. In contrast, the B1 receptor deficient mice are healthy, fertile, and normotensive *(55)*. In B1 knockout mice, bacterial lipopolysaccharide-induced hypotension is blunted, and there is a reduced accumulation of polymorphonuclear leukocytes in inflamed tissue. Tissue kallikrein knockout mice are unable to generate significant levels of kinins in most tissues and develop cardiovascular abnormalities early in adulthood despite normal blood pressure *(56)*. Collectively, these studies strongly support a role for the endogenous KKS in blood pressure homeostasis and cardiovascular function.

3.1. Antisense Inhibition of KKS in Central Regulation of Blood Pressure

Antisense inhibition strategy, based on interference of information flow from gene to protein, was used to explore the role of the central KKS in blood pressure regulation *(57,58)*. Acute intracerebroventricular (ICV) injection of antisense oligonucleotides for rat kininogen mRNA or kinin B2 receptor mRNA caused a rapid and significant blood pressure increase in SHR that returned to basal levels within 24 h *(57)*. Prolonged vasopressor effects were observed after repeated injections of antisense oligonucleotides. Mean blood pressure was not altered by intravenous injection of antisense oligonucleotide or by central injection of sense or scrambled oligonucleotide. Kininogen levels were significantly lower in the brain of SHR given antisense kininogen oligonucleotide compared with controls. Uptake of antisense oligonucleotides for rat kininogen or B2 receptor mRNA was detected in the hippocampus, thalamus, and hypothalamus periventricularis after the central injection of fluorescein isothiocyanate-conjugated antisense oligonucleotides. The role of brain kinin B1 receptor was further explored by central administration of an antisense oligonucleotide to rat kinin B1 receptor mRNA *(58)*. The use of B1 receptor antisense caused a significant reduction of blood pressure in SHR for more than 48 h, indicating that the activation of the brain B1 receptor by endogenous kinin metabolites may participate in the control of blood pressure. Collectively, these results indicated a differential role of B1 vs B2 receptors in central regulation of blood pressure.

3.2. Kallikrein–Kinin Administration on Blood Pressure

Intravenous infusion of tissue kallikrein or kinin results in a transient reduction of blood pressure that lasts only 1–2 minutes *(10)*. The short duration of tissue kallikrein–kinin in the circulation is due to the presence of tissue kallikrein inhibitors as well as kinin degrading enzymes in the blood vessels. Oral administration of purified pig pancreatic kallikrein has been shown to temporarily lower both the supine and upright blood pressure of hypertensive patients *(59–60)*. However, continuous oral kallikrein intake three times daily is required to maintain low blood pressure. The benefit of kallikrein in inducing blood pressure-lowering effect disappeared quickly on the termination of oral kallikrein intake. Therefore, somatic gene delivery that leads to continuous expression of a gene of interest for an extended period of time may be used as an alternative approach to circumvent this problem.

3.3. Systemic Gene Delivery of Human Tissue Kallikrein Reduces Blood Pressure in Genetically Hypertensive Rats

We employed gene transfer approaches to study the role of the KKS in hypertension, cardiovascular, and renal disease in animal models. To investigate the impact of supplying tissue kallikrein by gene delivery, we generated a series of human tissue kallikrein gene constructs under the control of the metallothionein metal response element, the albumin promoter, the Rous sarcoma virus 3′ long terminal repeat, or the cytomegalovirus promoter (CMV). Systemic delivery of the plasmid DNA constructs into SHR was effective in causing a prolonged reduction of blood pressure for 8 wk *(61,62)*. Local gene delivery via intramuscular, intraperitoneal, intra-portal vein, or ICV injections was also effective in inducing blood pressure-lowering effect in SHR *(62,63)*. The extent of blood pressure reduction was dependent on the dose of DNA injected, the gender of the animals, the promoter used in the gene construct, and the route of injection *(61–63)*. The kallikrein inhibitor aprotinin reversed the blood pressure-lowering effect in SHR receiving kallikrein gene transfer *(62)*. These results indicate that the hypotensive effect mediated by kallikrein gene delivery is mediated by the expression of functional kallikrein. The effect of kallikrein in inducing blood pressure reduction is mediated through the B2 receptor, as icatibant abolished kallikrein's blood pressure-lowering effect *(63)*. Although delivery of kallikrein in plasmid DNA, which can be administered repeatedly, produced a prolonged blood pressure reduction in hypertensive rats, the efficiency of cellular uptake and the expression of the transgene were low. To achieve high efficiency of gene transfer, we developed a replication-deficient adenoviral vector harboring the human kallikrein gene for somatic gene delivery.

3.4. Adenovirus-Mediated Kallikrein Gene Delivery Reduces Blood Pressure in Hypertensive Animal Models

Viral vectors are highly adapted to enter cells and to use the host machinery to synthesize foreign proteins. To achieve high-efficiency expression of tissue kallikrein in animal models, a transgene expression cassette containing the human tissue kallikrein cDNA under the control of the CMV promoter and 4F2 enhancer was inserted into an adenovirus vector and then transfected into human embryonic kidney (HEK) 293 cells. Expression of human tissue kallikrein was detected in the culture media by a specific enzyme-linked immunosorbant assay (ELISA). Incorporation of 4F2 enhancer increases gene expression more than 10-fold in cultured medium *(64)*. We have shown that a single intravenous injection of adenovirus encoding the human tissue kallikrein gene resulted in a profound reduction of blood pressure for weeks in SHR and in experimentally-induced hypertensive animal models including Dahl-SS, DOCA-salt, 2K1C, and 5/6 nephrectomy *(65–69)*, compared to rats injected with control adenovirus. In contrast, injection of the kallikrein gene had a minimal effect on blood pressure in control rats. The expression of recombinant human tissue kallikrein in rats following systemic or local gene delivery was detected by ELISA and immunohistochemistry, as well as by reverse transcription-polymerase chain reaction (RT-PCR) followed by Southern blot analysis. Immunoreactive human tissue kallikrein levels in rat sera or urine were highest at 3–5 d after adenovirus-mediated gene delivery and were still detectable at 24 d after injection *(65–69)*. Recombinant human tissue kallikrein was not detectable in the urine or sera of rats injected with control virus. Furthermore, our recent studies showed that systemic delivery of the kallikrein gene in fructose-induced hypertensive rats resulted in normalization of not only systolic blood pressure but also serum insulin levels, suggesting a protective role of the KKS against hypertension and associated insulin resistance in type 2 diabetes *(70)*. These beneficial effects were in conjunction with reduction in endothelin-1, endothelin-A receptor, and angiotensin II receptor type 1 expression, indicating a potential important role of the KKS in counter-balancing the vasoconstricting RAS and the endothelin system.

3.5. Hypertension and Cardiovascular Injury
by AAV-Mediated Kallikrein Gene Delivery

Adeno-associated virus (AAV) vector is attractive for long-term gene expression. However, the rate-limiting step in employing AAV gene delivery is the production of high titer-virus for in vivo studies. We have recently shown that a single intravenous injection of the recombinant AAV vector encoding the human tissue kallikrein gene into SHR resulted in a significant reduction of the systolic blood pressure from 2 weeks post gene delivery, and the blood-pressure lowering effect lasted for 20 weeks throughout the course of the experiments (71). Persistent expression of recombinant human kallikrein in rats was confirmed by ELISA and RT-PCR. Histological analysis showed remarkable amelioration of cardiovascular hypertrophy, renal injury, and collagen depositions in SHR receiving kallikrein gene transfer. In addition, reduced urinary albumin levels were detected following AAV-mediated kallikrein gene delivery. These studies showed that AAV-mediated delivery of the kallikrein gene rendered a long-term and stable reduction of hypertension and protected against renal injury and cardiac remodeling in the SHR model.

3.6. Proteomic Analysis of Renal Kallikrein Pathway
in Hypoxia-Induced Hypertension

Obstructive sleep apnea syndrome (OSAS), a disorder characterized by episodic hypoxia (EH), is a major public health problem. OSAS affects 4–5% of the general adult population and 1–2% of children in the United States. One of the major consequences of untreated OSAS is systemic hypertension. In addition to hypertension, OSAS has also been associated with both proteinuria and end-stage renal disease. A rat model of EH was used to obtain proteins from the kidney after EH induction, which were resolved by two-dimensional PAGE and then identified by MALDI-MS (72). Proteomic analysis showed that EH induces changes in renal protein expression consistent with the impairment of vasodilation mediated by kallikrein–kallistatin pathway. However, transgenic rats expressing human tissue kallikrein were protected from EH-induced hypertension. The results obtained from kallikrein transgenic rats reinforce the proteomic data. Therefore, EH-induced hypertension may result, in part, from altered regulation of the renal KKS.

4. KALLIKREIN–KININ-INDUCED TISSUE PROTECTION

4.1. Cardiac Infarction and Remodeling

Hypertensive individuals are more likely to develop other cardiovascular disorders such as peripheral vascular disease, coronary heart disease, congestive heart failure, and cerebrovascular diseases. Studies using ACE inhibitors clearly showed a protective effect of endogenous kinins in the development of cardiac hypertrophy and neointimal vascular injury (11,73). By employing transgenic and somatic gene transfer approaches, we demonstrated that the KKS plays an important role in cardiac protection. Overexpression of human tissue kallikrein in transgenic rats resulted in reduction of isoproterenol-induced cardiac hypertrophy and fibrosis, and these protective effects were abolished by icatibant (50). In addition, ablation of the B2 receptor gene in mice caused dilated cardiomyopathy followed by cardiac failure (54). Moreover, systemic delivery of adenovirus containing the tissue kallikrein gene attenuated blood pressure, cardiac hypertrophy, and fibrosis in pressure- and volume-overload hypertensive rat models such as SHR, 2K1C, Dahl-SS, and DOCA-salt rats *(65–69,74)*. Furthermore, kallikrein gene transfer reduced cardiac remodeling and apoptosis after myocardial infarction and delayed the progression of heart failure without changes in blood pressure *(75,76)*. In rats subjected to acute ischemia/ reperfusion (I/R), systemic delivery of the tissue kallikrein gene exerted cardiac protection by improving cardiac function and reducing myocardial infarction, the incidence of ventricular fibrillation, and apoptosis *(76,77)*. Icatibant abolished these beneficial effects, indicating a kinin-mediated event. Similar to systemic gene delivery, local delivery of the kallikrein gene significantly attenuated I/R-induced myocardial infarction and apoptosis in the left ventricle as detected by both terminal deoxynucleotidyl transferase-mediated dUTP nick end labeling (TUNEL) staining and DNA laddering. These results indicate that kallikrein–kinin not only plays an important role in the regulation of blood pressure homeostasis, but also in cardiovascular function by reducing ventricular remodeling, and heart failure and mortality associated with these conditions.

4.2. Salt- and Drug-Induced Renal Injuries

Chronic renal failure in humans can lead to end-stage renal disease, which eventually requires kidney transplant or dialysis. A high-salt diet can also cause extensive renal damage in Dahl-SS rats. Therefore, this is an excellent animal model for studying salt-induced renal damage in humans. A previous study showed that long-term infusion of purified rat tissue kallikrein via minipump attenuated glomerular sclerosis without affecting blood pressure in Dahl-SS rats on a high-salt diet *(78,79)*. The protective effect of kallikrein protein infusion was blocked by icatibant, indicating that the tissue kallikrein via kinin B2 receptor could exert a direct effect in protection against salt-induced renal lesions, independent of blood pressure reduction. Consistent with this finding, we showed that adenovirus-mediated kallikrein gene delivery enhanced renal function in Dahl-SS, 2K1C, and 5/6 nephrectomy hypertensive rats as evidenced by increases in renal blood flow, urine flow, glomerular filtration rates, electrolyte output, and urine excretion *(68,69,80)*. Moreover, kallikrein gene delivery not only attenuated salt-induced renal injury, but also partially reversed pre-existing renal lesions induced by high-salt loading *(80)*. This unique ability of kallikrein to repair renal tubular damage may have general implications, because we also observed a similar renal protection in normotensive rats with gentamycin-induced nephrotoxicity *(81)*. Our recent studies have shown that the protective effect of kallikrein on salt- and drug-induced renal injury was accompanied by reduced oxidative stress and inflammation, suggesting a potential role of the KKS in inhibiting oxidative stress and inflammation *(82,83)*.

4.3. Vascular Injury by Kallikrein Gene Delivery

We have shown that kallikrein gene transfer or kinin peptide inhibited the proliferation of cultured vascular smooth muscle cells *(84)*. Infection of the isolated aortic segments with adenovirus containing the human tissue kallikrein gene resulted in a time-dependent secretion of recombinant human kallikrein, which coincided with significant increases in NO and cGMP levels *(85)*. To further investigate the role of kallikrein–kinin in vascular injury, human tissue kallikrein gene was delivered locally into the rat left common carotid artery after balloon angioplasty. Kallikrein gene delivery resulted in a significant reduction in intima/media ratio at the injured vessel compared to the rats receiving control virus *(84,85)*. The inhibitory effect of kallikrein on neointima formation was blocked by L-NAME, an NO synthase inhibitor, and by icatibant, indicating a kinin–NO-dependent event. Moreover, systemic delivery of the kallikrein gene into a mouse model of arterial remodeling induced by permanent alteration in shear-stress conditions resulted in a reduction of neointima formation *(86)*. The protective action of kallikrein gene transfer was significantly reduced in kinin B2 knockout mice, but amplified in transgenic mice expressing human kinin B2 receptor, compared to wild-type mice *(86)*. In streptozotocin-induced diabetic mice, local delivery of the human tissue kallikrein gene halted the progression of microvascular rarefaction in hindlimb skeletal muscle by inhibiting apoptosis and promoting vascular regeneration *(87)*. Taken together, these results provide new insights into the role of the KKS in the vasculature and may have significant implications for therapeutic intervention in treating restenosis and atherosclerosis.

4.4. Hypertension-Induced Stroke

Hypertension is a critical factor in the development of stroke in humans and animal models. In stroke-prone spontaneously hypertensive rats (SHR-SP), high-salt intake accelerates the development of malignant hypertension *(88)*. In the brains of SHR-SP, fibrinoid necrosis and associated thrombosis primarily affect cerebral arterioles, leading to their obstruction and infarction, whereas cerebral hemorrhage is caused by micro-aneurysms *(89)*. A high dose of cerivastatin, a HMG-CoA reductase inhibitor, protected against hypertension-induced stroke and ameliorated stroke-associated symptoms, which were accompanied by reduced superoxide production and inflammatory cell infiltration to the stroke lesion in SHR-SP *(90)*. Lovastatin and simvastatin have also been shown to reduce brain injury during cerebral ischemia via upregulation of eNOS *(91)*. Moreover, a lethal form of hypertension develops in Dahl-SS rats fed a high-salt diet at an early age *(92)*. Pathological changes in the brain of Dahl-SS rats affected by stroke include hemorrhage, edema, and infarction. We showed that a single injection of adenovirus carrying the human tissue kallikrein gene into 4-wk-old Dahl-SS rats fed a high salt diet significantly reduced blood pressure elevation, stroke-induced mortality, and aortic hypertrophy, which was accompanied by increased cGMP levels, an indicator of NO formation *(92)*. These combined findings indicate that kallikrein–kinin through NO formation may play a protective role in stroke induced by hypertension.

4.5. Ischemic Stroke

Stroke is the third leading cause of death in the United States. Reperfusion injury is thought to play a critical role in the pathophysiology of cerebral ischemia. We showed that ICV injection of adenovirus containing the human tissue kallikrein gene significantly reduced neurological dysfunction and cerebral infarction after ischemia/reperfusion-induced brain injury *(93)*, and B2 receptor antagonism blocked these protective effects. A potential role of the kinin B1 receptor in ischemic injury has also been implicated. Kinin B1 receptor expression has been reported to be increased in the ischemic brain hemisphere after focal cerebral ischemia *(94)*. Moreover, a brief report showed that injection of a B1 receptor agonist into cerebroventricular space either prior to or at 3 h after cerebral ischemic injury significantly reduced cerebral infarct size at 24 h after middle cerebral artery occlusion (MCAO) *(95)*. Taken together, these results indicate

Table 1
Molecular Genetic Approaches: Tissue Kallikrein–Kinin System in Blood Pressure Regulation

Animal models	Blood pressure	Duration
Transgenic mice		
Human tissue kallikrein	↓	Lifetime
Human kinin B_2 receptor	↓	Lifetime
Transgenic rats		
Human tissue kallikrein	↓	Lifetime
Knockout mice		
Kinin B_2 receptor	↑	
Kinin B_1 receptor	No change	
Tissue kallikrein	No change	
Somatic delivery of the kallikrein gene in rats		
SHR	↓	6–8 wk
Dahl-SS	↓	4 wk
Two-kidney, one-clip	↓	4 wk
DOCA-salt	↓	4 wk
5/6 Nephroctomy	↓	5 wk
Fructose-induced diabetes	↓	4 wk
Antisense inhibition in SHR		
Kininogen	↑	24 h
Kinin B_2 receptor	↑	24 h
Kinin B_1 receptor	↓	4 d

that kallikrein–kinin, through kinin B2 and/or B1 receptor signaling, may play a protective role in ischemic brain injury. Stroke-induced neurological deficits and mortality are often associated with timing of treatment after the onset of stroke. Our recent studies showed that intravenous delivery of the kallikrein gene at 8 h and 3 d after MCAO significantly reduced neurological deficit scores and cerebral infarction. The results indicate that the blood–brain barrier is still open at 3 d after cerebral artery occlusion. Neuroprotection mediated by kallikrein was accompanied by the inhibition of inflammation and apoptosis and promoting the survival and growth of neuronal and endothelial cells. Similarly, a continuous supply of tissue kallikrein via protein infusion through a minipump protects against ischemia/reperfusion-induced neurological dysfunction and cerebral infarction after MCAO, and icatibant abolished these beneficial effects. These results indicate that kallikrein–kinin protects against cerebral ischemic injury after ishemic stroke by inhibiting inflammation and apoptosis, and promoting angiogenesis and neurogenesis.

5. MULTIPLE ROLES OF KALLIKREIN–KININ IN HYPERTENSION, CARDIOVASCULAR AND RENAL DISEASE, AND STROKE

Using strategies of transgenic and somatic gene transfer, as well as protein infusion approaches to achieve a continuous supply of kallikrein–kinin in vivo, we have shown that the KKS plays an important protective role in the development of hypertension in several animal models (Table 1). In addition to blood pressure reduction, kallikrein gene delivery or kallikrein protein infusion improves cardiac, renal and neurological functions,

Table 2
Kallikrein Gene Delivery or Protein Infusion Attenuates Cardiovascular
and Renal Injuries and Stroke in Hypertensive and Normotensive Animal Models

Rat models	Cardiac remodeling	Renal injury	Stenosis	Stroke
SHR	↓	–	–	–
Dahl-SS	↓	↓	–	↓
DOCA-Salt	↓	↓	–	–
2K1C	↓	↓	–	–
5/6 Nephrectomy	↓	↓	–	–
Angioplasty	–	–	↓	–
Myocardial I/R	↓	–	–	–
MCAO/reperfusion	–	–	–	↓

and protects against cardiovascular, renal and cerebral injuries in hypertensive and normotensive animal models with cardiovascular and renal diseases (Table 2). Our studies
demonstrated that kallikrein gene delivery exhibits beneficial effects in the heart, kidney, blood vessel, and brain in various animal models. These include blood pressure
reduction; attenuation of renal injury, cardiac infarction, and cardiac remodeling; inhibition of neointimal formation in blood vessels after balloon angioplasty; and reduction of
stroke-induced mortality and cerebral infarction. Taken together, our results indicate
that kallikrein–kinin therapy may have significant therapeutic potential for treating
cardiovascular and renal diseases induced by hypertension, ischemia/reperfusion and
high-salt intake.

ACKNOWLEDGMENTS

This work was supported by the National Institutes of Health grants HL-29397 and
DK-066350.

REFERENCES

1. Bhoola, K. D., Figueroa, C. D., and Worthy, K. (1992) Bioregulation of kinins: kallikreins, kininogens,
   and kininases. *Pharmacol. Rev.* **44,** 1–80.
2. Marceau, F. (1995) Kinin B1 receptors: a review. *Immunopharmacology* **30,** 1–26.
3. Regoli, D., Gobeil, F., Nguyen, Q. T., et al. (1994) Bradykinin receptor types and B2 subtypes. *Life
   Sci.* **55,** 735–749.
4. Regoli, D., Rhaleb, N. E., Drapeau, G., and Dion, S. (1990) Kinin receptor subtypes. *J. Cardiovasc.
   Pharmacol.* **15,** S30–S38.
5. Madeddu, P., Glorioso, N., Maioli, M., et al. (1991) Regulation of rat renal kallikrein expression by
   estrogen and progesterone. *J. Hypertens. Suppl.* **9,** S244–S245.
6. Rosewicz, S., Detjen, K., Logsdon, C. D., Chen, L. M., Chao, J., and Riecken, E. O. (1991) Glandular
   kallikrein gene expression is selectively down-regulated by glucocorticoids in pancreatic AR42J cells.
   Endocrinology **128,** 2216–2222.
7. Chao, J., Tillman, D. M., Wang, M. Y., Margolius, H. S., and Chao, L. (1986) Identification of a new
   tissue kallikrein-binding protein. *Biochem. J.* **239,** 325–331.
8. Zhou, G. X., Chao, L., and Chao, J. (1992) Kallistatin: a novel human tissue kallikrein inhibitor.
   Purification, characterization, and reactive center sequence. *J. Biol. Chem.* **267,** 25,873–25,880.

9. Chao, J., Chai, K. X., Chen, L. M., et al. (1990) Tissue kallikrein-binding protein is a serpin. I. Purification, characterization, and distribution in normotensive and spontaneously hypertensive rats. *J. Biol. Chem.* **265,** 16,394–16,401.
10. Chao, J., Stallone, J. N., Liang, Y.-M., Chen, L.-M., and Chao, L. (1997) Kallistatin is a potent new vasodilator. *J. Clin. Investig.* **100,** 11–17.
11. Linz, W. and Scholkens, B. A. (1992) Role of bradykinin in the cardiac effects of angiotensin-converting enzyme inhibitors. *J. Cardiovasc. Pharmacol.* **20,** S83–S90.
12. Martorana, P. A., Kettenbach, B., Breipohl, G., Linz, W., and Scholkens, B. A. (1990) Reduction of infarct size by local angiotensin-converting enzyme inhibition is abolished by a bradykinin antagonist. *Eur. J. Pharmacol.* **182,** 395–396.
13. Liu, Y. H., Yang, X. P., Sharov, V. G., et al. (1997) Effects of angiotensin-converting enzyme inhibitors and angiotensin II type 1 receptor antagonists in rats with heart failure. *J. Clin. Investig.* **99,** 1926–1935.
14. Abelous, J. E. and Bardier, E. (1909) Les substances hypotensives de l'urine humaine normale. *CR Soc. Biol. (Paris)* **66,** 511.
15. Frey, E. K. and Kraut, H. (1926) Uber einen von der Niere ausgeschiedenen die Herztatigkeit anregenden Stoff. *Hoppe Seylers Z Physiol. Chem.* **157,** 32.
16. Frey, E. K., Kraut, H., Werle, E., et al. (1968) *Das Kalikrein–Kinin system unnd seine inhibitoren.* Enke Verlag, Stuttgart.
17. Chao, J. and L. Chao. (1995) Biochemistry, regulation and potential function of kallistatin. *Biol. Chem. Hoppe-Seyler* **376,** 705–713.
18. Nustad, K., Pierce, J. V., and Vaaje, K. (1975) Synthesis of kalikreins by rat kidney slices. *Br. J. Pharamcol.* **53,** 229.
19. Elliot, R. and Nuzum, F. (1934) Urinary excretion of a depressor substance (kallikrein of Frey and Kraut) in arterial hypertension. *Endocrinology* **18,** 462–474.
20. Margolius, H. S., Geller, R. G., Pisano, J. J., et al. (1971) Altered urinary kallikrein excretion in human hypertension. *Lancet* **2,** 1063.
21. Keiser, H. R., Margolius, H. S., Brown, R., et al. (1976) Urinary kallikrein in patients with reno-vascular hypertension. In: *Chemistry and Biology of the Kallikrein–Kinin System in Health and Disease* (Pisano, J. J. and Austen, K. F., eds.), US Government Printing Office, Washington, DC, pp. 423–426.
22. Keiser, H. R., Geller, R. G., Margolius, H. S., et al. (1976) Urinary kallikrein in hypertensive animal models. *Fed. Proc.* **35,** 199.
23. Zinner, S. H., Margolius, H. S., Rosner, B., Keiser, H. R., and Kass, E. H. (1976) Familial aggregation of urinary kallikrein concentration in childhood: relation to blood pressure, race and urinary electrolytes. *Am. J. Epidemiol.* **104,** 124–132.
24. Margolius, H. S. (1989) Tissue kallikreins and kinins: regulation and roles in hypertensive and diabetic diseases. *Ann. Rev. Pharmacol. Toxicol.* **29,** 343–364.
25. Zinner, S. H., Margolius, H. S., Rosner, B., and Kass, E. H. (1978) Stability of blood pressure rank and urinary kallikrein concentration in childhood. *Circulation* **58,** 908–915.
26. Berry, T. D., Hasstedt, S. J., Hunt, S. C., et al. (1989) A gene for high urinary kallikrein may protect against hypertension in Utah kindreds. *Hypertension* **13,** 3–8.
27. Favaro, S., Baggio, B., Antonello, A., et al. (1975) Renal kallikrein content of spontaneously hypertensive rats. *Clin. Sci. Mol. Med.* **49,** 69–71.
28. Powers, C. A., Baer, P. G., and Nasjletti, A. (1984) Reduced glandular kallikrein-like activity in the anterior pituitary of the New Zealand genetically hypertensive rat. *Biochem. Biophys. Res. Commun.* **119,** 689–693.
29. Gilboa, N., Rudofsky, U. H., Phillips, M. I., and Magro, A. M. (1989) Modulation of urinary kallikrein and plasma renin activities does not affect established hypertension in the fawn-hooded rat. *Nephron* **51,** 61–66.
30. Maddedu, P., Varoni, M. V., Demontis, M. P., et al. (1997) Kallikrein–kinin system and blood pressure sensitivity to salt. *Hypertension* **29,** 471–477.
31. Bouhnik, J., Richoux, J. P., Huang, H., et al. (1992) Hypertension in Dahl salt-sensitive rats: biochemical and immunohistochemical studies. *Clin. Sci.* **83,** 13–22.
32. Woodley-Miller, C., Chao, J., and Chao, L. (1989) Restriction fragment length polymorphisms mapped in spontaneously hypertensive rats using kallikrein probes. *J. Hypertens.* **7,** 865–871.
33. Pravenec, M., Kren, V., Kunes, J., et al. (1991) Cosegregation of blood pressure with a kallikrein gene family. *Hypertension* **17,** 242–246.

34. Gavras, I. and Gavras, H. (1988) Anti-hormones and blood pressure: bradykinin antagonists in blood pressure regulation. *Kidney Int.* **34,** S60–S62.

35. Majima, M., Mizogami, S., Kuribayashi, Y., Katori, M., and Oh-ishi, S. (1994) Hypertension induced by a nonpressor dose of angiotensin II in kininogen-deficient rats. *Hypertension* **24,** 111–119.

36. Margolius, H. S., Horwitz, D., Geller, R. G., et al. (1974) Urinary kallikrein in normal subjects: relationships to sodium intake and sodium retaining steroids. *Circ. Res.* **35,** 812.

37. Horwitz, D., Margolius, H. S., and Keiser, H. R. (1975) Effects of potassium intake on urinary kallikrein and aldosterone excretion. (Abstract) *Clin. Res.* **23,** 221A.

38. Jin, L., Chao, L., and Chao, J. (1999) Potassium supplement upregulates the expression of renal kallikrein and bradykinin B_2 receptor in spontaneously hypertensive rats. *Am. J. Physiol.* **45,** F476–F484.

39. Ward, R. (1990) Familial aggregation and genetic epidemiology of blood pressure. In: *Hypertension: Pathophysiology, Diagnosis and Management* (Laragh, J. H. and Brenner, B. M., eds.), Raven, New York, pp. 81–100.

40. Elliott, P., Stamler, J., Nichols, R., et al. (1996) Intersalt revisited: further analyses of 24 hour sodium excretion and blood pressure within and across populations. Intersalt Cooperative Research Group. *BMJ* **312,** 1249–1253.

41. Alderman, M. H., Cohen, H., and Madhavan, S. (1998) Dietary sodium intake and mortality: the National Health and Nutrition Examination Survey (NHANES I). *Lancet* **351,** 781–785.

42. Roberts, W. C. (2001) High salt intake, its origins, its economic impact, and its effect on blood pressure. *Am. J. Cardiol.* **88(11),** 1338–1346.

43. Weinberger, M. H., Miller, J. H., Luft, F. C., Grim, C. E., and Fineberg, N. S. (1986) Definitions and characteristics of sodium sensitivity and blood pressure resistance. *Hypertension* **8(Suppl II),** 127–134.

44. Song, Q., Chao, J., and Chao, L. (1997) DNA polymorphisms in the 5′-flanking region of the human tissue kallikrein gene. *Human Genet.* **99,** 727–734.

45. Murphey, L. J., Eccles, W. K., Williams, G. H., and Brown, N. J. (2004) Loss of sodium modulation of plasma kallikreins in human hypertension. *J. Pharmacol. Exp. Ther.* **308,** 1046–1052.

46. Yu, H., Song, Q., Freedman, B. I., et al. (2002) Association of the tissue kallikrein gene promoter with ESRD and hypertension. *Kidney Int.* **61,** 1030–1039.

47. Wang, J., Xiong, W., Yang, Z., et al. (1994) Human tissue kallikrein induces hypotension in transgenic mice. *Hypertension* **23,** 236–243.

48. Song, Q., Chao, J., and Chao, L. (1996) High level of circulating human tissue kallikrein induces hypotension in a transgenic mouse model. *Clin. Exp. Hypertens.* **18,** 975–993.

49. Chao, J. and Chao, L. (1996) Functional analysis of human tissue kallikrein in transgenic mouse models. *Hypertension* **27,** 491–494.

50. Silva, J. A. Jr., Araujo, R. C., Baltatu, O., et al. (2000) Reduced cardiac hypertrophy and altered blood pressure control in transgenic rats with the human tissue kallikrein gene. *FASEB J.* **14,** 1858–1860.

51. Wang, D., Chao, J., and Chao, L. (1997) Hypotension in transgenic mice overexpressing human bradykinin B2 receptor. *Hypertension* **29,** 488–493.

52. Alfie, M. E., Yang, X., Hess, F., and Carretero, O. A. (1996) Salt-sensitive hypertension in bradykinin B2 receptor knockout mice. *Biochem. Biophys. Res. Commun.* **224,** 625–630.

53. Emanueli, C. and Madeddu, P. (1999) Role of the kallikrein–kinin system in the maturation of the cardiovascular phenotype. *Am. J. Hypertens.* **12,** 988–999.

54. Emanueli, C., Maestri, R., Corradi, D., et al. (1999) Dilated and failing cardiomyopathy in bradykinin B(2) receptor knockout mice. *Circulation* **100,** 2359–2365.

55. Pesquero, J. B., Araujo, R. C., Heppenstall, P. A., et al. (2000) Hypoalgesia and altered inflammatory responses in mice lacking kinin B1 receptors. *Proc. Natl Acad. Sci. USA* **97,** 8140–8145.

56. Meneton, P., Bloch-Faure, M., Hagege, A. A., et al. (2001) Cardiovascular abnormalities with normal blood pressure in tissue kallikrein-deficient mice. *Proc. Natl Acad. Sci. USA* **98,** 2634–2639.

57. Madeddu, P., Parpaglia, P. P., Glorioso, N., Chao, J., and Chao, L. (1996) Antisense inhibition of the brain kallikrein–kinin system. *Hypertension* **28,** 980–987.

58. Emanueli, C., Chao, J., Regoli, D., Chao, L., Ni, A., and Madeddu, P. (2000) The bradykinin B_1 receptor participates in the central regulation of blood pressure in spontaneously hypertensive rats. *Br. J. Pharmacol.* **126(8),** 1769–1776.

59. Ogawa, K., Ito, T., Bun, M., Mochizuki, M., and Satake, T. (1985) Effects of orally administered glandular kallikrein on urinary kallikrein and prostaglandin excretion, plasma immunoreactive prostanoids and platelet aggregation in essential hypertension. *Klin. Wochenschr.* **63,** 332–336.

60. Overlack, A., Stumpe, K. O., Kolloch, R., Ressel, C., and Krueck, F. (1981) Antihypertensive effect of orally administered glandular kallikrein in essential hypertension. Results of double blind study. *Hypertension* **3,** I18–I21.
61. Chao, J., Jin, L., Chen, L. M., Chen, V. C., and Chao, L. (1996) Systemic and portal vein delivery of human kallikrein gene reduces blood pressure in hypertensive rats. *Hum. Gene Ther.* **7,** 901–911.
62. Wang, C., Chao, L., and Chao, J. (1995) Direct gene delivery of human tissue kallikrein reduces blood pressure in spontaneously hypertensive rats. *J. Clin. Investig.* **95,** 1710–1716.
63. Xiong, W., Chao, J., and Chao, L. (1995) Muscle delivery of human tissue kallikrein gene reduces blood pressure in hypertensive rats. *Hypertension* **25,** 715–719.
64. Chao, J. and Chao, L. (2002) The role of adrenomedullin in cardiovascular and renal function. *Drug News Perspect* **15,** 511–518.
65. Jin, L., Zhang, J. J., Chao, L., and Chao, J. (1997) Gene therapy in hypertension: adenovirus-mediated kallikrein gene delivery in hypertensive rats. *Hum. Gene Ther.* **8,** 1753–1761.
66. Chao, J., Zhang, J., Lin, K. F., and Chao, L. (1998) Adenovirus-mediated kallikrein gene delivery attenuates hypertension, cardiac hypertrophy and renal injury in Dahl salt-sensitive rats. *Hum. Gene Ther.* **9,** 21–31.
67. Dobrzynski, E., Yoshida, H., Chao, J., and Chao, L. (1999) Adenovirus-mediated kallikrein gene delivery attenuates hypertension and protects against renal injury in deoxycorticosterone-salt rats. *Immunopharmacology* **44,** 57–65.
68. Yayama, K., Wang, C., Chao, L., and Chao, J. (1998) Kallikrein gene delivery attenuates hypertension and cardiac hypertrophy and enhances renal function in Goldblatt hypertensive rats. *Hypertension* **31,** 1104–1110.
69. Wolf, W. C., Yoshida, H., Agata, J., Chao, L., and Chao, J. (2000) Human tissue kallikrein gene delivery attenuates hypertension, renal injury, and cardiac remodeling in chronic renal failure. *Kidney Int.* **58,** 730–739.
70. Zhao, C., Wang, P., Xiao, X., et al. (2003) Gene therapy with human tissue kallikrein reduces hypertension and hyperinsulinemia in fructose-induced hypertensive rats. *Hypertension* **42,** 1026–1033.
71. Wang, T., Li, H., Zhao, C., et al. (2004) Recombinant adeno-associated virus-mediated kallikrein gene therapy reduces hypertension and attenuates its cardiovascular injuries. *Gene Therapy* **11,** 1342–1350.
72. Thongboonkerd, V., Gozal, E., Sachleben, L. R. Jr., et al. (2002) Proteomic analysis reveals alterations in the renal kallikrein pathway during hypoxia-induced hypertension. *J. Biol. Chem.* **277,** 34,708–34,716.
73. Farhy, R. D., Carretero, O. A., Ho, K. L., and Scicli, A. G. (1993) Role of kinins and nitric oxide in the effects of angiotensin converting enzyme inhibitors on neointima formation. *Circ. Res.* **72,** 1202–1210.
74. Bledsoe, G., Chao, L., and Chao, J. (2003) Kallikrein gene delivery attenuates cardiac remodeling and promotes neovascularization in spontaneously hypertensive rats. *Am. J. Physiol. Heart Circ. Physiol.* **285,** H1479–H1488.
75. Agata, J., Chao, L., and Chao, J. (2002) Kallikrein gene delivery improves cardiac reserve and attenuates remodeling after myocardial infarction. *Hypertension* **40,** 653–659.
76. Yoshida, H., Zhang, J. J., Chao, L., and Chao, J. (2000) Kallikrein gene delivery attenuates myocardial infarction and apoptosis after myocardial ischemia and reperfusion. *Hypertension* **35,** 25–31.
77. Yin, H., Chao, L., and Chao, J. (2001) Kallikrein–kinin protects against myocardial apoptosis after ischemia and reperfusion via activation of Akt-Bad-14-3-3 and Akt-GSK-3 signaling pathways. High Blood Pressure Council, September 23–26, 2001, Washington, DC, Abstract #P75, p. 66.
78. Uehara, Y., Hirawa, N., Kawabata, Y., et al. (1994) Long-term infusion of kallikrein attenuates renal injury in Dahl salt-sensitive rats. *Hypertension* **24,** 770–777.
79. Hirawa, N., Uehara, Y., Suzuki, T., et al. (1999) Regression of glomerular injury by kallikrein infusion in Dahl salt-sensitive rats is a bradykinin-B2-receptor-mediated event. *Nephron* **81,** 183–193.
80. Chao, J., Zhang, J. J., Lin, K. F., and Chao, L. (1998) Adenovirus-mediated kallikrein gene delivery reverses salt-induced renal injury in Dahl salt-sensitive rats. *Kidney Int.* **54,** 1250–1260.
81. Murakami, H., Yayama, K., Chao, L., and Chao, J. (1998) Human kallikrein gene delivery protects against gentamycin-induced nephrotoxicity in rats. *Kidney Int.* **53,** 1305–1313.
82. Zhang, J. J., Bledsoe, G., Kato, K., Chao, L., and Chao, J. (2004) Tissue kallikrein attenuates salt-induced renal fibrosis by inhibition of oxidative stress. *Kidney Int.* **66,** 722–732.
83. Bledsoe, G., Crickman, S., Xia, C. F., Murakami, H., Chao, L., and Chao, J. (2006) Kallikrein/kinin protects against gentamicin-induced nephrotoxicity by inhibition of inflammation and apoptosis. *Nephrol. Dial Transplant.* **21(3),** 624–633.

84. Murakami, H., Yayama, K., Miao, R. Q., Wang, C., Chao, L., and Chao, J. (1999) Kallikrein gene delivery inhibits vascular smooth muscle cell growth and neointima formation in the rat artery after balloon angioplasty. *Hypertension* **34,** 164–170.

85. Murakami, H., Miao, R. Q., Chao, L., and Chao, J. (1999) Adenovirus-mediated kallikrein gene transfer inhibits neointima formation via increased production of nitric oxide in rat artery. *Immunopharmacology* **44,** 137–143.

86. Emanueli, C., Salis, M. B., Chao, J., et al. (2000) Adenovirus-mediated human tissue kallikrein gene delivery inhibits neointima formation induced by interruption of blood flow in mice. *Arterioscler. Thromb. Vasc. Biol.* **20,** 1459–1466.

87. Emanueli, C., Salis, M. B., Pinna, A., et al. (2002) Prevention of diabetes-induced microangiopathy by human tissue kallikrein gene transfer. *Circulation* **106,** 993–999.

88. Takeda, Y., Yoneda, T., Demura, M., Furukawa, K., Miyamori, I., and Mabuchi, H. (2001) Effects of high sodium intake on cardiovascular aldosterone synthesis in stroke-prone spontaneously hypertensive rats. *J. Hypertens.* **19,** 635–639.

89. Richer, C., Vacher, E., Fornes, P., and Giudicelli, J. F. (1997) Antihypertensive drugs in the stroke-prone spontaneously hypertensive rat. *Clin. Exp. Hypertens.* **19,** 925–936.

90. Kawashima, S., Yamashita, T., Miwa, Y., et al. (2003) HMG-CoA reductase inhibitor has protective effects against stroke events in stroke-prone spontaneously hypertensive rats. *Stroke* **34,** 157–163.

91. Endres, M., Laufs, U., Huan, Z., et al. (1998) Stroke protection by 3-hydroxy-3-methylglutaryl (HMG)-CoA reductase inhibitors mediated by endothelial nitric oxide synthase. *Proc. Natl Acad. Sci. USA* **95,** 8880–8885.

92. Zhang, J. J., Chao, L., and Chao, J. (1999) Adenovirus-mediated kallikrein gene delivery reduces aortic thickening and stroke-induced death rate in Dahl salt-sensitive rats. *Stroke* **30,** 1925–1931.

93. Xia, C. F., Yin, H., Borlongan, C. V., Chao, L., and Chao, J. (2004) Kallikrein gene transfer protects against ischemic stroke by promoting glial cell migration and inhibiting apoptosis. *Hypertension* **43,** 1–8.

94. Sloan, K. E., Relton, J. K., Frew, E. M., and Whalley, E. T. (2001) Upregulation of kinin B1 receptor expression after cerebral ischemia in the rat. Society for Neuroscience Meeting, November 10–15, 2001, San Diego, CA, Abstract #332.7.

95. Frew, E. M., Relton, J. K., Sloan, K. E., and Whalley, E. T. (2001) Bradykinin B1 receptor activation protects against ischemic brain injury after transient MCAO in the rat. Society for Neuroscience Meeting, November 10–15, 2001, San Diego, CA, Abstract #332.8.

V   OTHER HORMONAL SYSTEMS AND HYPERTENSION

17 Physiology of Natriuretic Peptides and Their Receptors

Kailash N. Pandey

CONTENTS

1. INTRODUCTION

Initial discovery by de Bold et al. *(1)* demonstrated that atrial extracts contained natriuretic activity that led to isolate "atrial natriuretic factor/peptide (ANF/ANP)." ANP is the first described member in the natriuretic peptide (NP) hormone family, which elicits natriuretic, diuretic, vasorelaxant, and antimitogenic effects, all of which are largely directed to the reduction of fluid volume and blood pressure *(2,3)*. Later, two other members, brain natriuretic peptide (BNP) and C-type natriuretic peptide (CNP) were identified, which also exhibit biochemical and structural characteristics similar to ANP, but each derived from a separate gene *(4)*. Although ANP, BNP, and CNP have highly homologous structure, they bind to specific cell surface receptors and elicit some discrete biological functions *(3,5)*. Three subtypes of NP receptors, namely natriuretic peptide receptor-A, -B, and -C (NPRA, NPRB, and NPRC, respectively) have been identified. NPRA and NPRB contain an extracellular ligand binding domain, a single

From: *Contemporary Endocrinology: Hypertension and Hormone Mechanisms*
Edited by: R. M. Carey © Humana Press Inc., Totowa, NJ

transmembrane region, and cytoplasmic protein kinase-like homology domain (KHD) and guanylyl cyclase (GC) catalytic domain *(6,7)*. Interestingly, both ANP and BNP activate NPRA, which produces second messenger cGMP in response to hormone binding; however, CNP activates NPRB, which also produces cGMP, but all three natriuretic peptides indiscriminately bind to NPRC, which lacks GC catalytic activity *(5,8,9)*. NPRA serves as the principal receptor of ANP and BNP, and most of the physiological effects of these peptide hormones are triggered by generation of second messenger cGMP *(10,11)*. In the kidney, ANP increases glomerular filtration rate, suppresses Na^+-reabsorption at the collecting duct, and inhibits renin release. ANP also inhibits the secretion of aldosterone and vasopressin. These actions of ANP stimulate natriuresis and diuresis *(3)*. In the vasculature, ANP relaxes angiotensin II (ANG II) norepinephrine, and K^+-induced vascular smooth muscle cell contraction, causing immediate vasorelaxant effect *(3)*. The activity and expression of NPRA are regulated by a number of factors, including the ligand itself *(12–14)*. The studies with *Npr1* (coding for NPRA) gene-targeting in mice have revealed the hallmark significance of NPRA in the control of blood pressure and role in cardiovascular disease states *(15,16)*. Mice lacking NPRA develop severe cardiac hypertrophy, fibrosis, and dilatation, which are reminiscent of heart disease as seen in untreated human hypertensive patients *(15)*. The potential significance of CNP/NPRB is believed in vasodilation and localized to vasculature especially to vessel walls *(17)*. It is considered that regulated expression of CNP derived from endothelial cells targets NPRB on adjacent smooth muscle cells *(18)*. Thus, the principal role of CNP is considered as a direct vasodilator involved in the regulation of vascular tone through targeting of NPRB on smooth muscle cells in arteries and veins *(17,19)*. The objective of this current review is to summarize and document the previous findings and recent discoveries of natriuretic peptides and receptor systems with particular emphasis on cellular signaling, and physiological and pathological significance in control of blood pressure and cardiovascular homeostasis.

2. STRUCTURE AND MOLECULAR PROPERTIES OF NATRIURETIC PEPTIDES

ANP, primarily synthesized in the granules of heart atrium; BNP, initially isolated from the brain, but predominantly present in the heart and displays most variability in the primary structure; and CNP, isolated from porcine brain are highly conserved among the species *(4)*. All three NPs contain highly conserved residues with a 17-member disulfide ring but deviate from each other in flanking sequences. The primary structure deduced from cDNAs suggested that ANP is synthesized first as the 152-amino-acid prepro-ANP that contained sequences of active peptides in its carboxyl-terminal region, and major form of circulatory ANP is a 28-residue molecule *(20–22)*. Different lengths of sequences of ANP were synthesized in studies on structure–activity relationship, and it was indicated that the ring conformation of ANP molecule with a disulfide-bonded loop is essential for its activities *(3,23)*. Furthermore, the carboxyl-terminal sequence extending from the ring structure to Asn–Phe–Arg–Tyr is also required for the biological activity of ANP. The amino acid sequence of ANP is almost identical across the mammalian species, except at position 10 which is isoleucine in rat, mouse, and rabbit; however, in human, dog, and bovine, ANPs have methionine at this position *(23)*.

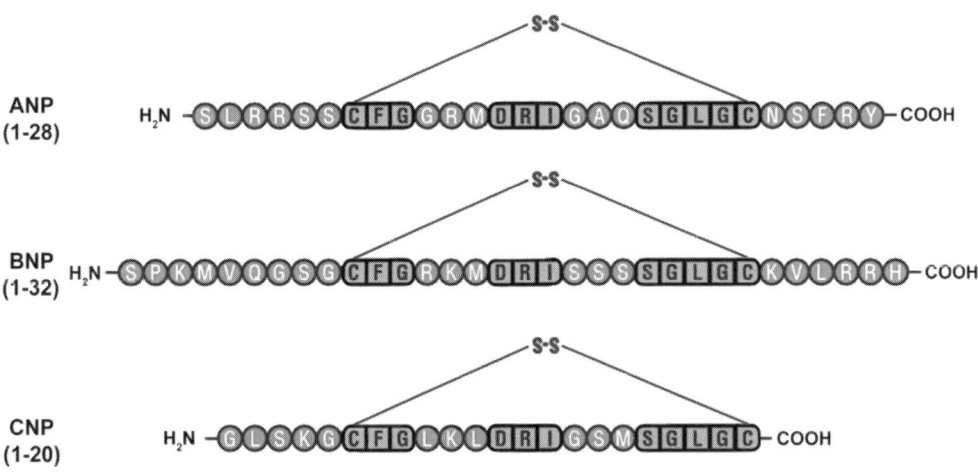

Fig. 1. Amino acid sequence and structure of natriuretic peptides. The sequence comparison of the mature human ANP, BNP, and CNP with conserved residues represented by darkened square boxes. The lines between the two cysteine residues in each natriuretic peptide (ANP, BNP, and CNP) indicate a 17-residue disulfide bridge, essential for biological activity. ANP, atrial natriuretic peptide; BNP, brain natriuretic peptide; and CNP, C-type natriuretic peptid.

The biologically active ANP is produced by proteolytic cleavage of pro-ANP molecule into the predominant 28-amino acid ANP (residues 99–126) and the inactive ANP (residues 1–98). The active form of ANP has disulfide-bonded loop between cysteine 105 and cysteine 121, essential for the biological activity *(3,23)*. All ANP analogs with natriuretic or diuretic activity share this common central ring structure *(24,25)*. Subsequently, BNP *(26)* and CNP *(27)* were both isolated from porcine brain extracts on the basis of their potent relaxant effects. Soon, it was established that BNP is predominantly synthesized and secreted from the heart *(28)*. Similarly, CNP is predominantly localized in the central nervous system and endothelial cells and is considered a noncirculatory natriuretic peptide hormone *(29)*. Like ANP, both BNP and CNP are synthesized from large precursor molecules and the mature bioactive peptides contain 17-residue loop bridged by an intramolecular disulfide bond. In essence, 11 of these amino acids are identical in biologically active ANP, BNP, and CNP; however, the amino- and carboxyl-terminus vary in length and composition (Fig. 1). Among the species, BNP exhibits most variability in primary structure, and both ANP and CNP are highly conserved across the species. The mechanisms of action of NPs in relation to their structure and physiology are not well understood. A large body of work has been accumulated to define the essential functional parameters of NPs to elicit the biological responsiveness.

3. SYNTHESIS AND SECRETION OF NATRIURETIC PEPTIDES

Indeed, the three natriuretic peptides ANP, BNP, and CNP have highly homologous structure, but they have distinct sites of synthesis. Both ANP and BNP are predominantly synthesized in the heart, and ANP concentrations range from 50- to 100-fold higher than BNP. The atrium is the primary site of synthesis for both hormones within the heart; however, ventricle also produces both ANP and BNP but at the level 100- to 1000-fold less than the atrium, respectively. It has been observed that the difference in the natriuretic peptide concentrations also correlate with mRNA levels *(30)*. Interestingly, the expression of both ANP and BNP increases dramatically in both the atrium and the ventricle in cardiac hypertrophy *(31,32)*, nevertheless, the ventricle becomes the primary site of synthesis and release for BNP. In patients with severe congestive heart failure (CHF), the concentrations of both ANP and BNP increase higher than control values; however, the BNP concentrations increase 10- to 50-fold higher than a comparative increase in ANP concentrations *(31)*. These findings indicated that ANP and BNP elicit distinct physiological and pathophyiological effects. In essence, ANP and BNP show similar hemodynamic responses, whereas BNP exerts a longer duration of action and causes enhanced rather than blunted natriuretic responses as compared with ANP *(32,33)*. On the contrary, it has also been shown that the amino-terminal pro-ANP is a better diagnostic tool than BNP to assess left ventricular systolic dysfunction *(34)*.

Cardiac atrium expresses almost 50- to 100- fold or even higher ANP mRNA levels as compared with extracardiac tissues *(35)*. Interestingly, higher ventricular ANP is present in the developing embryo and fetus, nevertheless, both mRNA and peptide levels of ANP decline rapidly during the prenatal period *(36)*. However, ANP gene expression in ventricle is postnatally reinducible in response to phenylephrine administration, after-load stress, and myocardial infarction *(37)*. Indeed, the mRNA levels of BNP are markedly lower than ANP in heart; however, the BNP concentrations are higher in the ventricle as compared with both neonatal and adult rat hearts, but the reduction in the ventricular expression of BNP is far less than ANP in the adult hearts *(38)*. Although the circulating BNP levels are far less than that of ANP levels in normal subjects, the increase in BNP concentrations in plasma can surpass the level of ANP in patients with CHF *(31,39,40)*. On the contrary, CNP does not seem to behave as a cardiac hormone and its levels are extremely low in the circulation *(41)*. CNP is largely present in the central nervous system *(42)* and in the vascular endothelial cells *(43–46)*. D-type natriuretic peptide (DNP) represents an additional member in the natriuretic peptide hormone family *(47,48)*. DNP is present in the venom of the green mamba (*Dendroaspis angusticeps*) as a 38-amino acid peptide molecule. In addition, a 32-amino acid peptide termed urodilatin (URO) is identical to C-terminal sequence of pro-ANP and appears to be present only in urine *(49,50)*. It was initially purified from human urine and is presumed to be only synthesized in the kidney *(51)*. URO is not present in the circulation and appears to be a unique intrarenal natriuretic peptide with unexplored physiological significance *(51,52)*.

4. IDENTIFICATION AND STRUCTURE DETERMINATION OF NATRIURETIC PEPTIDE RECEPTORS

Initial crosslinking and photoaffinity labeling studies showed the existence of ANP receptors with a wide range of molecular weight (M_r) of 60–180 kDa, and were identified by sodium dodecyl sulfate polyacrylamide gel electrophoresis (SDS-PAGE) and autoradiography from different cells and tissue types. Photoaffinity labeling studies showed the specific labeling of a single protein band of ANP receptor with apparent M_r of 125 kDa in plasma membranes of bovine adrenal cortex *(53)*, and with 135–140 kDa of kidney cortex *(54)*, Leydig tumor (MA-10) cells *(55)*, and neuroblastoma cells *(56)*.

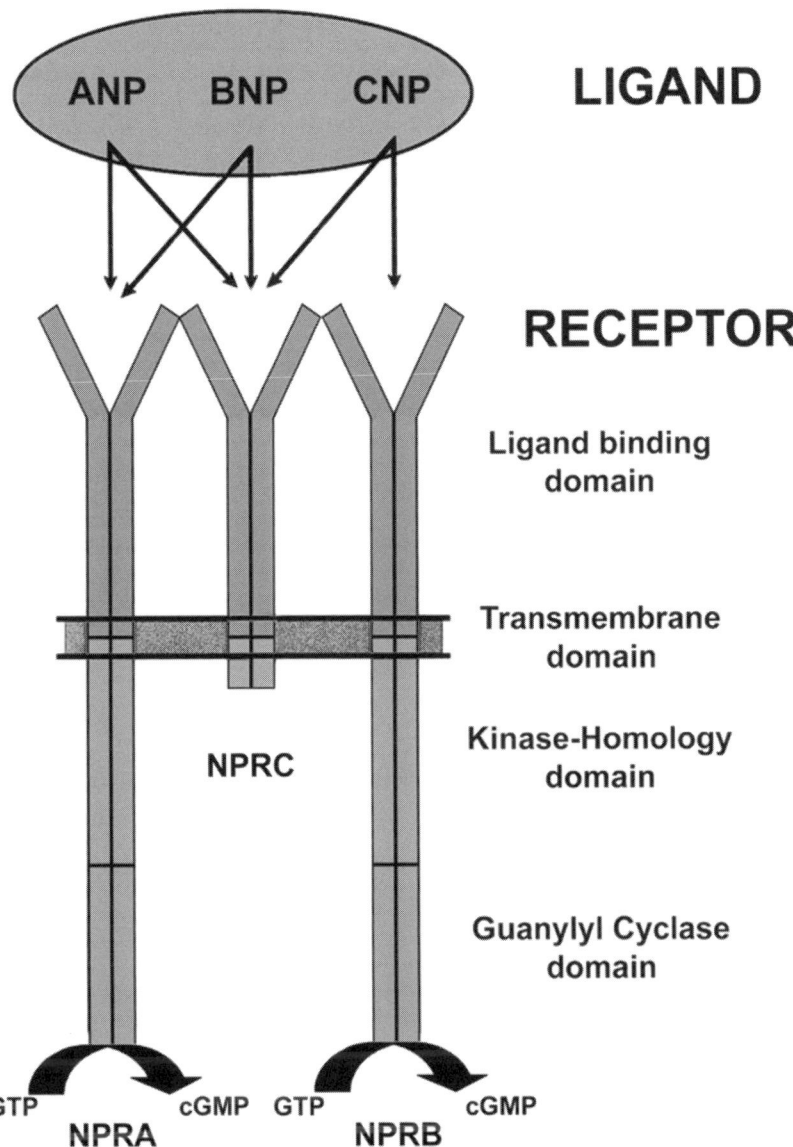

Fig. 2. Ligand specificity and transmembrane models for the natriuretic peptide receptors. A schematic representation of the natriuretic peptides to specifically activate the natriuretic peptide receptors; NPRA, NPRB, and NPRC as indicated. The solid lines connect the receptors with their preferred ligand. The ligand binding domains, transmembrane regions, and intracellular domains have been indicated. The NPRA and NPRB are shown to generate the second messenger cGMP. NPRA, natriuretic peptide receptor-A; NPRB, natriuretic peptide receptor-B; and NPRC, natriuretic peptide receptor-C.

In contrast, labeling of additional protein bands, including major radiolabeled protein species of the 60–70 kDa was reported by photoaffinity labeling or affinity crosslinking of ANP receptors in various plasma membrane preparations (57–59) or intact cultured cells (60). Subsequently, high-affinity binding sites for ANP were co-purified with particulate guanylyl cyclase (GC) activity, which indicated that both ANP binding and

Table 1
Soluble and Various Plasma Membrane Forms of Guanylyl Cyclases
With Respective Ligands and Prominent Tissue Distribution

Ligand	Guanylyl cyclases	Tissue-specific distribution
ANP/BNP	GC-A/NPRA	Kidney, adrenal glands, heart, lung vascular bed, ovary, testis, brain, and other tissues
CNP	GC-B/NPRB	Vascular bed, fibroblast, heart, lung adrenal gland, brain, ovary, and other tissues
Guanylin/ uroguanylin/ enterotoxin	GC-C	Colon, intestine, and kidney
Orphan	GC-D	Olfactory neuroepithelium
Orphan	GC-E	Retina, pineal gland
Orphan	GC-F	Retina
Orphan	GC-G	Skeletal muscle, lung, intestine, and kidney
Calcium-binding proteins	ROS-GC	Rod outer segment
Orphan	GC-Y-X1	Sensory neurons of C. elegans
NO, CO	Soluble cyclase	Smooth muscle, platelet, kidney, lung, and other tissues

GC activity reside in the 120- to 180-kDa receptor molecules *(61–65)*. The 70-kDa ANP receptor protein was also isolated and did not have GC catalytic activity *(66,67)*. Initially, ANP receptors were characterized based on the differential binding characteristics and ability to generate second messenger cGMP in response to various lengths of ANP peptides, truncated at the amino and/or carboxyl terminal of 28-residues ANP *(68–70)*. Based on the biological activity of different ANP analogs, ANP receptors were classified as biologically active and clearance or silent receptors *(71)*. Subsequently, different subtypes of ANP receptors were identified by photoaffinity and crosslinking, which appeared to be specific to different cell types *(69,72)*. Intriguing was the finding that, using photoaffinity labeling, three distinct types of natriuretic peptide receptors were classified in different cell types *(69)*. Biochemical, immunohistochemical, and molecular biological data indicated that natriuretic peptides and their receptors are quite widespread in their tissue distributions, suggesting pleiotropic actions at both systemic and local levels *(3,9,69,73,74)*.

Cloning and expression of cDNA led to identify and characterize the primary structure of three distinct subtypes of natriuretic peptide receptors (NPRs), which are currently designated as NPRA *(6,75–77)*, NPRB *(78,79)*, and NPRC *(80)*. The three receptor subtypes (NPRA, NPRB, and NPRC) constitute natriuretic peptide receptor family. The general topological structure of NPRA and NPRB is consistent with at least four distinct domains. As such, the entire coding region of both NPRA and NPRB is separated by a single transmembrane spanning region into extracellular ligand-binding domain and intracellular protein kinase-like homology domain, also referred to as kinase homology domain (KHD) and GC catalytic domain *(6,78)*. NPRA and NPRB are also referred to as GC-A and GC-B, respectively *(7)*. The extracellular ligand-binding domains of NPRA and NPRB show approx 44% sequence identity. Within the intracellular domains of both of these receptors, approx 250-amino acid region of the carboxyl-terminus portion constitutes GC catalytic domain. The KHD constitutes an approx 280-amino acid region that immediately follows the transmembrane spanning region of these receptor proteins. The GC catalytic region has the highest sequence similarity (88%) between NPRA and NPRB; however, KHD has only 60% sequence identity between these two receptors. Although >80% of the conserved amino acid residues that have been found in all protein kinases *(81)* are also present in NPRA and NPRB, the functional significance of this homology of KHD has not yet been established. Whether NPRA and NPRB contain intrinsic protein kinase activity for autophosphorylation or to phosphorylate other cellular proteins is not yet known. The comparison of the amino acid sequences indicates 62% identity among NPRA and NPRB proteins. Intracellular regions appear more highly conserved than extracellular domains of these two receptors (78 vs 43%). The nucleotide sequence in the kinase domain is less conserved between NPRA and NPRB than the sequence in the GC catalytic domain of these receptors.

The third member of the natriuretic peptide receptor family, NPRC, constitutes a large extracellular domain of 496-amino acids, a single transmembrane domain, and a very short 37-amino acid cytoplasmic tail that bears no homology domain of any other known receptor proteins. The extracellular region of NPRC is approx 30% identical to NPRA and NPRB. Ligand receptor binding studies have shown that NPRC has much less stringent specificity for structural variants of ANP than does NPRA or NPRB *(82)*. The extracellular domain of NPRC possesses two pairs of cysteine residues along with one isolated cysteine near the transmembrane domain, three potential signals for N-glycosylation, and several serines and threonines for the O-linked glycosylation sites *(80)*. Earlier, it was proposed that NPRC may function as a clearance receptor to remove natriuretic peptides from the circulation *(71)*; however, a number of studies provide the evidence that NPRC plays roles in biological action of natriuretic peptides *(83–85)* and clearance name carries only by a default nomenclature to NPRC.

The transmembrane GC receptors contain a single cyclase catalytic active site per polypeptide molecule; however, based on the structure modeling data *(86)*, two polypeptide chains seem to be required to activate the function of NPRA *(87–89)*. The dimerization region of the receptor has been suggested to be located between the KHD and GC catalytic domain that have been predicted to form an amphipathic alpha helix structure *(90)*. The NPRB has the overall domain structure similar to that of NPRA with binding selectivity to CNP, also generates the second messenger cGMP *(10,17,90–93)*. NPRA is the dominant form of the natriuretic peptide receptors found in peripheral organs and mediates most of the known actions of ANP and BNP. Whereas NPRB is localized mainly in the brain and vascular tissues, it is thought to mediate the actions of CNP in the central nervous systems and also in vascular bed.

There have been other members of the membrane-bound GC receptor family including the first cloned sea urchin GC receptor *(94)*, sea urchin egg peptide receptor *(95)*, heat-stable enterotoxin, and endogenous peptide guanylin and uroguanylin receptors *(10)*. Recently, additional members of GC family of receptors have been identified by homology-based cDNA library screening. Interestingly, those include retinal-GC or rod outer segment membrane GC (ROS-GC), or ret-GC receptor *(96,97)*, GC-D receptor in olfactory sensory neurons *(98)*, GC-E and GC-F receptors in eyes *(99)*; GC-G receptor in peripheral tissues such as lung, and GCY-X1 receptor in sensory neurons of *Caenorhabditis elegans* along with more than 29 other similar gene products that have been identified *(100,101)*. Most of these receptor proteins are considered orphan members of GC-coupled receptor family, as their ligands have not yet been identified. These orphan receptor proteins constitute overall molecular configuration similar to that of NPRA. The molecular cloning of the ROS-GC or retinal-GC showed that this subspecies GC receptors was distinct from the cell surface receptor subfamily and functions in transducing Ca^{2+} signals arising within the sensory neurons. The cloned enzyme was unresponsive to ANP and CNP, and showed minimal sequence identity (30%) with NPRA and NPRB *(11)*. This new subfamily of receptor is suggested to transduce the Ca^{2+} signals arising inside the sensory neurons of the retina instead of the transduction of the peptide signals arising outside the cells. Thus, it is expected that several of the members of GC receptor family could provide new and unexpected mechanism of functions in this emerging field of natriuretic peptide family of receptors.

5. TRANSMEMBRANE SIGNAL TRANSDUCTION MECHANISMS

Initial studies showed that ANP markedly increases cGMP in target tissues in a dose-related manner *(102–105)*. The production of cGMP is believed to result from ANP binding to the extracellular domain of NPRA, which probably allosterically regulates an increased specific activity of the receptor *(8,11,12,14,73,90)*. Previous findings have indicated that binding of ANP to the receptor by itself is probably not sufficient to stimulate GC catalytic activity and requires ATP *(106–108)*. Because the nonhydrolyzable analogs of ATP mimicked ANP effect, it was suggested that ATP acts directly by allosteric regulation of GC catalytic activity of NPRA. The ligand binding and the interaction of ATP with the KHD increase the cGMP production without affecting the affinity for the substrate *(106,109–111)*. Overexpression and isolation of NPRA demonstrated that GC catalytic domain cannot be activated by ANP alone without ATP-binding to KHD region of NPRA *(107,112,113)*. Further studies provided the essential evidence that ATP binding to KHD of the receptor is important for receptor effectors coupling of GC family of receptors *(11,108,114)*. Deletion of the KHD of NPRA and NPRB receptors also suggested that KHD represses the GC catalytic activity of these receptors *(5,115)*. Both NPRA and NPRB contain a glycine-rich ATP binding motif within the KHD which is known as glycine-rich cluster sequence *(108,111,116)*. It has been suggested that the glycine-rich sequence motif is critical in ATP binding and ANP signaling of NPRA family of receptors. The glycine-rich motif of receptor has also been named as the ATP-regulatory module (ARM) and the sequence of the motif includes: Gly–Arg–Gly–Ser–Asn–Tyr–Gly *(108)*. The similar counterpart glycine-rich sequence is also present in the NPRB cDNA sequence. Intriguing was the finding that respective glycine-rich sequence motif has been shown to be interchangeable, functionally identical and is critical in the ATP-dependent transduction activities of both NPRA and NPRB transmembrane receptors *(116)*. Furthermore, site-directed mutagenesis studies pointed out that the middle Gly in the glycine-rich region seems to be critical in both the formation of the ATP-binding pocket and signaling process of GC family of NP receptors *(116)*. These investigators suggested that there is a tight regulatory control of the transmission of intracellular signal of the receptor during the generation of second messenger cGMP *(11,117,118)*.

It has been suggested that the juxtamembrane hinge structure of NPRA undergoes a significant conformational change in response to ligand binding, and it may play an important role in the transmembrane signaling process *(119)*. The amino acid sequence near the transmembrane region is well conserved in NPRA that contains several closely located proline residues and a pair of cysteine residues. The mutation of one of the proline in this region renders the receptor to bind the ligand but blocks GC catalytic activity of the receptor *(119)*. Similarly, in the juxtamembrane hinge region, the elimination of disulfide bond by cysteine residues resulted in constitutive receptor activation. These findings suggested that juxtamembrane hinge region structure of NPRA may play a critical role in receptor activation and signal transduction mechanisms of GC-coupled receptors. It has also been suggested that glycosylation is essential for ligand binding activity of NPRA *(120–122)*. On the contrary, one study suggested that glycosylation is not essential for ANP binding of NPRA *(123)*. On the other hand in GC-C receptor, all N-linked glycosylation consensus sites have been mutated individually by site-directed mutagenesis to check proper stability and ligand binding which indicated that certain sites might be important for receptor stability *(124)*. The glycosylation sites from GC-coupled receptors are mapped onto the NPRA binding domain structure and have been found to be scattered on the surface of the receptor with the exception of the hormone binding site and dimer interface of the receptor *(125)*. The glycosylation sites in GC-coupled receptors have been implicated to be important for proper folding and stability of the receptor proteins *(120,126,127)*. However, the role of glycosylation sites in the ligand binding of the receptor has not been provided. Nevertheless, the glycosylation of the extracellular domain of NP receptors can be considered of significant importance for receptor orientation and packaging on the cell surface similar to that of other plasma membrane proteins *(128)*. However, it should be noted that there is no appreciable conservation of the precise position of the glycosylation sites within the members of GC-receptor family. Clearly, more experimentation is needed to confirm the functional role of glycosylation in transmembrane signaling of GC-coupled receptors.

The heterogeneity of NP receptors and their diverse cellular distribution suggest that different mechanisms might be involved in the cellular action of NPs *(9,83,129,130)*. ANP has been shown to stimulate the formation of inositol phosphates in cultured vascular smooth muscle cells *(131,132)*, however, in the inner medullary collecting duct cells and in the smooth muscle tissue, ANP stimulated the stimulation of inositol phosphates at lower dosages, and inhibited the generation of these metabolites at higher dosages which increase generation of cGMP *(133,134)*. It has also been shown that ANP inhibits the thrombin-induced synthesis and release of endothelin in cultured rat aortic endothelial cells by blocking the phosphoinositide breakdown *(135,136)*. Murine Leydig tumor (MA-10) cells predominantly overexpress NPRA and treatment of these cells with ANP dramatically decreases the hydrolysis of phosphoinositides *(137)*. The H-8, a specific inhibitor of cGMP-dependent protein kinase, reversed the inhibitory effect of ANP on the generation of inositol phosphates, supporting the involvement of cGMP-dependent protein kinase in this process *(138)*. ANP has also been shown to inhibit both autophosporylation and enzymatic activity of protein kinase C (PKC) in different cell systems *(139–143)*. It is not yet known if the ANP-dependent inhibitory effects on the phosphoinositide metabolism and PKC autophosphorylation and/or enzyme activity are exerted in a composite manner to negatively regulate the phosphoinositide, Ca^{2+}, and PKC cascade system. It is also possible that the effect of ANP is transmitted to block the inositoltrisphosphate (IP3) and Ca^{2+} signaling pathways independently in response to a particular agonist stimulation. It has been suggested that potassium channels can be stimulated by ANP through the activation of PKGs which require ATP and can also be activated by G proteins (144). However, the possible involvement of potassium channels in the ANP-dependent inhibitory response on the generation of inositol phosphates remains to be investigated. It has been shown that NPRC plays a mediatory role in the adenylyl cyclase signal transduction system involving the inhibitory guanine nucleotide-regulatory proteins (G proteins) in aorta (145) and brain (146). Furthermore, ANP has also been shown to interact with phospholipase C via NPRC involving G proteins (134). It has been shown that GTPγS synergistically enhanced the effect of ANP on GC catalytic activity (138,147).

6. INTERNALIZATION, DOWNREGULATION, AND DESENSITIZATION OF NATRIURETIC PEPTIDE RECEPTORS

Internalization and sequestration of hormone receptors have been implicated to play important roles in the process of receptor downregulation. It is anticipated that NPRA is downregulated in response to ANP activation that could be mediated by receptor internalization, sequestration, and metabolic degradation (9,14,118,129). Stoichiometric analyses of the metabolic processing of ANP/NPRA complexes in Leydig tumor (MA-10) cells and PC-12 cells containing endogenous receptors (9,55,148,149), and in COS-7 cells as well as human embryonic kidney-293 (HEK-293) cells expressing recombinant receptors (14,118,129), provided the evidence that a large population of the bound ligand–receptor complexes are internalized, processed intracellularly and degraded products are released into culture medium. Lysosomotropic agents inhibited the degradation of ANP, suggesting that ANP was metabolized in lysosomes. Similarly, studies utilizing PC-12 cells have also indicated that ANP–NPRA complexes are internalized and sequestered into the intracellular compartments (148). On the other hand, it was indicated that in renomedullary interstitial as well as in mesangial cells, ANP–NPRA complexes were not processed intracellularly (150). These authors suggested that a rapid dissociation of ligand–receptor complexes seems to take place upon ANP binding to NPRA at 37°C and intact ligand is released into culture medium. However, it is difficult to some extent to contemplate the findings of those previous studies because the dissociation of ligand was carried out in medium containing high concentrations of unlabeled ANP to preclude the rebinding of dissociated ligand to receptors. The cells utilized in those previous studies, contained more than one receptor subtypes including both NPRA and NPRC (150). Although it has been earlier indicated that in neuroblastoma cell, the bound ligand to NPRA was degraded and released by a neutral metalloendopeptidase on plasma membrane (151). Nevertheless, further studies have not been carried out to confirm those previous results.

The kinetic studies of metabolic processing of ANP involving NPRC that does not contain GC catalytic activity has been reported by several investigators utilizing vascular smooth muscle cells (152–159). The downregulation of NPRC has been shown in cultured vascular smooth muscle cells which predominantly contain this receptor protein

(156,157,159,160–163). The downregulation of NPRC seems to be associated with increased internalization of the ligand–receptors complexes involving receptor-mediated endocytotic mechanisms *(157,164)*. It has been suggested that a portion of the receptor population recycles back to the plasma membrane and newly synthesized receptors reconstitute the receptor population *(157)*. The downregulation of NPRA has also been observed and reported in PC-12 cells containing endogenous receptors *(148)* and in COS-7 and HEK-293 cells containing recombinant receptors *(14,118)*. Thus, down-regulation of NP receptors by ligand-dependent internalization plays an important role in NP receptor signaling and function. The carboxyl-terminal deletion studies of NPRA have suggested that specific sites in the GC catalytic domain and KHD seem to play a critical role in the endocytosis and sequestration of GC-coupled receptor proteins *(118)*. It should be mentioned that a number of studies have also shown that after prolonged treatment of cultured cells with ANP, both receptor density and GC activity are decreased with simultaneous decrease in mRNA levels *(13,165–167)*. In addition, trans-forming growth factor-β1 (TGF-β1), ANG II, and endothelin have also been shown to reduce NPRA mRNA levels in cultured cells *(165,168,169)*. Some of these studies have established that a decrease in mRNA levels of NPRA correlated well with repressed transcriptional activity of NPRA.

It has been suggested that NPRA exists in the phosphorylated state and the addition of ANP causes a decrease in the phosphate contents as well as reduction in the ANP-dependent GC catalytic activity *(170)*. The apparent mechanism of desensitization of NPRA is in contrast to many other cell-surface receptors that appear to be desensitized by phosphorylation *(171–176)*. The initial findings also suggested that ANP seems to stimulate phosphorylation of its GC-coupled receptor protein *(139,177–179)*. Interestingly, the later studies indicated that ANP stimulates the phosphorylation of NPRA which may be essential for receptor activation *(180,181)*. A protein of 55 kDa has been identified that binds specifically to the KHD of NPRA that has been impli-cated in the desensitization of this receptor protein *(182)*. It should be noted that the apparent mechanism of desensitization of NPRA via dephosphorylation is in contrast to G protein-coupled receptors, which seem to be desensitized by a mechanism involving phosphorylation *(174,175)*.

It has recently been indicated that cGMP-dependent protein kinase (PKG), a serine–threonine kinase is capable of phosphorylating NPRA in vitro *(183)*. These authors suggested that PKG is recruited to the plasma membrane after ANP treatment and increases the GC catalytic activity of NPRA. It was further suggested that PKG translocation was ANP-dependent but not nitric oxide dependent. Thus ANP-dependent NPRA–PKG interaction may provide an important mechanism for cGMP-dependent signaling and regulation of receptor function and sensitivity in target cells. However, much remains to be known about the exact molecular regulatory mechanisms of desensitization and signaling pathways of NPRA, which may involve more than one process.

7. RENAL HEMODYNAMICS AND VASCULAR FUNCTIONS

ANP action is perceived to facilitate the excretion of salt and water with an increase in glomerular filtration rate *(3,184–189)*. Renal sites of ANP action include inner medullary collecting duct, glomerulus, and mesangial cells *(190–193)*. The intracellular actions of ANP in renal cells include the stimulation of GC activity and reduction in adenylyl cyclase and phospholipase C activities, sodium influx, and reduced calcium concentrations *(3,83)*. The increased production of cGMP at ANP concentrations affecting renal functions correlates with the effects of dibutyryl-cGMP, which prevents mesangial cell contraction in response to ANG II *(194)*. The most compelling evidence supporting a role for cGMP in mediating the renal effects of ANP was obtained with selective NPRA antagonists, A71915 and HS-121-1, to eliminate the renal effect of infused ANP, including the elevation of urinary cGMP *(195,196)*. These studies established that ANP effect in kidney is largely mediated by cGMP through the activation of NPRA. ANP markedly lowers renin secretion from kidney and also affects plasma renin concentrations *(184,187,197,198)*. Ample experimental data have established that ANP plays an important role in regulation of renal function by its vasodilatory and natriuretic responses and its ability to counteract the renin–angiotensin–aldosterone system (RAAS) in a tissue-specific manner *(187)*. Attempts have been made to define physiological responses in kidney by infusing the exogenous ANP *(199)*. Cardiac appendectomy has been used to prevent ANP release; however, the problem in this setting is that the missing normal cardiac function results in a lack of physiological reflexes that are normally elicited by atrial components *(200)*. Another approach has used monoclonal antibodies against circulating ANP; however, problems are related to nonspecific effect of the antibody or antigen complexes. One of the classical approaches has been taken to specifically inhibit the signaling pathway of NPRA to block cGMP production. Although two compounds, A71917 and HS-140-1, have been shown to diminish the effect of ANP by antagonizing NPRA, however, these compounds do not completely inhibit NPRA activity *(151,201)*. A number of factors influence kidney's ability to excrete sodium and water *(202–205)*. Activation of natriuretic peptides (ANP, BNP) enhances the pressure–natriuresis relationship and reduces atrial pressures. It has also been suggested that chloride-mediated feedback control of NPRA occurs in the kidney and plays a role in ANP-mediated natriuresis *(206)*. Initial as well as recent studies have shown that ANP–NPRA system suppresses renin and decreases blood pressures *(16,184,197,198,207)*.

Gene-targeting strategies in mice provide novel approaches in the study of the physiological responses corresponding to gene-dosage in vivo *(208,209)*. Gene-targeted mice carrying gene disruption or gene duplication have provided strong support for the physiological roles of natriuretic peptides and their receptor systems in kidney function *(15,16,198,210–216)*. The studies with *Npr1* (coding for NPRA) gene-disrupted mice demonstrated that at birth, the absence of NPRA allows greater renin and ANG II levels and increased renin mRNA expression compared with the wild-type mice *(198)*. However, at 3–16 wk of age, both circulating and kidney renin and ANG II levels were decreased dramatically in Npr1 homozygous null mutant mice as compared with wild-type control mice. This decrease in renin activity in adult null mutant mice is implicated because of progressive elevation in arterial pressure leading to inhibition of renin synthesis and release from the kidney juxtaglomerular cells. It has been suggested that increased levels of ANP released into the plasma in response to blood volume expansion is attributed to be mainly responsible for the natriuretic and diuretic responses *(199,203)*. It has also been shown that both ANP and acute blood volume expansion act on the kidney through a similar saturable mechanism *(16,212)*. Recent studies have examined the quantitative contributions and possible mechanisms mediating the responses of varying numbers of *Npr1* gene copies by determining the renal plasma flow (RPF), glomerular filtration rate (GFR), urine flow, and sodium excretion patterns following blood volume expansion in *Npr1* homozygous null mutant (0-copy), wild-type (2-copy), and gene-duplicated (4-copy) mice in an *Npr1* gene-dose-dependent manner *(16)*. By using whole blood, hemodilution did not occur and plasma protein levels were not reduced. Although the blood volume expansion stimulated the release of ANP in all three *Npr1* genotypes of mice, significant functional responses (RPF, GFR, and sodium excretion) occurred only in wild-type (2-copy) and gene-duplicated (4-copy) mice but not in homozygous null mutant (0-copy) mice. These findings demonstrated that the ANP–NPRA axis is primarily responsible for mediating the renal hemodynamic and sodium excretory responses to intravascular blood volume expansion. ANP responses to volume expansion led to the significantly lesser excretion of sodium and water in 0-copy null mutant mice and significantly greater excretory responses along with reduced tubular reabsorption in 4-copy gene-duplicated mice as compared with 2-copy wild-type mice. Similarly, during the volume expansion, urinary cGMP concentration was significantly lower in null mutant mice and greater in 4-copy gene-duplicated mice. These findings established that NPRA is a hallmark receptor, which plays a critical role in mediating the natriuresis, diuresis, and renal hemodynamic responses to acute blood volume expansion.

ANP inhibits aldosterone synthesis and release from adrenal glomerulosa cells *(3,217)* suggesting that this ANP action could be physiologically important, which probably accounts for natriuretic and diuretic effects. The established biochemical and cellular effects of ANP within adrenal glomerulosa cells include the activation of GC activity and potassium channel conductance, whereas T-type calcium channels conductance and adenylyl cyclase activity are suppressed *(83)*. The NPRA antagonist HS-142-1 eliminated ANP effects to suppress the aldosterone synthesis and to elevate cGMP production in bovine adrenal glomerulosa cells, providing additional evidence for the involvement of NPRA in the inhibition of ANP-dependent aldosterone secretion *(218)*. However, the correlative evidence that cGMP suppresses the aldosterone secretion was challenged by the observation that aldosterone release was maintained in the presence of cGMP analogs such as dibutyryl-cGMP or 8-bromo-cGMP *(3,219)*. Further studies suggested that ANP acts via NPRA in the adrenal gland to increase cGMP concentrations, resulting in an activation of cAMP-dependent phosphodiesterases, which decrease both cAMP and aldosterone concentrations in adrenal glands *(220)*.

The studies on the effect of ANP either in intact aortic rings or in cultured vascular smooth muscle cells have always reported an elevation in cGMP. The correlative evidence between ANP-induced cGMP accumulation and vasodilation has suggested the role of cGMP as the second messenger of dilator responses to ANP *(3,13,83)*. ANP as well as cGMP analogs have been found to reduce the agonist-induced increases in cytosolic Ca^{2+} concentrations *(221,222)*. It has been reported that cGMP activates sarcolemmal Ca^{2+}-ATPase, and this mechanism may be important in the ANP-induced decreases in cytosolic Ca^{2+} in vascular smooth muscle cells *(223,224)*. Nevertheless, it is anticipated that the ultimate effect of ANP in vascular smooth muscle cells could be because of the production of cGMP and the activation of cGMP-dependent protein kinases *(143,222)*.

8. ANTIGROWTH AND ANTIPROLIFERATIVE EFFECTS

ANP has been shown to act as a growth suppressor in a variety of cell types including kidney *(225–229)*, heart *(13)*, neurons *(230,231)*, thymus *(232)*, and vasculature *(29,226,231,233–237)*. ANP also inhibits mitogen activation of fibroblasts *(238)*. Interestingly, cGMP analogs mimicked the antiproliferative action of ANP, thus it is considered that ANP exerts the antimitogenic effects largely through the second messenger cGMP *(229,222,236,239)*. ANP has been shown to inhibit collagen synthesis in cardiac fibroblasts *(240)* and also it inhibits hypertrophy in primary cultures of cardiac myocytes *(241–243)*. Similarly, PKG has been shown to suppress extracellular matrix production in vascular smooth muscle cells *(244)*. The expression of ANP and BNP genes is greatly augmented in hypertrophied hearts, which supports the notion that autocrine and/or paracrine effects of ANP–BNP signal play an important role against pathological cardiac hypertrophy in disease states *(242,245)*. The mechanisms of signaling pathways which elicit antimitogenic effect of ANP–NPRA are not yet well characterized. However, both GC-linked NP receptors, NPRA, and NPRB, as well as GC-unlinked NP receptor, NPRC, have been suggested to play a role in ANP-dependent antimitogenic responses *(229,236,246,247)*. Previous studies have demonstrated that ANP inhibits ANG II- and platelet-derived growth factor (PDGF)-dependent MAPK activity in different tissues and cell types *(229,246,247)*. However, the involvement of specific ANP receptor subtypes in the inhibitory effects of ANP on the agonist-stimulated MAPK activity is controversial. Clearly more experimentation is needed to delineate the underlying mechanisms of the antiproliferative effect of ANP in target cells. ANP has been shown to inhibit MAPK activity after stimulation with mitogenic agents; however, the actual mechanism of its inhibitory effect is not well understood. Previous studies have indicated that ANP exerts an inhibitory effect on MAPK activity in kidney mesangial cells in a cGMP-dependent manner *(227)*. However, in astroglial cells, ANP was shown to inhibit extracellular-regulated MAPK (Erk1/2) activity through NPRC *(246)*. In contrast, recent findings have indicated that des-(Cys[105]–Cys[121])-ANP, a ligand selective to NPRC, did not inhibit basal or serum-stimulated MAPK and DNA synthesis in fibroblasts, however, CNP, which acts through NPRB, potently inhibited MAPK activity in fibroblast cells in a cGMP-dependent manner *(238)*. It has been postulated that cGMP-dependent signaling mechanisms of NPRA are initiated probably at the level of gene transcription; however, the exact nature of this activation remains to be elucidated *(13)*. A previous report also indicated that cGMP and PKG signaling increased the MAPK activity in contractile rat vascular smooth muscle cells *(248)*. However, the mechanisms by which cGMP/PKG leads to the activation of MAPKs are unclear. Similarly, cAMP- and cGMP-dependent protein kinases have also been shown both to inhibit as well as to activate MAPK pathways, depending on the cell types and culture conditions *(249)*.

In addition to its antimitogenic effect, ANP has been shown to induce apoptosis in cultured vascular smooth muscle cells and in neonatal rat cardiac myocytes *(250,251)*. ANP-induced apoptotic effect was mimicked by 8-bromo-cGMP, a membrane-permeable analog of cGMP, and by nitroprusside, an activator of soluble guanylyl cyclase. Furthermore, ANP effect was potentiated by a cGMP-specific phosphodiesterase inhibitor zaprinast. It was indicated that norepinephrine, a myocyte growth effector, inhibited ANP-induced apoptosis via activation of β-adrenergic receptor and elevation of cAMP

(251). The existence of a complementary ANP-mediated mechanism to inhibit cell growth is not surprising. The inhibition of cell proliferation is often accompanied by an increased probability of apoptosis, whereas growth-promoting agents tend to promote cell growth and proliferation. For instance, ANG II inhibits apoptosis, in contrast, ANP and nitric oxide, both potently inhibit cell growth and proliferation and induce apoptosis *(251,252)*. It has been suggested that the antiapoptotic Bcl-2 homologue Mcl-1 might serve as an important target in ANP-induced apoptosis of cardiac myocytes. The Bcl-2 homologue Mcl-1 was initially identified as a protein which was upregulated during the differentiation of monocytoid cell line ML-1 cells *(253–255)*. Interestingly, Mcl-1 is expressed at high levels in heart *(251,256)*. However, more experiments are needed to establish a direct causal relationship between ANP effect and apoptosis.

9. ROLE IN PATHOPHYSIOLOGY OF HYPERTENSION AND CARDIOVASCULAR DISORDERS

In response to an increase in atrial distension, ANP is released into the circulation and mediates natriuretic, diuretic, and vasorelaxant effects. High levels of endogenous ANP are thought to compensate the condition of patients with heart failure by reducing preload and afterload. Evidence suggests that a high plasma ANP–BNP level is a prognostic predictor in humans with heart failure *(257–259)*. Studies with ANP-deficient genetic strains of mice demonstrated that a defect in the ANP synthesis can cause hypertension *(210)*. The blood pressures of homozygous null mutant animals were elevated by 8–12 mmHg when they were fed with standard or intermediate salt diets. Heterozygous animals showed normal blood pressures and normal amount of circulatory ANP, however, they became hypertensive and blood pressure was elevated by 20–27 mmHg if these animals were fed with high salt diets *(207,210,260)*. Those previous findings clearly demonstrated that genetically reduced production of ANP can lead to salt-sensitive hypertension. On the other hand, the disruption of *Npr1* gene indicated that the blood pressure of homozygous mutant mice remained elevated and unchanged in response to either minimal or high salt diets *(211)*. These investigators suggested that NPRA may exert its major effect at the level of vasculature and probably does so independently of salt. On the contrary, Oliver et al. *(213)* reported that disruption of *Npr1* gene resulted in chronic elevation of blood pressure in mice fed with high salt diets. Indeed, more studies are needed to clarify the relationship between salt-sensitivity and blood pressures in *Npr1* gene-targeted mice.

Transgenic mice overexpressing ANP developed sustained hypotension with arterial pressure that was 25–30 mmHg lower than their nontransgenic siblings *(189,207,261)*. A recent study demonstrated that somatic delivery of ANP gene in spontaneously hypertensive rat (SHR) induced a sustained reduction of systemic blood pressure, raising the possibility of using ANP as therapeutic agent for treatment of human hypertension *(262)*. Genetic mouse models with disruption of both ANP and NPRA genes have provided strong support for the role of this hormone-receptor system in the regulation of arterial pressure and other physiological functions *(15,16,198,207,210–214,216,263)*. Therefore, the genetic defects that reduce the activity of ANP and its receptor system can be considered as candidate contributors to essential hypertension and CHF *(16,210, 212,216,264,265)*. Interestingly, complete absence of NPRA causes hypertension in mice and leads to altered renin and ANG II levels, cardiac hypertrophy, and lethal vascular events similar to those seen in untreated human hypertensive patients *(15,16,198)*. In contrast, increased expression of NPRA reduces the blood pressure and increases the second messenger cGMP, corresponding to the increasing number of *Npr1* gene copies *(16,213,214)*.

ANP affects blood pressure directly through its natriuretic, diuretic, and vasodilatory actions *(187)*. It also affects blood pressure indirectly, for example, by inhibiting the RAAS, which is known to cause hypertension and cardiovascular diseases, if excessively stimulated *(266)*. Genetic defects that reduce the activity or influence the ANP–NPRA system greatly contribute to the development of hypertension. The mechanistic role of ANP–NPRA system in counteracting the pathophysiology of hypertension is not well understood. Although the expression of ANP and BNP is markedly increased in patients with hypertrophic or failing heart, it is unclear if the NP system is activated to play a protective role by reducing the detrimental effects of high blood pressure caused by sodium retention and fluid volume, inhibiting the RAAS, or it is simply a consequence of the hypertrophic changes occurring in heart. Recent studies indicated that intrarenal renin in newborn *Npr1* homozygous null mutant pups (2 days after birth) was 2.5-fold higher than in 2-copy wild-type counterparts *(198)*. However, adult (16-wk) hypertensive *Npr1* null mutant mice showed 50–70% reduction in plasma renin concentrations and renal renin contents as compared with wild-type control animals. In contrast, the adrenal renin contents and mRNA expression levels were elevated approx 1.5- to 2.0-fold in adult homozygous null mutant mice than wild-type mice. However, the factors that modulate renin gene expression in the adrenal gland have not been clearly identified. Together, the studies in both SHR and *Npr1* gene-knockout hypertensive mouse models suggest that in hypertension, both kidney and circulatory renin concentrations are decreased, however, as a compensatory event, the adrenal renin is increased *(198)*. Thus in light of those previous findings, it can be suggested that ANP–NPRA system may play a key regulatory role in the synthesis and maintenance of both systemic and tissue levels of RAAS components in both physiological and pathological conditions.

Studies in patients with chronic CHF have suggested that their plasma ANP levels decreased, whereas plasma cGMP levels increased significantly from femoral artery to the femoral vein, however, in patients with mild CHF, the plasma cGMP level correlated with ANP level *(257)*. Furthermore, these authors suggested that among patients with severe CHF, plasma cGMP levels reached a plateau despite high levels of plasma ANP, and the molar ratio of cGMP production to ANP in peripheral circulation was significantly lower than those in patients with mild CHF. The findings of those previous studies further indicated that downregulation of NPRA may also occur in the peripheral vascular bed of patients with chronic severe CHF. On the other hand, it is widely believed that ANP concentrations are markedly increased both in cardiac tissues and in plasma of CHF patients *(258,259)*. In hypertrophied heart, ANP and BNP genes are overexpressed, suggesting that autocrine and/or paracrine effects of natriuretic peptides predominate and might serve as an endogenous protective mechanism against maladaptive pathological cardiac hypertrophy *(242,243,265)*. Inactivation of either ANP or *Npr1* gene in mice increases the cardiac mass to a great extent *(15,210)*. A significant inverse relationship has been found between myocardial ANP mRNA expression or peptide levels and increases in left ventricular cardiac mass *(245)*. Those previous findings suggested that ANP expression plays a protective role in hypertrophied heart. Cosegregation analysis of genetic crosses suggested a protective role for ANP against ventricular hypertrophy *(245)*. Those previous findings demonstrated that low ventricular ANP gene expression can be linked genetically to high cardiac mass independently of blood pressure that is consistent with a protective role for ANP against left ventricular cardiac hypertrophy. Furthermore, it has been shown that functional alterations of ANP promoter are linked to cardiac hypertrophy in progenies of crosses between Wistar–Kyoto (WKY) and Wistar–Kyoto-derived hypertensive (WKYH) rats *(267)*. These authors suggested that a single nucleotide polymorphism altered the transcriptional activity of ANP gene promoter, and implicated that ANP may protect cardiomyocytes against hypertrophy as a strong candidate gene for the determination of left ventricular mass. Based on these findings it is speculated that a similar mutation in the NPRA might be of potential significance to elicit the cardiac hypertrophy in human population in that ANP–NPRA-dependent cGMP may play a critical role in the protection against ventricular cardiac hypertrophy and CHF.

10. CONCLUSIONS

The discovery of ANP was rapidly followed by a rapid advancement of research on both basic and clinical aspects of NPs and their receptor system. Thus far, three related NPs and three distinct receptors have been identified and cloned that have advanced our knowledge toward understanding the control of high blood pressure, hypertension, and cardiovascular disorders to a great extent. Biochemical and molecular studies have been advanced to examine receptor function and signaling mechanisms and the role of second messenger cGMP in physiology and pathophysiology of hypertension, renal hemodynamics, and cardiovascular functions. Tools have been developed to examine receptor internalization, downregulation and/or desensitization of both GC-coupled and GC-uncoupled NP receptors in different cell systems. The development of gene-knockout and gene-duplication mouse models along with transgenic mice have provided a framework for understanding both the physiological and pathophysiological importance of NPs and their receptors and the signaling pathways involved in their mechanisms of action in hypertension and cardiovascular disease states. Although a considerable progress has been made, the transmembrane signal transduction mechanisms of NPs and their receptors remain unresolved. Future challenges should include the identification and characterization of cellular targets of NPs and second messenger cGMP including cytosolic and nuclear proteins, role in gene transcription, cell growth and proliferation, apoptosis, and differentiation. A more vigorous study of the crosstalk with other signaling mechanisms needs to be pursued systematically. Now, NPs are considered as circulating markers of CHF, however, their therapeutic potential for the treatment of cardiovascular diseases such as hypertension, renal insufficiency, cardiac hypertrophy, CHF, and stroke is still lacking. Indeed, the alternative avenues of investigations need to be undertaken, as we are at the initial stage of the molecular therapeutic and pharmacogenomic implications.

ACKNOWLEDGMENTS

I thank Mrs. Kamala Pandey for her assistance during the preparation of this review. The research in the author's laboratory is supported by the grants from the National Institutes of Health (HL 57531 and HL 62147) and Louisiana Health Excellence Fund.

REFERENCES

1. de Bold, A. J., Borenstein, H. B., Veress, A. T., and Sonnenberg, H. (1981) A rapid and potent natriuretic response to intravenous injection of atrial myocardial extract in rats. *Life Sci.* **28**, 89–94.
2. de Bold, A. J. (1985) Atrial natriuretic factor: a hormone produced by the heart. *Science* **230**, 767–770.
3. Brenner, B. M., Ballerman, B. J., Gunning, M. E., and Zeidel, M. L. (1990) Diverse biological actions of atrial natriuretic peptide. *Physiol. Rev.* **70**, 665–699.
4. Rosenzweig, A. and Seidman, C. E. (1991) Atrial natriuretic factor and related peptide hormones. *Annu. Rev. Biochem.* **60**, 229–255.
5. Koller, K. J., deSauvage, F. J., Lowe, D. G., and Goeddel, D. V. (1992) Conservation of the kinase-like regulatory domain is essential for activation of the natriuretic peptide receptor guanylyl cyclase. *Mol. Cell. Biol.* **12**, 2581–2590.
6. Pandey, K. N. and Singh, S. (1990) Molecular cloning and expression of murine guanylate cyclase/atrial natriuretic factor receptor cDNA. *J. Biol. Chem.* **265**, 12,342–12,348.
7. Garbers, D. L. (1992) Guanylyl cyclase receptors and their endocrine paracrine and autocrine ligands. *Cell* **71**, 1–4.
8. Drewett, J. G. and Garbers, D. L. (1994) The family of guanylyl cyclase receptors and their ligands. *Endocr. Rev.* **15**, 135–162.
9. Pandey, K. N. (1996) Vascular action: natriuretic peptide receptor. In: *Contemporary Endocrinology: Endocrinology of the Vasculature* (Sowers, J. R., ed.), Humana, Totawa, NJ, pp. 255–267.
10. Lucas, K. A., Pitari, G. M., Kazerounian, S., et al. (2000) Guanylyl cyclases and signaling by cGMP. *Pharmacol. Rev.* **52**, 375–413.
11. Sharma, R. K. (2002) Evolution of the membrane guanylate cyclase transduction system. *Mol. Cell. Biochem.* **230**, 3–30.
12. Pandey, K. N. (1993) Stoichiometric analysis of internalization recycling and redistribution of photoaffinity labeled guanylyl cyclase/atrial natriuretic factor receptors in cultured murine Leydig tumor cells. *J. Biol. Chem.* **268**, 4382–4390.
13. Cao, L. and Gardner, D. G. (1995) Natriuretic peptides inhibit DNA synthesis in cardiac fibroblast. *Hypertension* **25**, 227–234.
14. Pandey, K. N., Nguyen, H. T., Sharma, G. D., Shi, S.-J., and Kreigel, A. M. (2002) Ligand-regulated internalization trafficking and down-regulation of guanylyl cyclase/atrial natriuretic peptide receptor-A in human embryonic kidney 293 cells. *J. Biol. Chem.* **277**, 4618–4627.
15. Oliver, P. M., Fox, J. E., Kim, R., et al. (1997) Hypertension cardiac hypertrophy and sudden death in mice lacking natriuretic peptide receptor-A. *Proc. Natl Acad. Sci. USA* **94**, 14,730–14,735.
16. Shi, S. J., Vellaichamy, E., Chin, S. Y., Smithies, O., Navar, L. G., and Pandey, K. N., Natriuretic peptide receptor A mediates renal sodium excretory responses to blood volume expansion. *Am. J. Physiol.* **285**, F694–F702.
17. Lowe, D. G. (1997) The guanylyl cyclase-B receptor. In: *Contemporary Endocrinology: Natriuretic Peptides in Health and Disease* (Samson, W. K. and Levin, E. R., eds.), Humana, Totowa, NJ, pp. 35–50.
18. Suga, S., Nakao, K., Hosoda, K., et al. (1992) Receptor selectivity of natriuretic peptide family atrial natriuretic peptide, brain natriuretic peptide and C-type natriuretic peptide. *Endocrinology* **130**, 229–239.
19. Hama, N., Itoh, H., Shirakami, G., et al. (1994) Detection of C-type natriuretic peptide in human circulation and marked increase of plasma CNP level in septic shock patients. *Biochem. Biophys. Res. Commun.* **198**, 1177–1182.
20. Maki, M., Takayanagi, R., Misono, K., Pandey, K. N., Tibbetts, C., and Inagami, T. (1984) Structure of rat atrial natriuretic factor precursor deduced from cDNA sequence. *Nature* **309**, 722–724.
21. Yamanaka, M., Greenburg, B., Johnson, L., et al. (1984) Cloning and sequence analysis of the cDNA for the rat atrial natriuretic factor precursor. *Nature* **309**, 719–722.
22. Atlas, S. A., Kleinert, H. D., Camargo, M. J., Januszewicz, A., and Sealey, J. E. (1984) Purification sequencing and synthesis of natriuretic and vasoactive rat atrial peptide. *Nature* **309**, 717–719.
23. Inagami, T. (1989) Atrial natriuretic factor. *J. Biol. Chem.* **264**, 3043–3046.
24. Misono, K. S., Fukumi, H., Grammer, R. T., and Inagami, T. (1984) Rat atrial natriuretic factor: complete amino acid sequence and disulfide linkage essential for biological activity. *Biochem. Biophys. Res. Commun.* **119**, 524–529.

25. Schiller, P. W., Bellini, F., Dionne, G., et al. (1986) Synthesis and activity of atrial natriuretic peptide (ANP) analogs with reduced ring size. *Biochem. Biophys. Res. Commun.* **138,** 880–886.

26. Sudoh, T., Minamino, N., Kangawa, K., and Matsuo, H. (1988) Brain natriuretic peptide-32: N-terminal six amino acid extended form of brain natriuretic peptide identified in porcine brain. *Biochem. Biophys. Res. Commun.* **155,** 726–732.

27. Sudoh, T., Minamino, N., Kangawa, K., and Matsuo, H. (1990) C-type natriuretic peptide (CNP): a new member of natiuretic peptide family identified in porcine brain. *Biochem. Biophys. Res. Commun.* **168,** 863–870.

28. Philips, R. A., Ardeljan, M., Shimabukuro, S., ct al. (1991) Normalisation of left ventricular mass and associated changes in neurohormones and atrial natriuretic peptide after 1 year of sustained nifedipine therapy for severe hypertension. *J. Am. Card.* **17,** 1595–1602.

29. Suga, S., Nakao, K., Hosoda, K., et al. (1992) Phenotype-related alteration in expression of natriuretic peptide receptors in aortic smooth muscle cells. *Circ. Res.* **71,** 34–39.

30. Kojima, M., Minamino, N., Kangawa, K., and Matsuo, H. (1989) Cloning and sequence analysis of cDNA encoding a precursor for rat brain natriuretic peptide. *Biochem. Biophys. Res. Commun.* **159,** 1420–1426.

31. Mukoyama, M., Nakao, K., Hosoda, K., et al. (1991) Brain natriuretic peptide as a novel cardiac hormone in humans: evidence for an exquisite dual natriuretic peptide system ANP and BNP. *J. Clin. Invest.* **87,** 1402–1412.

32. Yoshimura, M., Yasue, H., Morita, E., et al. (1991) Hemodynamic renal and hormonal responses to brain natriuretic peptide infusion in patients with congestive heart failure. *Circulation* **84,** 1581–1588.

33. Omland, T., Aakvaag, A., Banarjee, V. V., et al. (1996) Plasma brain natriuretic peptide as an indicator of left ventricular systolic function and long-term survival after acute myocardial infarction: comparison with plasma atrial natriuretic peptide and N-terminal proatrial natriuretic peptide. *Circulation* **93,** 1963–1969.

34. McDonagh, T. A., Robb, S. D., Murdoch, D. R., et al. (1998) Biochemical detection of left-ventricular systolic dysfunction. *Lancet* **351,** 9–13.

35. Gardner, D. G., Deschepper, C. F., Ganong, W. F. (1986) Extra atrial expression of the gene for atrial natriuretic factor. *Proc. Natl Acad. Sci. USA* **83,** 6697–6701.

36. Cameron, V. A., Aitken, G. D., Ellmers, L. J., Kennedy, M. A., and Espiner, E. A. (1996) The sites of gene expression of atrial, brain and C-type natriuretic peptides in mouse fetal development: temporal changes in embryos and placenta. *Endocrinology* **137,** 817–824.

37. Larsen, T. H. and Saetersdal, T. (1993) Regional appearance of atrial natriuretic peptide in the ventricles of infarcted rat hearts Virchows Arch B Cells. *Pathol. Incl. Mol. Pathol.* **64,** 309–314.

38. Glembotski, C. C. (1997) Cellular and molecular biology of B-type natriuretic peptide. In: *Contemporary Endocrinology: Natriuretic Peptides in Health and Disease* (Samson, W. K. and Levin, E. R.), vol. 5, Humana, Totawa, NJ, pp. 95–106.

39. Hanford, D. S. and Glembotski, C. C. (1996) Stabilization of the B-type natriuretic peptide mRNA in cardiac myocytes by alpha-adrenergic receptor activation: potential roles for protein kinase C and mitogen-activated protein kinase. *Mol. Endocrinol.* **10,** 1719–1727.

40. Hanford, D. S., Thuerauf, D. J., Murray, S. F., and Glembotski, C. C. (1994) Brain natriuretic peptide is induced by α_1-adrenergic agonists as a primary response gene in cultured rat cardiac myocytes. *J. Biol. Chem.* **269,** 26,227–26,233.

41. Igaki, T., Itoh, H., Suga, S., et al. (1996) C-type natriuretic peptide in chronic renal failure and its action in humans. *Kidney Int.* **49,** S144–S147.

42. Ogawa, Y., Nakao, K., Nakagawa, O., et al. (1992) C-type natriuretic peptide: characterization of the gene and peptide. *Hypertension* **19,** 809–813.

43. Suga, S., Nakao, K., Itoh, H., et al. (1992) Endothelial production of C-type natriuretic peptide and its marked augmentation by transforming growth factor-beta: possible existence of "vascular natriuretic peptide system". *J. Clin. Invest.* **90,** 1145–1149.

44. Suga, S., Itoh, H., Komatsu, Y., et al. (1993) Cytokine-induced C-type natriuretic peptide (CNP) secretion from vascular endothelial cells—evidence for CNP as a novel autocrine/paracrine regulator from endothelial cells. *Endocrinology* **133,** 3038–3041.

45. Tamura, N., Ogawa, Y., Yasoda, A., Itoh, H., Saito, Y., Nakao, K. (1996) Two cardiac natriuretic peptide genes (atrial natriuretic peptide and brain natriuretic peptide) are organized in tandem in the mouse and human genomes. *J. Mol. Cell. Cardiol.* **28,** 1811–1815.

46. Chen, H. H. and Burnett, J. C. Jr. (1998) C-type natriuretic peptide: the endothelial component of the natriuretic peptide system. *J. Cardiovas. Pharmacol.* **32,** S22–S28.

47. Schweitz, H., Vigne, P., Moinier, D., Frelin, C. H., and Lazdunski, M. (1992) A new member of the natriuretic peptide family is present in the venom of the green mamba (*Dendroaspis angusticeps*). *J. Biol. Chem.* **267,** 13,928–13,932.

48. Lisy, O., Jougasaki, M., Heublein, D. M., et al. (1999) Renal actions of synthetic Dendroaspis natriuretic peptide. *Kidney Int.* **56,** 502–508.

49. Schulz-Knappe, P., Forssmann, K., Herbst, F., Hock, D., Pipkorn, R., and Forssmann, W. D. (1988) Isolation and structural analysis of "urodilatin" a new peptide of the cardiodilatin (ANP)-family extracted from human. *Urine Klin. Wochenschr.* **66,** 752–759.

50. Feller, S. M., Magert, H. J., Schulz-Knappe, P., et al. (1990) Urodilatin (hANF 95-126)—characteristics of a new atrial natriuretic factor peptide. In: *Atrial Natriuretic Factor* (Struthers, A., ed.), Blackwell, Oxford, UK, pp. 209–226.

51. Goetz, K. L. (1991) Renal natriuretic peptide (urodilatin?) and atriopeptin: evolving concepts. *Am. J. Physiol.* **261,** F921–F932.

52. Saxenhofer, H., Roselli, A., Weidmann, P., et al. (1990) Urodilatin a natriuretic factor from kidneys can modify renal and cardiovascular function in men. *Am. J. Physiol.* **259,** F832–F838.

53. Misono, K. S., Grammer, R. T., Rigby, J. W., and Inagami, T. (1985) Photoaffinity labeling of atrial natriuretic factor receptor in bovine and rat adrenal cortical membranes. *Biochem. Biophys. Res. Commun.* **130,** 994–1001.

54. Yip, C. C., Laing, L. P., and Flynn, T. G. (1985) Photoaffinity labeling of atrial natriuretic factor receptors of rat kidney cortex plasma membranes. *J. Biol. Chem.* **260,** 8229–8232.

55. Pandey, K. N., Inagami, T., Misono, K. S. (1986) Atrial natriuretic factor receptor on cultured Leydig tumor cells: ligand binding and photoaffinity labeling. *Biochemistry* **25,** 8467–8472.

56. Pandey, K. N., Misono, K. S., Takayanagi, R., Pavlou, S., and Inagami, T. (1987) Atrial natriuretic factor receptor in neuroblastoma cells of ganglionic origin: binding characteristics and photoaffinity labeling. *J. Neuro. Chem.* **48,** 1544–1552.

57. Hirose, S., Akiyama, F., Shinjo, M., Ohno, H., and Murakami, K. (1985) Solubilization and molecular weight estimation of atrial natriuretic factor receptor from bovine adrenal cortex. *Biochem. Biophys. Res. Commun.* **130,** 574–579.

58. Vandlen, R. L., Arcuri, K. E., and Napier, M. A. (1985) Identification of a receptor for atrial natriuretic factor in rabbit aorta membranes by affinity cross-linking. *J. Biol. Chem.* **260,** 10,889–10,892.

59. Meloche, S., Ong, H., Cantin, M., and De Lean, A. (1986) Affinity cross-linking of atrial natriuretic factor to its receptor in bovine adrenal zona glomerulosa. *J. Biol. Chem.* **261,** 1525–1528.

60. Schenk, D. B., Phelps, M. N., Porter, J. G., Scarborough, R. M., McEnroe, G. A. and Lewicki, J. A. (1985) Identification of the receptor for atrial natriuretic factor on cultured vascular cells. *J. Biol. Chem.* **260,** 14,887–14,890.

61. Kuno, T., Andresen, J. W., Kamisaki, Y., et al. (1986) Co-purification of an atrial natriuretic factor receptor and particulate GC from rat lung. *J. Biol. Chem.* **261,** 5817–5823.

62. Paul, A. K., Marala, R. B., Jaiswal, R. K., and Sharma, R. K. (1987) Co-existence of guanylate cyclase and atrial natriuretic factor receptor in 180 kDa protein. *Science* **235,** 1224–1227.

63. Takayanagi, R., Inagami, T., Snajdar, R. M., Imada, T., Tamura, M., and Misono, K. S. (1987) Two distinct forms of receptors for atrial natriuretic factor in bovine adrenocortical cells: purification ligand binding and peptide mapping. *J. Biol. Chem.* **262,** 12,104–12,113.

64. Meloche, S., McNicoll, N., Liu, B., Ong, H., and DeLean, A. (1988) Atrial natriuretic factor R1 receptor from bovine adrenal glomerulosa: purification characterization and modulation by amiloride. *Biochemistry* **27,** 8151–8158.

65. Marala, R. B. and Sharma, R. K. (1988) Characterization of atrial-natriuretic factor-coupled membrane guanylate cyclase from rat and mouse testes. *Biochem. J.* **251,** 301–304.

66. Schenk, D. B., Phelps, M. N., Porter, J. G., Fuller, F., Cordell, B., and Lewicki, J. A. (1987) Purification and subunit composition of atrial natriuretic peptide receptor. *Proc. Natl Acad. Sci. USA* **84,** 5121–5125.

67. Takayanagi, R., Snajdar, R. M., Imada, T., et al. (1987) Purification and characterization of two types of atrial natriuretic factor receptors from bovine adrenal cortex: guanylate cyclase-linked and cyclase-free receptors. *Biochem. Biophys. Res. Commun.* **144,** 244–250.

68. Leitman, D. C., Andresen, L. W., Kuno, T., Kamisaki, Y., Chang, J. K., and Murad, F. (1986) Identification of multiple binding sites for atrial natriuretic factor by affinity cross-linking in cultured endothelial cells. *J. Biol. Chem.* **261,** 11,650–11,655.

69. Pandey, K. N., Pavlou, S. N., and Inagami, T. (1988) Identification and characterization of three distinct atrial natriuretic factor receptors: evidence for tissue-specific heterogeneity of receptor subtypes in vascular smooth muscle kidney tubular epithelium and Leydig tumor cells by ligand binding photoaffinity labeling and tryptic proteolysis. *J. Biol. Chem.* **263**, 13,406–13,413.

70. Scarborough, R. M., McEnroe, G. A., Arfsten, A., Kang, L. L., Schwartz, K., and Lewicki, J. A. (1988) D-amino acid-substituted atrial natriuretic peptide analogs reveal novel receptor recognition requirements. *J. Biol. Chem.* **263**, 16,818–16,822.

71. Maack, T., Suzuki, M., Almeida, F. A., et al. (1987) Physiological role of silent receptors of atrial natriuretic factor. *Science* **238**, 675–678.

72. Leitman, D. C., Andresen, J. W., Catalano, R. M., Waldman, S. A., Tuan, J. J., and Murad, F. (1988) Atrial natriuretic peptide binding cross-linking and stimulation of cyclic GMP accumulation and particulate guanylate cyclase activity in cultured cells. *J. Biol. Chem.* **263**, 3720–3728.

73. Pandey, K. N. (1997) Physiology of the natriuretic peptides: gonadal function. In: *Contemporary Endocrinology: Natriuretic Peptides in Health and Disease* (Samson, W. K. and Levin, E. R., eds.), Humana, Totawa, NJ, pp. 171–191.

74. Levin, E. R., Gardner, D. G., and Samson, W. K. (1998) Natriuretic peptides. *N. Engl. J. Med.* **339**, 321–328.

75. Chinkers, M., Garbers, D. L., Chang, M. S., et al. (1989) A membrane form of guanylate cyclase is an atrial natriuretic peptide receptor. *Nature* **338**, 78–83.

76. Lowe, D. G., Chang, M.-S., Hellmis, R., et al. (1989) Human atrial natriuretic peptide receptor defines a new paradigm for second messenger signal transduction. *EMBO J.* **8**, 1377–1384.

77. Marala, R. B., Duda, T., Goraczniak, R. M., and Sharma, R. K. (1992) Genetically tailored atrial natriuretic factor-dependent guanylate cyclase: immunological and functional identity with 180 kDa membrane guanylate cyclase and ATP signaling site. *FEBS Lett.* **296**, 254–258.

78. Schulz, S., Singh, S., Bellet, R. A., et al. (1989) The primary structure of a plasma membrane guanylate cyclase demonstrates diversity within this new receptor family. *Cell* **58**, 1155–1162.

79. Chang, M. S., Lowe, D. G., Lewis, M., Hellmis, R., Chen, E., and Goeddel, D. V. (1989) Differential activation by atrial and brain natriuretic peptides of two different receptor guanylate cyclases. *Nature* **341**, 68–72.

80. Fuller, F., Porter, J. G., Arfsten, A. E., et al. (1988) Atrial natriuretic peptide clearance receptor: complete sequence and functional expression of cDNA clones. *J. Biol. Chem.* **263**, 9395–9401.

81. Hanks, S. K., Quinn, A. M., and Hunter, T. (1988) The protein kinase C family conserved features and deduced phylogeny of the catalytic domains. *Science* **241**, 42–52.

82. Bovy, P. R. (1990) Structure activity in the atrial natriuretic peptide (ANP) family. *Med. Res. Rev.* **10**, 115–142.

83. Anand-Srivastava, M. B. and Trachte, G. J. (1993) Atrial natriuretic factor receptor and signal transduction mechanisms. *Pharmacol. Rev.* **45**, 455–497.

84. Palaparti, A., Li, Y., and Anand-Srivastava, M. B. (2000) Inhibition of atrial natriuretic peptide (ANP) C receptor expression by antisense oligonucleotides in A10 vascular smooth muscle cells is associated with attenuation of ANP-C receptor mediated inhibition of adenylyl cyclase. *Biochemical. J.* **346**, 312–320.

85. Zhou, H. and Murthy, K. S. (2003) Identification of the G-protein activation sequence of the single-transmembrane natriuretic peptide receptor C (NPR-C). *Am. J. Cell. Physiol.* **284**, C1255–C1261.

86. van den Akker, F., Zang, X., Miyagi, H., Huo, X., Misono, K. S., and Yee, V. C. (2000) Structure of the dimerized hormone-binding domain of a guanylyl cyclase-coupled receptor. *Nature* **406**, 101–104.

87. Wilson, E. M. and Chinkers, M. (1995) Identification of sequences mediating guanylyl cyclase dimerization. *Biochemistry* **34**, 4696–4701.

88. Yang, R. B. and Garbers, D. L. (1997) Two eye guanylyl cyclase are expressed in the same photo-receptor cells and form homomers in preference to heteromers. *J. Biol. Chem.* **272**, 13,738–13,742.

89. Labrecque, J., McNicoll, N., Marquis, M., and De Lean, A. (1999) A disulfide-bridged mutant of natriuretic peptide receptor-A displays constitutive activity: role of receptor dimerization in signal transduction. *J. Biol. Chem.* **274**, 9752–9759.

90. Garbers, D. L. and Lowe, D. G. (1994) Guanylyl cyclase receptors. *J. Biol. Chem.* **269**, 30,714–30,744.

91. Lowe, D. G., Klisak, I., Sparkes, R. S., Mohandas, T., and Goeddel, D. V. (1990) Chromosomal distribution of three members of the human natriuretic peptide receptor/guanylyl cyclase gene family. *Genomics* **8**, 304–312.

92. Koller, K. J., Lowe, D. G., Bennett, G. L., et al. (1991) Selective activation of the B natriuretic peptide receptor by C-type natriuretic peptide (CNP). *Science* **252,** 120–123.

93. Duda, T. and Sharma, R. K. (1995) ATP modulation of the ligand binding and signal transduction activities of the type C natriuretic peptide receptor guanylate cyclase. *Mol. Cell. Biochem.* **152,** 179–183.

94. Singh, S., Lowe, D. G., Thorpe, D. S., et al. (1988) Membrane guanylate cyclase is a cell-surface receptor with homology to protein kinases. *Nature* **334,** 708–712.

95. Thorpe, D. S., and Garbers, D. L. (1989) The membrane form of guanylate cyclase: homology with a subunit of the cytoplasmic form of the enzyme. *J. Biol. Chem.* **264,** 6545–6549.

96. Goraczniak, R. M., Duda, T., Sitaramayya, A., and Sharma, R. K. (1994) Structural and functional characterization of the rod outer segment membrane guanylate cyclase. *Biochem. J.* **302,** 455–461.

97. Lowe, D. G., Dizhoor, A. M., Liu, K., et al. (1995) Cloning and expression of a second photoreceptor-specific membrane retina guanylyl cyclase (RetGC) RetGC-2. *Proc. Natl Acad. Sci. USA* **92,** 5535–5539.

98. Fulle, H. J., Vassar, R., Foster, D. C., Yang, R. B., Axel, R., and Garbers, D. L. (1995) A receptor guanylyl cyclase expressed specifically in olfactory sensory neurons. *Proc. Natl Acad. Sci. USA* **92,** 3571–3575.

99. Yang, R. B., Foster, D. C., Garbers, D. L., and Fulle, H. J. (1995) Two membrane forms of guanylyl cyclase found in the eye. *Proc. Natl Acad. Sci. USA* **92,** 602–606.

100. Yu, S., Avery, L., Baude, E., and Garbers, D. L. (1997) Guanylyl cyclase expression in specific sensory neurons: a new family of chemosensory receptors. *Proc. Natl Acad. Sci. USA* **94,** 3384–3387.

101. Baude, E. J., Arora, V. K., Yu, S., Garbers, D. L., and Wedel, B. J. (1997) The cloning of a *Caenorhabditis elegans* guanylyl cyclase and the construction of a ligand-sensitive mammalian/nematode chimeric receptor. *J. Biol. Chem.* **272,** 16,035–16,039.

102. Hamet, P., Tremblay, J., Pang, S. C., et al. (1984) Effect of native and synthetic atrial natriuretic factor on cyclic GMP. *Biochem. Biophys. Res. Commun.* **123,** 515–527.

103. Waldman, S. A., Rappoport, R. M., and Murad, F. (1984) Atrial natriuretic factor selectively activates particulate guanylyl cyclase and elevates cyclic GMP in rat tissues. *J. Biol. Chem.* **259,** 14,332–14,334.

104. Pandey, K. N., Kovacs, W. J., and Inagami, T. (1985) The inhibition of progesterone secretion and the regulation of cyclic nucleotides by atrial natriuretic factor in gonadotropin responsive murine Leydig tumor cells. *Biochem. Biophys. Res. Commun.* **133,** 800–806.

105. Tremblay, J., Gertzer, R., Vinay, P., Pang, S. C., Beliveau, R. and Hamet, P. (1985) The increase of cGMP by atrial natriuretic factor correlates with the distribution of particulate guanylate cyclase. *FEBS Lett.* **181,** 17–22.

106. Kurose, H., Inagami, T., and Ui, M. (1987) Participation of adenosine 5′- triphosphate in the activation of membrane-bound guanylate cyclase by the atrial natriuretic factor. *FEBS Lett.* **219,** 375–379.

107. Chinkers, M., Singh, S., and Garbers, D. L. (1991) Adenine nucleotides are required for activation of rat atrial natriuretic peptide receptor/guanylyl cyclase expressed in a baculovirus system. *J. Biol. Chem.* **266,** 4088–4093.

108. Goraczniak, R. M., Duda, T., and Sharma, R. K. (1992) A structural motif that defines the ATP-regulatory module of guanylate cyclase in atrial natriuretic factor signaling. *Biochem. J.* **282,** 533–537.

109. Chang, C.-H., Kohse, K. P., Chang, B., et al. (1990) Characterization of ATP-stimulated guanylyl cyclase activation in rat lung membranes. *Biochem. Biophys. Acta* **1052,** 159–165.

110. Gazzano, H., Wu, H. I., and Waldman, S. A. (1991) Adenine nucleotide regulation of particulate guanylate cyclase from rat lung. *Biochem. Biophys. Acta* **1077,** 99–106.

111. Duda, T., Goraczniak, R. M., and Sharma, R. K. (1991) Site-directed mutational analysis of a membrane guanylate cyclase cDNA reveals the atrial natriuretic factor signaling site. *Proc. Natl Acad. Sci. USA* **88,** 7882–7886.

112. Larose, L., McNicoll, N., Ong, H., and De Lean, A. (1991) Allosteric modulation by ATP of the bovine adrenal natriuretic factor R1 receptor functions. *Biochemistry* **30,** 8990–8995.

113. Wong, S. K., Ma, C. P., Foster, D. C., Chen, A. Y., and Garbers, D. L. (1995) The guanylyl cyclase-A receptor transduces an atrial natriuretic peptide/ATP activation signal in the absence of other proteins. *J. Biol. Chem.* **270,** 30,818–30,822.

114. Duda, T., Goraczniak, R. M., and Sharma, R. K. (1993) Core sequence of ATP regulatory module in receptor guanylate cyclases. *FEBS Lett.* **315,** 143–148.

115. Chinkers, M. and Garbers, D. L. (1989) The protein kinase of the ANP receptor is required for signaling. *Science* **245,** 1392–1394.

116. Duda, T., Goraczniak, R. M., and Sharma, R. K. (1993) The glycine residue of ATP regulatory module in receptor guanylate cyclases that is essential in natriuretic factor signaling. *FEBS Lett.* **335,** 309–314.

117. Sharma, R. K., Duda, T., and Sitaramayya, A. (1994) Plasma membrane guanylate cyclase is a multimodule transduction system. *Amino Acids* **7,** 117–127.

118. Pandey, K. N., Kumar, R., Li, M., and Nguyen, H. (2000) Functional domains and expression of truncated atrial natriuretic peptide receptor-A: the carboxyl-terminal regions direct the receptor internalization and sequestration in COS-7 cells. *Mol. Pharm.* **57,** 259–267.

119. Huo, X., Abe, T., and Misono, K. S. (1999) Ligand binding-dependent limited proteolysis of the atrial natriuretic peptide: juxtamembrane hinge structure essential for transmembrane signal transduction. *Biochemistry* **38,** 16,941–16,951.

120. Lowe, D. G. and Fendly, B. M. (1992) Human natriuretic peptide receptor-A guanylyl cyclase: hormone cross-linking and antibody reactivity distinguish receptor glycoforms. *J. Biol. Chem.* **267,** 21,691–21,697.

121. Fenrick, R., Bouchard, N., McNicoll, N., and De Lean, A. (1997) Glycosylation of asparagines 24 of the natriuretic peptide receptor-B is crucial for the formation of a competent ligand binding domain. *Mol. Cell. Biochem.* **173,** 25–32.

122. Fenrick, R., McNicoll, N., and De Lean, A. (1996) Glycosylation is critical for natriuretic peptide receptor-B function. *Mol. Cell. Biochem.* **165,** 103–109.

123. Miyagi, M., Zhang, X., and Misono, K. S. (2000) Glycosylation sites in the atrial natriuretic peptide receptor oligosaccharide structures are not required for hormone binding. *Eur. J. Biochem.* **267,** 5758–5768.

124. Hesegawa, M., Hidaka, Y., Wada, A., Hirayama, T., and Shimonishi, Y. (1999) The relevance of N-linked glycosylation to the binding of a ligand to guanylate cyclase C. *Eur. J. Biochem.* **263,** 338–346.

125. van den Akker, F. (2001) Structural insights into the ligand binding domains of membrane bound guanylyl cyclases and natriuretic peptide receptors. *J. Mol. Biol.* **311,** 923–937.

126. Koller, K. J., Lipari, M. T., and Goeddel, D. V. (1993) Proper glycosylation and phosphorylation of the type A natriuretic peptide receptor are required for hormone-stimulated guanylyl cyclase activity. *J. Biol. Chem.* **268,** 5997–6003.

127. Heim, J. M., Singh, S., and Gerzer, R. (1996) Effect of glycosylation on cloned ANF-sensitive guanylyl cyclase. *Life Sci.* **59,** L61–L68.

128. Wormald, M. R. and Dwek, R. A. (1999) Glycoproteins: glycan presentation and protein-fold stability. *Struct. Fold Des.* **7,** R155–R160.

129. Pandey, K. N. (2001) Dynamics of internalization and sequestration of guanylyl cyclase/atrial natriuretic peptide receptor-A. *Can. J. Physiol. Pharmacol.* **79,** 631–639.

130. Pandey, K. N. (2002) Intracellular trafficking and metabolic turnover of ligand-bound guanylyl cyclase/atrial natriuretic peptide receptor-A into subcellular compartments. *Mol. Cell. Biochem.* **230,** 61–72.

131. Resink, T. J., Scott-Burden, T., Baur, U., Jones, C. R., and Buhler, F. R. (1988) Atrial natriuretic peptide induces breakdown of phosphatidylinositol phosphates in cultured vascular smooth muscle cells. *Eur. J. Biochem.* **172,** 499–505.

132. Hirata, M., Chang, C. M., and Murad, F. (1989) Stimulatory effect of atrial natriuretic factor on phosphoinositide hydrolysis in cultured bovine aortic smooth muscle cells. *Biochem. Biophys. Acta* **1010,** 346–351.

133. Teitelbaum, I., Strasheim, A., and Berl, T. (1990) Epidermal growth factor-stimulated phosphonositide hydrolysis in cultured rat inner medullary collecting tubule cells regulation by G protein calcium and protein kinase. *C. J. Clin. Investig.* **85,** 1044–1050.

134. Berl, T., Mansour, J., and Teitelbaum, I. (1991) ANP stimulates phospholipase C in cultured RIMCT cells: roles of protein kinases and G proteins. *Am. J. Physiol.* **29,** F590–F595.

135. Hu, R. M., Levin, E. R., Pedram, A., and Frank, H. J. (1993) Insulin increases the production and secretion of endothelin from cultured bovine endothelial cells. *Diabetes* **42,** 351–358.

136. Emori, T., Hirata, Y., Imai, T., Eguchi, S., Kanno, K., and Marumos, F. (1993) Cellular mechanism of natriuretic peptides-induced inhibition of endothelin-1 biosynthesis in rat endothelial cells. *Endocrinology* **133,** 2474–2480.

137. Khurana, M. L. and Pandey, K. N. (1996) Atrial natriuretic peptide inhibits the phosphoinositide hydrolysis in murine Leydig tumor cells. *Mol. Cell. Biochem.* **158,** 97–105.

138. Khurana, M. L. and Pandey, K. N. (1995) Catalytic activation of guanylate cyclase/atrial natriuretic factor receptor by combined effects of ANF and GTPγS in plasma membranes of Leydig tumor cells. *Arch. Biochem. Biophys.* **316,** 392–398.

139. Pandey, K. N. (1989) Stimulation of protein phosphorylation by atrial natriuretic factor in plasma membranes of bovine adrenal cortical cells. *Biochem. Biophys. Res. Commun.* **163,** 988–994.

140. Pandey, K. N. (1994) Atrial natriuretic factor inhibits the phosphorylation of protein kinase C in plasma membrane preparations of cultured Leydig tumor cells. *J. Androlo.* **15,** 100–109.

141. Pandey, K. N. (1994) Atrial natriuretic factor inhibits autophosphorylation of protein kinase C and a 240 kDa protein in plasma membranes of bovine adrenal glomerulosa cells: involvement of cGMP-dependent and -independent signal transduction mechanisms. *Mol. Cell. Biochem.* **141,** 103–111.

142. Kumar, R., von Geldern, T., Calle, R., and Pandey, K. N. (1356) Overexpression of protein kinase C-α and negative regulation by atrial natriuretic peptide receptor-A in transfected murine Leydig tumor cells. *Biochem. Biophys. Acta* **1356,** 221–228.

143. Kumar, R., Cartledge, W. A., Lincoln, T. M., and Pandey, K. N. (1997) Expression of guanylyl cyclase-A/atrial natriuretic peptide receptor blocks the activation of protein kinase C in vascular smooth muscle cells: role of cGMP and cGMP-dependent protein kinase. *Hypertension* **28,** 528–534.

144. White, R. E., Lee, A. B., Shcherbatko, A. D., Lincoln, T. M., Schonbrunn, A., and Armstrong, D. L. (1993) Potassium channel stimulation by natriuretic peptides through cGMP-dependent dephosphorylation. *Nature* **361,** 263–266.

145. Anand-Srivastava, M. B., Srivastava, A., and Cantin, M. J. (1987) Pertussis toxin attenuates atrial natriuretic factor-mediated inhibition of adenylate cyclase. *J. Biol. Chem.* **262,** 4931–4934.

146. Drewett, J. G., Ziegler, R. J., and Trachte, G. J. (1992) Neuromodulatory effects of atrial natriuretic peptides correlate with an inhibition of adenylate cyclase but not an activation of guanylate cyclase. *J. Pharmacol. Exp. Ther.* **260,** 689–696.

147. Khurana, M. L. and Pandey, K. N. (1994) Modulation of guanylate cyclase-coupled atrial natriuretic factor receptor activity by mastoparan and ANF in murine Leydig tumor cells: role of G-proteins. *Biochem. Biophy. Acta* **1224,** 61–67.

148. Rathinavelu, A. and Isom, G. E. (1991) Differential internalization and precessing of atrial natriuretic factor B and C receptors in PC-12 cells. *Biochem. J.* **276,** 493–497.

149. Rathinavelu, A., and Isom, G. E. (1993) Lysosomal delivery of ANP receptors following internalization of PC-12 cells. *Life Sci.* **53,** 1007–1014.

150. Koh, G. Y., Nussenzweig, D. R., Okolicany, J., Price, D. A., and Maack, T. (1992) Dynamics of atrial natriuretic factor-guanylate cyclase receptors and receptor-ligand complexes in cultured glomerular mesangial and renomedullary interstitial cells. *J. Biol. Chem.* **267,** 11,987–11,994.

151. Delporte, C., Poloczek, P., Tastenoy, M., Winard, J., and Christopher, J. (1992) Atrial natriuretic peptide binds to ANP-R 1 receptors in neuroblastoma cells or is degraded extracellularly at the Ser-Phe bond. *Eur. J. Pharmacol.* **227,** 247–256.

152. Hirata, Y., Takata, S., Tomita, M., and Takaichi, S. (1985) Binding internalization and degradation of atrial natriuretic peptide in cultured vascular smooth muscle cells of rat. *Biochem. Biophys. Res. Commun.* **132,** 976–984.

153. Napier, M., Arcuri, K., and Vandlen, R. (1986) Binding and internalization of atrial natriuretic factor by high-affinity receptors in A10 smooth muscle cells. *Arch. Biochem. Biophys.* **248,** 516–522.

154. Murthy, K. K., Thibault, G., and Cantin, M. (1989) Binding and intracellular degradation of atrial natriuretic factor by cultured vascular smooth muscle cells. *Mol. Cell. Endocrinol.* **67,** 195–206.

155. Nussenzveig, D. R., Lewicki, J. A., and Maack, T. (1990) Cellular mechanisms of the clearance function of type-C receptors of atrial natriuretic factor. *J. Biol. Chem.* **265,** 20,952–20,958.

156. Cahill, P. A., Redmond, E. M., and Keenan, A. K. (1990) Vascular atrial natriuretic factor receptor subtypes are not independently regulated by atrial peptides. *J. Biol, Chem.* **265,** 21,896–21,906.

157. Pandey, K. N. (1992) Kinetic analysis of internalization recycling and redistribution of atrial natriuretic factor-receptor complex in cultured vascular smooth muscle cells: ligand-dependent receptor down-regulation. *Biochem. J.* **288,** 4382–4390.

158. Cohen, D., Koh, G. Y., Nikonova, L. N., Porter, J. G., and Maack, T. (1996) Molecular determinants of the clearance function of type-C receptor of natriuretic peptides. *J. Biol. Chem.* **271,** 9863–9869.

159. Anand-Srivastava, M. B. (2000) Down-regulation of atrial natriuretic peptide ANP-C receptor is associated with alteration in G-protein expression in A10 smooth muscle cells. *Biochemistry* **39,** 6503–6513.

160. Neuser, D. and Bellermann, P. (1986) Receptor binding cGMP stimulation and receptor desensitization by atrial natriuretic peptides in cultured A10 vascular smooth muscle cells. *FEBS Lett.* **209,** 347–351.

161. Hirata, Y., Hirose, S., Takada, S., Takagi, Y., and Matsubara, H. (1987) Down-regulation of atrial natriuretic peptide receptor and cyclic GMP response in cultured rat vascular smooth muscle cells. *Eur. J. Pharmacol.* **135,** 439–442.

162. Roubert, P., Lonchampt, M. O., Chabrier, P. E., Plas, P., Goulin, J., and Braquet, P. (1987) Down-regulation of atrial natriuretic factor receptors and correlation with cGMP stimulation in rat cultured vascular smooth muscle cells. *Biochem. Biophys. Res. Commun.* **148,** 61–67.

163. Hughes, R. J., Struthers, R. S., Fong, A. M., and Insel, P. A. (1987) Regulation of the atrial natriuretic peptide receptor on a smooth muscle cell. *Am. J. Physiol.* **253,** C809–C816.

164. Hirata, Y., Takata, S., Takagi, Y., Matsubara, H., and Omae, T. (1986) Regulation of atrial natriuretic peptide receptors in cultured vascular smooth muscle cells of rat. *Biochem. Biophys. Res. Commun.* **138,** 405–412.

165. Fujio, N., Gossard, F., Bayard, F., and Tremblay, J. (1994) Regulation of natriuretic peptide receptor A and B expression by transforming growth factor-β_1 in cultured aortic smooth muscle cells. *Hypertension* **23,** 908–913.

166. Hum, D., Besnard, S., Sanchez, R., et al. (2004) Characterization of a cGMP-response element in the guanylyl cyclase/natriuretic peptide receptor A gene promoter. *Hypertension* **43,** 1270–1278.

167. Cao, L., Chen, S. C., Humphreys, M. H., and Gardner, D. G. (1998) Ligand-dependent regulation of NPR-A gene expression in inner medullary collecting duct cells. *Am. J. Physiol.* **275,** F119–F125.

168. Garg, R. and Pandey, K. N. (2003) Angiotensin II-mediated negative regulation of Npr1 promoter activity and gene expression. *Hypertension* **41,** 730–736.

169. Chen, Y. O. and Gardner, D. G. (2003) Endothelin inhibits NPR-A and stimulates eNOS gene expression in rat IMCD cells. *Hypertension* **41,** 675–681.

170. Potter, L. R. and Garbers, D. L. (1992) Dephosphorylation of the guanylyl cyclase-A receptor causes desensitization. *J. Biol. Chem.* **267,** 14,531–14,534.

171. Sibley, D. R., Benovic, J. L., Caron, M. G., and Lefkowitz, R. J. (1987) Regulation of transmembrane signaling by receptor phosphorylation. *Cell* **48,** 913–933.

172. Hugnir, R. I. and Greengard, P. (1990) Regulation of neurotransmitter receptor desensitization by protein phosphorylation. *Neuron* **5,** 555–567.

173. Goodman, O. B. Jr., Krupnick, J. G., Santini, F., et al. (1996) β-arrestin acts as a clathrin adaptor in endocytosis of the β_2-adrenergic receptor. *Nature* **383,** 447–450.

174. Zhang, J., Ferguson, S. S., Barak, L. S., et al. (1997) Molecular mechanisms of G protein-coupled signaling: role of G protein-coupled receptor kinases and arrestins in receptor desensitization and resensitization. *Receptors Channels* **5,** 193–199.

175. Lefkowitz, R. J., Pitcher, J., Krueger, K., and Daaka, Y. (1998) Mechanisms of β-adrenergic receptor desensitization and resensitization. *Adv. Pharmacol.* **42,** 416–420.

176. Sorkin, A. and von Zastrow, M. (2002) Signal transduction and endocytosis: close encounters of many kinds. *Nature Rev. Mol. Cell. Biol.* **3,** 600–614.

177. Ballerman, B. J., Marala, R. B., Sharma, R. K. (1988) Characterization and regulation by protein kinase C of renal glomerular atrial natriuretic peptide receptor-coupled guanylate cyclase. *Biochem. Biophys. Res. Commun.* **157,** 755–761.

178. Duda, T. and Sharma, R. K. (1990) Regulation of guanylate cyclase activity by atrial natriuretic factor and protein kinase C. *Mol. Cell. Biochem.* **93,** 179–184.

179. Larose, L., Rondeau, J. J., Ong, H., and De Leans, A. (1992) Phosphorylation of atrial natriuretic factor R1 receptor by serine/threonine protein kinases: evidence for receptor regulation. *Mol. Cell. Biochem.* **115,** 203–211.

180. Foster, D. C. and Garbers, D. L. (1998) Dual role for adenine nucleotides in the regulation of the atrial natriuretic peptide receptor guanylyl cyclase-A. *J. Biol. Chem.* **273,** 16,311–16,318.

181. Potter, L. R. and Hunter, T. (1998) Phosphorylation of the kinase homology domain is essential for activation of the A-type natriuretic peptide receptor. *Mol. Cell. Biol.* **18,** 2164–2172.

182. Chinkers, M. (1994) Targeting of a distinctive protein serine phosphatase to the protein kinase-like domain of the atrial natriuretic peptide receptor. *Proc. Natl Acad. Sci. USA* **91,** 11,075–11,079.

183. Airhart, N., Yang, Y. F., Roberts, C. T. Jr., and Silberbach, M. (2003) Atrial natriuretic peptide induces natriuretic peptide receptor-cGMP-dependent protein kinase interaction. *J. Biol. Chem.* **278,** 38,693–38,698.

184. Burnett, J. C. Jr., Granger, J. P., and Opgenorth, T. J. (1984) Effects of synthetic atrial natriuretic factor on renal function and renin release. *Am. J. Physiol.* **247,** F863–F866.

185. Camarago, M. J., Kleinert, H. D., Atlas, S. A., Sealey, J. E., Laragh, J. H., and Maack, T. (1984) Ca^{2+} -dependent hemodynamic and natriuretic effects of atrial extract in isolated rat kidney. *Am. J. Physiol.* **246,** F447–F456.

186. Freeman, R. H., Davis, J. O., and Vari, R. C. (1985) Renal response to atrial natriuretic factor in conscious dogs with caval constriction. *Am. J. Physiol.* **248,** R495–R500.

187. Meyer, M. and Forsmann, W. G. (1997) Renal actions of atrial natriuretic peptide. In: *Natriuretic Peptides in Health and Disease* (Samson, W. K. and Levin, E. R., eds.), Humana, Totawa, NJ, pp. 147–170.

188. Villrreal, D. and Freeman, R. H. (1997) Natriuretic peptides and salt sensitivity In: *Contemporary Endocrinology: Natriuretic Peptides in Health and Disease* (Samson, W. K. and Levin, E. R., eds.), Humana, Totowa, NJ, pp. 239–258.

189. Melo, L. G., Steinhelper, M. E., Pang, S. C., Tse, Y., and Ackermann, U. (2000) ANP in regulation of arterial pressure and fluid-electrolyte balance: lessons from genetic mouse models. *Physiol. Genomics* **3,** 45–58.

190. Nonguchi, H., Knepper, M. A., and Mangiello, V. C. (1987) Effects of atrial natriuretic factor on cyclic guanosine monophosphate and cyclic adenosine monophosphate accumulation in micro-dissected nephron segments from rats. *J. Clin. Investig.* **79,** 500–507.

191. Kremer, S., Troyer, D., Kreisberg, J., and Skorecki, K. (1988) Interaction of atrial natriuretic peptide-stimulated guanylyl cyclase and vasopressin-stimulated calcium signaling pathways in the glomerular mesangial cells. *Arch. Biochem. Biophys.* **260,** 763–767.

192. Light, D. B., Schwiebert, E. M., Karlson, K. H., and Stanton, B. A. (1989) Atrial natriuretic peptide inhibits a cation channel in renal inner medullary collecting duct cells. *Science* **243,** 383–385.

193. Cermak, R., Kleta, R., Forssman, W. G., and Schlatter, E. (1996) Natriuretic peptides increase a K^+ conductance in rat mesangial cells. *Pflugers Arch.* **431,** 571–577.

194. Appel, R. G. (1990) Mechanism of atrial natriuretic factor-induced inhibition of rat mesangial cell mitogenesis. *Am. J. Physiol.* **259,** E312–E318.

195. von-Geldern, T. W., Budzik, G. P., Dillon, T. P., et al. (1990) Atrial natriuretic peptide antagonists: biological evaluation and structural correlations. *Mol. Pharmacol.* **38,** 771–778.

196. Sano, T., Morishita, Y., Matsuda, Y., and Yamada, K. (1992) Pharmacological profile of HS-142-1 a novel nonpeptide atrial natriuretic peptide antagonist of microbial origin I Selective inhibition of the actions of natriuretic peptides in anesthetized rats. *J. Pharmacol. Exp. Ther.* **260,** 825–831.

197. Obana, K., Naruse, N., Naruse, K., et al. (1985) Synthetic rat atrial natriuretic factor inhibits in vitro and in vivo rennin secretion in rats. *Endocrinology* **117,** 1282–1284.

198. Shi, S.-J., Nguyen, H. T., Sharma, G. D., Navar, L. G., and Pandey, K. N. (2001) Genetic disruption of atrial natriuretic peptide receptor-A alters renin and angiotensin II levels. *Am. J. Physiol.* **281,** F665–F673.

199. Paul, R. V., Ferguson, T., and Navar, L. G. (1988) ANF secretion and renal responses to volume expansion with equilibrated blood. *Am. J. Physiol.* **255,** F936–F943.

200. Schwab, T. R., Edwards, B. S., Heublein, D. M., and Burnett, J. C. Jr. (1986) Role of atrial natriuretic peptide in volume-expansion natriuresis. *Am. J. Physiol.* **251,** R310–R313.

201. Ohyama, Y., Miyamoto, R., Morishita, Y., et al. (1992) Stable expression of natriuretic peptide receptors: effects of HS-142-1 a non-peptide ANP antagonist. *Biochem. Biophys. Res. Commun.* **189,** 336–342.

202. Anderson, J. V., Christofides, N. D., and Bloom, S. R. (1986) Plasma release of atrial natriuretic peptide in response to blood volume expansion. *J. Endorinol.* **109,** 9–13.

203. Antunes-Rodrigues, J., Machado, B. H., Andrade, H. A., et al. (1992) Carotid aortic and renal baroreceptors mediate the atrial natriuretic peptide release induced by blood volume expansion. *Proc. Natl Acad. Sci. USA* **89,** 6829–6831.

204. Navar, L. G. and Hamm, L. L. (1999) The kidney in blood pressure regulation. in *Atlas of Diseases of Kidney. Hypertension and the Kidney* (Wilcox, C. S., ed.), Vol. 3, Current Medicine, Inc., Philadelphia, PA, pp. 1–22.

205. McCann, S. M., Gutkowska, J., and Antunes-Rodrigues, J. (2003) Neuroendocirne control of body fluid homeostasis. *Braz. J. Med. Biol. Res.* **36,** 165–181.

206. Misono, K. S. (2000) Atrial natriuretic factor binding to its receptor is dependent on chloride concentration: a possible feedback control mechanism in renal salt regulation. *Circ. Res.* **86,** 1135–1139.

207. Melo, L. G., Veress, A. T., Ackerman, U., et al. (1999) Chronic regulation of arterial blood pressure in ANP transgenic and knockout mice: role of cardiovascular sympathetic tone. *Cardiovasc. Res.* **43,** 437–441.

208. Takahashi, N. and Smithies, O. (1999) Gene-targeting approaches to analyzing hypertension. *J. Am. Soc. Nephrol.* **10**, 1598–1605.

209. Kim, H. S., Lu, G., John, S. W. M., Maeda, N., and Smithies, O. (2002) Molecular phenotyping for analyzing subtle genetic effects in mice: application to an angiotensinogen gene titration. *Proc. Natl Acad. Sci. USA* **99**, 4602–4607.

210. John, S. W., Krege, J. H., Oliver, P. M., et al. (1995) Genetic decreases in atrial natriuretic peptide and salt-sensitive hypertension. *Science* **267**, 679–681.

211. Lopez, M. J., Wong, S. K.-F., Kishimoto, I., et al. (1995) Salt-resistant hypertension in mice lacking the guanylyl cyclase-A receptor for atrial natriuretic peptide. *Nature* **378**, 65–68.

212. Kishimoto, I., Dubois, S. K., and Garbers, D. L. (1996) The heart communicates with the kidney exclusively through the guanylyl cyclase-A receptor: acute handling of sodium and water in response to volume expansion. *Proc. Natl Acad. Sci. USA* **93**, 6215–6219.

213. Oliver, P. M., John, S. W., Purdy, K. E., et al. (1998) Natriuretic peptide receptor 1 expression influences blood pressures of mice in a dose-dependent manner. *Proc. Natl Acad. Sci. USA* **95**, 2547–2551.

214. Pandey, K. N., Oliver, P. M., Maeda, N., and Smithies, O. (1999) Hypertension associated with decreased testosterone levels in natriuretic peptide receptor-A gene-knockout and gene-duplicated mutant mouse models. *Endocrinology* **11**, 5112–5119.

215. Matsukawa, N., Grzesik, W. J., Takahashi, N., et al. (1999) The natriuretic peptide clearance receptor locally modulates the physiological effects of the natriuretic peptide system. *Proc. Natl Acad. Sci. USA* **96**, 7403–7408.

216. Holtwick, R., Baba, H. A., Ehler, E., et al. (2002) Left but not right cardiac hypertrophy in atrial natriuretic peptide receptor-deficient mice is prevented by angiotensin type 1 receptor antagonist losartan. *J. Cardiovasc. Pharmacol.* **40**, 725–734.

217. Atarashi, K., Mulrow, P. J., Franco-Sanenz, R., Snajdar, R., and Rapp, J. (1984) Inhibition of aldosterone production by an atrial extract. *Science* **224**, 992–994.

218. Oda, S., Sano, T., Morishita, Y., and Matsuda, Y. (1992) Pharmacological profile of HS-142-1 a novel nonpeptide atrial natriuretic peptide (ANP) antagonist of microbial origin II Restoration by HS-142-1 of ANP-induced inhibition of aldosterone production in adrenal glomerulosa cells. *J. Pharmacol. Exp. Ther.* **263**, 241–245.

219. Barrett, P. O. and Isales, C. M. (1988) The role of cyclic nucleotides in atrial natriuretic peptide-mediated inhibition of aldosterone secretion. *Endocrinology* **122**, 2790–2795.

220. MacFarland, R. T., Zelus, B. D., and Beavo, J. A. (1991) High concentrations of a cGMP-stimulated phosphodiesterase mediate ANP-induced decreases in cAMP and steroidogenesis in adrenal glomerulosa cells. *J. Biol. Chem.* **266**, 136–142.

221. Hassid, A. (1986) Atriopeptin II decreases cytosolic free Ca^{2+} in cultured vascular smooth muscle cells. *Am. J. Physiol.* **251**, C681–C686.

222. Lincoln, T. M., Komalavilas, P., and Cornwell, T. L. (1994) Pleiotropic regulation of vascular smooth muscle tone by cyclic GMP-dependent protein kinase. *Hypertension* **243**, 383–385.

223. Rashatwar, S. S., Cornwell, T. L., and Lincoln, T. M. (1987) Effect of 8-bromo cGMP on Ca^{2+}-ATPase by cGMP dependent protein kinase. *Proc. Natl Acad. Sci. USA* **84**, 5685–5689.

224. Cornwell, T. L. and Lincoln, T. M. (1989) Regulation of intracellular Ca^{2+} levels in cultured vascular smooth muscle cells: reduction of Ca^{2+} by atriopeptin and 8-bromo-cyclic GMP is mediated by cyclic GMP-dependent protein kinase. *J. Biol. Chem.* **264**, 1146–1155.

225. Johnson, A., Lermioglu, F., Garg, U. C., Morgan-Boyd, R., and Hassid, A. (1988) A novel biological effect of atrial natriuretic peptide hormone inhibition of mesangial cell mitogenesis. *Biochem. Biophys. Res. Commun.* **152**, 893–897.

226. Appel, R. G. (1992) Growth-regulatory properties of atrial natriuretic factor. *Am. J. Physiol.* **262**, F911–F918.

227. Sugimoto, T., Kikkawa, R., Haneda, M., and Shigeta, Y. (1993) Atrial natriuretic peptide inhibits endothelin-1 induced activation of mitogen-activated protein kinase in cultured rat mesangial cells. *Biochem. Biophys. Res. Commun.* **195**, 72–78.

228. Isono, M., Haneda, M., Maeda, S., Omatsu-Kanbe, M., and Kikkawa, R. (1998) Atrial natriuretic peptide inhibits endothelin-1-induced activation of JNK in glomerular mesangial cells. *Kidney* **53**, 1133–1142.

229. Pandey, K. N., Nguyen, H. T., Li, M., and Boyle, J. W. (2000) Natriuretic peptide receptor-A negatively regulates mitogen-activated protein kinase and proliferation of mesangial cells: role of cGMP-dependent protein kinase. *Biochem. Biophys. Res. Commun.* **271**, 374–379.

230. Hu, R. M. and Levin, E. R. (1994) Astrocyte growth is regulated by neuropeptides through Tis 8 and basic fibroblast growth factor. *J. Clin. Investig.* **93**, 1820–1827.

231. Biesiada, E., Razandi, M., and Levin, E. R. (1996) Egr-1 activates basic fibroblast growth factor transcription. *J. Biol. Chem.* **271**, 18,576–18,581.

232. Vollmer, A. M., Schmidt, K. N., and Schulz, R. (1996) Natriuretic peptide receptors on rat thymocytes: inhibition of proliferation by atrial natriuretic peptide. *Endocrinology* **137**, 1706–1713.

233. Abell, T. J., Richards, A. M., Ikram, H., Espiner, E. A., and Yandle, T. (1989) Atrial natriuretic factor inhibits proliferation of vascular smooth muscle cells stimulated by platelet-derived growth factor. *Biochem. Biophys. Res. Commun.* **160**, 1392–1396.

234. Itoh, H., Pratt, R. E., and Dzau, V. (1990) Atrial natriuretic polypeptide inhibits hypertrophy of vascular smooth muscle cells. *J. Clin. Investig.* **86**, 1690–1697.

235. Morishita, R., Gibbons, G. H., Pratt, R. E., et al. (1994) Autocrine and paracrine effects of atrial natriuretic peptide gene transfer on vascular smooth muscle and endothelial cellular growth. *J. Clin. Investig.* **94**, 824–829.

236. Hutchinson, H. G., Trinadade, P. T., Cunanan, D. B., Wu, C. F., and Pratt, R. E. (1997) Mechanisms of natriuretic-peptide-induced growth inhibition of vascular smooth muscle cells. *Cardiovasc. Res.* **35**, 158–167.

237. Suhasini, M., Li, H., Lohmann, S. M., Boss, G. R., and Pilz, R. B. (1998) Cyclic-GMP-dependent protein kinase inhibits the Ras/mitogen-activated protein kinase pathway. *Mol. Cell. Biol.* **18**, 6983–6994.

238. Chrisman, T. D. and Garbers, D. L. (1999) Reciprocal antagonism coordinates C-type natriuretic peptide and mitogen-signaling pathways in fibroblasts. *J. Biol. Chem.* **274**, 4293–4299.

239. Dzau, V. J. (1993) The role of mechanical and hormonal factors in growth regulation of vascular smooth muscle cells and cardiac myocytes. *Curr. Opin. Neph. Hypertens.* **2**, 27–32.

240. Redondo, J., Bishop, J. E., and Wilkins, M. R. (1998) Effect of atrial natriuretic peptide and cyclic GMP phosphodiesterase inhibition on collagen synthesis by adult cardiac fibroblasts. *Br. J. Pharm.* **124**, 1455–1462.

241. Calderone, A., Thaik, C. M., Takahashi, N., Chang, D. L. F., and Colucci, W. S. (1998) Nitric oxide atrial natriuretic peptide and cyclic GMP inhibit the growth-promoting effects of norepinephrine in cardiac myocytes and fibroblasts. *J. Clin. Investig.* **101**, 812–818.

242. Silberbach, M., Gorenc, T., Hershberger, R. E., Stork, P. J. S., Steyger, P. S., and Roberts, C. T. Jr. (1999) Extracellular signal-regulated protein kinase activation is required for the anti-hypertrophic effect of atrial natriuretic factor in neonatal rat ventricular myocytes. *J. Biol. Chem.* **274**, 24,858–24,864.

243. Horio, T., Nishikimi, T., Yoshihara, F., Matsuo, H., Takishita, S., and Kangawa, K. (2000) Inhibitory regulation of hypertrophy by endogenous atrial natriuretic peptide in cultured cardiac myocytes. *Hypertension* **35**, 19–24.

244. Dey, N. B., Boerth, N. J., Murphy-Ullrich, J. E., Chang, P. L., Prince, C. W., and Lincoln, T. M. (1998) Cyclic GMP-dependent protein kinase inhibits osteopontin and thrombospondin production in rat aortic smooth muscle cells. *Circ. Res.* **82**, 139–146.

245. Masciotra, S., Picard, S., and Deschepper, C. F. (1999) Cosegregation analysis in genetic crosses suggests a protective role for atrial natriuretic factor against ventricular hypertrophy. *Circ. Res.* **84**, 1453–1458.

246. Prins, B. A., Weber, M. J., Hu, R.-M., Pedram, A., Daniels, M., and Levin, E. R. (1996) Atrial natriuretic peptide inhibits mitogen-activated protein kinase through the clearance receptor: potential role in the inhibition of astrocyte proliferation. *J. Biol. Chem.* **271**, 14,156–14,162.

247. Sharma, G. D., Nguyen, H. T., Antonov, A. S., Gerrity, R. G., van Geldern, T. W., and Pandey, K. N. (2002) Negative regulation of mitogen-activated protein kinase (ERK 2 and p38[MAPK]) in cultured human vascular smooth muscle cells. *Mol. Cell. Biochem.* **233**, 165–173.

248. Komalavilas, P., Shah, P. K., Jo, H., and Lincoln, T. M. (1999) Activation of mitogen-activated protein kinase pathways by cyclic GMP and cyclic GMP-dependent protein kinase in contractile vascular smooth muscle cells. *J. Biol. Chem.* **274**, 34,301–34,309.

249. Bornfeldt, K. E. and Krebs, E. G. (1999) Crosstalk between protein kinase A and growth factor receptor signaling pathways in arterial smooth muscle. *Cell. Signal.* **11**, 465–477.

250. Trindade, P., Hutchinson, H. G., Pollman, M. J., Gibbons, G. H., and Pratt, R. E. (1995) Atrial natriuretic peptide (ANP) and C-type natriuretic peptide (CNP) induce apoptosis in vascular smooth muscle cells (VMSC). *Circulation* **92**, 1–696.

251. Wu, C. F., Bishopric, N. H., and Pratt, R. E., Atrial natriuretic peptide induces apoptosis in neonatal rat cardiac myocytes. *J. Biol. Chem.* **272,** 14,860–14,866.

252. Pollman, M. J., Yamada, T., Horiuchi, M., and Gibbons, G. H. (1996) Vasoactive substances regulate vascular smooth muscle cell apoptosis. *Circ. Res.* **79,** 748–756.

253. Kozopas, K. M., Yang, T., Buchan, H. L., Zhou, P., and Craig, R. W. (1993) MCLI a gene expressed in programmed myeloid cell differentiation has sequence similarity to BCL2. *Proc. Natl Acad. Sci.* **90,** 3516–3520.

254. Oltvai, Z. N., Milliman, C. L., and Korsmeyer, S. J. (1993) Bcl-2 hetereodimerizes in vivo with a conserved homolog Bax that accelerates programmed cell death. *Cell* **74,** 609–619.

255. Kiefer, M. C., Brauer, M. J., Powers, V. C., et al. (1995) Modulation of apoptosis by the widely distributed Bcl-2 homologue Bak. *Nature* **374,** 736–739.

256. Krajewski, S., Bodrug, S., Krajewski, M., et al. (1995) Immunohistochemical analysis of Mcl-1 protein in human tissues. *Am. J. Pathol.* **146,** 1309–1319.

257. Tsutamoto, T., Kanamari, T., Morigami, N., Sugimoto, Y., Yamaoka, O., and Kinoshita, M. (1993) Possibility of down-regulation of atrial natriuretic peptide receptor coupled to gyanylate cyclase in peripheral vascular beds of patients with chronic severe heart failure. *Circulation* **87,** 70–75.

258. Wei, C.-M., Heublein, D. M., Perrella, M. A., et al. (1993) Natriuretic peptide system in human heart failure. *Circulation* **88,** 1004–1009.

259. Chen, H. H. and Burnett, J. C. Jr. (1999) The natriuretic peptides in heart failure. *Proc. Assoc. Am. Phys.* **111,** 406–416.

260. Melo, L. G., Veress, A. T., Chong, C. K., Pang, S. C., Flynn, T. G., and Sonnenberg, H. (1998) Salt-sensitive hypertension in ANP knockout mice: potential role of abnormal plasma renin activity. *Am. J. Physiol.* **274,** R255–R261.

261. Steinhelper, M. E., Cochran, K. L., and Field, L. J. (1990) Hypotension in transgenic mice expressing atrial natriuretic factor fusion genes. *Hypertension* **16,** 301–307.

262. Lin, X., Hanze, J., Heese, F., Sodmann, R., and Lang, R. E. (1995) Gene expression of natriuretic peptide receptors in myocardial cells. *Circ. Res.* **77,** 750–758.

263. Holtwick, R., Gotthardt, M., Skryabin, B., et al. (2002) Smooth muscle-selective deletion of guanylyl cyclase-A prevents the acute but not chronic effects of ANP on blood pressure. *Proc. Natl Acad. Sci. USA* **99,** 7142–7147.

264. Zhao, L., Long, L., and Morrell, N. W. (1999) NPRA-deficient mice show increased susceptibility to hypoxia-induced pulmonary hypertension. *Circulation* **99,** 605–607.

265. Knowles, J. W., Esposito, G., Mao, L., and Smithies, O. (2001) Pressure independent enhancement of cardiac hypertrophy in natriuretic peptide receptor-A deficient mice. *J. Clin. Investig.* **107,** 975–984.

266. Navar, L. G. (1997) The kidney in blood pressure regulation and development of hypertension. *Med. Clin. North Am.* **81,** 1165–1198.

267. Deschepper, C. F., Masciotra, S., Zahabi, A., Boutin-Ganache, I., Picard, S., and Reudelhuber, T. L. (2001) Function alterations of the Nppa promoter are linked to cardiac ventricular hypertrophy in WKY/WKHA rat crosses. *Circ. Res.* **88,** 223–228.

18 Sex Steroids and Hypertension

Andrew P. Miller and Suzanne Oparil

1. INTRODUCTION

There is a sexual dimorphism in the development of cardiovascular disease (CVD) in humans *(1,2)*. The prevalence of total CVD, defined as coronary heart disease (CHD), congestive heart failure, stroke, and hypertension, is much lower in premenopausal women than in age-matched men, but rises quickly in women after the fifth decade to surpass that of men at later ages *(2)*. Epidemiologic and observational studies of menopausal hormone therapy associate a lower risk of CHD development and CVD mortality with hormone treatment *(3–9)*. Based on this evidence and an extensive volume of mechanistic studies from in vitro and animal research, it was thought that ovarian hormones, principally estrogens, were vasoprotective. However, because large randomized controlled trials of menopausal hormone therapy have demonstrated no cardiovascular benefit and some evidence of harm (increased CHD, stroke, and thromboembolic events in women assigned to some hormone treatments), this concept of estrogenic vasoprotection has been called into question *(10–13)*.

Similar to the pattern for CVD, there is a striking age-dependent sexual dimorphism in the prevalence of hypertension [Fig. 1; *(2)*]. In early adulthood, hypertension [defined as systolic blood pressure (BP) ≥ 140 mmHg and/or diastolic BP ≥ 90 mmHg] is less common among women than men. However, after the fifth decade of life, the incidence of hypertension increases more rapidly in women than in men, with the prevalence of hypertension in women equal to or exceeding that in men during the sixth decade. Although women have lower systolic BP levels than men during early adulthood, the

From: *Contemporary Endocrinology: Hypertension and Hormone Mechanisms*
Edited by: R. M. Carey © Humana Press Inc., Totowa, NJ

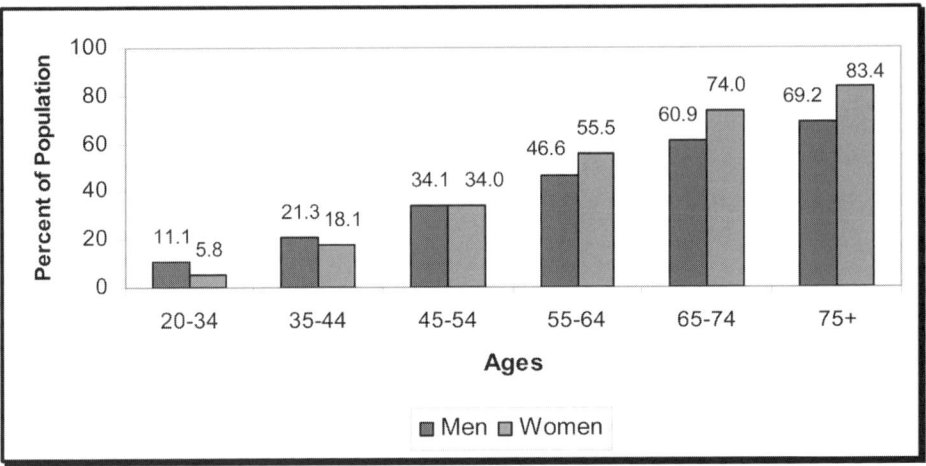

Prevalence of High Blood Pressure in Americans by Age and Sex NHANES: 1999-2002

Fig. 1. Prevalence of high blood pressure in Americans (age 20 yr and above) by age and sex (NHANES 1999–2002). (From ref. 2 accessed on: 2 Feb 2007 at http://www.americanheart.org/downloadable/heart/11050481905292005Statcharts.ppt)

opposite is true after the sixth decade. Regardless of age, diastolic BP tends to be slightly lower in women than in men (14–16).

A large body of fundamental evidence implicates sex steroids as vasoactive substances, modulators of vascular remodeling and injury responses, regulators of other vasoactive hormones, and participants in the coagulation cascade. In this chapter, we will focus on the effects of estrogens, progestins, and androgens on normal BP regulation and on the pathophysiology of hypertension. Special attention will be given to newer evidence offering insight into the complexity of sex steroid metabolism and into the age-dependent changes in vascular responses to sex steroids.

2. SEX HORMONES AND BLOOD PRESSURE

2.1. Estrogens

To account for the observed sexual dimorphism, sex steroids have been implicated as effectors of BP regulation in animals and humans (17–19). Endogenous estradiol tends to lower BP. Observational studies of BP through the menstrual cycle have demonstrated that BP is lower when estradiol levels peak during the luteal phase than when they are at their nadir during the follicular phase (20–22). Further, the menopause is associated with a significant increase in BP in cross-sectional studies (23). In a prospective study of BP in premenopausal, perimenopausal, and postmenopausal women, an age-independent 4–5 mmHg increase in systolic BP was found in postmenopausal women (24). Additional support for BP lowering effects comes from the observation that BP is reduced when endogenous estradiol levels become elevated during pregnancy (25). Interestingly though, BP reductions are maximal during the first and second trimesters of pregnancy when estradial levels are increased 8- to 15-fold; BP rises during the third trimester when estradiol levels increase to over 180-fold, suggesting that other factors regulate BP during pregnancy.

Data on the BP effects of hormone interventions (contraceptive estrogens or estrogenic preparations in menopausal hormone therapy) have been inconsistent, with reports of neutral BP (26,27), lowering BP (28–32), and elevating BP effects (13,33–35). In the Postmenopausal Estrogen/Progestin interventions (PEPI) trial, which enrolled 875 healthy normotensive early postmenopausal women, assignment to conjugated equine estrogen (CEE, 0.625 mg/d) ± a progestin did not impact systolic or diastolic BP when compared with placebo controls (26). In contrast, when transdermal estradiol was administered at physiologic doses to healthy postmenopausal women in two studies that evaluated ambulatory BP, active treatment significantly lowered nocturnal systolic, diastolic and mean BP (3–7 mmHg) when compared with placebo (30,31). The observational study component of the Women's Health Initiative (WHI-OS) collected data on risk factors for CVD, including BP, from 98,705 women aged 50–79 yr, the largest multiethnic, best characterized cohort of postmenopausal women ever studied (33). WHI-OS found that current hormone use was associated with a 25% greater likelihood of having hypertension compared with past use or no prior use. Further, among 5310 postmenopausal women randomized to CEE (0.625 mg/d) compared to a placebo group as part of the randomized controlled trial component of WHI, there was a 1.1-mmHg increase from baseline in systolic BP at 1 yr of follow up that persisted throughout the 6.8 yr of follow up (13). There was no difference in diastolic BP between treatment groups.

Although many studies included small numbers of subjects and lacked comparative controls, use of oral contraceptive agents has been associated with development of hypertension (15). Since the initial report associating the development of hypertension with oral contraceptive use (34), several investigators have noted elevated BP in a subgroup of women taking these agents, with an improvement in BP on withdrawal (15). In one report of 22 patients referred after a development of hypertension temporally associated with initiation of oral contraceptives, use of these agents was associated with increased plasma renin activity and aldosterone excretion, with improvement in these hormone levels and in BP within weeks of oral contraceptive withdrawal (35). In the Nurses' Health Study II (NHS II), a prospective cohort study of 68,297 premenopausal women free of CVD, the multivariate risk for the development of hypertension among the current users of oral contraceptives compared with never-users was 1.8 (CI 1.5–2.3) (36). Absolute risk was small, however (only 41.5 cases of hypertension per 10,000 person-years could be attributed to oral contraceptive use), and risk decreased quickly with a cessation of contraceptive use [past users had only a slightly increased risk (RR, 1.2; CI, 1.0–1.4) compared with never users]. In summary, these data support a general conclusion that contraceptive estrogens increase BP, conjugated equine estrogen has little effect on BP, and estradiol probably lowers BP (19).

2.2. Progestins

Similar to estrogens, the effects of progestins on BP appear to be dependent on the type of progestin. Natural progesterone has been associated with BP lowering or neutral effects. Higher levels of progesterone correlate with lower systolic but not diastolic BP during the second and third trimesters of pregnancy (37). In a crossover study of 15 postmenopausal women assigned to placebo or transdermal estradiol ± intravaginal progesterone, addition of progesterone did not affect the nocturnal BP lowering seen with estradiol compared with placebo treatment *(31)*. Similarly, the nonandrogenic medroxyprogesterone acetate (MPA) appears to have BP neutral or lowering effects. In a double-blind, crossover study of 29 postmenopausal women assigned to 4 wk of CEE and placebo or increasing doses of MPA, there was a dose-dependent decrease in ambulatory daytime diastolic and mean BPs for those women assigned to the progestin compared with placebo *(38)*.

In contrast, most studies of the synthetic progestins for contraception or hormone therapy have revealed a BP-elevating effect. Oral contraceptives in particular appear to precipitate or accelerate hypertension *(15)*. Data from NHS II support a role for progestins in contraceptive-induced hypertension. When risk of developing hypertension was assessed based on progestin potency, compared with never-users of contraceptives, women who took low, medium, and high progestational potency preparations had a multivariate risk of 1.6 (CI = 1.0–2.2), 2.5 (CI = 1.8–3.4), and 2.0 (CI = 1.4–3.0), respectively *(36)*. This pro-hypertensive effect was better tested in a study of two oral contraceptives that both contained 30 μg ethinyl estradiol, but two doses of the progestin levonororgestrel (150 and 250 μg) *(39)*. In this study, a dose-dependent response of BP to the progestin component was demonstrated.

2.3. Androgens

Compared to the female sex steroids, much less is known about the effects of androgens on BP *(19,40)*. Lower serum levels of testosterone and androstenedione have been described in men with hypertension, supporting the hypothesis that androgens may be vasoprotective *(41,42)*. However, these studies are subject to confounding by other factors known to affect androgen levels, most notably ageing and stress *(43,44)*.

When the hypothesis that androgens lower BP was tested in longitudinal and cross-sectional studies, an association with BP has not been consistently demonstrated. In a subgroup of 66 men from the Multiple Risk Factor Intervention Trial (MRFIT), testosterone levels were followed over 13 yr *(45)*. Greater longitudinal decreases in testosterone correlated positively with increases in cardiovascular risk factors, including a more atherogenic lipid profile, behavioral stress, and tobacco use; however, no association was found with BP. Likewise, in the larger Rotterdam Study, levels of androgens [dihydroepiandrosterone sulfate (DHEAS), total and bioavailable testosterone (TT and BT)] did not correlate significantly with BP in 1032 nonsmoking men and women, whereas lower levels of androgens did associate in an age-adjusted analysis with more obesity, insulin resistance and aortic atherosclerosis in men *(46)*. In a cross-sectional study of 400 independently living men (aged 40–80 yr), one standard deviation increase in TT and BT levels correlated with a reduced risk of the metabolic syndrome (including the individual components of waist circumference and fasting glucose level), but did not correlate significantly with BP [OR, 0.83 (0.65–1.07) and 0.95 (0.73–1.23) for TT and BT, respectively] *(47)*. Finally, in the Tromso Study, sex hormone levels and resting BP were examined in a cross-sectional study including 1548 men, aged 25–84 yr *(48)*. In the age-adjusted analysis, lower testosterone and sex hormone-binding globulin levels correlated significantly with higher systolic BP ($p < 0.001$). When corrected for body mass index, this relationship persisted ($p < 0.001$ and $p = 0.002$ for testosterone and sex hormone-binding gloubulin, respectively). Thus, the overall evidence suggests a possible reducing or neutral effect for endogenous androgens on BP. This hypothesis remains to be tested, however, in randomized controlled trials with androgens as interventions *(40)*.

3. VASCULAR EFFECTS OF ESTROGENS

Most of the vascular effects of estrogens are mediated by the activation of estrogen receptors (ERs), which are expressed in most cell types that influence vascular function, including vascular smooth muscle cells (VSMCs), endothelial cells, and leukocytes *(49–53)*. Two major ER subtypes, ER-α and ER-β, have been described *(54,55)* and have been shown in transfection experiments to regulate both distinct and common target genes *(56)*. Interestingly, of the functional categories of estrogen-regulated genes, most numerous were those encoding cytokines and inflammatory factors, signal transduction factors, and adhesion/cytoskeletal molecules. Both ER-α and ER-β are expressed in the vasculature *(57)*, and many of the effects of estrogens, including their protective effects in the setting of vascular injury, have been attributed to the activation of ER-α *(58)*. Subsequent studies have revealed a more complex pattern of ER subtype-dependent and cell-specific actions of estrogens to promote vascular repair: activated ER-α stimulates endothelial cell migration and proliferation, whereas activated ER-β inhibits migration and proliferation of VSMCs *(59)*.

Activation of ERs has been described in the classic sex steroid pathway: (1) estrogen diffuses directly through the plasma membrane, and (2) forms an estrogen–ER complex (an ER dimer), then (3) the activated complex translocates to the nucleus, (4) in which it binds to estrogen response elements (EREs) and stimulates transcription or gene suppression [Fig. 2; *(60)*]. Microarray technology has characterized the genes affected by estrogens in MCF-7 cells; of note, estradiol turns off 70% of the genes it affects in this breast cancer cell line *(61)*. Transcriptional profiling of estrogen-related gene expression in vascular cells is ongoing in a number of laboratories, including our own.

A nongenomic pathway for estrogen actions has been proposed, whereby estrogens interact with signal-generating receptors bound to the plasma membrane and elicit rapid effects on vascular cells *(60)*. The acute vasodilator effects of estrogens, discussed below, appear to be mediated in this manner via ERs expressed in both endothelial and VSMCs [Fig. 3; *(60)*].

3.1. Effects of Estrogens on Vascular Tone

Estrogens have both acute and chronic effects on vascular tone. The former are too rapid to be mediated by regulation of gene transcription and occur by a nongenomic mechanism, whereas the latter are mediated by ERs acting as transcription factors to effect specific vascular gene expression. Acutely, estrogens produce vasodilation by interacting with an ER-α subpopulation in caveolae of endothelial cells *(51)*, which rapidly activate the mitogen-activated protein kinase (MAPK) and phosphatidylinositol 3-kinase (PI3K)/Akt-kinase pathways *(62,63)* and, thus, directly increase endothelial nitric oxide synthase (eNOS) activity [Fig. 3; *(60)*]. This endothelial-dependent pathway is augmented by an additional endothelial-independent pathway, in which

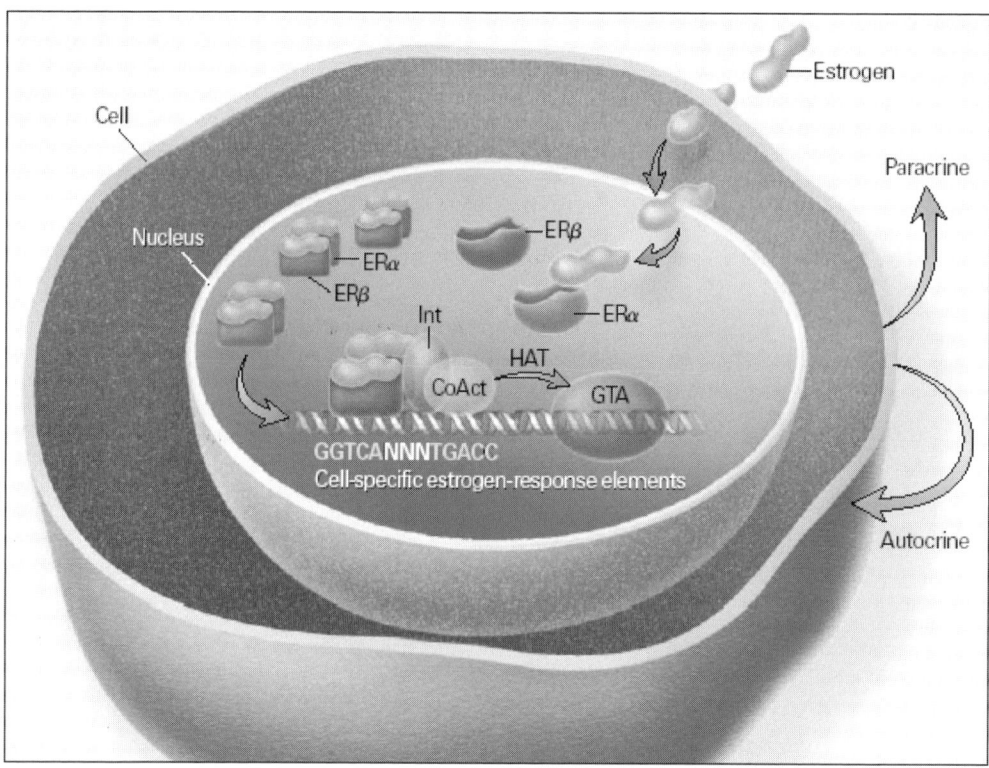

Fig. 2. Mechanism of estrogen-receptor (ER) activation of gene expression. In the classical steroid pathway, estrogen enters target cells by passive diffusion and binds to high-affinity intracellular receptors. ER-α and -β act as transcriptional factors that undergo conformational changes after ligand binding. The estrogen–ER complexes form dimers and then bind to specific sites in the control regions of their target genes (estrogen-response elements). The complexes associate with several proteins capable of activating the general transcriptional apparatus (GTA), the multiprotein complex containing RNA polymerase that transcribes DNA into RNA. These ER-associated proteins include coactivator proteins (CoAct) and general integrators of transcription (Int). ER-associated proteins may have enzymatic functions as well, such as histone acetyltransferase (HAT) activity. Estrogen receptors may also suppress the transcription of selected target genes by interacting with corepressors. Reproduced with permission from ref. 60.

estradiol opens Ca^{2+}- and voltage-activated K^+ channels in endothelial-denuded porcine coronary arteries and in isolated VSMCs in vitro (64). Together, these pathways provide the fundamental basis for the observation that exogenous estradiol dilates brachial and coronary arteries in postmenopausal women and in men (65–67).

Longer term, estrogen induces changes in vascular tone by mediating expression of genes for the synthesis of vasodilator molecules, including prostacyclin and nitric oxide. Prostacyclin production is increased in response to 17β-estradiol in rat aortic SMCs in culture via increases in both cyclooxygenase and prostacyclin synthetase activities (68). In a mouse model of atherosclerosis (LDL receptor knockout), estradiol upregulates cyclooxygenase-2-derived prostacyclin production through an ER-α-dependent mechanism that accounts for much of its atheroprotective effect in this model (69). Nitric oxide production is effected by genomic as well as nongenomic

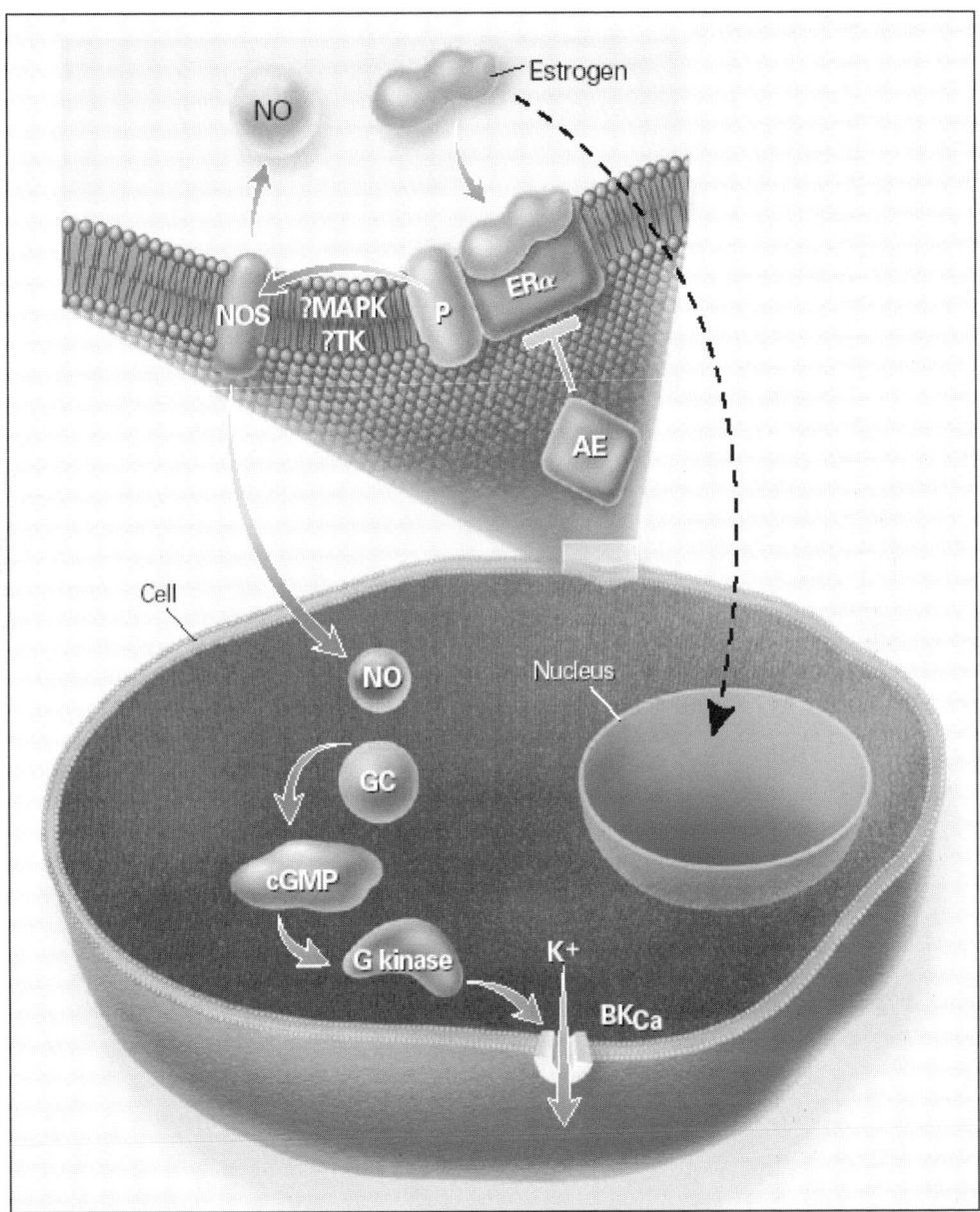

Fig. 3. Rapid, nongenomic pathways of estrogen–estrogen receptor actions. Estrogen causes rapid activation of nitric oxide synthase (NOS) in a manner that does not require new gene transcription. In endothelial cells (upper portion of figure), this occurs by a novel action of an estrogen receptor (ER)-α subpopulation in caveolae *(51)*, is blocked by antiestrogens (AE), and may require a class of receptor-associated proteins (P) distinct from those that act with the receptors to mediate changes in transcription. The result is rapid activation of endothelial NOS, through signal-transduction pathways involving the mitogen-activated protein kinase (MAPK) and phosphatidylinositol 3-kinase/Akt-kinase pathways *(60,61)*. In vascular smooth-muscle cells (lower portion of figure), estrogen rapidly activates calcium-activated potassium channels (BKCa), which hyperpolarize and relax smooth-muscle cells *(62)*. BKCa activation in vascular smooth muscle occurs through a pathway that is dependent on nitric oxide (NO) and cyclic guanosine monophosphate (cGMP). GC denotes guanylate cyclase, G kinase cGMP-dependent protein kinase, and TK tyrosine kinase. Reproduced with permission from ref. *60*.

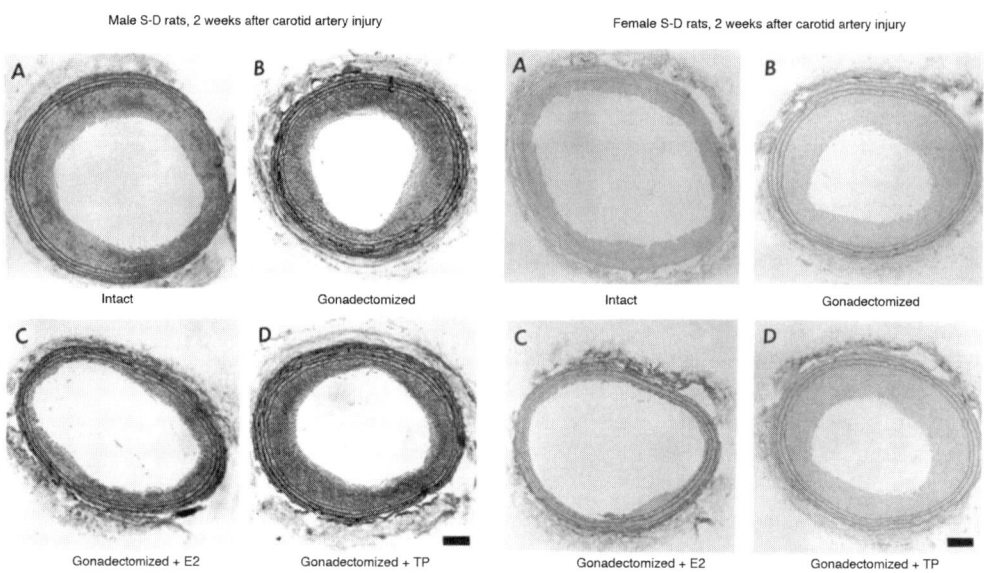

Fig. 4. Representative light micrographs of right common carotid arteries from male (left) and female (right) Sprague–Dawley rats 14 d after balloon injury. Balloon-injured right carotid arteries from (**A**) an intact rat, (**B**) a gonadectomized rat, (**C**) a gonadectomized plus 17β-estradiol-treated (E2) rat, and (**D**) a gonadectomized plus testosterone-treated (TP) rat. Bar = 100 μm. Reproduced with permission from ref. *80.*

pathways. Expression of eNOS and neuronal NOS (nNOS) is upregulated during pregnancy and by exogenous estradiol administration in the guinea pig *(70)*. These mechanisms support the observations that long-term administration of estrogens increases acetylcholine-induced vasodilation in coronary arteries of nonhuman primates *(71,72)*, postmenopausal women *(73,74)*, and male-to-female transsexuals *(75,76)*.

3.2. Effects of Estrogens on Vascular Remodeling

The effects of estrogens on vascular injury responses and vascular remodeling have been well characterized (reviewed in refs. *19,77*) and will be discussed only briefly here because they are only indirectly involved in the pathogenesis of hypertension. In animal models, there is a sexual dimorphism in the response to vascular injury (female < male), providing evidence that estrogens protect against neointima formation [Fig. 4; *(78–81)*] and promote re-endothelialization *(82)*. This vasoprotective effect is mediated by an ER-dependent mechanism *(83)* and is elicited in the first 72 h after injury *(84)*. Our laboratory has characterized an early anti-inflammatory mechanism for estradiol-induced inhibition of the acute neointimal response to endoluminal vascular injury, with potent inhibition of inflammatory mediator expression *(85)* and leukocyte infiltration *(86)* of the injured blood vessel in the first 24 h after injury. Additionally, estradiol attenuates adventitial fibroblast activation and myofibroblast transformation in the same injury model *(87,88)*.

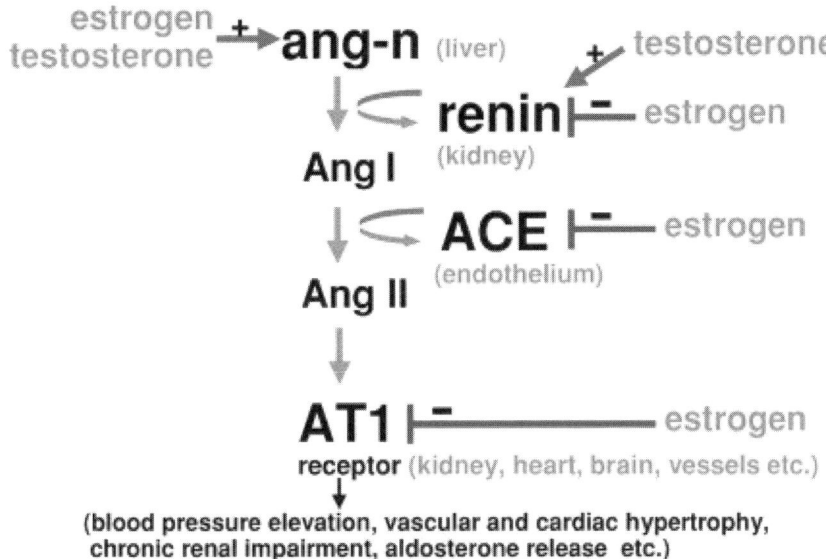

Fig. 5. The influence of estrogen and testosterone on the cascade leading to angiotensin II formation and subsequent receptor activation. Reproduced with permission from ref. *80.*

3.3. Effects of Estrogens on Vasoactive Hormones / Local Mediators

Estrogens modulate the production of numerous vasoactive factors, including homocysteine, endothelin, and components of the renin–angiotensin–aldosterone system. Homocysteine has been shown to induce VSMC growth and endothelial damage, and is an independent marker of cardiovascular risk *(89–91).* In clinical studies, estrogens consistently lower circulating homocysteine levels in postmenopausal women *(92–95).* Whether this effect represents biological inhibition of homocysteine production or an indirect result of estrogen-induced changes in albumin metabolism is a topic of controversy *(96).* Endothelin-1 has been implicated in postmenopausal hypertension by the observations that hypertensive postmenopausal women have higher circulating levels than normotensives and that levels increase after menopause *(97,98).* Further, estrogen therapy has been directly associated with decreases in circulating endothelin-1 levels in postmenopausal women *(98,99).* Estradiol inhibits endothelial cell production of endothelin-1 in response to serum and angiotensin II (AII) stimulation *(100),* apparently by an ER-independent mechanism *(101).* Estradiol also inhibits the damaging actions of endothelin-1 on VSMCs, including MAPK activation and mitogen-stimulated c-fos and c-myc expression *(102).* Taken together, the effects of estradiol on homocysteine and endothelin-1 appear to promote endothelial and VSMC health.

Gender differences in various components of the renin–angiotensin–aldosterone cascade, including important estrogenic modulation of angiotensinogen production and renin, angiotensin-converting enzyme (ACE), and angiotensin AT-1 receptor expression, have been observed [reviewed in ref. *(103)*; Fig. 5]. The synthesis of angiotensinogen in hepatocytes is stimulated by estrogen *(104),* probably by binding to an ERE in the angiotensinogen gene promoter *(105).* This pro-hypertensive effect of estrogen on the initial step of the cascade opposes its inhibitory actions on downstream components.

The presence of endogenous estrogen and the use of estrogen replacement therapy are associated with lower levels of plasma renin and ACE activity *(104,106–111)*. Renin levels are lower in women than in men, and in postmenopausal women receiving estrogen therapy than in those not receiving estrogen *(106,107)*.

Serum ACE activity also decreases in response to estrogen administration in postmenopausal women *(107,108)*, nonhuman primates *(109)*, and normotensive or hypertensive rats *(110,111)*. Additionally, estrogen induces the production of the heptapeptide Ang 1–7, a potent vasodilator and inhibitor of SMC growth *(111)*. Further, estrogen appears to downregulate the expression of AT-1 receptors, a final step in the cascade that is responsible for many of the harmful effects of the renin–angiotensin–aldosterone system. In rat aortic tissue and in isolated VSMCs, removal of estrogen (by ovariectomy or by adjusting the composition of the culture media) leads to the overexpression of AT-1 receptors compared with controls (by 187 and 160%, respectively) *(112)*. This effect is reversed by estrogen supplementation. Likewise, estrogen treatment has been shown to reduce angiotensin-induced aldosterone secretion in ovariectomized rats *(113)*. This effect appears to be mediated by a post-transcriptional mechanism by which estradiol interferes with ribosomal efficiency for AT-1 receptor translation *(114)*. Taken together, these studies support a dichotomous action of estrogen on the renin–angiotensin–aldosterone system, whereby it increases the initial substrate (angiotensinogen) but inhibits the generation and biological action of the active hormones (angiotensin II and aldosterone) (Fig. 5).

3.4. Effects of Estrogens on Sodium Handling: Renal and CNS Mechanisms

Female sex hormones protect against salt-induced increases in BP, at least in part by increasing the sensitivity of the pressure–natriuresis relationship and augmenting renal excretion of sodium *(115)*. Studies carried out in normotensive women during the menstrual cycle, during use of oral contraceptives, and after menopause show that the pressure–natriuresis relationship is steep in young women during all phases of the menstrual cycle and during oral contraceptive use, indicating insensitivity to salt; however, the pressure–natriuresis curve is shifted to the right in menopausal women, indicating that BP becomes salt-sensitive after the menopause (Fig. 6). Mechanistic studies support estrogen as the sex steroid that mediates this effect. In a genetic salt-sensitive rat model (Dahl salt-sensitive), ovariectomy elicits development of hypertension, which is prevented by estrogen replacement or by feeding a very low sodium diet *(116)*. Ovariectomy is associated with a twofold increase in renal AT_1 receptor expression that can be reversed with estrogen treatment in this model.

Salt-sensitivity is mediated by marked activation of the central and peripheral nervous systems in estrogen-depleted environments *(117)*. Studies in spontaneously hypertensive rats (SHR) demonstrate a sexual dimorphism such that young female SHR have lower BP and an attenuated response to high dietary salt compared with age-matched males *(118)*. When subjected to ovariectomy and removal of dietary phytoestrogens, these animals demonstrate salt-sensitive hypertension (rise in BP > 40 mmHg in response to a high-salt diet) that is reversed with hexamethonium-induced ganglionic blockade indicating the dependence on the sympathetic nervous system *(119)*.

The mechanism of this neurally mediated salt-sensitive hypertension has been elucidated in an elegant series of studies carried out in male SHRs *(120–136)*. In this

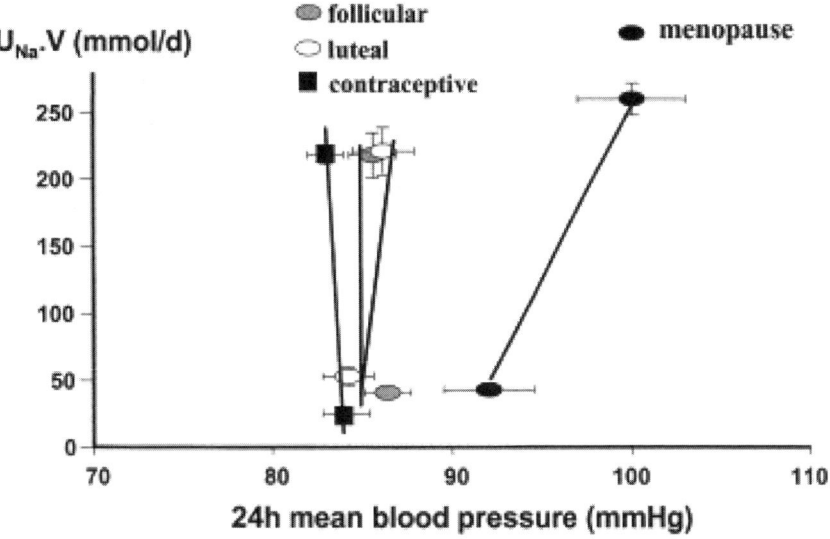

Fig. 6. Pressure–natriuresis relationship in normotensive women during the normal menstrual cycle, during the use of oral contraceptives, and after menopause. All women received randomly a diet low in sodium (40 mmol Na/d) and high in sodium (250 mmol Na/d) for 1 wk. Blood pressure was measured over 24 h using ambulatory blood pressure monitoring. Reproduced with permission from ref. *115*.

model, dietary salt supplementation increases BP by reducing norepinephrine release from nerve terminals in the anterior hypothalamic area (AHA), thus reducing the activation of sympathoinhibitory neurons in the AHA (Fig. 7). This, in turn, results in an increased sympathetic outflow and higher BP. Two mechanisms have been shown to contribute to this effect: (1) reduced noradrenergic input into AHA via baroreflex pathways, and (2) local inhibition of norepinephrine release in AHA by the inhibitory neuromodulator atrial natriuretic peptide (ANP). Studies employing microinjection of a blocking monoclonal antibody to ANP directly into the AHA and the nucleus tractus solitarius (NTS) demonstrated for the first time that endogenous ANP in the brain is functionally active in the tonic control of BP and baroreflex sensitivity in the SHR but plays a lesser role in the normotensive Wistar–Kyoto (WKY) control. In the WKY, excitation of NTS neurons by baroreflex afferents leads to the activation of sympathoinhibitory neurons in NTS and AHA, strong inhibition of sympathetic nervous system outflow, and a decrease in BP. In SHR, brain ANP acts at the levels of the NTS and the AHA to perturb this baroreflex regulatory pathway. ANP tonically activates sympathoinhibitory neurons in the caudal NTS of SHR, thereby restraining the rise in BP, and tonically inhibits baroreflex responsiveness to alterations in BP. Thus, ANP appears to act at a number of sites in brain to facilitate the development and maintenance of sympathetically mediated hypertension in the SHR model.

Importantly, the robust pressor response to dietary salt supplementation that is seen in male SHR and is absent from young intact females, appears with ageing such that 13-mo-old ("middle-aged") females manifest marked salt sensitivity (~40 mmHg increase in BP in response to dietary salt supplementation) *(137)*. In contrast, when estradiol was removed from the environment by ovariectomy and dietary restriction

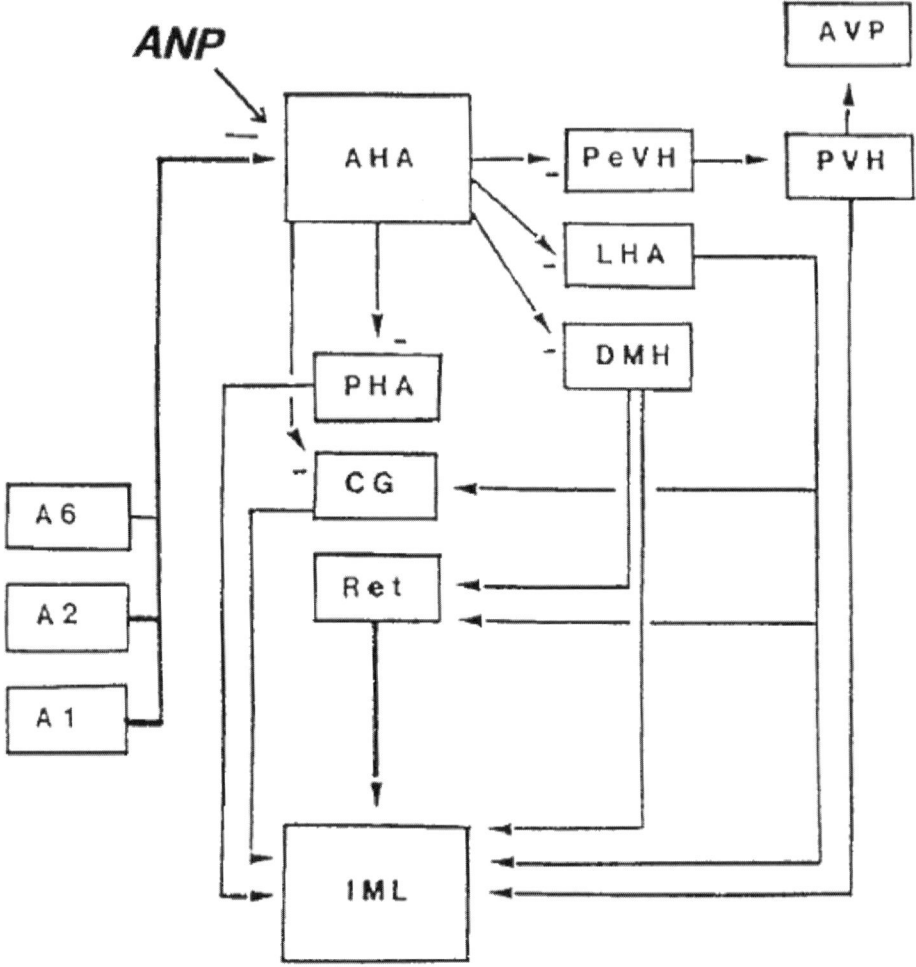

Fig. 7. Schematic representation of the major noradrenergic projections to the anterior hypothalamic area and the major direct and indirect projection from anterior hypothalamic area to "pressor" nuclei. In SHR, increased activity of the inhibitory neuromodulator ANP in anterior hypothalamic area and reduced input from baroreceptor afferents synapsing in brain stem nuclei reduce norepinephrine release in anterior hypothalamic area, resulting in reduced inhibitory control of sympathetic outflow. Dashes (–) indicate synaptic inhibition; A1, A2, A6, brainstem noradrenergic nuclei; AHA anterior hypothalamic area; AVP, arginine vasopressin release; CG, central gray of the midbrain; DMH, dorsomedial nucleus of the hypothalamus; IML, preganglionic sympathetic nucleus; LHA, lateral hypothalamic area; PeVH, periventricular; PHA, posterior hypothalamic area; PVH, paraventricular hypothalamic nucleus; Ret, medullary reticular formation. Reproduced with permission from ref. *120.*

of phytoestrogens, a slightly greater pressor response was observed (~50 mmHg). Likewise, in the AHA of middle-aged SHR, there was an accompanying decrease in norepinephrine to salt supplementation that resembles that of the male. Similar to the BP effect, there is a small but significant effect of estradiol on this large decrease in norepinephrine release.

Collectively, these studies support the concept that menopause precipitates salt sensitivity in the ageing female population, contributing to the rapid increase in prevalence of hypertension in this group. The clinical implication of this interpretation is that diuretic therapy is of paramount importance in hypertensive postmenopausal women, consistent with many current guidelines *(138–140)*.

4. VASCULAR EFFECTS OF PROGESTINS

Progesterone receptors (PRs), like ERs, exist in two isoforms, PR-A and PR-B, and have both genomic and nongenomic functions *(141)*. Structurally, the two forms differ only in that PR-B contains an additional 164 amino acid N-terminal extension, and both are derived from the same gene by the use of two promoters, whose activation is regulated by estrogen *(141,142)*. Interestingly, PR-A functions as a repressor of PR-B activity, as well as of the transcriptional activity of estrogen, glucocorticoid, androgen, and mineralocorticoid receptors, in many cell lines *(143)*. Although studied extensively in reproductive tissues, PR expression in vascular tissues has been identified *(144)*, but not yet well characterized *(142)*.

4.1. Effects of Progestins on Vascular Tone

The progestins generally antagonize the effects of estrogen on vascular tone. Although native progesterone has minimal effects on endothelium-dependent and endothelium-independent relaxation of arteries in vivo and in vitro, coadministration of progesterone with estrogen blunts both modes of vasodilator response to the latter hormone *(145, 146)*. The synthetic progestin MPA appears to be a more potent antagonist of estrogen than native progesterone. In ovariectomized monkeys, MPA, but not progesterone, reduced or completely abolished endothelium-dependent vasorelaxation in response to administration of conjugated equine estrogen in doses comparable to those administered to humans *(147)*. Likewise, in ovariectomized monkeys subjected to coronary vasospasm induced by direct stimulation, progesterone + estradiol protected, whereas MPA + estradiol failed to protect against vasospasm *(148)*.

Data from in vitro studies of human umbilical vein endothelial cells support differential effects of progesterone and MPA *(149)*. In this cell type, progesterone stimulates eNOS activity, does not alter the stronger stimulatory effects of estradiol on eNOS, and augments estradiol-induced ERK1/2 phosphorylation and Akt phosphorylation. In contrast, MPA does not alter eNOS activity, blunts estradiol-induced increases in eNOS activity, and reduces estradiol-dependent ERK1/2 phosphorylation. Thus, progesterone and MPA are not equivalent because they have distinct direct biological effects on vasoactive mediators and intracellular signaling pathways, as well as differential effects on the actions of estradiol.

4.2. Effects of Progestins on Vascular Remodeling

Similar to their effects on vascular tone, progesterone may be protective whereas MPA antagonizes the modulatory effects of estrogen on vascular remodeling in response to various stresses, including mechanical injury, thereby producing unfavorable effects on the vascular injury response. Native progesterone has a dose-dependent inhibitory effect on DNA synthesis and proliferation in rat aortic SMCs in vitro *(150)*. This effect occurs at physiologic doses and is mediated by the reductions in cyclin A and E mRNA levels. In the setting of vascular injury in our laboratory, we found that exogenous native progesterone, administered alone and with estradiol, had variable effects on neointima formation, with a net null effect on the actions of coadministered estrogen in rat carotid arteries (unpublished data). We attributed these observations to variable partial conversion of exogenous progesterone to estrogen by the rat. In contrast, MPA had no independent biological effect, but did blunt the antiproliferative and anti-inflammatory effects of estradiol in the balloon-injured carotid artery of the ovariectomized rat *(81,86,151)*. Our laboratory has also demonstrated that, although MPA alone has no effect on neointima formation after acute endoluminal injury in carotid arteries of gonadectomized rats of both sexes *(151)*, it greatly increases neointima formation in injured arteries of intact female rats to near levels in males *(81)*. When coadminstered with estradiol to ovariectomized female rats, MPA abolishes estrogen-induced inhibition of neointima formation *(151)* and completely blocks acute anti-inflammatory responses to estradiol *(86)*. The latter effect of MPA may be mediated by its demonstrated interference with nuclear factor-κB suppression by other steroids such as glucocorticoids *(149)*.

4.3. Effects of Progestins on the Renin–Angiotensin–Aldosterone System and Renal Sodium Handling

Limited data support a possible stimulatory effect for progesterone on components of the renin–angiotensin–aldosterone system and suggest that progesterone may be a competitive inhibitor of mineralocorticoid receptors. In women undergoing stimulation for in vitro fertilization, there is a positive relationship between progesterone levels and plasma renin activity during and after ovulation, as well as throughout pregnancy, if successfully conceived *(152)*. Progesterone, injected subcutaneously, increases plasma renin activity and aldosterone levels in vivo in Sprague–Dawley rats and increases baseline and angiotensin II-stimulated aldosterone production in vitro in isolated zona glomerulosa cells *(153)*. Conversely, progesterone has been shown to competitively bind mineralocorticoid receptors with a similar affinity as aldosterone, and presumably as an antagonist, in rodents and guinea pigs *(154)*.

When administered to humans, progesterone produces a natriuresis *(155,156)*. Originally ascribed to competitive inhibition of aldosterone *(157)*, further studies revealed a mineralocorticoid-independent effect *(156)*. More recent data suggest a direct action for progesterone in the distal nephron: progesterone increases calcium reabsorption and sodium excretion in the distal but not proximal tubule of the rabbit kidney, and progesterone receptors are found in the distal nephron but not in the proximal tubules *(158)*. Whether these effects can be extrapolated to other progestins (e.g., MPA) is of yet unknown.

5. VASCULAR EFFECTS OF ANDROGENS

There is a sexual dimorphism in BP that is mainly due to androgens. In major rat models of hypertension (Dahl salt-sensitive, SHR, deoxycorticosterone acetate-induced, and New Zealand genetically hypertensive), BP is consistently higher in males than in females *(159,160)*. When subjected to gonadectomy, young male, but not female, SHRs are protected from hypertension development, a finding that is reversed by testosterone administration to gonadectomized rats of both the sexes *(18,19,160)*. Removing the androgen receptor (AR), as in the testicular feminization syndrome *(161)*, or blocking

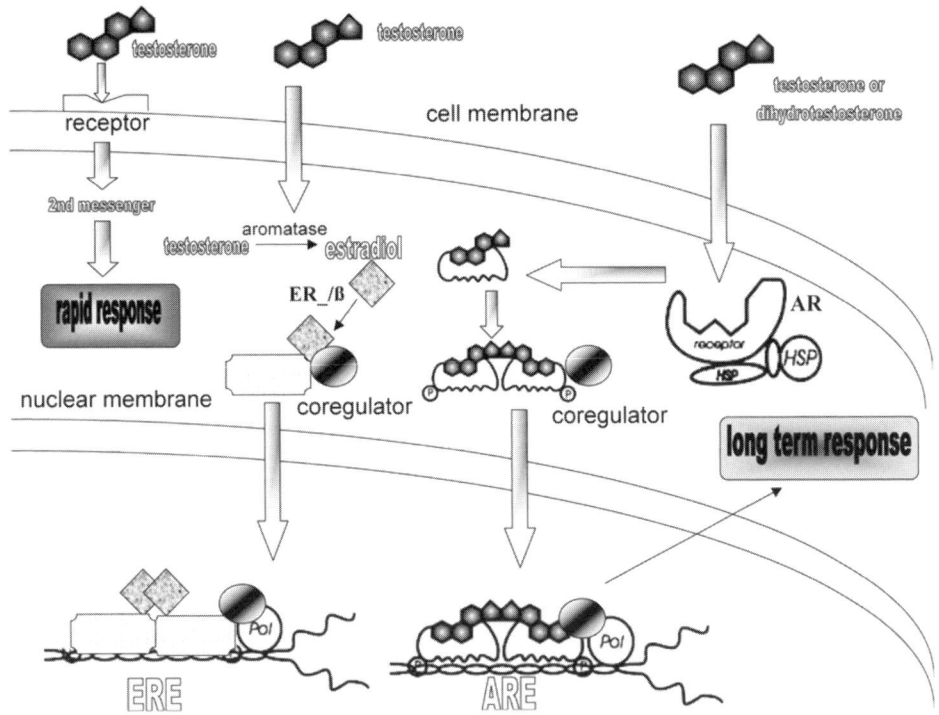

Fig. 8. Nongenomic and genomic androgen mechanisms. *Left*: Nongenomic effects of testosterone, which are triggered by binding to a still uncharacterized (nonclassical) membrane receptor. This activates second messengers, including calcium and protein kinases, which produce typically rapid responses. Genomic effects are depicted in the *middle* and on the *right*. Testosterone (or other aromatizable synthetic androgens) crosses the cell membrane to be converted to estradiol (or the aromatic synthetic analog) by aromatase, which then binds to and activates ER-α or ER-β. *Right*: DHT (or other nonaromatizable androgens) enters the cell to bind and activate the AR. Ligand-bound ER or AR dissociate their heat-shock protein (HSP), undergo conformational changes, dimerize, and translocate into the nucleus in which they bind to specific sites known as estrogen response elements (ERE) or androgen response elements (ARE) located within the DNA of target nuclear genes to produce long-term genomic effects of testosterone. Reproduced with permission from ref. *159.*

it with the AR antagonist flutamide *(162)* results in loss of gender differences in BP, suggesting that this effect is mediated by ARs.

The AR is almost ubiquitously expressed and has been characterized in endothelial and VSMCs *(159,163,164)*. Similar to the female sex steroids, testosterone has both genomic and nongenomic effects via interactions with its receptor [Fig. 8; *(159)*]. The classical pathway of genomic action occurs by testosterone binding to a single copy of the AR with subsequent effects on expression of other genes. This genomic pathway is modulated by a number of coregulators, proteins that activate or repress transcription. The nongenomic pathway is thought to be mediated by an as yet uncharacterized membrane-bound AR *(165)*. Testosterone can undergo metabolic conversion in tissues via 5α-reductase to form dihydrotestosterone (DHT), which acts on AR, or via aromatization to estradiol, which acts on ER-α/β *(159)*. Although only a small fraction (<5%) of total testosterone is shuttled through these pathways, they serve to amplify [DHT has a higher binding affinity for and slower dissociation rate from AR *(166)*] and to diversify its actions *(159)*.

5.1. Effects of Androgens on Vascular Tone

Studies using flow-mediated dilation (FMD) as an outcome have demonstrated dose-dependent effects of testosterone on vascular tone. At higher doses, testosterone has been shown to dilate normal canine arteries *(167)* and to increase FMD of brachial arteries in men *(168,169)*. However, within the physiological range, both endogenous and exogenous testosterone impair endothelium-dependent vasodilation. Men with prostate cancer treated with castration demonstrate enhanced brachial artery FMD in comparison with matched-eugonadal controls *(170)*. Likewise, hypogonadal men have greater basal FMD than matched eugonadal controls, and testosterone substitution at physiological levels significantly decreases FMD in the hypogonadal group *(171)*. Whether this effect is mediated by the nongenomic, genomic, or aromatase pathway is yet to be determined *(159)*.

Testosterone has been shown to have bidirectional effects on substances that affect vascular tone. Short-term testosterone administration at higher doses in the canine coronary artery induces vasodilation by increasing endothelium-derived nitric oxide *(167)*. Testosterone induces increases in cross-sectional area, average coronary peak flow velocity, and coronary blood flow in epicardial and resistance arteries, whereas pretreatment with L-NAME to block nitric oxide synthesis decreases this response. In the canine coronary microcirculation, testosterone opens ATP-sensitive K^+ channels to induce hyperemia, an effect that is blocked by pretreatment with glybenclamide *(167)*. In contrast to these acute vasodilator effects, testosterone has been shown to increase thromboxane A_2 receptor density in cultured rat aortic SMCs *(172)* and in rat aortae *(173)*. Functionally, this increase in receptor numbers results in increased contractile responsiveness to thromboxane A_2 in vitro and in vivo *(173,174)*. In addition, testosterone has been shown to increase contractile responsiveness to endothelin-1 in porcine coronary artery rings ex vivo *(175)*. Together, these findings support an overall minor effect for testosterone on vascular tone, with conflicting potential mechanisms of action.

5.2. Effects of Androgens on Vascular Remodeling

Testosterone *per se* has little effect on vascular injury responses and vascular remodeling. Our laboratory has shown that orchiectomy with or without testosterone replacement does not alter the intact male phenotype of a robust neointimal response 2 wk after endoluminal injury of the rat carotid artery [Fig. 4; *(81)*]. However, testosterone does appear to antagonize the vasoprotective effects of estradiol in this model. Against a background of endogenous testosterone, the vascular injury response is unaffected by estradiol treatment, whereas in the gonadectomized male with an identical dose-schedule of estradiol administration, neointima formation is attenuated and the injury response is converted to resemble that of the intact female. Thus, crosstalk at some level must permit testosterone to inhibit the vasoprotective effects of estrogen. Importantly, recent evidence suggests that testosterone may induce vascular inflammation *(163)*, an effect that opposes the actions of estradiol *(85,86)* and may account for the absence of estrogen-induced vasoprotection in the intact male animal. Further investigation is needed to elucidate the mechanism of this interesting and potentially important hormonal interaction.

5.3. Effects of Androgens on the Kidney
and the Renin–Angiotensin–Aldosterone System

Studies in animal models have shown that the effects of androgens on BP are mediated, at least in part, via the kidney *(18,19)*. In rat models, the presence of androgens corre-lates with development of glomerular injury, glomerulosclerosis, proteinuria, and decreased glomerular filtration rate *(176)*. Similar to the absence of estrogen in menopause, the presence of testosterone shifts the pressure–natriuresis relationship to the right. For example, male SHRs demonstrate a blunted natriuretic response to increased BP, and this relationship is corrected by castration *(177)*. Likewise, testosterone treatment of ovariectomized SHRs results in a rightward shift of the pressure–natriuresis relationship and the development of hypertension *(177)*. This effect may be elicited by the activation of ARs in the kidney, which are found predominantly in the proximal tubule of the nephron *(18,162)*.

The effect on pressure–natriuresis has been related to testosterone-induced changes in the renin–angiotensin–aldosterone system (Fig. 5). Our laboratory has demonstrated that activation of the renin–angiotensin–aldosterone system contributes to androgen-dependent hypertension in the SHR. BP, plasma renin activity, and hepatic angiotensinogen RNA levels are higher in intact male than in intact female SHRs; gonadectomy retards the deve-lopment of hypertension and lowers plasma renin activity and angiotensinogen levels; and testosterone replacement of the gonadectomized male restores the pattern of the intact male *(160)*. Consistent with these observations, others have demonstrated a dose-dependent stimulatory effect of testosterone on plasma renin activity in castrated male Sprague–Dawley rats *(177)*. Likewise, gender differences in ACE expression have been related to androgens. In mice, ACE levels (RNA and protein) are higher in the myocardium of males than females; this discrepancy increases as the animals age; and castration markedly reduces male ACE levels *(178)*. Thus, evidence from animal studies supports the concept that testosterone enhances renin–angiotensin–aldosterone system activity, favors renal sodium retention, and elevates BP.

6. SEX STEROID METABOLISM

Both female and male sex steroids are subject to metabolic transformation. As mentioned previously, a small percentage of the body's testosterone enters the aromatase pathway to become estradiol. Thus, some of the vascular actions of testosterone might, in fact, be mediated by estradiol *(19)*. Similarly, estradiol undergoes sequential meta-bolism to catecholestradiols and methoxyestradiols that have intrinsic biologic activity that may be mediated by ER-independent pathways. For example, 2-methoxyestradiol, a product of catechol-O-methyltransferase metabolism, has no affinity for ERs but is a more potent inhibitor of glomerular endothelial cell proliferation (invoked as a mechanism of glomerulosclerosis) than estradiol *(179)*. Although yet in its infancy, research into the actions of sex steroid metabolites should provide valuable insights into the complexity that underlies sex steroid biology.

7. AGEING AND HORMONAL RESPONSE

Age-related change in sex steroid, especially estrogen, responsiveness is a topic of intense current interest. The sexual dimorphism in CVD is clearly age-dependent.

Premenopausal women are protected from the development of hypertension and CVD, whereas the prevalence of these disorders increases rapidly in elderly women [Fig. 1; *(2)*]. The findings of preclinical studies in animal models and observational studies in which hormone therapy is initiated during the perimenopausal period provide strong evidence that estrogen protects against CVD. These observations stand in conflict with the results of large clinical trials enrolling elderly postmenopausal women that demonstrate no benefit and potential harm for menopausal hormone therapy on cardiovascular endpoints *(10–13)*. The search for an explanation for age-dependent changes in sex steroid responsiveness in women has led to fundamental studies in ageing animal models.

Estrogen-induced modulation of sympathetic tone and prevention of salt-induced hypertension in the SHR are blunted in a middle-aged model *(137)*. Likewise, favorable effects of estradiol on vascular tone in the SHR are attenuated with advancing age. Wynne et al. assessed effects of estradiol-induced endothelium-dependent and -independent relaxation after phenylephrine contraction in vascular strips from aortae of young adult (12-wk-old) and ageing (16-mo-old) intact female SHR *(180)*. Nitrite/nitrate production, Ca^{2+} influx (by $^{45}Ca^{2+}$ uptake), and ER-α and -β expression (by Western blot) were also assessed. There was a statistically nonsignificant trend for reduced ER-α and -β expressions in the aortae of aging rats. Both endothelium-dependent and -independent relaxations were significantly blunted in the aging compared with young rats, with evidence for decreased nitrite–nitrate production and Ca^{2+} influx after E2 treatment in the ageing animals. This study provides additional evidence that vascular responsiveness to E2 may be blunted with ageing.

Several lines of evidence suggest that ER expression may decrease in the vasculature and in the brain with advancing age. Losordo et al. evaluated postmortem coronary artery specimens from premenopausal ($n = 18$; age 31.6 ± 1.9 yr) and postmenopausal ($n = 21$; age 71.8 ± 2.3 yr) women for ER expression by immunohistochemistry *(50)*. Although the study focused on the negative association of atherosclerosis with ER expression in individual vessels, the coronary arteries of postmenopausal women were less likely on the whole to be ER-positive than those of premenopausal women (43 vs 61%, respectively; $p = 0.34$), independent of atherosclerotic lesion formation. Similarly, age-specific decreases in ER-α and -β expressions have been demonstrated in brain regions from 11–12-mo-old compared with 3–4-mo-old female Sprague–Dawley rats *(181)*. Further research in animal models of postmenopausal hypertension is ongoing *(182,183)*.

A possible mechanism of the loss of estrogen responsiveness associated with ageing is DNA methylation *(184)*. A major mechanism for the downregulation of gene expression is methylation of cytosine- and guanine-rich areas in the promoter regions of genes, so called "CpG islands." This promoter-associated CpG-island methylation has been associated with permanent inactivation of gene transcription. Using Southern blot analysis, investigators have shown an age-related increase in ER-α methylation in vascular tissues *(184)*. Whether methylation of ERs can explain the very important ageing effect on hormone responsiveness or whether other mechanisms, such as alternative splicing and post-translational modification of ERs, may be at play is yet to be determined.

8. CONCLUSIONS

There is an age-dependent sexual dimorphism in the development of hypertension. Compared to postmenopausal women and men, premenopausal women are protected against hypertension. In animal studies, estradiol tends to dilate resistance vessels, in part by stimulating the generation of vasodilator prostaglandins, including prostacyclin, and nitric oxide. Further, estradiol has favorable effects on vascular tone and vascular remodeling through excitatory actions on endothelial cells, inhibitory actions on VSMCs, and anti-inflammatory actions on multiple cell types in the acutely and chronically injured artery. Importantly, estrogen modulates salt-sensitivity through direct effects on the kidney and renin–angiotensin–aldosterone system, as well as by attenuating salt-induced activation of the sympathetic nervous system through a reduction in anterior hypothalamic nucleus norepinephrine release. Progestins appear to inhibit these actions of estrogens, though native progesterone may have minor vasorelaxant and natriuretic effects. Testosterone has largely pro-hypertensive properties, but diverse actions through aromatization and the 5α-reductase pathways make its net effect somewhat unpredictable. Greater awareness of sex-specific differences in CVD, along with recent controversies regarding the risks and benefits of menopausal hormone therapy, have increased attention to these important health issues.

REFERENCES

1. Glendy, R. E., Levine, S. A., and White, P. D. (1937) Coronary disease in youth: comparison of 100 patients under 40 with 300 persons past 80. *JAMA* **109**, 1775–1781.
2. American Heart Association. (2004) *Heart Disease and Stroke Statistics—2005 Update*. American Heart Association, Dallas, TX.
3. Stampfer, M. J. and Colditz, G. A. (1991) Estrogen replacement therapy and coronary heart disease: a quantitative assessment of the epidemiologic evidence. *Prev. Med.* **20**, 47–63.
4. Psaty, B. M., Heckbert, S. R., Atkins, D., et al. (1994) The risk of myocardial infarction associated with the combined use of estrogens and progestins in postmenopausal women. *Arch. Intern. Med.* **154**, 1333–1339.
5. Grodstein, F., Stampfer, M. J., Manson, J. E., et al. (1996) Postmenopausal estrogen and progestin use and the risk of cardiovascular disease. *N. Engl. J. Med.* **335**, 453–461.
6. Sourander, L., Rajala, T., Makinen, J., Erkkola, R., and Helenius, H. (1998) Cardiovascular and cancer morbidity and mortality and sudden cardiac death in postmenopausal women on oestrogen replacement therapy. *Lancet* **352**, 1965–1969.
7. Grodstein, F., Stampfer, M. J., Falkeborn, M., Naessen, T., and Persson, I. (1999) Postmenopausal hormone therapy and risk of cardiovascular disease and hip fracture in a cohort of Swedish women. *Epidemiology* **5**, 476–480.
8. Varas-Lorenzo, C., Garcia-Rodriguez, L. A., Perez-Gutthalm, S., and Duque-Oliart, A. (2000) Hormone replacement and incidence of acute myocardial infarction: a population-based nested case–control study. *Circulation* **101**, 2572–2578.
9. Henderson, B. E., Paganini-Hill, A., and Ross, R. K. (1991) Decreased mortality in users of estrogen replacement therapy. *Arch. Intern. Med.* **151**, 75–78.
10. Hulley, S., Grady, D., Bush, T., et al. for the Heart and Estrogen/progestin Replacement Study (HERS) Research Group. (1998) Randomized trial of estrogen plus progestin for secondary prevention of coronary heart disease in postmenopausal women. *JAMA* **280**, 605–613.
11. Grady, D., Herrington, D., Bittner, V., et al. for the HERS Research Group. (2002) Cardiovascular disease outcomes during 6.8 years of hormone therapy: heart and estrogen/progestin replacement study follow-up (HERS II). *JAMA* **288**, 49–57.
12. Rossouw, J. E., Anderson, G. L., Prentice, R. L., et al. for the writing group for the Women's Health Initiative Investigators. (2002) Risks and benefits of estrogen plus progestin in healthy post-menopausal women: principal results from the Women's Health Initiative randomized controlled trial. *JAMA* **288**, 321–333.
13. Anderson, G. L., Limacher, M., Assaf, A. R., et al. for the Women's Health Initiative Steering Committee. (2004) Effects of conjugated equine estrogen in postmenopausal women with hysterectomy: the Women's Health Initiative randomized controlled trial. *JAMA* **291**, 1701–1712.

14. Burt, V. L., Whelton, P., Roccella, E. J., et al. (1995) Prevalence of hypertension in the US adult population: results from the Third National Health and Nutrition Examination Survey, 1988–1991. *Hypertension* **25,** 305–313.
15. Rosenthal, T. and Oparil, S. (2000) Hypertension in women. *J. Hum. Hypertens.* **14,** 691–704.
16. Calhoun, D. and Oparil, S. (2003) Gender and blood pressure. In: *Hypertension Primer* (Izzo, J. L. and Black, H. R., eds.), 3rd edn, Lippincott, Williams & Wilkins, Baltimore, MD, pp. 253–257.
17. August, P. and Oparil, S. (1999) Hypertension in women. *J. Clin. Endocrinol. Metab.* **84,** 1862–1866.
18. Reckelhoff, J. F. (2001) Gender differences in the regulation of blood pressure. *Hypertension* **37,** 1199–1208.
19. Dubey, R. K., Oparil, S., Imthurn, B., and Jackson, E. K. (2002) Sex hormones and hypertension. *Cardiovasc. Res.* **53,** 688–708.
20. Dunne, F. P., Barry, D. G., Ferriss, J. B., Grealy, G., and Murphy, D. (1991) Changes in blood pressure during the normal menstrual cycle. *Clin. Sci.* **81,** 515–518.
21. Karpanou, E. A., Vyssoulis, G. P., Georgoudi, D. G., Toutouza, M. G., and Toutouzas, P. K. (1993) Ambulatory blood pressure changes in the menstrual cycle of hypertensive women: significance of plasma renin activity values. *Am. J. Hypertens.* **6,** 654–659.
22. Chapman, A. B., Zamudio, S., Woodmansee, W., et al. (1997) Systemic and renal hemodynamic changes in the luteal phase of the menstrual cycle mimic early pregnancy. *Am. J. Physiol.* **273,** F777–F782.
23. Staessen, J. A., Celis, H., and Fagard, R. (1998) The epidemiology of the association between hypertension and menopause. *J. Hum. Hypertens.* **12,** 587–592.
24. Staessen, J. A., Ginocchio, G., Thijs, L., and Fagard, R. (1997) Conventional and ambulatory blood pressure and menopause in a prospective population study. *J. Hum. Hypertens.* **11,** 507–514.
25. Siamopoulos, K. C., Papinkolaou, S., Elisaf, M., Theodorou, J., Pappas, H., and Papanikolaou, N. (1996) Ambulatory blood pressure monitoring in normotensive pregnant women. *J. Hum. Hypertens.* **10,** S51–S54.
26. PEPI Trial Writing Group. (1995) Effects of estrogen or estrogen/progestin regimens on heart disease risk factors in postmenopausal women: the postmenopausal estrogen/progestin interventions (PEPI) trial. *JAMA* **273,** 199–208.
27. Schunkert, H., Danser, A. H., Hense, H. W., Derkx, F. H., Kurzinger, S., and Riegger, G. A. (1997) Effects of estrogen replacement therapy on the renin–angiotensin system in postmenopausal women. *Circulation* **95,** 39–45.
28. Mercuro, G., Zoncu, S., Pilia, I., Lao, A., Melis, G. B., and Cherchi, A. (1997) Effects of acute administration of transdermal estrogen on postmenopausal women with systemic hypertension. *Am. J. Cardiol.* **80,** 652–655.
29. Mercuro, G., Zoncu, S., Piano, D., et al. (1998) Estradiol-17β reduces blood pressure and restores the normal amplitude of the circadian blood pressure rhythm in postmenopausal hypertension. *Am. J. Hypertens.* **11,** 909–913.
30. Cagnacci, A., Rovati, L., Zanni, A., Malmusi, S., Facchinetti, F., and Volpe, A. (1999) Physiological doses of estradiol decrease nocturnal blood pressure in normotensive postmenopausal women. *Am. J. Physiol. Heart Circ. Physiol.* **276,** H1355–H1360.
31. Seely, E. W., Walsh, B. W., Gerhard, M. D., and Williams, G. H. (1999) Estradiol with or without progesterone and ambulatory blood pressure in postmenopausal women. *Hypertension* **33,** 1190–1194.
32. Butkevich, A., Abraham, C., and Phillips, R. A. (2000) Hormone replacement therapy and 24-hour blood pressure profile of postmenopausal women. *Am. J. Hypertens.* **13,** 1039–1041.
33. Wassertheil-Smoller, S., Anderson, G., Psaty, B. M., et al. (2000) Hypertension and its treatment in postmenopausal women: baseline data from the women's health initiative. *Hypertension* **36,** 780–789.
34. Woods, J. W. (1967) Oral contraceptives and hypertension. *Lancet* **2,** 653–654.
35. Crane, M. G., Harris, J. J., and Winsor, W. 3rd. (1971) Hypertension, oral contraceptive agents, and conjugated estrogens. *Ann. Intern. Med.* **74,** 13–21.
36. Chasan-Taber, L., Willett, W. C., Manson, J. E., et al. (1996) Prospective study of oral contraceptives and hypertension among women in the United States. *Circulation* **94,** 483–489.
37. Kristiansson, P. and Wang, J. X. (2001) Reproductive hormones and blood pressure during pregnancy. *Hum. Reprod.* **16,** 13–17.
38. Harvey, P. J., Molloy, D., Upton, J., and Wing, L. M. (2001) Dose response effect of cyclical medroxy-progesterone on blood pressure in postmenopausal women. *J. Hum. Hypertens.* **15,** 313–321.

39. Khaw, M. T. and Peart, W. S. (1982) Blood pressure and contraceptive use. *Br. Med. J.* **285**, 403–407.
40. Rhoden, E. L. and Morgentaler, A. (2004) Risks of testosterone-replacement therapy and recommendations for monitoring. *N. Engl. J. Med.* **350**, 482–492.
41. Hughes, G. S., Mathur, R. S., and Margollus, H. S. (1989) Sex steroid hormones are altered in essential hypertension. *J. Hypertens.* **7**, 181–187.
42. Phillips, G. B., Jing, T. Y., Resnick, L. M., Barbagallo, M., Laragh, J. H., and Sealey, J. E. (1993) Sex hormones and hemostatic risk factors for coronary heart disease in men with hypertension. *J. Hypertens.* **11**, 699–702.
43. Mohr, B. A., Guay, A. T., O'Donnell, A. B., and McKinlay, J. B. (2005) Normal, bound and nonbound testosterone levels in normally ageing men: results from the massachusetts male ageing study. *Clin. Endocrinol.* **62**, 64–73.
44. Kalin, M. F. and Zumhoff, B. (1990) Sex hormones and coronary artery disease: a review of clinical studies. *Steroids* **55**, 330–352.
45. Zmuda, J. M., Cauley, J. A., Kriska, A., Glynn, N. W., Gutai, J. P., and Kuller, L. H. (1997) Longitudinal relation between endogenous testosterone and cardiovascular disease risk factors in middle-aged men: a 13-year follow-up of former multiple risk factor intervention trial participants. *Am. J. Epidemiol.* **146**, 609–617.
46. Hak, A. E., Witteman, J. C., de Jong, F. H., Geerlings, M. I., Hofman, A., and Pols, H. A. (2002) Low levels of endogenous androgens increase the risk of atherosclerosis in elderly men: the Rotterdam study. *J. Clin. Endocrinol. Metab.* **87**, 3632–3639.
47. Muller, M., Grobbee, D. E., den Tonkelaar, I., Lamberts, S. W., and van der Schouw, Y. T. (2005) Endogenous sex hormones and metabolic syndrome in aging men. *J. Clin. Endocrinol. Metab.* **90(5)**, 2618–2623.
48. Svartberg, J., von Muhlen, D., Schirmer, H., Barrett-Connor, E., Sundfjord, J., and Jorde, R. (2004) Association of endogenous testosterone with blood pressure and left ventricular mass in men: the Tromso study. *Eur. J. Endocrinol.* **150(1)**, 65–71.
49. Karas, R. H., Patterson, B. L., and Mendelsohn, M. E. (1994) Human vascular smooth muscle cells contain functional estrogen receptor. *Circulation* **89**, 1943–1950.
50. Losordo, D. W., Kearney, M., Kim, E. A., Jekanowski, J., and Isner, J. M. (1994) Variable expression of the estrogen receptor in normal and atherosclerotic coronary arteries of premenopausal women. *Circulation* **89**, 1501–1510.
51. Chambliss, K. L., Yuhanna, I. S., Mineo, C., et al. (2000) Estrogen receptor alpha and endothelial nitric oxide synthase are organized into a functional signaling module in caveolae. *Circ. Res.* **87**, E44–E52.
52. Lantin-Hermoso, R. L., Rosenfeld, C. R., Yuhanna, I. S., German, Z., Chen, Z., and Shaul, P. W. (1997) Estrogen acutely stimulates nitric oxide synthase activity in fetal pulmonary artery endothelium. *Am. J. Physiol.* **273**, L119–L126.
53. Stefano, G. B., Cadet, P., Breton, C., et al. (2000) Estradiol-stimulated nitric oxide release in human granulocytes is dependent on intracellular calcium transients: evidence of a cell surface estrogen receptor. *Blood* **95**, 3951–3958.
54. Walter, P., Green, S., Greene, G., et al. (1985) Cloning of the human estrogen receptor cDNA. *Proc. Natl Acad. Sci. USA* **82**, 7889–7893.
55. Kuiper, G. G. J. M., Enmark, E., Pelto-Huikko, M., Nilsson, S., and Gustafsson, J. A. (1996) Cloning of a novel receptor expressed in rat prostate and ovary. *Proc. Natl Acad. Sci. USA* **93**, 5925–5930.
56. Stossi, F., Barnett, D. H., Frasor, J., Komm, B., Lyttle, C. R., and Katzenellenbogen, B. S. (2004) Transcriptional profiling of estrogen-regulated gene expression via estrogen receptor (ER) α or ERβ in human osteosarcoma cells: distinct and common target genes for these receptors. *Endocrinology* **145**, 3473–3486.
57. Hodges, Y. K., Tung, L., Yan, X. D., Graham, D., Horwitz, K. B., and Horwitz, L. D. (2000) Estrogen receptors α and β: prevalence of estrogen receptor β mRNA in human vascular smooth muscle and transcriptional effects. *Circulation* **101**, 1792–1798.
58. Pare, G., Krust, A., Karas, R. H., et al. (2002) Estrogen receptor-alpha mediates the protective effects of estrogen against vascular injury. *Circ. Res.* **90**, 1087–1092.
59. Geraldes, P., Sirois, M. G., and Tanguay, J. F. (2003) Specific contribution of estrogen receptors on mitogen-activated protein kinase pathways and vascular cell activation. *Circ. Res.* **93**, 399–405.
60. Mendelsohn, M. E. and Karas, R. H. (1999) The protective effects of estrogen on the cardiovascular system. *N. Engl. J. Med.* **340**, 1801–1811.

61. Frasor, J., Danes, J. M., Komm, B., Chang, K. C., Lyttle, C. R., and Katzenellenbogen, B. S. (2003) Profiling of estrogen up- and down-regulated gene expression in human breast cancer cells: insights into gene networks and pathways underlying estrogenic control of proliferation and cell phenotype. *Endocrinology* **144,** 4562–4574.

62. Haynes, M. P., Sinha, D., Strong Russell, K., et al. (2000) Membrane estrogen receptor engagement activates endothelial nitric oxide synthase via the PI3-kinase-Akt pathway in human endothelial cells. *Circ. Res.* **87,** 677–682.

63. Simoncini, T., Hafezi-Moghadam, A., Brazil, D. P., Ley, K., Chin, W. W., and Liao, J. K. (2000) Interaction of oestrogen receptor with the regulatory subunit of phosphatidylinositol-3-OH kinase. *Nature* **407,** 538–541.

64. White, R. E., Darkow, D. J., and Lang, J. L. (1995) Estrogen relaxes coronary arteries by opening BKCa channels through a cGMP-dependent mechanism. *Circ. Res.* **77,** 936–942.

65. Reis, S. E., Gloth, S. T., Blumenthal, R. S., et al. (1994) Ethinyl estradiol acutely attenuates abnormal coronary vasomotor responses to acetylcholine in postmenopausal women. *Circulation* **89,** 52–60.

66. Gilligan, D. M., Badar, D. M., Panza, J. A., Quyyumi, A. A., and Cannon, R. O. 3rd. (1994) Acute vascular effects of estrogen in postmenopausal women. *Circulation* **90,** 786–791.

67. Blumenthal, R. S., Heldman, A. W., Brinker, J. A., et al. (1997) Acute effects of conjugated estrogens on coronary blood flow response to acetylcholine in men. *Am. J. Cardiol.* **80,** 1021–1024.

68. Chang, W. C., Nakao, J., Orimo, H., and Murota, S. I. (1980) Stimulation of prostaglandin cyclo-oxygenase and prostacyclin synthetase activities by estradiol in rat aortic smooth muscle cells. *Biochem. Biophys. Acta* **620,** 472–479.

69. Egan, K. M., Lawson, J. A., Fries, S., et al. (2004) COX-2-derived prostacyclin confers athero-protection on female mice. *Science* **306,** 1954–1957.

70. Weiner, C. P., Lizasoain, I., Baylis, S. A., Knowles, R. G., Charles, I. G., and Moncada, S. (1994) Induction of calcium-dependent nitric oxide synthases by sex hormones. *Proc. Natl Acad. Sci. USA* **91,** 5212–5216.

71. Williams, J. K., Adams, M. R., and Klopfenstein, H. S. (1990) Estrogen modulates responses of atherosclerotic coronary arteries. *Circulation* **81,** 1680–1687.

72. Williams, J. K., Honoré, E. K., and Adams, M. R. (1997) Contrasting effects of conjugated estrogens and tamoxifen on dilator responses of atherosclerotic epicardial coronary arteries in nonhuman primates. *Circulation* **96,** 1970–1975.

73. Herrington, D. M., Braden, G. A., Williams, J. K., and Morgan, T. M. (1994) Endothelial-dependent coronary vasomotor responsiveness in postmenopausal women with and without estrogen replacement therapy. *Am. J. Cardiol.* **73,** 951–952.

74. Roque, M., Heras, M., Roig, E., et al. (1998) Short-term effects of transdermal estrogen replacement therapy on coronary vascular reactivity in postmenopausal women with angina pectoris and normal results on coronary angiograms. *J. Am. Coll. Cardiol.* **31,** 139–143.

75. McCrohon, J. A., Walters, W. A., Robinson, J. T., et al. (1997) Arterial reactivity is enhanced in genetic males taking high dose estrogens. *J. Am. Coll. Cardiol.* **29,** 1432–1436.

76. New, G., Timmins, K. L., Duffy, S. J., et al. (1997) Long-term estrogen therapy improves vascular function in male to female transsexuals. *J. Am. Coll. Cardiol.* **29,** 1437–1444.

77. Chen, Y. F. and Oparil, S. (1998) Effects of sex steroids in vascular injury. In: *Endocrinology of Cardiovascular Function* (Levin, E. R. and Nadler, J. L., eds.), Kluwer Academic, Boston, MA, pp. 45–59.

78. Foegh, M., Asotra, S., Howell, M., and Ramwell, P. (1994) Estradiol inhibition of arterial neointimal hyperplasia after balloon injury. *J. Vasc. Surg.* **19,** 722–726.

79. Sullivan, T. R., Karas, R. H., Aronovitz, M., et al. (1995) Estrogen inhibits the response-to-injury in a mouse carotid artery model. *J. Clin. Investig.* **96,** 2482–2488.

80. Chen, S. J., Li, H., Durand, J., Oparil, S., and Chen, Y. F. (1996) Estrogen reduces myointimal proliferation after balloon injury of rat carotid artery. *Circulation* **93,** 577–584.

81. Oparil, S., Levine, R. L., Chen, S. J., Durand, J., and Chen, Y. F. (1997) Sexually dimorphic response of the balloon injured rat carotid artery to hormone treatment. *Circulation* **95,** 1301–1307.

82. White, C. R., Shelton, J., Chen, S. J., et al. (1997) Estrogen restores endothelial cell function in an experimental model of vascular injury. *Circulation* **96,** 1624–1630.

83. Bakir, S., Mori, T., Durand, J., Chen, Y. F., Thompson, J. A., and Oparil, S. (2000) Estrogen-induced vasoprotection is estrogen receptor dependent: evidence from the balloon-injured rat carotid artery model. *Circulation* **101,** 2342–2344.

84. Mori, T., Durand, J., Chen, Y., Thompson, J. A., Bakir, S., and Oparil, S. (2000) Effects of short-term estrogen treatment on the neointimal response to balloon injury of rat carotid arteries. *Am. J. Cardiol.* **85,** 1276–1279.

85. Miller, A. P., Feng, W., Xing, D., et al. (2004) Estrogen modulates inflammatory mediator expression and neutrophil chemotaxis in injured arteries. *Circulation* **110,** 1664–1669.

86. Xing, D., Miller, A., Novak, L., Rocha, R., Chen, Y. F., and Oparil, S. (2004) Estradiol and progestins differentially modulate leukocyte infiltration after vascular injury. *Circulation* **109,** 234–241.

87. Li, G., Chen, Y. F., Greene, G. L., Oparil, S., and Thompson, J. A. (1999) Estrogen inhibits vascular smooth muscle cell-dependent adventitial fibroblast migration in vitro. *Circulation* **100,** 1639–1645.

88. Li, G., Chen, S. J., Oparil, S., Chen, Y. F., and Thompson, J. A. (2000) Direct in vivo evidence demonstrating neointimal migration of adventitial fibroblasts after balloon injury of rat carotid arteries. *Circulation* **101,** 1362–1365.

89. Wall, R. T., Harlan, J. M., Harkar, L. A., and Striker, G. E. (1980) Hyperhomocysteine-induced endothelial cell injury in vitro: a model for the study of vascular injury. *Thromb. Res.* **18,** 1113–1121.

90. Tsai, J. C., Perrella, M. A., Yoshizumi, M., et al. (1994) Promotion of vascular smooth muscle cell growth by homocysteine: a link to atherosclerosis. *Proc. Natl Acad. Sci. USA* **91,** 6369–6375.

91. Boushey, C. J., Beresford, S. A., Omenn, G. S., and Motulsky, A. G. (1995) A quantitative assessment of plasma homocysteine as a risk factor for vascular disease: probable benefits of increasing folic acid intakes. *JAMA* **274,** 1049–1057.

92. van der Mooren, M. J., Wouters, M. G., Blom, H. J., Schellekens, L. A., Eskes, T. K., and Rolland, R. (1994) Hormone replacement therapy may reduce high serum homocysteine in postmenopausal women. *Eur. J. Clin. Investig.* **24,** 733–736.

93. Mijatovic, V., Kenemans, P., Netelenbos, C., et al. (1998) Postmenopausal oral 17β-estradiol continuously combined with dydrogesterone reduces fasting serum homocysteine levels. *Fertil. Steril.* **69,** 876–882.

94. Barnabei, V. M., Phillips, T. M., and Hsia, J. (1999) Plasma homocysteine in women taking hormone replacement therapy: the postmenopausal estrogen/progestin interventions (PEPI) trial. *J. Womens Health Gend. Based Med.* **8,** 1167–1172.

95. van Baal, W. M., Smolders, R. G. V., van der Mooren, M. J., Teerlink, T., and Kenemans, P. (1999) Hormone replacement therapy and plasma homocysteine level. *Obstet. Gynecol.* **94,** 485–491.

96. Smolders, R. G., de Meer, K., Kenemans, P., Jakobs, C., Kulik, W., and van der Mooren, M. J. (2005) Oral estradiol decreases plasma homocysteine, vitamin B_6 and albumin in postmenopausal women, but does not change the whole body homocysteine remethylation and transmethylation flux. *J. Clin. Endocrinol. Metab.* **90(4),** 2218–2224.

97. Komatsumoto, S. and Nara, M. (1995) Changes in the level of endothelin-1 with aging. *Nippon Ronen Igakki Zasshi* **32,** 664–669.

98. Wilcox, J., Hatch, I., Gentzshein, E., Sanczyk, F., and Lobo, R. (1997) Endothelin levels decrease after oral and nonoral estrogen in postmenopausal women with increased cardiovascular risk factors. *Fertil. Steril.* **67,** 273–277.

99. Ylikorkala, O., Orpana, A., Puolakka, J., Pyorala, T., and Viinikka, L. (1995) Postmenopausal hormonal replacement decreases plasma levels of endothelin-1. *J. Clin. Endocrinol. Metab.* **80,** 3384–3387.

100. Morey, A. K., Razandi, M., Pedram, A., Hu, R. M., Prins, B. A., and Levin, E. R. (1998) Oestrogen and progesterone inhibit the stimulated production of endothelin-1. *Biochem. J.* **330,** 1097–1105.

101. Dubey, R. K., Jackson, E. K., Keller, P. J., Imthurn, B., and Rosselli, M. (2001) Estradiol metabolites inhibit endothelin synthesis by and estrogen receptor-independent mechanism. *Hypertension* **37,** 640–644.

102. Morey, A. K., Pedram, A., Razandi, M., et al. (1997) Estrogen and progesterone inhibit vascular smooth muscle proliferation. *Endocrinology* **138,** 3330–3339.

103. Fischer, M., Baessler, A., and Schunkert, H. (2002) Renin angiotensin system and gender differences in the cardiovascular system. *Cardiovasc. Res.* **53,** 672–677.

104. Klett, C., Ganten, D., Hellmann, W., et al. (2002) Regulation of angiotensinogen synthesis and secretion by steroid hormones. *Endocrinology* **130,** 3660–3668.

105. Feldmer, M., Kaling, M., Takahashi, S., Mullins, J. J., and Ganten, D. (1991) Glucocorticoid- and estrogen-responsive elements in the 5′-flanking region of the rat angiotensinogen gene. *J. Hypertens.* **9,** 1005–1012.

106. Danser, A. H., Derkx, F. H., Schalekamp, M. A., Hense, H. W., Riegger, G. A., and Schunkert, H. (1998) Determinants of interindividual variation of renin and prorenin concentrations: evidence for a sexual dimorphism of (pro)renin levels in humans. *J. Hypertens.* **16,** 853–862.

107. Schunkert, H., Danser, A. H., Hense, H. W., Derkx, F. H., Kurzinger, S., and Riegger, G. A. (1997) Effects of estrogen replacement therapy on the renin–angiotensin system in postmenopausal women. *Circulation* **95**, 39–45.

108. Proudler, A. J., Ahmed, A. I., Crook, D., Fogelman, I., Rymer, J. M., and Stevenson, J. C. (1995) Hormone replacement therapy and serum angiotensin-converting enzyme activity in postmenopausal women. *Lancet* **346**, 89–90.

109. Brosnihan, K. B., Weddle, D., Anthony, M. S., Heise, C., Li, P., and Ferrario, C. M. (1997) Effects of chronic hormone replacement on the renin–angiotensin system in cynomolgus monkeys. *J. Hypertens.* **15**, 719–726.

110. Dean, S. A., Tan, J., O'Brien, E. R., and Leenen, F. H. H. (2005) 17β-estradiol downregulates tissue angiotensin-converting enzyme and ANG II type 1 receptor in female rats. *Am. J. Physiol. Regul. Integr. Comp. Physiol.* **288**, R759–R766.

111. Brosnihan, K. B., Li, P., Ganten, D., and Ferrario, C. M. (1997) Estrogen protects transgenic hypertensive rats by shifting the vasoconstrictor–vasodilator balance of RAS. *Am. J. Physiol. Regul. Integr. Comp. Physiol.* **273**, R1908–R1915.

112. Nickenig, G., Baumer, A. T., Grohe, C., et al. (1998) Estrogen modulates AT_1 receptor gene expression in vitro and in vivo. *Circulation* **97**, 2197–2201.

113. Roesch, D. M., Tian, Y., Zheng, W., Shi, M., Verbalis, J. G., and Sandberg, K. (2000) Estradiol attenuates angiotensin-induced aldosterone secretion in ovariectomized rats. *Endocrinology* **141**, 4629–4636.

114. Wu, Z., Maric, C., Roesch, D. M., Zheng, W., Verbalis, J. G., and Sandberg, K. (2003) Estrogen regulates adrenal angiotensin AT_1 receptors by modulating AT_1 receptor translation. *Endocrinology* **144**, 3251–3261.

115. Pechere-Bertschi, A. and Burnier, M. (2004) Female sex hormones, salt, and blood pressure regulation. *Am. J. Hypertens.* **17**, 994–1001.

116. Harrison-Bernard, L. M., Schulman, I. H., and Raij, L. (2003) Postovariectomy hypertension is linked to increased renal AT_1 receptor and salt sensitivity. *Hypertension* **42**, 1157–1163.

117. Carlson, S. H., Roysomutti, S., Peng, N., and Wyss, J. M. (2001) The role of the central nervous system in NaCl-sensitive hypertension in spontaneously hypertensive rats. *Am. J. Hypertens.* **14**, 155S–162S.

118. Calhoun, D. A., Zhu, S. T., Chen, Y. F., and Oparil, S. (1995) Gender and dietary NaCl in spontaneously hypertensive and Wistar–Kyoto rats. *Hypertension* **26**, 285–289.

119. Fang, Z., Carlson, S. H., Chen, Y. F., Oparil, S., and Wyss, J. M. (2001) Estrogen depletion induces NaCl-sensitive hypertension in female spontaneously hypertensive rats. *Am. J. Physiol. Regul. Integr. Comp. Physiol.* **281**, R1934–R1939.

120. Oparil, S., Chen, Y. F., Berecek, K., Calhoun, D., and Wyss, J. M. (1995) The role of the central nervous system in hypertension. In: *Hypertension: Pathophysiology, Diagnosis and Management* (Laragh, J. H. and Brenner, B. M., eds.), Raven, New York, pp. 713–740.

121. Oparil, S., Chen, Y. F., Peng, N., and Wyss, J. M. (1996) Anterior hypothalamic norepinephrine, atrial natriuretic peptide, and hypertension. *Front Neuroendocrinol.* **17**, 212–246.

122. Wyss, J. M., Chen, Y. F., Jin, H., Gist, R., and Oparil, S. (1987) Spontaneously hypertensive rats exhibit reduced hypothalamic noradrenergic input after NaCl loading. *Hypertension* **10**, 313–320.

123. Chen, Y. F., Meng, Q. C., Wyss, J. M., Jin, H., and Oparil, S. (1988) High NaCl reduces hypothalamic norepinephrine turnover in hypertensive rats. *Hypertension* **11**, 55–62.

124. Oparil, S., Chen, Y.-F., Meng, Q., Yang, R.-H., Jin, H., and Wyss, M. (1988) The neural basis of salt sensitivity in the rat: altered hypothalamic function. *Am. J. Med. Sci.* **295**, 360–362.

125. Jin, H., Chen, Y. F., Yang, R. H., Meng, Q. C., and Oparil, S. (1988) Impaired release of atrial natriuretic factor in NaCl loaded spontaneously hypertensive rats. *Hypertension* **11**, 739–744.

126. Wyss, J. M., Yang, R., Jin, H., and Oparil, S. (1988) Hypothalamic microinjection of alpha2-adrenoceptor agonists causes greater sympathoinhibition in spontaneously hypertensive rats on high NaCl diets. *J. Hypertens.* **6**, 805–813.

127. Jin, H., Chen, Y. F., Yang, R. H., and Oparil, S. (1989) Atrial natriuretic factor in NaCl-sensitive and NaCl-resistant spontaneously hypertensive rats. *Hypertension* **14**, 404–412.

128. Yang, R. H., Jin, H., Chen,Y. F., Wyss, J. M., and Oparil, S. (1990) Blockade of endogenous anterior hypothalamic atrial natriuretic peptide with monoclonal antibody lowers blood pressure in spontaneously hypertensive rats. *J. Clin. Investig.* **86**, 1985–1990.

129. Chen, C. W., Chen, Y. F., Meng, Q. C., Wyss, J. M., and Oparil, S. (1991) Decreased norepinephrine release in anterior hypothalamus of NaCl-sensitive spontaneously hypertensive rats during high NaCl intake. *Brain Res.* **565,** 135–141.

130. Calhoun, D. A., Wyss, J. M., and Oparil, S. (1991) High NaCl diet enhances arterial baroreceptor reflex in NaCl-sensitive spontaneously hypertensive rats. *Hypertension* **17,** 363–368.

131. Jin, H., Yang, R. H., Chen, Y. F., Wyss, J. M., and Oparil, S. (1991) Altered stores of atrial natriuretic peptide in specific brain nuclei of NaCl-sensitive spontaneously hypertensive rats. *Am. J. Hypertens.* **4,** 449–455.

132. Jin, H., Yang, R. H., Wyss, J. M., and Oparil, S. (1991) Intrahypothalamic clonidine infusion prevents NaCl-sensitive hypertension in spontaneously hypertensive rats. *Hypertension* **18,** 224–229.

133. Jin, H., Yang, R. H., Calhoun, D. A., Wyss, J. M., and Oparil, S. (1992) Atrial natriuretic peptide modulates baroreceptor reflex in spontaneously hypertensive rat. *Hypertension* **20,** 374–379.

134. Yang, R. H., Jin, H., Wyss, J. M., Chen, Y. F., and Oparil, S. (1992) Pressor effect of blocking atrial natriuretic peptide in nucleus tractus solitarii. *Hypertension* **19,** 198–205.

135. Nakamura, Y., Calhoun, D. A., Chen, Y. F., Wyss, J. M., and Oparil, S. (1993) Excitatory sympathetic reflex in NaCl-sensitive spontaneously hypertensive rats. *Hypertension* **22,** 285–291.

136. Zhu, S. T., Chen, Y. F., Wyss, J. M., et al. (1996) Atrial natriuretic peptide blunts arterial baroreflex in spontaneously hypertensive rats. *Hypertension* **27,** 297–302.

137. Peng, N., Clark, J. T., Wei, C. C., and Wyss, J. M. (2003) Estrogen depletion increases blood pressure and hypothalamic norepinephrine in middle-aged spontaneously hypertensive rats. *Hypertension* **41,** 1164–1167.

138. Chobanian, A. V., Bakris, G. L., Black, H. R., et al. (2003) Seventh report of the joint national committee on prevention, detection, evaluation, and treatment of high blood pressure. *Hypertension* **42,** 1206–1252.

139. Chalmers, J., MacMahon, S., Mancia, G., et al. (1999) World Health Organization– International Society of Hypertension guidelines for the management of hypertension: Guidelines Sub-committee of the World Health Organization. *Clin. Exp. Hypertens.* **21,** 1009–1060.

140. Cifkova, R., Erdine, S., Fagard, R., et al. for the ESH/ESC Hypertension Guidelines Committee. (2003) Practice guidelines for primary care physicians: 2003 ESH/ESC hypertension guidelines. *J. Hypertens.* **21,** 1779–1786.

141. Li, X. and O'Malley, B. W. (2003) Unfolding the action of progesterone receptors. *J. Biol. Chem.* **41,** 39,261–39,264.

142. Turgeon, J. L., McDonnell, D. P., Martin, K. A., and Wise, P. M. (2004) Hormone therapy: physiological complexity belies therapeutic simplicity. *Science* **304,** 1269–1273.

143. Giangrande, P. H. and McDonnell, D. P. (1999) The A and B isoforms of human progesterone receptor: two functionally different transcription factors encoded by a single gene. *Recent Prog. Horm. Res.* **54,** 291–313.

144. Ingegno, M. D., Money, S. R., Thelmo, W., et al. (1988) Progesterone receptors in the human heart and great vessels. *Lab. Invest.* **59,** 353–356.

145. Miller, V. M. and Vanhoutte, P. M. (1991) Progesterone and modulation of endothelium-dependent responses in canine coronary arteries. *Am. J. Physiol.* **261,** R1022–R1027.

146. Jiang, C. W., Sarrel, P. M., Lindsay, D. C., Poole-Wilson, P. A., and Collins, P. (1992) Progesterone induces endothelium-independent relaxation of rabbit coronary artery in vitro. *Eur. J. Pharmacol.* **211,** 163–167.

147. Williams, J. K., Honore, E. K., Washburn, S. A., and Clarkson, T. B. (1994) Effects of hormone replacement therapy on reactivity of atherosclerotic coronary arteries in cynomolgous monkeys. *J. Am. Coll. Cardiol.* **24,** 1757–1761.

148. Miyagawa, K., Rosch, J., Stanczyk, F., and Hermsmeyer, K. (1997) Medroxyprogesterone interferes with ovarian steroid protection against coronary vasospasm. *Nat. Med.* **3,** 324–327.

149. Simoncini, T., Mannella, P., Fornari, L., et al. (2004) Differential signal transduction of progesterone and medroxyprogesterone acetate in human endothelial cells. *Endocrinology* **145,** 5745–5756.

150. Lee, W. S., Harder, J. A., Yoshizumi, M., Lee, M. E., and Haber, E. (1997) Progesterone inhibits arterial smooth muscle cell proliferation. *Nat. Med.* **3,** 1005–1008.

151. Levine, R. L., Chen, S. J., Durand, J., Chen, Y. F., and Oparil, S. (1996) Medroxyprogesterone attenuates estrogen-mediated inhibition of neointima formation after balloon injury of the rat carotid artery. *Circulation* **94,** 2221–2227.

152. Sealy, J. E., Itskovitz-Eldor, J., Rubattu, S., et al. (1994) Estradiol- and progesterone-related increases in the renin–aldosterone system: studies during ovarian stimulation and early pregnancy. *J. Clin. Endocrinol. Metab.* **79,** 258–264.

153. Braley, L. M., Menachery, A. I., Yao, T., Mortensen, R. M., and Williams, G. H. (1996) Effect of progesterone on aldosterone secretion in rats. *Endocrinology* **137,** 4773–4778.

154. Myles, K. and Funder, J. W. (1996) Progesterone binding to mineralocorticoid receptors: in vitro and vivo studies. *Am. J. Physiol.* **270,** E601–E607.

155. Landau, R. L., Bergenstal, D. M., Lugibihl, K., and Kascht, M. E. (1955) The metabolic effects of progesterone in man. *J. Clin. Endocrinol.* **15,** 1194–1215.

156. Oparil, S., Ehrlich, E. N., and Lindheimer, M. D. (1975) Effect of progesterone on renal sodium handling in man: relation to aldosterone excretion and plasma renin activity. *Clin. Sci. Mol. Med.* **49,** 139–147.

157. Landau, R. L. and Lugibihl, K. (1958) Inhibition of the sodium retaining influence of aldosterone by progesterone. *J. Clin. Endocrinol.* **18,** 1237–1245.

158. Brunette, M. G. and Leclerc, M. (2002) Renal action of progesterone: effect on calcium reabsorption. *Mol. Cell Endocrinol.* **194,** 183–190.

159. Liu, P. Y., Death, A. K., and Handelsman, D. J. (2003) Androgens and cardiovascular disease. *Endocr. Rev.* **24,** 313–340.

160. Chen, Y. F., Naftilan, A. J., and Oparil, S. (1992) Androgen-dependent angiotensinogen and renin messenger RNA expression in hypertensive rats. *Hypertension* **19,** 456–463.

161. Ely, D. L., Salisbury, R., Hadi, D., Turner, M., and Johnson, M. L. (1991) Androgen receptor and the testes influence hypertension in a hybrid rat model. *Hypertension* **17,** 1104–1110.

162. Reckelhoff, J. F., Zhang, H., Srivastava, K., and Granger, J. P. (1999) Gender differences in hypertension in spontaneously hypertensive rats: role of androgens and androgen receptor. *Hypertension* **34,** 920–923.

163. Death, A. K., McGrath, K. C., Sader, M. A., et al. (2004) Dihydrotestosterone promotes vascular cell adhesion molecule-1 expression in male human endothelial cells via a nuclear factor-κB-dependent pathway. *Endocrinology* **145,** 1889–1897.

164. Liu, P. Y., Christian, R. C., Ruan, M., Miller, V. M., and Fitzpatrick, L. A. (2005) Correlating androgen and estrogen steroid receptor expression with coronary calcification and atherosclerosis in men without known coronary artery disease. *J. Clin. Endocrinol. Metab.* **90,** 1041–1046.

165. Heinlein, C. A. and Chang, C. (2002) The roles of androgen receptors and androgen-binding proteins in nongenomic androgen actions. *Mol. Endocrinol.* **16,** 2181–2187.

166. Grino, P. B., Griffin, J. E., and Wilson, J. D. (1990) Testosterone at high concentrations interacts with the human androgen receptor similarly to dihydrotestosterone. *Endocrinology* **26,** 1165–1172.

167. Chou, T. M., Sudhir, K., Hutchison, S. J., et al. (1996) Testosterone induces dilation of canine coronary conductance and resistance arteries in vivo. *Circulation* **94,** 2614–2619.

168. Ong, P. J., Patrizi, G., Chong, W. C., Webb, C. M., Hayward, C. S., and Collins, P. (2000) Testosterone enhances flow-mediated brachial artery reactivity in men with coronary artery disease. *Am. J. Cardiol.* **85,** 269–272.

169. Kang, S. M., Jang, Y., Kim, J. Y., et al. (2002) Effect of oral administration of testosterone on brachial arterial vasoreactivity in men with coronary artery disease. *Am. J. Cardiol.* **89,** 862–864.

170. Herman, S. M., Robinson, J. T., McCredie, R. J., Adams, M. R., Boyer, M. J., and Celermajer, D. S. (1997) Androgen deprivation is associated with enhanced endothelium-dependent dilatation in adult men. *Arterioscler. Thromb. Vasc. Biol.* **17,** 2004–2009.

171. Zitzmann, M., Brune, M., and Nieschlag, E. (2002) Vascular reactivity in hypogonadal men is reduced by androgen substitution. *J. Clin. Endocrinol. Metab.* **87,** 5030–5037.

172. Masuda, A., Mathur, R., and Haluska, P. V. (1991) Testosterone increases thromboxane A_2 receptors in cultured rat aortic smooth muscle cells. *Circ. Res.* **69,** 638–643.

173. Matsuda, K., Ruff, A., Morinelli, T. A., Mathur, R. S., and Haluska, P. V. (1994) Testosterone increases thromboxane A_2 receptor density and responsiveness in rat aorta and platelets. *Am. J. Physiol.* **267,** H887–H893.

174. Schror, K., Morinelli, T. A., Masuda, A., Matsuda, K., Mathur, R. S., and Halushka, P. V. (1994) Testosterone treatment enhances thromboxane A2 mimetic induced coronary artery vasoconstriction in guinea pigs. *Eur. J. Clin. Investig.* **24,** 50–52.

175. Teoh, H., Quann, A., Leung, S. W. S., and Man, R. Y. K. (2000) Differential effects of 17β-estradiol and testosterone on the contractile responses of procine coronary arteries. *Br. J. Pharmacol.* **129,** 1301–1308.

176. Baylis, C. (1994) Age-dependent glomerular damage in the rat: dissociation between glomerular injury and both glomerular hypertension and hypertrophy: male gender as a primary risk factor. *J. Clin. Investig.* **94,** 1823–1829.

177. Reckelhoff, J. F., Zhang, H., and Granger, J. P. (1998) Testosterone exacerbates hypertension and reduces pressure–natriuresis in male spontaneously hypertensive rats. *Hypertension* **31,** 435–439.

178. Freshour, J. R., Chase, S. E., and Vikstrom, K. L. (2002) Gender differences in cardiac ACE expression are normalized in androgen-deprived male mice. *Am. J. Physiol. Heart Circ. Physiol.* **283,** H1997–H2003.

179. Xiao, S., Gillespi, D. G., Baylis, C., Jackson, E. K., and Dubey, R. K. (2001) Effects of estradiol and its metabolites on glomerular endothelial nitric oxide synthesis and mesangial cell growth. *Hypertension* **37,** 645–650.

180. Wynne, F. L., Payne, J. A., Cain, A. E., Reckelhoff, J. F., and Khalil, R. A. (2004) Age-related reduction in estrogen receptor-mediated mechanisms of vascular relaxation in female spontaneously hypertensive rats. *Hypertension* **43,** 405–412.

181. Wilson, M. E., Roswell, K. L., Kashon, M. L., et al. (2002) Age differentially influences estrogen receptor-α (ERα) and estrogen receptor-β (ERβ) gene expression in specific regions of the rat brain. *Mech. Ageing Dev.* **123,** 593–601.

182. Fortepiani, L. A., Zhang, H., Racusen, L., Roberts, L. J., and Reckelhoff, J. F. (2003) Characterization of an animal model of postmenopausal hypertension in spontaneously hypertensive rats. *Hypertension* **41,** 640–645.

183. Hinojosa-Laborde, C., Craig, T., Zheng, W., Ji, H., Haywood, J. R., and Sandberg, K. (2004) Ovariectomy augments hypertension in aging female Dahl salt-sensitive rats. *Hypertension* **44,** 405–409.

184. Post, W. S., Goldschmidt-Clermont, P. J., Wilhide, C. C., et al. (1999) Methylation of the estrogen receptor gene is associated with aging and atherosclerosis in the cardiovascular system. *Cardiovasc. Res.* **43,** 985–991.

19   The Lipoxygenase System in the Vasculature and Hypertension

Naftali Stern and Michael L. Tuck

1. INTRODUCTION

Lipoxygenase (LO) enzymes play a role in the secretion of blood pressure modulating hormones, especially renin and aldosterone. LO products are also generated by cells comprising the arterial wall *per se*, or by cell types interacting with the vascular lining, i.e., polymorphonuclear leukocytes, monocytes, macrophages, lymphocytes, and platelets. Although the physiologically important LO metabolites are all products of fatty acid oxidation, mainly of arachidonic and linoleic acid, they are rather diverse in terms of origin, biosynthetic sequence and biological effects: some act as paracrine or autocrine hormones, by binding to specific receptors and eliciting local responses through defined signaling routes; others are merely intracellular signaling molecules mediating the effects of hormones such as angiotensin II or endothelin, growth factors such as PDGF or cytokines such as interleukin (IL)-4; still others are metabolites whose role and mode of action in the vasculature remain poorly defined. LO products, then, may affect blood

From: *Contemporary Endocrinology: Hypertension and Hormone Mechanisms*
Edited by: R. M. Carey © Humana Press Inc., Totowa, NJ

pressure directly as independent vasoactive compounds, or indirectly, either as cellular signaling tools in stimulus response coupling for hormone release or as local agents, which modify arterial structure, mediate vascular inflammatory processes, and contribute to atherosclerosis.

2. THE LO FAMILY

The LO enzymes are a family of dioxygenases, which catalyze the conversion of polyunsaturated fatty acids into conjugated hydroperoxides. Arachidonic (eicosatetraenoic, C20:4), linoleic (octadecadienoic, C18:2), and linolenic (octadecatrienoic, C18:3) acids are the most important substrates for LOs in mammals. Traditionally, LOs have been classified by a single enzyme property, i.e., their positional specificity, referring to the carbon number on the fatty acid structure that they preferentially oxygenate: 5 lipoxygenase (5LO), 12 lipoxygenase (12LO) and 15 lipoxygenase (15LO). Although this classification still dominates the field, it is utterly insufficient to reflect the diversity of mammalian LOs and their phylogenetic relatedness on one hand and the inconsistency in functional specificity of phylogenetically related enzymes across various mammalian species on the other hand.

In general, mammalian LOs can be now divided into four classes: (a) 5LOs; (b) platelet-type 12LOs; (c) reticulocyte 12/15LOs; (d) epidermis-type LOs. Examples of common confusion in identity include the human epidermis-type 15LO (also referred to as 15LO type 2), whose murine ortholog is an arachidonic acid 8LO (variance in positional specificity of closely related genes); the close relation and high sequence homology between the human reticulocyte-type 15LO and the porcine leukocyte-type 12LO, despite differences in positional specificity (12 vs 15); and the fact that the epidermis-type 12LO, the epidermis type 15LO and the platelet type 12LO can each convert arachidonic acid into either 12- or 15HPETE (albeit at different proportions), but do *not* belong to the 12/15LO family *(1–3)*. Table 1 summarizes the current classification of LO enzymes and outlines the most important forms in mammalian cells.

3. VASCULAR LO METABOLITES

3.1. The 5LO Metabolites and Their Actions in the Vasculature

The 5LO must be activated by a related peptide known as 5 lipoxygenase activating protein (PLAP), which has three transmembrane-spanning regions and two hydrophilic loops. Both 5LO and 5LO-activating protein (FLAP) are required for eicosanoid production. Most of the FLAP is associated with the nuclear membrane, and some with endoplasmic reticulum. FLAP may function as a membrane anchor for 5LO or as a membrane-independent activator of 5LO, perhaps as a substrate transfer protein that binds arachidonic acid or other fatty acid substrates for 5LO activity. 5LO resides in the cytosol in a resting cell, but associates with the cytosolic membranes or nuclear membrane once the cell is activated *(4)*.

The major biosynthetic events in the generation of 5LO metabolites are illustrated in Fig. 1 *(5)*. 5LO introduces first an active oxygen to carbon 5 of arachidonic acid, resulting in the formation of 5HPETE. This unstable derivative is either reduced to 5HETE, or converted to leukotriene A4 (LTA4). Leukotriene A4, in turn, can be channeled by LTA4 hydrolase to form leukotriene B$_4$ (LTB$_4$). Alternatively, LTA4 can be conjugated

Table 1
Classification of Mammalian Lipoxygenase (LO) Enzymes Including Common Forms
Representing the Four Mammalian LO Subfamilies

12/15LO	Platelet-type 12LO	Epidermis-type LOs	5LO
Rabbit 15LO		Human epidermis 12(R)LO	Human 5LO
Human 15LO-type 1	Human platelet 12LO	Human epidermis 15LO (15LO type 2)	Hamster 5LO
Porcine leukocyte 12LO		Mouse epidermis 8LO	Rat 5LO
Mouse leukocyte 12LO	Mouse platelet 12LO	Mouse epidermis 12(R)LO	Mouse 5LO

with glutathione into one of the cysteinyl leukotrienes termed LTC_4, LTD_4, or LTE_4, as shown in Fig. 1. The synthesis of LTC_4 is catalyzed intracellularly by LTC_4 synthetase, whereas LTD_4 and LTE_4 can be generated from LTC_4 extracellularly.

The 5HETE was shown to increase endothelial cell growth via activation of Jak/STAT and phosphatidylinositol 3-kinase/Akt signaling, leading to induction of expression of basic fibroblast growth factor 2 (6), but is otherwise understudied as a vasoactive compound. A membrane binding site for 5HETE was identified in human neutrophils (PMN). Several properties of the presumed action of 5HETE in neutrophils, such as mobilization of Ca^{2+}, and alteration in the binding of GTP gamma S to the membrane suggest that 5HETE acts by a downregulatable, G protein-linked mechanism distinct from LTB_4 receptors (7).

LTB_4, and the cysteinyl (cys) derivatives of leukotrienes, LTC_4, LTD_4, and LTE_4 display strong proinflammatory activities in cardiovascular tissues. LTB_4 is generated mainly in neutrophils and macrophages and, upon its release, it increases chemotaxis for neutrophils; enhances neutrophil adhesion to endothelial cells; interferes with the anti-adhesive effect of aspirin; and augments vascular permeability. LTB_4 also increases inflammatory responses indirectly, by stimulating the formation of other proinflammatory mediators, i.e., IL-1, IL-2, INF-γ by T-lymphocytes (5,8). As would be expected for a system that generates proinflammatory compounds, the 5LO pathway is abundantly expressed in macrophages, foam cells and inflammatory cells (dendritic cells, mast cells, and neutrophilic granulocytes) in atherosclerotic lesions of the aorta, coronary and carotid arteries. Further, the number of 5LO expressing cells markedly increased in advanced lesions (9,10).

Currently, there are four presumed LT-activated, seven-transmembrane domain-, G protein-coupled receptors for leukotrienes, of which two apparently mediate LTB_4 actions and are termed BLT-Rs. The other two receptors bind LTD_4 and LTC_4, and are referred to as $cysLT_1$-R and $cysLT_2$-R. $CysLT_1$-R is expressed mainly in macrophages and blood leukocytes (11) and can be blocked by a group of classical CysLT1 antagonists including MK571, ICI198615 and pobilukast (12). $CysLT_2$-R is expressed in endothelial cells, can be antagonized by the nonselective cystLTr blocker BAYu9773, and is strongly upregulated by IL-4. Recent evidence suggests that both $cysLT_1$-R and $cysLT_2$-R receptors are expressed in rat VSMC and that the $cysLT_1$-R is the dominant form in these cells (13). A third CysLT receptor can be activated only by LTC_4 and LTD_4. In light of the increased expression of 5LO in atherosclerotic lesions, it has been postulated that leukocytes, endothelial cells, and T-cell might interact in self- as well as

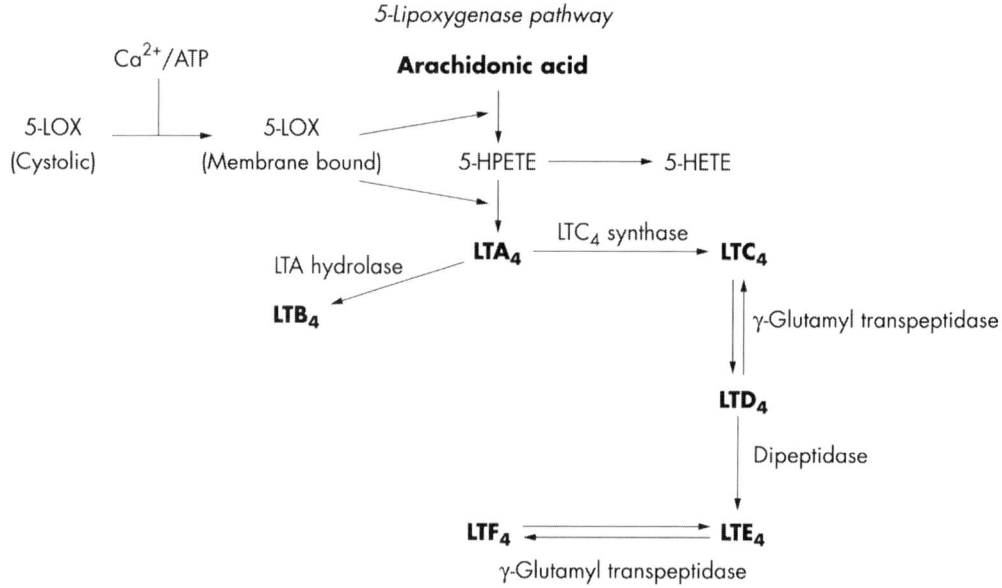

Fig. 1. The 5-lipoxygenase pathway and its major biosynthetic products (from ref. 5).

mutually enhancing inflammatory cross talk: LTs originating in macrophages or poly-morphonuclear cells might activate cysLT$_1$-Rs in an autocrine or paracrine manner (Fig. 2). Leukotrienes from these cells may also activate cysLT$_2$-Rs on endothelial cells and cysLT$_1$-Rs on T-lymphocytes in a paracrine fashion *(11)*. Additionally, VSMC and endothelial cells can also produce leukotrienes, at least under conditions such as hyper-tension, diabetes, and NO deficiency *(14–16)*, and are, thus, a potential source of agonists for the activation of cysLT$_1$-R-expressing macrophages that already migrated into subendothelial space or the media of the arterial wall. In human atherosclerotic plaques both CysLT1 and CysLT2 receptors are expressed *(10)*. In addition to their role as inflammatory promoters, cysteinyl-leukotrienes may also exert direct vasoactive effects and were shown to induce either vasoconstriction or vasodilation, in a species and/or vascular bed dependent manner *(17–21)*. In human saphenous veins, LTC$_4$ and LTD$_4$ induce vasodilation at very low doses and elicit vasoconstriction at higher doses, whereas coronary arteries appear unresponsive to either LTC$_4$ or LTD$_4$ *(12,20)*. In con-trast, in human atherosclerotic coronary arteries, LTC$_4$ and LTD$_4$ elicit a dose-related constrictor effect *(20)*. When administered systemically, though, LTD$_4$ increases blood pressure in rats in a dose-related fashion *(22)*. LTC$_4$, LTD$_4$, and LTE$_4$ also induce vaso-constriction in distal segments of pulmonary arteries and in the mesenteric bed *(17)*. Consistent with the possibility that cysteinyl-leukotrienes directly affect the contractile state of VSMC is the observation in cultured rat artery smooth muscle cells that LTD$_4$ and LTC$_4$ dose-dependently increased intracellular calcium concentration, which could be attenuated by montelukast, a selective type 1 CysLTs receptor antagonist *(13)*.

However, under well-defined experimental conditions it appears that at least some of the leukotriene-induced vasoconstriction is endothelium dependent. In one study, selective type 1 CysLTs receptor antagonists dose dependently prevented acetylcholine-induced contraction elicited in an endothelium-dependent preparation exposed to indomethacin

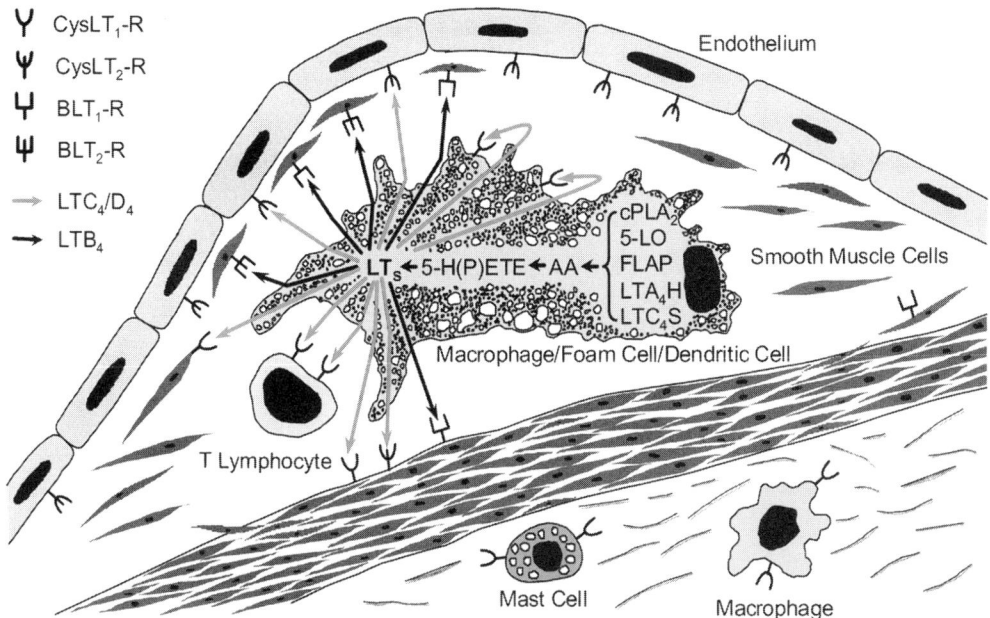

Fig. 2. Macrophage-vascular cell cross-talk mediated via leukotrienes (from ref. *11*).

and precontracted with phenylephrine *(13)*. In some instances, endothelium dependent vasodilation may also depend on some 5LO products, as illustrated by the observation that substance P induced endothelium-dependent relaxation in monkey and dog coronary arteries can be inhibited by the 5LO inhibitor AA861 *(23)*.

There is also cumulative evidence suggesting that abnormal vasculature, such as presumably exists in hypertension and diabetes, exhibits increased formation of and/or sensitivity to various leukotrienes. Indeed, under stressful vascular conditions, excessive vascular leukotrienes generation can be turned on by vasopressor hormones, a mechanism that is turned off when the offensive factor (e.g., correction of hyperglycemia in diabetes) is removed. Indeed, such increased production of leukotrienes can also contribute to altered regulation of blood pressure. For example, in L-NAME hypertensive rats, 5LO blockade with MK-886 ameliorates hypertension. Aortic tissue from L-NAME hypertensive rats increases the release of cysteinyl leukotrienes in response to norepinephrine, and norepinephrine-induced contraction of aortic rings from such L-NAME-treated rats (but not from control rats) can be attenuated by pretreatment with a 5LO inhibitor, a CysLT1 receptor antagonist or by a dual CysLT1/CysLT2 receptor antagonist *(16)*. In normal rats, angiotensin II-induced vasoconstriction appears not to depend on the 5LO system and is not associated with changes in leukotriene generation. However, in aortas from the (mRen-2)27 transgenic rats, which overexpress renin and develop hypertension, angitensin II induced a large increase in CysLT formation and either the 5LO inhibitor AA861 or the CysLT1 receptor antagonist MK571 attenuated the contractile response to angiotensin II *(24)*. Likewise, angiotensin II increased cysteinyl leukotriene production only in aortas from SHR but not from the normotensive genetic control WKY *(14)*, and neutralization of the 5LO axis either by the selective 5LO inhibitor AA-861 or the cysteinyl leukotriene receptor antagonist MK-571 significantly reduced the vasoconstrictor responses to angiotensin II only in arterial preparations from SHR *(14,25)*. Finally, cysteinyl leukotrienes also participate in angiotensin II-induced contraction in diabetic rats, presumably another example of impaired vascular function, but not in control rats or in diabetic rats treated with insulin via receptors distinct from the classical CysLT1 and CysLT2 receptors *(15)*. Collectively these data indicate that abnormal vasculature overproduces leukotrienes, at least in response to angiotensin II, and that these products then contribute to angiotensin II-dependent arterial tone. It is noteworthy that both atherosclerosis, as emerges from human studies, and abnormal arterial functional status, such as seen in the hypertensive and diabetic animal models, are linked to 5LO activation. Therefore the potential for cross-amplification of 5LO when hypertension and atherosclerotic lesions coexist requires testing.

3.2. The 12-, 12/15-, and 15LO and Their Products

3.2.1. EICOSANOIDS GENERATED BY 12-, OR 12/15LO

A number of active metabolites can be generated by 12- or 12/15LOs, including 12HPETE and 12HETE (by dioxygenation of C12); 15HPETE and 15HETE (by dioxygenation of C15); 13-hydroperoxyoctadecadienoic acid (HPODE) and 13-hydroxy-octadecadienoic (HODE) [by dioxygenation of C13 of linoleic acid] as well as hepoxillins and lipoxins (LXs), which are discussed in subsequent sections. There are two major forms of 12LOs, the platelet-type and the leukocyte-type. In man, the platelet type is expressed predominantly in platelets *(3)* but recent data indicate that it is also expressed in human endothelial cell *(26)*. Additionally, variant isoform of platelet-type 12LO is expressed in human VSMC *(27)*. The leukocyte type, which is extremely close to the human reticulocyte-type 15LO, and is hence designated as 12/15LO, is expressed in the human adrenal zona glomerulosa, human monocytes as well as in VSMC *(3,28,29)*.

Both the platelet- and leukocyte-type 12LOs contain 14 exons, but they are nonhomologous (65%) and encode proteins whose enzymatic properties differ significantly from each other *(3)*. The platelet-12LO preferentially metabolizes C20 fatty acids and is nearly inactive on C18 fatty acids, whereas the leukocyte type enzymes has a broad substrate specificity and can oxygenate C18 and also C22 acids at considerable efficiency *(1,3)*. Therefore, 13HODE, a product of linoleic acid metabolism can only be generated by the 12/15LO (and also by 15LO), but not by the platelet type 12LO. The platelet-type 12LO is also hardly capable of oxygenating esterified fatty acids or fatty acids complexed into membranes or lipoproteins, whereas the 12/15LO enzymes can use such fatty acids as substrates *(1,3)*. Finally, the 12/15LO enzymes undergo product-dependent suicidal inactivation, whereas the platelet-type enzymes do not *(1,3)*.

3.2.2. EICOSANOIDS GENERATED BY 15LOS

As already indicated, 15LO activity resulting in the formation of 15HPETE, 15HETE, 13HPODE, or 13HODE can be displayed by two enzyme types: (a) the human reticulocyte 15LO that is, in fact, practically equivalent to the 12/15LO (leukocyte type) and is also referred to as 15LO type 1; (b) the epidermis type 15LO, also referred to as 15LO type 2 *(29)*. Currently, 12/15LO is reportedly expressed in human monocytes and zona glomerulosa cells, whereas the expression of 15LO type 2 in man is documented in the prostate, lung, skin, esophagus, and cornea *(28,30,31)*. Although both 12- and 15HETE can be generated by the 12/15LO (15LO type 1), 12HETE is apparently still the dominant product of most 12/15LOs *(3)*. Relating this basic concept to observations in vascular tissue, it is noteworthy that normal rabbit aortas synthesize 12HETE as the principal LO metabolite whereas atherosclerotic aortas from both cholesterol-fed and Watanabe heritable hyperlipidemic rabbits show major and selective increases in the synthesis of 15HETE *(32)*. Studies of human atherosclerotic tissue also find evidence for 15LO expression *(33)* or enzymatic activity (i.e., the formation of 15HETE or 13HODE *(34,35)*. Because arachidonic acid is substrate to the formation of both 12- and 15HETE, such dominance of 15HETE formation would be impossible to explain unless a predominantly 15HETE generating system has been turned on. One possible explanation is that 15HETE thus formed is the product of the cyclooxygenase pathway of arachidonate metabolism *(36)*, though no direct support for this in vascular tissue exists. The other possibility, which is supported by recent finding from our laboratory, is that human vascular cells also express 15LO type 2 *(37)*.

4. VASCULAR RECEPTORS AND CELLULAR TARGETS FOR THE ACTION OF 12-, 12/15- AND 15LO PRODUCTS

With the exception of well-characterized receptors for leukotrienes, which are discussed in the section on 5LO, cellular receptors for 12- and 15LO products are vaguely defined and specific receptor antagonists for their action are not available. The existence of receptor(s) is not required to explain the actions of HETEs as intracellular signaling molecules but would be expected in instances in which they operate as independent bioactive molecules. One report suggested that the mono-HETEs 5(S)-, 12(R)-, 12(S)- and 15(S)-HETE can interact with the TXA2/PGH2 receptor because these metabolites inhibited binding of a radiolabeled thromboxane ligand to this receptor *(38)*. Lewis lung carcinoma and human skin Langerhans cells have predominantly cytosolic high affinity binding sites for 12HETE *(3)*, but how these scarce data pertain to the vascular effects of HETEs is unclear. The interaction of LO-derived HETEs with some well recognized "noneicosanoid" receptors, as reviewed in the following section, provides partial explanation, at best, for the multiple biological effects of these eicosanoids.

4.1. PPARα

Although neither 12- nor 15HETE apparently activates PPARα *(39)*, certain non-classical LO metabolites can serve as PPARα agonists. 2-Arachidonylglycerol (2-AG), an arachidonate metabolite shown to bind to cannabinoid receptors, can be metabolized by both 15LO-1 and 15LO-2 to a 15-hydroxyeicosatetraenoic acid glyceryl ester (15HETE-G), which, in turn, can activate PPARα *(40)*. PPARα can also bind LTB$_4$ *(41)*, and this interaction has been proposed as a coregulatory route for LTB$_4$ signaling, aimed to exert a moderating effect on inflammation, thus counterbalancing the multiple proinflammatory effects of this eicosanoid.

4.2. PPARγ

Many fatty acids, including some LO products such as 15HETE and 13HODE, can bind and activate PPARγ, but a clear HETE-dependent biological response elicited by this mechanism has been shown in just a few instances *(42,43)*. Other intracellular ligands, though, such as the cyclooxygenase product 15-deoxyΔ^{12,14}-PJ$_2$ *(44)*, may bind more avidly to PPARγ than LO metabolites. The LO products 13HODE and 15HETE may be particularly potent activators of PPARγ in macrophages, thus suggesting a potential cell specificity in terms of the interaction between LO products and PPARγ *(45)*. Further, there are downstream differences in coactivator recruitment by PPARγ/ cis-retinoic acid receptor heterodimers, which depend on the type of ligand bound to PPARγ: the effects of the LO metabolites 13HODE and 15HETE on PPARγ are amplified by the coactivator CREB-binding protein, whereas the effect of 15-deoxyΔ^{12,14}-PJ$_2$ is preferentially enhanced by steroid receptor coactivator-1 *(45)*. In the process of implantation in mice, progesterone has been recently shown to indirectly activate PPARγ by stimulation of 12/15LO, thus supplying 12HETE, 15HETE, and 13HODE as ligands for PPARγ *(46)*. Thus, LO products, especially 15HETE and 13HODE, as well as 12HETE, appear to activate PPARγ in a cell- and function-specific manner. Of particular importance for vascular disease is the finding that these LO products can activate PPARγ even when they are seeded within LDL particles *(45)*.

4.3. VR1

The vanilloid receptor 1, VR1, is a receptor for capsaicin expressed in unmyelinated axon terminals known as C-fibers. Activation of the VR1 receptor, apparently located on perivascular sensory nerves, elicits a vasodilator action associated with, and dependent on the local release of the calcitonin gene-related peptide (CGRP), a peptide known for its potent VSMC relaxing effect *(47)*. Many fatty acids can activate VR1 receptors, including LO derived eicosanoids such as 12HPETE, 15HPETE, 5HETE, 15HETE, and LTB$_4$ *(48)*, but how such potential interactions affect vascular function is currently unknown. Bradykinin released during tissue injury can activate 12LO. Since bradykinin is known to activate VR1, this effect may be transduced indirectly, via the induction of 12LO activity, providing 12HETE as a ligand for this receptor *(49)*.

4.4. Role of 12HETE and Other 12- or 15LO Metabolites in VSMC Signaling

Much more is known on how 12HETE signals through various VSMC transduction cascades than on any other 12- or 15LO metabolite. 12HETE is involved in agonist-mediated increases in VSMC Ca^{2+} *(50,51)*, which impacts on cell contractility, but may also facilitate associated signaling for more delayed effects such as growth. LO inhibitors blunt the rise in intracellular calcium elicited by angiotensin II [Arg8]-vasopressin and endothelin, and the calcium response to angiotensin can be restored by the addition of 12HETE, but not 5- or 15HETE *(50,51)*, via mechanisms which suggest that 12HETE contributes to the release of Ca^{2+} from intracellular pools *(51,52)*. The 15LO metabolite 13HODE was shown to increase calcium fixing into cultured VSMC *(53)*. In VSMC from canine basilar arteries, 12HETE increases the generation rate of diacylglycerol, a product of phospholipase C *(54)*. In cultured VSMC, 12HETE, and 15HETE, which are generated from arachidonic acid released by norepinephrine-stimulated cytosolic cPLA$_2$-activity, are critical for tyrosine kinase-dependent activation (phosphorylation) of phospholipase D *(55)*. 12HETE also affects the RAC1/PAK1/MEKK1/SEK1/JNK/c-JUN pathway, which regulates cell growth. In this respect, 12HETE activates MAPK *(56)*, probably by upstream activation of PAK1 *(57)*. Indeed, either 12- or 15HETE can activate p38 MAPK and, accordingly, p38 MAPK activation elicited by either norepinephrine or angiotensin II can be attenuated by LO inhibitors *(56,58)*. In rat renal mesangial cells

12HETE leads to activation of p38MAPK and its target transcription factor cAMP-responsive element-binding protein *(59)*.

There is some evidence suggesting that LO products (other than eicosanoids of the 5LO lineage) may exert potential proinflammatory vascular effects via activation of NF-κB. 13HODE, a 15LO product of linoleic acid metabolism, induces MCP-1 and VCAM expression in VSMC via an NF-κB dependent mechanism *(60–63)*. The production of 13HODE in endothelial cells can be increased by LDL, presumably via induction of 12/15LO activity, thus providing the effector molecule to elicit such inflammatory reaction in the neighboring VSMC *(62)*. As a balancing effect, however, overexpression of 15LO in rabbit aortic VSMC actually inhibited the expression of cell adhesion molecules (CAM) and rendered the cells refractory to IL-1 stimulation *(63)*. This unexpected outcome likely results from oxidation of protein thiols of the signaling system by the excess of 15LO-derived hydroperoxy products. Thus, 15LO products can feed back and inhibit the proinflammatory signals set in motion by the very same metabolites.

5. LO PATHWAY PRODUCTS AFFECT ARTERIAL WALL STRUCTURE

Increased arterial pressure may result from alteration in arterial wall structure. LO-controlled mechanisms apparently contribute to impaired integrity of the endothelial lining, increased VSMC population and arterial wall hypertrophy, excessive formation of matrix proteins and atherosclerosis, which may interfere with vasorelaxant mechanisms, increase arterial wall rigidity, decrease large and small artery compliance, and facilitate the evolution of hypertension.

5.1. HETEs Increase Monocyte–Endothelial
and Monocyte–VSMC Interaction and Adhesion

12HETE increases the expression of vascular matrix proteins such as fibronectin *(59)*, induces endothelial cell retraction and increases integrin alpha V beta 3 surface expression, which may promote adhesion of inflammatory leukocytes to the endothelium *(64)*. The increased adhesion of monocytes to endothelial cells in diabetic *db/db* mice is mediated through 12/15LO products *(65)*. This is mediated, at least in part, by HETE-induced increases in the expression of adhesion molecules in endothelial cells. Indeed, in human umbilical vein endothelial cells both 15HPETE and 12HETE were reported to induce surface expression of a subset of CAM, ICAM-1, ELAM-1, and VCAM-1, in association with increased binding activity of the transcription factor, NF-κB, to the consensus motif common to the CAM genes in the nuclear extracts of these cells *(66)*. In contrast, Huang et al. *(67)* reported that 15HPETE and 15HETE inhibited the expression of TNFα-induced endothelial cell intercellular adhesion molecule-1, E-selectin, and vascular cellular adhesion molecule-1 in human endothelial cells. As indicated in the preceding section, however, 13HODE, another 15LO product, albeit of linoleic rather than arachidonic acid metabolism, induces MCP-1 and VCAM expression in VSMC via an NF-κB dependent mechanism *(60,61)*. Both pro- and counter-inflammatory responses, then, may be induced by the same LO pathway.

Transgenic mice overexpressing the murine 12/15LO gene, develop early atherosclerotic lesions, namely, fatty streaks, and their endothelial cells display increased binding capacity for monocytes, in association with enhanced ICAM-1 expression *(68)*. Not only endothelial cells, but also VSMC can activate the 12/15LO pathway to enhance monocyte adhesion, such that the monocytes can bind to subendothelial VSMC or VSMC exposed by endothelial injury. Treatment of human aortic VSMC (HVSMC) with angiotensin II or PDGF-BB significantly increased their binding to human monocytic THP-1 cells and to peripheral blood monocytes. This depended on 12/15LO or cyclooxygenase-2 activation and was apparently mediated via monocyte beta(1)- and beta(2)-integrins. Consistent with a role for 12/15LO pathway in enhancing VSMC's ability to bind monocytes is also the finding that VSMC derived from 12/15LO knockout mice displayed reduced binding to mouse monocytic cells. *(69)*. Counterbalancing some of these proinflammatory effects, 12(S)-hydroperoxyeicosapentaenoic acid (12(S)-HpEPE), 15(S)-HpEPE as well as the 5LO pathway product LTD5 were shown to inhibit IL-1β-induced expression of prostaglandin H synthase 2 (PGHS-2) in human pulmonary microvascular endothelial cells. Because PGHS-2 is responsible for overproduction of the prostaglandins (PGs) at inflammatory sites, these effects can potentially limit inflammatory responses *(70)*.

5.2. Platelet–Vascular Interactions and Vascular Disease: Role of Platelet 12LO and Platelet-Derived 12HETE

Platelets express the platelet type 12LO and comprise the largest source of circulating 12HETE. Collagen and collagen-related peptide, to which platelets are exposed following endothelial injury and denudation, rapidly increase 12HETE synthesis in platelets via the collagen receptor glycoprotein VI and activation of src-tyrosine kinases, PI3-kinase, mobilization of Ca^{2+}, and translocation of platelet 12LO. This effect is negatively regulated by platelet endothelial cell adhesion molecule (PECAM-1) and PKC *(71)*. There is evidence that platelet derived 12HETE is not merely a by-product of platelet activation but rather plays an important role in coagulation. In experimentally stenosed and endothelium-injured canine coronary arteries, inhibition of platelet 12HETE generation markedly attenuated platelet aggregation and thus may reduce coronary thrombosis in vivo *(72)*. Platelet-derived 12HETE can also interact with VSMC, as detailed in the following section.

5.3. LO Products Affect Vascular Cell Growth
5.3.1. 12LO AND VSMC GROWTH

Several lines of evidence suggest a role for LO pathways in vascular smooth muscle cell cycle. First, a number of reports indicated that LO inhibitors attenuated VSMC growth *(73–77)*. 12HETE *per se* increases VSMC proliferation and migration *(73)*. Further, LO blocker-induced inhibition of VSMC proliferation and migration could be reversed by direct addition of the 12HETE *(74)*. Second, the expression of 12/15LO was increased in balloon-injured arteries *(75)*, and the myointimal cell proliferation, which evolves in response to this injury, could be reduced by 12LO ribozymes or pharmacological inhibitors *(75–77)*. Finally, VSMC derived from 12/15LO knockout mice respond to angiotensin II- or PDGF-BB with diminished incorporation of ^{3}H-thymidine and ^{3}H-leucine *(78)*. LO products appear to accelerate cell growth via activation of MAP-kinase *(56,79)*, but other effects of 12HETE on cell signaling regulating elements such as recruitment of intracellular calcium *(50,51)* or activation of extra cellular-regulated protein kinase (ERK1/2), protein kinase C (PKC), phosphatidylinositol 3-kinase (PI3 kinase) and Src kinase *(80)* may all affect cell growth.

LO-dependent mechanisms may be also actively involved in the prevention of VSMC apoptosis. Nishio et al. *(81)* reported that the nonspecific LO blocker NDGA increased apoptotic indices in cultured rat VSMC exposed to phenylephrine in association with decreased Bcl-2 expression and apoptosis could be partially reversed by 15HETE. We have recently found that the LO inhibitor baicalein induced an increase in cell death in human VSMC secondary to an apoptotic process operating via the mitochondrial apoptotic pathway, which could be averted by the addition of 12HETE. Further, the transfection of VSMC with two different platelet type 12LO antisense constructs also resulted in apoptotic cell death *(82)*.

5.3.2. The 12- and 12/15LO Products Induce Fibroblast and VSMC Hypertrophy

Although several investigators have pointed out that HETEs, particularly 12HETE are mediators of cell growth, in other studies induction of cell hypertrophy was seen. In fibroblasts overexpressing 12LO, there was an increase in cell protein content and enlargement in cell size, in association with increased fibronectin and collagen deposition *(83)*. In porcine VSMC, 12HETE and 13HODE were shown to induce cell hypertrophy *(84)*. Why some VSMC respond to 12HETE by increase in size though others begin to proliferate is unclear but is likely related to culture conditions, phase in the cell cycle and the cell phenotype ("contractile" vs "secretory") of the cell.

5.4. Oxidative Stress in the Arterial Wall and HETEs

There is a complex relationship among LO enzymes, their products, and oxidative stress. First, LOs generate intermediary hydroperoxy metabolites such as 12H[P]ETE and 1512H[P]ETE, which can release reactive oxygen intracellularly, thereby increasing oxidative stress, unless they are reduced by phospholipid hydroperoxide glutathione peroxidase. The potential impact of these hydroperoxy derivatives is illustrated by the observation that 15HPETE induced a concentration-dependent loss of cardiomyocytes membrane integrity, which could be prevented by oxygen scavenging *(85)*. There is also evidence that 15HPETE directly induces damage in endothelial cell and adversely affects their ability to release t-PA and bind antithrombin III, though increasing the release of PAI-I *(86)*, all of which can be prevented by antioxidants. Second, LO products such as 5HPETE and LTB$_4$ are required for lysophosphatidic acid-stimulated H(2)O(2) release such as seen in keratinocyte-derived HaCaT cells *(87)*. Other LO products, including hydroperoxyoctadecadienoic acid (HPODE) and hydroperoxyeicosatetraenoic acid (HPETE), as well as cholesterol linoleate hydroperoxides can serve as "seeding molecules" which enter LDL particles, thereby rendering them particularly sensitive to further oxidation *(88)*. The 15LO product 13HODE, is a potent pro-oxidant in this setting, capable of accelerating the generation of biologically active oxidized phospholipids, which in turn increase monocyte adhesion *(88)*. Third, under hyperglycemic conditions, increased oxidative stress *per se* stimulates the expression of 12/15LO or 15LO. For example, after exposure of cultured bovine coronary artery endothelial cells to the hydrogen peroxide-generating system of glucose–glucose oxidase, the synthesis of the arachidonic acid metabolite 15HETE is strongly increased *(89)*. Fourth, angiotensin II increases oxidative stress, in part, via 5LO activity. It is well-established that angiotensin II-induced reactive oxygen species (ROS) formation is mediated, in part, through NAD[P]H-oxidase derived superoxide anions. A recent study in VSMC showed that angiotensin II also induces the generation of LTB_4, which then activates NAD[P]H-oxidase, leading to ROS. The entire process can be inhibited by 5LO blockade (90). Finally, 12/15LO serves as a catalytic sink for NO, such that monocytes and VSMC show increased consumption of NO if 12/15LO is not blocked (91). Because NO counterbalances ROS within the cells, this would result in a net increase in cellular oxidative stress. Further, the loss of NO might impair major NO-related protective mechanisms such as vasodilation, inhibition of VSMC growth and of leukocyte and platelet adhesion, thus collectively facilitating the evolution of hypertension and vascular disease.

6. HETEs AS DIRECT VASOACTIVE AGENTS AND THE ROLE OF LOs IN ARTERIAL TONE AND CONTRACTILITY

6.1. The Effects of HETES on Arterial Tone Depend on the Particular Vascular Bed Examined

Both 12HETE and 15HETE have been reported to induce either vasoconstrictor or vasodepressor effects. In the rat mesenteric arteries, both 12HETE and 12HPETE induced a concentration-dependent vasodilation. Of interest is the finding that small mesenteric arteries primarily produced 12HETE (92). 12HETE was also reported to elicit potent relaxation and hyperpolarization of porcine coronary microvessels (93). The mechanism underlying these vasodilator effects of 12HETE have not been studied but there is independent evidence that 12HETE can mediate, in part, and directly augment IL-1β-stimulated nitrite production and iNOS in cultured VSMC (94).

12HETE can also directly induce arterial constriction in some arterial systems, although it appears to be more important as a mediator of angiotensin II-dependent vasoconstriction. In isolated renal arcuate arteries of the dog, 12(S)-HETE acted as a vasoconstrictor, but the vasopressor effects of 12(R)-HETE were more prominent (95). In a renal juxtamedullary preparation, 12(S)-HETE caused a graded decrease in afferent arteriolar caliber, which could be blocked by L-type calcium channel inhibition (96). In isolated canine basilar artery segments (97) but not in the anesthetized rabbit cerebral arterioles (98), 12HPETE produced transient contraction of the artery segment whereas 12HETE had a much lower potency.

Much like the discordant direct effects of 12HETE, 15HETE may induce either vasoconstriction or vasodilation, depending on the particular vascular preparation. Indeed, when studied by a single group of investigators in several different arterial preparations from different animal species, 15HPETE or 15HETE were shown to elicit either vasodilation or vasoconstriction, depending on the specific arteries in question (99). It is therefore of interest that two independent studies reported that 15HETE was a constrictor in pulmonary arteries (100,101). Two additional reports supported a vasopressor role for 15HETE: in one study 15HETE elicited contractile responses in guinea pig cerebral arteries (102) and in the second investigation, 15HETE impaired acetylcholine-induced relaxation in rat aortic rings (103).

In contrast to these latter effects of 15HETE, several other metabolites of 15(or 12/15-)LO appear to reduce arterial tone in a number of different experimental settings.

13-Hydroxyoctadecadienoic acid (13HODE) and 13-hydroperoxyoctadecadienoic acid (13HPODE), induced dose-dependent relaxation of prostaglandin (PG) F2α-precontracted porcine coronary rings that persisted in the de-endothelialized vessels, thus suggesting a direct effect of these metabolites on vascular smooth muscle cells *(104)*. In the rabbit aorta, endothelial 15LO converts arachidonic acid into several vasoactive metabolites, two of which, 11,12,15-trihydroxyeicosatrienoic acid (THETA) and 15-hydroxy-11,12-epoxyeicosatrienoic acid (HEETA), have distinct vasodilatory properties. The biosynthesis of these additional "endothelium-derived relaxing factors," involves first 15LO metabolism of arachidonic acid, followed by further modification by cytochrome P450 isomerases, possibly CYP2J2 *(105,106)*. The production of these vasodilatory compounds is subject to upregulation by IL-13, which increases 15LO expression and activity *(107)*. The vasodilatory effect of the endothelium-derived 11,12,15-trihydroxyeicosatrienoic acid is mediated through activation of VSMC apamin-sensitive K^+ channels, leading to membrane hyperpolarization *(108)*. 11,12,15-Trihydroxyeicosatrienoic acid also contributes to acetylcholine dependent relaxation in the rabbit aorta *(109)*.

6.2. Role of LO Metabolites in Angitensin II-Induced Vasoconstriction

6.2.1. ROLE OF 12LO

Studies in the adrenal zona glomerulosa were the first to indicate that 12HETE is an important signaling molecule for angiotensin II-induced biological responses *(110,111,112)*. Several structurally unrelated LO inhibitors attenuated angiotensin II-induced vasoconstriction both in vivo and in vitro in rat and human preparations *(113,114)*. Angiotensin II increased 12LO expression, and 12- and 15HETE secretion in cultured porcine and human vascular smooth muscle cells *(28,115)*. Angiotensin II-induced calcium transients in VSMC are inhibited by several LO blockers, but the intracellular calcium response to angiotensin II under these conditions can be restored by the addition of 12HETE *(50,51)*. Recent observations in the renal microvasculature corroborate these findings that renal microvessels express both platelet-type 12LO and leukocyte-type 12LO. Angiotensin II was shown to increase renal microvascular 12HETE production, and 12HETE *per se* induced vasoconstriction in this system in association with an increase in myocyte [Ca2+]i. Further, the vasoconstrictor response of the afferent arteries to 12HETE was abolished during L-type calcium channel inhibition *(96)*.

6.2.2. ROLE OF CYSTEINYL-LEUKOTRIENES

As already discussed, there is evidence that angiotensin-II mediated vasoconstriction depends, in part, on increased secretion of CysLT, which apparently takes place when the vasculature is subjected to some functional distress such as hypertension, NO deficiency or exposure to high glucose. Under these conditions 5LO inhibition or CysLT1 receptor blockade attenuates angiotensin II-dependent vasoconstriction *(14,15, 24,25)*. Neither the increase in CysLTs nor the dependence of angiotensin II-induced vasoconstriction on 5LO-derived CystLTs is seen in normal rats or blood vessels. These results suggest that both diabetes and the hypertensive state are linked to activation of the 5LO system, which is further stimulated by angiotensin II.

6.2.3. ROLE OF THE CYTOCHROME P450 PRODUCT 20HETE

In addition to the stimulatory effect of Ang II on 12HETE and in hypertensive rats, on cysteinyl-leukotrienes as well, Ang II also markedly increases the formation of 20HETE, a product of the cytochrome p450 epoxygenase in renal vasculature *(116)*, and this metabolite also contributes to angiotensin II-induced vasoconstriction in the kidney. Indeed, it has been shown that 20HETE is a potent constrictor of renal and cerebral arteries, acting by VSMC depolarization through the blockade of Ca^{2+}-activated K^+ (K_{Ca}) channels *(117,118)*. 20HETE also plays an important role in tubuloglomerular feedback control of glomerular filtration rate (GFR) and in the renal vasoconstrictor response to endothelin (ET), vasopressin and Ang II *(119)*.

7. REGULATION OF LO ENZYMES

7.1. Angiotensin II

In porcine VSMC, human aortic smooth muscle cell, and rat mesangial cells, angiotensin II treatment increases 12LO mRNA expression and 12HETE *(28,59,115)*. Administration of the AT1 receptor blocker losartan diminishes leukocyte type 12LO expression in the renal tissue of neonatal rats *(120)*. Some of the most important biological effects elicited by angiotensin II in the vasculature are mediated by the induction of 12LO products, including vasoconstriction *(114)*, cell growth *(59)*, LDL oxidation *(121)*, and fibronectin formation *(59)*.

7.2. Diabetes and High Glucose

High glucose increases 12- and/or 12/15LO expression in endothelial cells and VSMC *(115,122,123)*. The attained rise in LO products, particularly in 12HETE, appears to mediate some of the known effects of hyperglycemia on vascular cells such as increased growth, migration, chemotaxis and macrophage adhesion. The augmented response to various agonists, which occurs in hyperglycemia, may be also related to LO induction. For example, phenylephrine induces a more pronounced proliferative response under high glucose conditions, which is aborted by LO inhibition *(73)*. Glucose-induced LO stimulation is not restricted to overproduction of 12HETE. In the rabbit, basal and acetylcholine (ACh)-stimulated release of 15HETE was significantly increased in the aorta of diabetic animals. Further, incubation of aortic segments from normal rabbits in high glucose medium caused a significant increase in basal and ACh-stimulated release of 15HETE, which was mainly, but not exclusively secondary to increased endothelial production of this prostanoid *(124)*.

7.3. Cytokines

7.3.1. IL-4

IL-4 down-regulates 5LO and upregulates 15LO type 1 expression in dendritic cells, which are lymphoid antigen-presenting cells capable of initiating immune responses in naive lymphocytes *(125)*. IL-4 also upregulates 12/1515LO activity such that the generated LO products serve as ligands for PPARγ1 in human blood monocytes. The activation of PPARγ1 by LO metabolites elicits a host of downstream effects such as increased expression of a macrophage scavenger receptor, CD36 or suppression of IL-2 production *(125–127)*. Indeed, the 15LO products 13HODE and 15HETE directly stimulated the expression of CD36 in macrophages *(126)*. Because 15LO can oxidize various lipid moieties, cytokine induced 15LO expression may increase LDL oxidation in hematopoietic cells interacting with vascular lining. Also, by increasing macrophage 12/15LO expression/activity, IL-4 can induce the formation of ligands for PPARγ (such as 13HODE) expressed in other cell types comprising the vascular–blood interface. One example to that effect is the finding that IL-4 modulates T cell function by suppressing IL-2 production through LO-derived products, which activate PPARγ *(127)*.

7.3.2. IL-13

IL-13, a cytokine secreted by Th2 lymphocytes, is capable of inducing the expression of 15LO in primary human monocytes *(128)* and in rabbit aortic endothelial cells *(129)*.

It is noteworthy that 12/15LOs and phospholipid hydroperoxide glutathione peroxidases are opposite enzymes balancing the intracellular concentration of hydroperoxy lipids. There appears to be an inverse regulation of 12/15LOs and hydroperoxy-lipid-reducing enzymes by IL-4 and -13, such that both cytokines increase 12/15LO expression and suppress phospholipid hydroperoxide glutathione peroxidase expression in human monocytes *(130)*. This concomitant alteration may facilitate 12/15LO dependent LDL oxidation, whereas depriving cells from one of the neutralizing mechanisms for hydroperoxy lipids.

7.3.3. ESTROGEN

In human umbilical vein endothelial cells, estradiol increased the activity of 15LO by 320%. The effect was probably nongenomic, as it could be reproduced by E2 complexed to BSA, such that entry of the steroid molecule to the cell was not possible *(131)*.

7.4. Lipoxins

LO interaction products, or lipoxins (LXs), are trihydroxytetraene-containing eicosanoids that can be generated at the vascular–luminal interface as a result of platelet–leukocyte and/or endothelial cell interactions. The basic principle is that transcellular biosynthesis takes place as a sequence of two consecutive fatty acid metabolizing enzymes, LO and cyclooxygenase or two LO enzymatic reactions, such that a product of one cyclooxygenase or LO pathways in one cell type is transferred for further metabolism by another LO pathway in a different cell type. 5LOX, 12LOX and 15LOX pathways can all participate in the biosynthesis of LXs. In humans, LXs are formed in vivo during multi-cellular responses such as inflammation, atherosclerosis, and in asthma. The generated specific tetraene-containing products function as inflammation stop signals, acting directly to down regulate key steps in leukocyte trafficking and prevent leukocyte-mediated acute tissue injury, or indirectly, by blocking the effects of proinflammatory leukotrienes (e.g., LXA_4 and LXB_4 antagonize LTB_4) *(132,133)*. In addition to their actions in inflammatory cells, LXA_4 and LXB_4 have been reported to stimulate prostacyclin secretion, increase endothelial-dependent vasodilation and inhibit endothelial cell P-selectin expression and hyperadhesiveness induced by LTs *(132–134)*. On the other hand, LXA_4 reportedly increases the expression and activity of the procoagulant tissue factor in endothelial cells and monocytes *(135)*. One recognized example in which all these various properties of LXs might interact with multiple other LO-derived eicosanoids is the documented in vivo generation

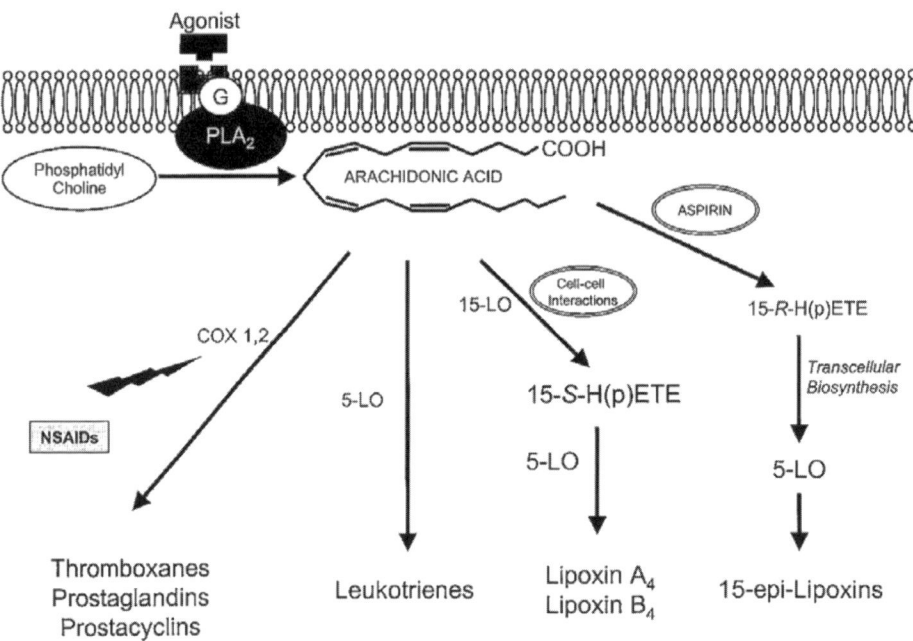

Fig. 3. The major biosynthetic routes of lipoxin formation from arachidonic acid: interactive action of lipoxygenase and cylooxygenase enzymes. The combination of two LOs (5-, 12-, or 15LO) on the same arachidonic acid molecule produces lipoxins. Aspirin can trigger the production of epimeric lipoxins through acetylation of COX-2, yielding 15-epi-H(p)ETEs, which are then converted to lipoxins by transcellular biosynthesis using 5LO from neutrophils. (From ref. *185*)

of LX after percutaneous transluminal coronary angioplasty *(136)*. During experimental acute renal failure, LXs attenuate the adhesion and transmigration of polymorpho-nuclear cells, increase the activation of monocytes, and promote the phagocytosis of apoptotic neutrophils by macrophages *(137)*. They also reduce mesangial cell proli-feration by inhibiting PDGF receptor tyrosine kinase activity and attenuation of VEGF-driven angiogenesis *(138,139)*.

Of interest are recent results indicating that aspirin's mechanism of action also involves the shunting of prostanoid metabolism from prostaglandin E2 into the generation of carbon 15 epimers of LX, or 15-epi-LX, also referred to as aspirin-triggered lipoxins (ATL). ATL mimic the effects of native LX. ATL formation requires the acetylation of COX2 by aspirin (acetyl-salicylic-acid). Inhibition of ATL formation interferes with the anti-adhesive effects of aspirin *(5,140–142)*.

Diet-derived fatty acids can also undergo transcellular reactions, resulting in the formation of bioactive LX-like compounds. In human endothelial cells treated with aspirin, COX-2 is upregulated and it converts C20:5 omega-3 to 18R-hydroxyeicos-apentaenoic acid (HEPE) and 15R-HEPE. Each can be used by polymorphonuclear leukocytes to generate separate classes of novel trihydroxy-containing mediators, including 5-series 15R-LX(5) and 5,12,18R-triHEPE, which are potent inhibitors of human polymorphonuclear leukocyte transendothelial migration and infiltration in vivo. The generation of these diet-derived "lipoxin analogs" also offers a new explanation for the apparent vasculoprotective effect of dietary omega-3 fatty acids *(143)*.

Although the vasodilator effect of LXs has been recognized nearly two decades ago *(144)*, this effect may be system-specific, as LXA_4 and LXB_4 were shown to constrict the mesenterial tree *(145)*. LXA_4 and LXB_4 were also shown to increase prostacyclin secretion in human endothelial cells *(136)*, which might explain, in part, their vasodilator and cell growth moderating effects. The overall significance of these effects for cardio-vascular pathophysiology and blood pressure regulation awaits elucidation.

Membrane lipoxin receptors (ALX), apparently of the seven transmembrane domains family, are expressed in leukocytes and endothelial cells In addition to these specific LX receptors, there is evidence that LXs and CysLTs such as LTD_4 interact on a "shared receptor," apparently the CysLT1 receptor. Finally, some short peptide ligands can also interact with ALX: indeed the LX receptor may bind a lipid ligand (LX) and a peptide ligand at different sites within the receptor structure *(146)*.

7.5. Hepoxillins

Hepoxillins are monohydroxy-epoxy metabolites of arachidonic acid generated from 12HPETE, either nonenzymatically, in the presence of hemoglobin as a catalyst, or by "hepoxillin synthases" *(3)*. Recently, a novel metabolite of this group, trioxilin C(3) [8,9,12-trihydroxyeicosatrienoic acid] was isolated from rabbit aorta homogenates when 12LO was supplied exogenously. Trioxilin C(3) apparently has potent vasodilator effects *(147)*.

8. LOs AND ATHEROGENESIS

8.1. Atherosclerosis and the 5LO Pathway

Although a fairly recently appreciated player in atherosclerosis, the 5LO pathway is currently the focus of increasing attention with respect to the evolution of athero-sclerotic vascular disease. First, 5LO was abundantly expressed in atherosclerotic lesions of apoE(-/-) and LDLR(-/-) deficient mice *(148)* as well as in human atherosclerotic arteries *(9)*. Further, 5LO expression apparently correlates with the severity of athero-sclerotic lesion in man *(9)*. Second, even the absence of just one of the two 5LO alleles confers significant resistance to atherosclerosis in a classical atherosclerosis-prone model such as the LDL receptor deficient mouse *(148)*. Third, bone marrow from 5LO(+/−) mice transplanted into LDLR(−/−) , induced a significant reduction in athero-sclerosis, thus implicating macrophage wild type 5LO as a culprit in the atherogenic process *(148)*. Fourth, an antagonist of the 5LO metabolite LTB_4 reduced monocyte adhesions and atherosclerotic surface area in apoE$^{-/-}$ as well as LDLr$^{-/-}$ mice *(149)*. Finally, two independent population studies have recently indicated a link between the 5LO system and vascular disease. One report concluded that specific variant genotypes of the 5LO gene are significantly associated with increased atherosclerotic burden in human subjects as assessed by carotid intima-media thickness and increases plasma C-reactive protein *(150)*. In another report, a four-marker single-nucleotide polymorphism (SNP) haplotype in the locus spanning the gene encoding FLAP was associated with a twofold greater risk of myocardial infarction and stroke in Iceland. Another haplotype in the same locus was associated with myocardial infarction in individuals from the UK. The asso-ciation in this study between this at risk haplotype and increased production of leukotriene B_4 by activated neutrophils from male subjects was of critical functional importance *(151)*.

8.2. The 12-, 12/15- and 15LO: Role in Lipid Modification

The 12-, 12/15- or 15LO products can be released in the vicinity of the arterial lining by platelets, monocytes, endothelial cells and VSMC, particularly in response to platelet aggregation, angiotensin II, elevated glucose, inflammation or mechanical arterial wall stress. An example to the latter is the finding that the synthesis of both 12- and 15HETE is dramatically increased in experimentally stenosed canine coronary arteries (152). The release of 5- and 12HETE is also augmented in myocardium subjected to ischemia (153). A variety of cellular targets in the arterial wall may be affected by these eicosanoids, and their formation is also not inconsequential for circulating or subendothelial LDL particles. 13HPODE and 15HPETE dramatically enhance the nonenzymatic oxidation of both 1-palmitoyl-2-arachidonoyl-sn-glycero-3-phosphocholine (PAPC) and cholesteryl linoleate in LDL particles. The oxidation products of PAPC, in turn, markedly increase monocyte adhesion to the endothelium. The pro-oxidant effect of 13HPODE and 15HPETE is substantially augmented once their concentration in LDL has reached a critical mass. Under these conditions, 13HPODE and 15HPETE are approximately two orders of magnitude more potent (on a molar basis) than hydrogen peroxide in causing the formation of biologically active oxidized phospholipids from PAPC. Because the presence of 13HPODE and 15HPETE in LDL greatly enhances LDL's susceptibility to further oxidation, they are referred to as "seeding molecules." HDL from normal individuals, but not from patients with coronary artery disease, inhibits LDL oxidation by artery wall cells and attenuates the proadhesive effect of the oxidized PAPC. One mechanism by which this protective effect of HDL is exerted is by removal of seeding molecules, such as the LO products 13HPODE and 15HPETE by Apo-A1 from LDL particles (26,154). In addition to role of 13HPODE in LDL modification, this 15LO product also impacts VSMC, in which it induces MCP-1 and VCAM expression via an NF-κB dependent mechanism (60,61).

Further support for the key role of LO in atherogenesis is provided by observations that disruption of the 12/15LO gene results in a sizable decrease in atherosclerosis in apo-E deficient mice or LDL receptor deficient mice. (155,156). Consistent with this concept is also the finding that in LDL receptor-deficient mice, targeted overexpression of 15LO in the vascular endothelium resulted in acceleration of early atherosclerosis (157).

LO-dependent lipid oxidation and uptake in various cell types involved in atherosclerosis can be accelerated by a number of circulating agents or locally released cytokines in an endocrine, paracrine or autocrine manner. For example, in mouse peritoneal macrophages and human monocytes, angiotensin II induced an increase in 12LO expression and activity. In addition, pretreatment with angiotensin II increased in a dose-, and AT-1 receptor-dependent manner the ability of mouse derived monocytes to modify LDL, resulting in greater chemotactic activity for monocytes, typical of minimally modified LDL. (28,121). In cultured porcine VSMC, angiotensin II , PDGF and IL-1, IL-4 and IL-8 increase leukocyte type 12LO mRNA expression and activity (158). The critical role of oxygen supply for the LO-driven oxidative modification of LDL is demonstrated by the finding that transient experimental anemia, which is accompanied by a long-lasting overexpression of the reticulocyte-type 15LOX protects cholesterol-fed rabbits from lipid deposition in the aortic wall (159).

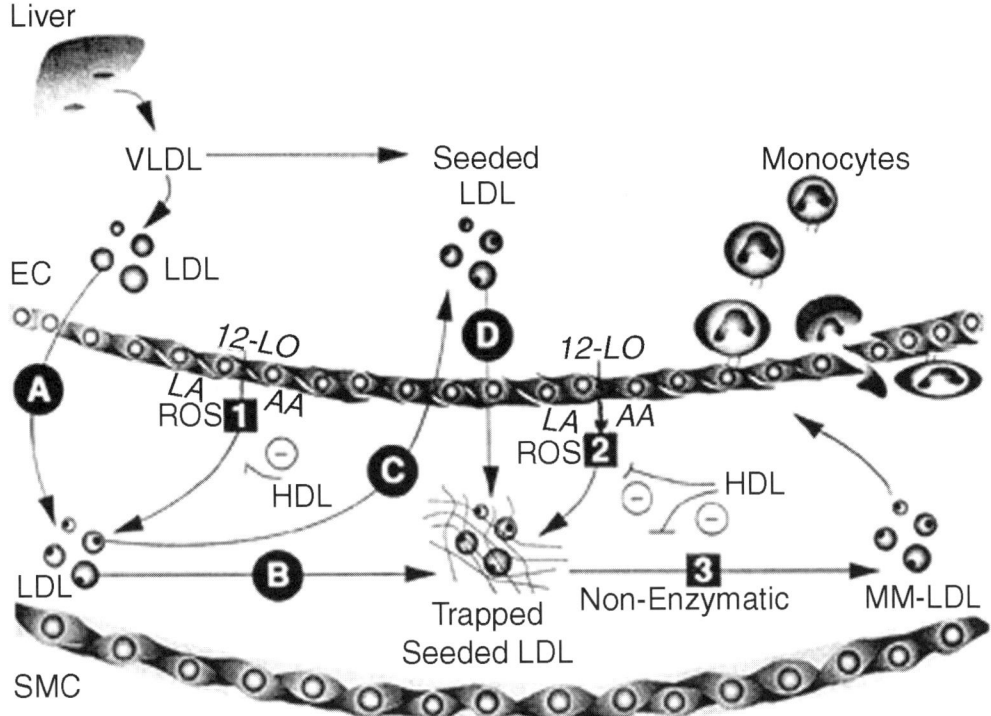

Fig. 4. A three-step model for LDL oxidation by artery wall cells. **Step 1**: LDL is seeded in the liver, microcirculation or in the subendothelial space by molecules generated secondary to LO action or from other sources. **Step 2**: LDL is trapped in the artery wall and receives further seeding molecules. Also, the artery wall cells generate and transfer ROS to the trapped seeded LDL. **Step 3**: When a critical level of seeding molecules relative to phospholipids is reached in the LDL, a nonenzymatic oxidation process generates oxidized PAPC products that induce NF-B activation, monocyte binding, MCP-1 production and M-CSF production, and that are present in mildly oxidized LDL (MM-LDL, minimally modified LDL) (from ref. *26*).

9. LO-DEPENDENT MECHANISMS MODULATE THE RENIN–ANGIOTENSIN ALDOSTERONE AXIS

12HETE and 15HETE inhibit the release of renin from rat renal cortical slices *(160)*. Further, angiotensin II-dependent inhibition of renin release, an important control mechanism that limits excessive stimulation of the renin angiotensin axis, is mediated via induction the 12LO pathway, as evidenced by increased production of 12HETE *(161,162)*. In agreement with the concept that LO products suppress renin secretion, 12HETE, 15HETE as well as 12HPETE and 15HPETE were also shown to inhibit prostacyclin-stimulated synthesis of renin in mesangial cell in vitro *(163)*. There is evidence that renal glomeruli express 12/15LO *(164)*, presumably the enzyme affecting renin secretion.

Several lines of evidence implicate the 12LO system as a mediator of angiotensin II-induced aldosterone secretion. First, angiotensin II increases the release of 12- and 15HETE in rat and human adrenal glomerulosa cells. Second, several structurally unrelated LO inhibitors block aldosterone, but not potassium- or ACTH-dependent aldosterone production. Finally, 12HETE can restore the effect of angiotensin II on aldosterone generation in LO-blocked glomerulosa cells *(110,111)*. In contrast, 5HETE inhibits angiotensin-II induced aldosterone synthesis *(112)*.

The administration of LO inhibitors in vivo resulted in a large and surprisingly concordant increases in both plasma renin (PRC) and aldosterone concentration *(165)*: not only PRC *(165,166)*, but also plasma aldosterone (Stern N, unpublished observation) increased. The increase in PRC was not because of the hypotensive effect of LO inhibitors, as it persisted even when the drop in blood pressure was inhibited by coinfusion with norepinephrine. In rats receiving chronic treatment with a LO inhibitor, PRC failed to decline in response to a high salt diet. In renal cortical slices from rats on high salt diet, 12HETE release was markedly increased, suggesting that 12HETE participates in inhibition of renin secretion during salt overload. These observations suggest a dominant physiological role for the 12LO system as a tonic inhibitor of renin release, particularly during dietary sodium overload.

10. SYMPATHETIC ACTIVITY AND THE LO SYSTEM

Several nonselective LO inhibitors can block the secretion of catecholamines from human neuroblastoma and pheochromocytoma cell lines *(167,168)* and cultured chromaffin cell *(169)* in vitro. Whether or not this reflects physiologically significant dependence of catecholamine release is unknown. The administration of LTD_4 increased systemic arterial pressure in SHR, in association with a three- to sixfold increase in plasma epinephrine and norepinephrine concentrations, which was followed by a prolonged hypotensive phase *(170)*.

11. LO IN HYPERTENSION

11.1. SHR

In mesenteric arteries in female SHR, generation of LO products appears to rise with age in parallel to the increasing blood pressure. There is also a sexual dimorphism in LO activity such that the production of LO-derived metabolites is much higher in female than in male SHR *(171)*. Further, in hypertensive rats, arachidonic acid may be preferentially converted into LO products that possess dominant vasopressor effects, as arachidonic acid elicited a constrictor effect in aortic rings, which was attenuated by the LO inhibitor baicalein *(172)*. More specific examination of LO products in SHR revealed that platelet 12HETE, plasma 12HETE as well as 12HETE release from aortic tissue was higher in SHR compared with WKY rats. Further, several lipoxygenase blockers including phenidone, CDC, ETI and panaxynol acutely reduce blood pressure in SHR *(166,173–176)*. The reduction in blood pressure induced by LO blockers was much more prominent in SHR than in WKY rats. Moreover, following the administration of 12LO blockers such as CDC and ETI, plasma 12HETE levels declined in parallel to the observed fall in blood pressure *(166,173)*. There is also evidence that early institution of LO blockers therapy markedly attenuates the evolution of high blood pressure in SHR *(173,177)*. Finally, the administration of the nonselective LO blocker phenidone in stroke-prone SHR with proteinuria and established hypertension arrested the progression of protein excretion and prevented the appearance of stroke *(178)*. Collectively, these studies clearly establish that 12LO are increased in platelets, serum, and vascular tissue from SHR.

Although angiotensin II-induced vasopressor response in vitro and in vivo appear to be mediated via 12LO-dependent mechanisms both in normotensive and hypertensive rats (SHR), a role for 5LO-derived eicosanoids in angiotensin II-dependent vaso-constriction is seen only in SHR. First, angiotensin II, acting through AT(1) receptor, induced a marked increase in cysteinyl leukotriene production in both intact and de-endothelialized aortic rings from SHR but not from WKY *(14)*. Second, the CysLT1 receptor antagonist MK571 significantly reduced the contractile effects of angiotensin II, but this effect, however, depended on the presence of the endothelium *(14,25)*. Third, in the mesenteric bed of SHR, the selective 5LO inhibitor AA-861 attenuated the vaso-constrictor responses to angiotensin II *(25)*. Fourth, cysteinyl leukotrienes, particularly LTD_4, induced a contractile response only in aortic rings from SHR, but not from WKY rats *(14)*, and LTC_4, LTD_4 and LTE_4 elicited a larger vasoconstrictor response in the mesenteric bed in SHR than in WKY rats *(25)*. Finally, LTD_4 induces a larger vasopressor response in SHR than in WKY rats *(22)*. Taken together these results suggest that leukotrienes are synthesized in vascular tissue, probably in VSMC, and that they play a role in blood pressure regulation in SHR. There is also an increased arterial response to cys-leukotrienes. Moreover, the increased sensitivity to Ang II in SHR results, in part, from angiotensin II-dependent formation of cysteinyl-leukotrienes, which is not seen in normotensive animals.

11.2. Effect of LO Inhibitors on BP

Overall, LO inhibitors lower blood pressure in either high renin (renovascular hypertensive rat) *(179)*; or normal renin models of hypertension (SHR) *(173–176)*, but not in low renin, hypervolemic models such as the DOCA salt hypertensive rat *(179)*. It is of interest that masoprocol, a nonselective LO inhibitor not only effectively lowered blood pressure in rats with fructose-induced hypertension, but also corrected the hyperinsulinemia, hypertriglyceridemia, and elevated circulating fatty acids seen in this model *(180)*. This beneficial metabolic influence of masoprocol may stem from non-LO related effects, such as direct anti-lipolytic action of this agent *(181)*, such that the correction of abnormal metabolism could lead to blood pressure normalization. It is likewise possible, however, that the "metabolic syndrome" in this model, leads to increased 12LO activity in a fashion similar to the stimulatory effect of overt diabetes and high glucose on 12LO. Under such putative conditions, masoprocol may normalize enhanced arterial 12LO in fructose-induced hypertension, thus resulting in blood pressure lowering.

There may be a role for prostacyclin production in the hypotensive effect of LO blockers. Potentially, LO blockade may shunt arachidonic acid metabolism to the cyclooxygenase pathway, thus resulting in increased prostacyclin production. In support of this mechanism is the observation that blood pressure of hypertensive rats pretreated with indomethacin was not affected by the same LO blockers shown to exert a hypo-tensive response when used alone (i.e., baicalein and cinnamyl-3,4-dihydroxy-α-cyano-cinnamate). Moreover, in hypertensive rats in which the LO blocker baicalein had decreased blood pressure, the administration of rabbit serum containing antibodies against 5,6-dihydro-PGI2, partially reversed the response to baicalein. Collectively, these data suggest that PGI2 contributes to the acute antihypertensive effect of baicalein in rats with angiotensin II-induced hypertension *(182)*.

11.3. Human Hypertension

Given the large database available on LO products in the vasculature, surprisingly little is known on the various LO systems in human hypertension. In one study, urinary 12HETE excretion as well as basal, but not thrombin-induced platelet production of 12HETE was much higher in individuals with essential hypertension than in normal subjects. This was associated with increased platelet-type 12LO protein expression in platelets from hypertensive subjects *(183)*. In contrast, although 12HETE is the major eicosanoid secreted by the human placenta, levels of released 12HETE are lower in placentas from hypertensive pregnancies *(184)*, presumably reflecting impaired placental structural integrity or subnormal blood supply in this setting.

REFERENCES

1. Kuhn, H. and Borchert, A. (2002) Regulation of enzymatic lipid peroxidation: the interplay of peroxidizing and peroxide reducing enzymes. *Free Radic. Biol. Med.* **33**, 154–172.
2. Funk, C. D., Chen, X. S., Johnson, E. N., and Zhao, L. (2002) Lipoxygenase genes and their targeted disruption. *Prostaglandins Other Lipid. Mediat.* **68–69**, 303–312.
3. Yamamoto, S., Suzyki, H., and Yesda, N. (1997) Arachidonate 12-lipoxygenase. *Prog. Lipid Res.* **36**, 23–41.
4. Radmark, O. P. (2000) The molecular biology and regulation of 5-lipoxygenase. *Am. J. Respir. Crit. Care Med.* **161**, S11–S15.
5. Martel-Pelletier, J., Lajeunesse, D., Reboul, P., and Pelletier, J. P. (2003) Therapeutic role of dual inhibitors of 5-LOX and COX, selective and non-selective non-steroidal anti-inflammatory drugs. *Ann. Rheum. Dis.* **62**, 501–509.
6. Zeng, Z. Z., Yellaturu, C. R., Neeli, I., and Rao, G. N. (2002) 5(S)-hydroxyeicosatetraenoic acid stimulates DNA synthesis in human microvascular endothelial cells via activation of Jak/STAT and phosphatidylinositol 3-kinase/Akt signaling, leading to induction of expression of basic fibroblast growth factor 2. *J. Biol. Chem.* **277**, 41,213–41,219.
7. O'Flaherty, J. T. and Rossi, A. G. (1993) 5-hydroxyicosatetraenoate stimulates neutrophils by a stereo-specific, G protein-linked mechanism. *J. Biol. Chem.* **268**, 14,708–14,714.
8. Rocha, P. N., Plumb, T. J., and Coffman, T. M. (2003) Eicosanoids: lipid mediators of inflammation in transplantation. *Semin. Immunopathol.* **25**, 215–227.
9. Spanbroek, R., Gräbner, R., Lötzer, K., et al. (2003) Expanding expression of the 5-lipoxygenase pathway within the arterial wall during human atherogenesis. *Proc. Natl Acad. Sci. USA* **100**, 1238–1243.
10. Fiorucci, S., Distrutti, E., Mencarelli, A., et al. (2003) Evidence that 5-lipoxygenase and acetylated cyclooxygenase 2-derived eicosanoids regulate leukocyte-endothelial adherence in response to aspirin. *Br. J. Pharmacol.* **139**, 1351–1359.
11. Lotzer, K., Spanbroek, R., Hildner, M., et al. (2003) Differential leukotriene receptor expression and calcium responses in endothelial cells and macrophages indicate 5-lipoxygenase-dependent circuits of inflammation and atherogenesis. *Arterioscler. Thromb. Vasc. Biol.* **23**, e32–e36.
12. Norel, X. and Brink, C. (2004) The quest for new cysteinyl-leukotriene and lipoxin receptors: recent clues. *Pharmacol. Ther.* **103**, 81–94.
13. Mazzetti, L., Franchi-Micheli, S., and Nistri, S. (2003) The ACh-induced contraction in rat aortas is mediated by the Cys Lt1 receptor via intracellular calcium mobilization in smooth muscle cells. *Br. J. Pharmacol.* **138**, 707–715.
14. Stanke-Labesque, F., Devillier, P., Veitl, S., Caron, F., Cracowski, J. L., and Bessard, G. (2001) Cysteinyl leukotrienes are involved in angiotensin II-induced contraction of aorta from spontaneously hypertensive rats. *Cardiovasc. Res.* **49**, 152–160.
15. Hardy, G., Stanke-Labesque, F., Peoc'h, M., et al. (2001) Cysteinyl leukotrienes modulate angiotensin II constrictor effects on aortas from streptozotocin-induced diabetic rats. *Arterioscler. Thromb. Vasc. Biol.* **21**, 1751–1758.

16. Stanke-Labesque, F., Hardy, G., Caron, F., Cracowski, J. L., and Bessard, G. (2003) Inhibition of leukotriene synthesis with MK-886 prevents a rise in blood pressure and reduces noradrenaline-evoked contraction in L-NAME-treated rats. *Br. J. Pharmacol.* **140,** 186–194.

17. Berkowitz, B. A., Zabko-Potapovich, B., Valocik, R., and Gleason, J. G. (1984) Effects of the leukotrienes on the vasculature and blood pressure of different species. *J. Pharmacol. Exp. Ther.* **229,** 105–112.

18. Labat, C., Oritz, J. L., Norel, X., et al. (1992) A second cysteinyl lekotriene receptor in human lung. *J. Pharmacol. Exp. Ther.* **263,** 800–805.

19. Allen, S. P., Chester, A. H., Dashwood, M. R., Tadjkarimi, S., Piper, P. J., and Yacoub, M. H. (1994) Preferential vasoconstriction to cysteinyl leukotrienes in the human saphenous vein compared with the internal mammary artery. Implication for graft performance. *Circulation* **90,** 515–524.

20. Allen, S., Dashwood, M., Morrison, K., and Yacoub, M. H. (1998) Differential lekotriene constrictor responses in human atherosclerptic coronary arteries. *Circulation* **97,** 2406–2413.

21. Lawson, D. L., Mehta, J. L., Mehta, P., and Nichols, W. W. (1989) Endothelium-dependent relaxation of rat aortic rings by leukotriene D4: importance of the magnitude of preload. *Eicosanoids* **2,** 175–181.

22. Zukovska-Grojec, Z., Bayorh, M. A., Kopin, I. J., and Feurstein, G. (1985) Overall and regional hemodynamic effects of leukotriene D4 in spontaneously hypertensive rats. *Hypertension* **7,** 507–513.

23. Fujioka, H., Ayajiki, K., Shinozaki, K., Toda, N., and Okamura, T. (2002) Mechanisms underlying endothelium-dependent, nitric oxide- and prostanoid-independent relaxation in monkey and dog coronary arteries. *Naunyn Schmiedebergs Arch. Pharmacol.* **366,** 488–495.

24. Stanke-Labesque, F., Hardy, G., Vergnaud, S., et al. (2002) Involvement of cysteinyl leukotrienes in angiotensin II-induced contraction in isolated aortas from transgenic (mRen-2)27 rats. *J. Hypertens.* **20,** 263–272.

25. Shastri, S., McNeill, J. R., Wilson, T. W., Poduri, R., Kaul, C., and Gopalakrishnan, V. (2001) Cysteinyl leukotrienes mediate enhanced vasoconstriction to angiotensin II but not endothelin-1 in SHR. *Am. J. Physiol. Heart Circ. Physiol.* **281,** H342–H349.

26. Navab, M., Hama, S. Y., Anantharamaiah, G. M., et al. (2000) Normal high density lipoprotein inhibits three steps in the formation of mildly oxidized low density lipoprotein: steps 2 and 3. *J. Lipid Res.* **41,** 1495–1508.

27. Limor, R., Weisinger, G., Gilad, S., et al. (2001) A novel form of platelet-type 12-lipoxygenase mRNA in human vascular smooth muscle cells. *Hypertension* **38,** 864–871.

28. Kim, J. A., Gu, J. L., Natarajan, R., Berliner, J. A., and Nadler, J. L. A. (1995) leukocyte type of 12-lipoxygenase is expressed in human vascular and mononuclear cells. Evidence for upregulation by angiotensin II. *Arterioscler. Thromb. Vasc. Biol.* **15,** 942–948.

29. Kuhn, H., Walther, M., and Kuban, R. J. (2002) Mammalian arachidonate 15-lipoxygenases structure, function and biological implications. *Prostaglandins Other lipid Mediat.* **68–69,** 263–290.

30. Gu, J. L., Natarajan, R., Ben-Ezra, J., et al. (1994) Evidence that a leukocyte type of 12-lipoxygenase is expressed and regulated by angiotensin II in human adrenal glomerulosa cells. *Endocrinology* **134,** 70–77.

31. Gonzalez, A. L., Roberts, R. L., Massion, P. P., Olson, S. J., Shyr, Y., and Shappell, S. B. (2004) 15-Lipoxygenase-2 expression in benign and neoplastic lung: an immunohistochemical study and correlation with tumor grade and proliferation. *Hum. Pathol.* **35,** 840–849.

32. Simon, T. C., Makheja, A. N., and Bailey, J. M. (1989) Formation of 15-hydroxyeicosatetraenoic acid (15-HETE) as the predominant eicosanoid in aortas from Watanabe Heritable Hyperlipidemic and cholesterol-fed rabbits. *Atherosclerosis* **75,** 31–38.

33. Yla-Herttuala, S., Rosenfeld, M. E., Parthasarathy, S., et al. (1991) Gene expression in macrophage-rich human atherosclerotic lesions. 15-lipoxygenase and acetyl low density lipoprotein receptor messenger RNA colocalize with oxidation specific lipid-protein adducts. *J. Clin. Investig.* **87,** 1146–1152.

34. Belkner, J., Wiesner, R., and Kuhn, H. (1992) Identification of oxidatively modified lipids in athero-sclerotic lesions of human aortas. *Agents Actions Suppl.* **37,** 78–84.

35. Kuhn, H., Heydeck, D., Hugou, I., and Gniwotta, C. (1997) In vivo action of 15-lipoxygenase in early stages of human atherogenesis. *J. Clin. Investig.* **99,** 888–893.

36. Thuresson, E. D., Lakkides, K. M., and Smith, W. L. (2002) PGG2, 11R-HPETE and 15R/S-HPETE are formed from different conformers of arachidonic acid in the prostaglandin endoperoxide H synthase-1 cyclooxygenase site. *Adv. Exp. Med. Biol.* **507,** 67–72.

37. Limor, R., Kaplan, M., Weisinger, G., Knoll, E., and Stern, N. (2004) Aldosterone increases 12 lipoxygenase expression and LDL oxidation in human vascular smooth muscle cell: a novel mechanism for aldosterone-induced vasculopathy. International Society of Hypertension, Sao Paolo, Brazil, February 2004 (Abstract).

38. Mais, D. E., Saussy, D. L. Jr., Magee, D. E., and Bowling, N. L. (1990) Interaction of 5-HETE, 12-HETE, 15-HETE and 5,12-diHETE at the human platelet thromboxane A2/prostaglandin H2 receptor. *Eicosanoids* **3,** 121–124.

39. Yu, K., Bayona, W., Kallen, C. B., et al. (1995) Differential activation of peroxisome proliferator-activated receptors by eicosanoids. *J. Biol. Chem.* **270,** 23,975–23,983.

40. Kozak, K. R., Gupta, R. A., and Moody, J. S. (2002) 15-Lipoxygenase metabolism of 2-arachidonyl-glycerol. Generation of a peroxisome proliferator-activated receptor alpha agonist. *J. Biol. Chem.* **277,** 23,278–23,286.

41. Devchand, P. R., Keller, H., Peters, J. M., Vazquez, M., Gonzalez, F. J., and Wahli, W. (1996) The PPARalpha-leukotriene B4 pathway to inflammation control. *Nature* **384,** 39–43.

42. Huang, J. T., Welch, J. S., Ricote, M., et al. (1999) Interleukin-4-dependent production of PPAR-gamma ligands in macrophages by 12/15-lipoxygenase *Nature* **400,** 378–382.

43. Shappell, S. B., Gupta, R. A., Manning, S., et al. (2001) 15S-Hydroxyeicosatetraenoic acid activates peroxisome proliferator-activated receptor gamma and inhibits proliferation in PC3 prostate carcinoma cells. *Cancer Res.* **15,** 61,497–61,503.

44. Linscheid, P., Keller, U., Blau, N., Schaer, D. J., and Muller, B. (2003) Diminished production of nitric oxide synthase cofactor tetrahydrobiopterin by rosiglitazone in adipocytes. *Biochem. Pharmacol.* **15,** 65,593–65,598.

45. Wigren, J., Surapureddi, S., Olsson, A. G., Glass, C. K., Hammarstrom, S., and Soderstrom, M. (2003) Differential recruitment of the coactivator proteins CREB-binding protein and steroid receptor coactivator-1 to peroxisome proliferator-activated receptor gamma/9-cis-retinoic acid receptor heterodimers by ligands present in oxidized low-density lipoprotein. *J. Endocrinol.* **177,** 207–214.

46. Li, Q., Cheon, Y. P., Kannan, A., Shanker, S., Bagchi, I. C., and Bagchi, M. K. (2004) A novel pathway involving progesterone receptor, 12/15-lipoxygenase-derived eicosanoids, and peroxisome proliferator-activated receptor gamma regulates implantation in mice. *J. Biol. Chem.* **279,** 11,570–11,581.

47. Zygmunt, P. M., Petersson, J., and Andersson, D. A. (1999) Vanilloid receptors on sensory nerves mediate the vasodilator action of anandamide. *Nature* **400,** 452–457.

48. Hwang, S. W., Cho, H., Kwak, J., et al. (2000) Direct activation of capsaicin receptors by products of lipoxygenases: endogenous capsaicin-like substances. *Proc. Natl Acad. Sci. USA* **97,** 6155–6160.

49. Shin, J., Cho, H., Hwang, S. W., et al. (2002) Bradykinin-12-lipoxygenase-VR1 signaling pathway for inflammatory hyperalgesia. *Proc. Natl Acad. Sci. USA* **99,** 10,150–10,155.

50. Saito, F., Hori, M. T., Berger, M., et al. (1992) 12-Lipoxygenase products modulate calcium signals in vascular smooth muscle cells. *Hypertension* **20,** 138–143.

51. Stern, N., Yanagawa, N., Saito, F., et al. (1993) Potential role of 12-hydroxyeicosatetraenoid acid in angiotensin II-induced calcium signal in rat glomerulosa cells. *Endocrinology* **133,** 843–847.

52. Kanda, H., Hori, M. T., Golub, M. S., and Tuck, M. L. (2001) Inhibitors of arachidonic acid metabolism have variable effects on calcium signaling pathways. *Am. J. Hypertens.* **14,** 248–253.

53. Stoll, L. L., Morland, M. R., and Spector, A. A. (1994) 13-HODE increases intracellular calcium in vascular smooth muscle cells. *Am. J. Physiol.* **266(4),** C990–C996.

54. Ohta, S., Nishihara, J., Oka, Y., Todo, H., Kumon, Y., and Sakaki, S. (1995) Possible mechanism to induce protein kinase C-dependent arterial smooth muscle contraction after subarachnoid haemorrhage. *Acta Neurochir. (Wien)* **137,** 217–225.

55. Parmentier, J. H., Muthalif, M. M., Saeed, A. E., and Malik, K. U. (2001) Phospholipase D activation by norepinephrine is mediated by 12(s)-, 15(s)-, and 20-hydroxyeicosatetraenoic acids generated by stimulation of cytosolic phospholipase a2. Tyrosine phosphorylation of phospholipase d2 in response to norepinephrine. *J. Biol. Chem.* **276,** 15,704–15,711.

56. Wen, Y., Nadler, J. L., Gonzales, N., Scott, S., Clauser, E., and Natarajan, R. (1996) Mechanisms of ANG II-induced mitogenic responses: role of 12-lipoxygenase and biphasic MAP kinase. *Am. J. Physiol.* **271(4),** C1212–C1220.

57. Wen, Y., Gu, J., Knaus, U. G., Thomas, L., Gonzales, N., and Nadler, J. L. (2000) Evidence that 12-lipoxygenase product 12-hydroxyeicosatetraenoic acid activates p21-activated kinase. *Biochem. J.* **349(2),** 481–487.

58. Kalyankrishna, S. and Malik, K. U. (2003) Norepinephrine-induced stimulation of p38 mitogen-activated protein kinase is mediated by arachidonic acid metabolites generated by activation of cytosolic phospholipase A(2) in vascular smooth muscle cells. *J. Pharmacol. Exp. Ther.* **304,** 761–772.

59. Reddy, M. A., Adler, S. G., Kim, Y. S., et al. (2002) Interaction of MAPK and 12-lipoxygenase pathways in growth and matrix protein expression in mesangial cells. *Am. J. Physiol. Renal Physiol.* **283,** F985–F994.

60. Dwarakanath, R. S., Sahar, S., Reddy, M. A., Castanotto, D., Rossi, J. J. and Natarajan R. (2004) Regulation of monocyte chemoattractant protein-1 by the oxidized lipid, 13-hydroperoxyoctadeca-dienoic acid, in vascular smooth muscle cells via nuclear factor-kappa B (NF-kappa B). *J. Mol. Cell Cardiol.* **36,** 585–950.

61. Natarajan, R., Reddy, M. A., Malik, K. U., Fatima, S., and Khan, B. V. (2001) Signaling mechanisms of nuclear factor-kappab-mediated activation of inflammatory genes by 13-hydroperoxyoctadeca-dienoic acid in cultured vascular smooth muscle cells. *Arterioscler. Thromb. Vasc. Biol.* **21,** 1408–1413.

62. Derian, C. K. and Lewis, D. F. (1992) Activation of 15-lipoxygenase by low density lipoprotein in vascular endothelial cells. Relationship to the oxidative modification of low density lipoprotein. *Prostaglandins Leukot. Essent. Fatty Acids* **45,** 49–57.

63. Banning, A., Schnurr, K., Bol, G. F., et al. (2004) Inhibition of Basal and interleukin-1-induced vcam-1 expression by phospholipid hydroperoxide glutathione peroxidase and 15-lipoxygenase in rabbit aortic smooth muscle cells. *Free Radic. Biol. Med.* **36,** 135–144.

64. Tang, D. G., Chen, Y. Q., Diglio, C. A., and Honn, K. V. (1993) Protein kinase C-dependent effects of 12(S)-HETE on endothelial cell vitronectin receptor and fibronectin receptor. *J. Cell. Biol.* **121,** 689–704.

65. Hatley, M. E., Srinivasan, S., Reilly, K. B., Bolick, D. T., and Hedrick, C. C. (2003) Increased production of 12/15 lipoxygenase eicosanoids accelerates monocyte/endothelial interactions in diabetic db/db mice. *J. Biol. Chem.* **278,** 25,369–25,375.

66. Sultana, C., Shen, Y., Rattan, V., and Kalra, V. K. (1996) Lipoxygenase metabolites induced expression of adhesion molecules and transendothelial migration of monocyte-like HL-60 cells is linked to protein kinase C activation. *J. Cell. Physiol.* **167,** 477–487.

67. Huang, Z. H., Bates, E. J., Ferrante, J. V., et al. (1997) Inhibition of stimulus-induced endothelial cell intercellular adhesion molecule-1, E-selectin, and vascular cellular adhesion molecule-1 expression by arachidonic acid and its hydroxy and hydroperoxy derivatives. *Circ. Res.* **80,** 149–158.

68. Reilly, K. B., Srinivasan, S., Hatley, M. E., et al. (2004) 12/15-Lipoxygenase activity mediates inflammatory monocyte/endothelial interactions and atherosclerosis in vivo. *J. Biol. Chem.* **279,** 9440–9450.

69. Cai, Q., Lanting, L., and Natarajan, R. (2004) Growth factors induce monocyte binding to vascular smooth muscle cells: implications for monocyte retention in atherosclerosis. *Am. J. Physiol. Cell Physiol.* **287,** C707–C714.

70. Ait-Said, F., Elalamy, I., Werts, C., et al. (2003) Inhibition by eicosapentaenoic acid of IL-1beta-induced PGHS-2 expression in human microvascular endothelial cells: involvement of lipoxygenase-derived metabolites and p38 MAPK pathway. *Biochim. Biophys. Acta* **1631,** 77–84.

71. Coffey, M. J., Jarvis, G. E., Gibbins, J. M. (2004) Platelet 12-lipoxygenase activation via glycoprotein VI: involvement of multiple signaling pathways in agonist control of H(P)ETE synthesis. *Circ. Res.* **94,** 1598–1605.

72. Katoh, A., Ikeda, H., Murohara, T., Haramaki, N., Ito, H., and Imaizumi, T. (1998) Platelet-derived 12-hydroxyeicosatetraenoic acid plays an important role in mediating canine coronary thrombosis by regulating platelet glycoprotein IIb/IIIa activation. *Circulation* **98,** 2891–2898.

73. Nishio, E. and Watanabe, Y. (1997) Role of the lipoxygenase pathway in phenylephrine-induced vascular smooth muscle cell proliferation and migration. *Eur. J. Pharmacol.* **336,** 267–273.

74. Huang, H. C., Wang, H. R., and Hsieh, L. M. (1994) Antiproliferative effect of baicalein, a flavonoid from a Chinese herb, on vascular smooth muscle cell. *Eur. J. Pharmacol.* **251,** 91–93.

75. Natarajan, R., Pei, H., Gu, J. L., Sarma, J. M., and Nadler, J. (1999) Evidence for 12-lipoxygenase induction in the vessel wall following balloon injury. *Cardiovasc Res.* **41,** 489–499.

76. Fujita, H., Saito, F., Sawada, T., Kushiro, T., Yagi, H., and Kanmatsuse, K. (1999) Lipoxygenase inhibition decreases neointimal formation following vascular injury. *Atherosclerosis* **147,** 69–75.

77. Gu, J. L., Pei, H., Thomas, L., et al. (2001) Ribozyme-mediated inhibition of rat leukocyte-type 12-lipoxygenase prevents intimal hyperplasia in balloon-injured rat carotid arteries. *Circulation* **103,** 1446–1414.

78. Reddy, M. A., Kim, Y. S., Lanting, L., and Natarajan, R. (2003) Reduced growth factor responses in vascular smooth muscle cells derived from 12/15-lipoxygenase-deficient mice. *Hypertension* **41,** 1294–1300.

79. Rao, G. N., Baas, A. S., Glasgow, W. C., Eling, T. E., and Runge, M. S. (1994) Alexander: activation of mitogen-activated protein kinases by arachidonic acid and its metabolites in vascular smooth muscle cells. *J. Biol. Chem.* **269,** 32,586–32,591.

80. Szekeres, C. K., Trikha, M., and Honn, K. V. (2002) 12(S)-HETE, pleiotropic functions, multiple signaling pathways. *Adv. Exp. Med. Biol.* **507,** 509–515.

81. Nishio, E. and Watanabe, Y. (1997) The regulation of mitogenesis and apoptosis in response to the persistent stimulation of alpha1-adrenoceptors: a possible role of 15-lipoxygenase. *Br. J. Pharmacol.* **122,** 1516–1522.

82. Weisinger, G., Hirsch, M., Knoll, E., Limor, R., and Stern, N. (2003) Pharmacological inhibition and anti-sense knockout of the platelet type 12 lipoxygenase induce apoptosis in human vascular smooth muscle cells. 18th Meeting of the American Society of Hypertension, May 20th, New York.

83. Wen, Y., Gu, J., Peng, X., Zhang, G., and Nadler, J. (2003) Overexpression of 12-lipoxygenase and cardiac fibroblast hypertrophy. *Trends Cardiovasc. Med.* **13,** 129–136.

84. Reddy, M. A., Thimmalapura, P. R., Lanting, L., Nadler, J. R., Fatima, S., and Natarajan, R. (2002) The oxidized lipid product, 12-(s) hydroxyeicosatetraenoic acid, induces hypertrophy and fibronectin transcription in vascular smooth muscle cells via p38MAPK and CREB activation. *J. Biol. Chem.* **277,** 9920–9928.

85. Thollon, C., Iliou, J. P., Cambarrat, C., Robin, F., and Vilaine, J. P. (1995) Nature of the cardiomyocyte injury induced by lipid hydroperoxides. *Cardiovasc. Res.* **30,** 648–655.

86. Soeda, S., Honda, O., Fujii, N., and Shimeno, H. (1997) Effect of 15-hydroperoxyeicosatetraenoic acid on the fibrinolytic factor release and the antithrombin binding of vascular endothelial cells. *Biol. Pharm. Bull.* **20,** 15–19.

87. Sekharam, M., Cunnick, J. M., and Wu, J. (2000) Involvement of lipoxygenase in lysophosphatidic acid-stimulated hydrogen peroxide release in human HaCaT keratinocytes. *Biochem. J.* **346(3),** 751–758.

88. Navab, M., Berliner, J. A., Subbanagounder, G., et al. (2001) HDL and the inflammatory response induced by LDL-derived oxidized phospholipids. *Arterioscler. Thromb. Vasc. Biol.* **21,** 481–488.

89. Callahan, K. S. and Garcia, J. G. (1994) Oxidant exposure stimulates cultured coronary artery endothelial cells to release 15-HETE: differential effects on PGI2 and 15-HETE synthesis. *J. Lab. Clin. Med.* **124,** 569–578.

90. Luchtefeld, M., Drexler, H., and Schieffer, B. (2003) 5-Lipoxygenase is involved in the angiotensin II-induced NAD(P)H-oxidase activation. *Biochem. Biophys. Res. Commun.* **308,** 668–672.

91. Coffey, M. J., Natarajan, R., Chumley, P. H., et al. (2001) Catalytic consumption of nitric oxide by 12/15-lipoxygenase: inhibition of monocyte soluble guanylate cyclase activation. *Proc. Natl Acad. Sci. USA* **98,** 8006–8011.

92. Miller, A. W., Katakam, P. V., Lee, H. C., Tulbert, C. D., Busija, D. W., and Weintraub, N. L. (2003) Arachidonic acid-induced vasodilation of rat small mesenteric arteries is lipoxygenase-dependent. *J. Pharmacol. Exp. Ther.* **304,** 139–144.

93. Zink, M. H., Oltman, C. L., Lu, T., et al. (2001) 12-lipoxygenase in porcine coronary microcirculation: implications for coronary vasoregulation. *Am. J. Physiol. Heart Circ. Physiol.* **280,** H693–H704.

94. Hashimoto, T., Kihara, M., Yokoyama, K., et al. (2003) Lipoxygenase products regulate nitric oxide and inducible nitric oxide synthase production in interleukin-1beta stimulated vascular smooth muscle cells. *Hypertens. Res.* **26,** 177–184.

95. Ma, Y. H., Harder, D. R., Clark, J. E., and Roman, R. J. (1991) Effects of 12-HETE on isolated dog renal arcuate arteries. *Am. J. Physiol.* **261(2),** H451–H456.

96. Yiu, S. S., Zhao, X., Inscho, E. W., and Imig, J. D. (2003) 12-Hydroxyeicosatetraenoic acid participates in angiotensin II afferent arteriolar vasoconstriction by activating L-type calcium channels. *J. Lipid Res.* **44,** 2391–2399.

97. Nishiyama, M., Okamoto, H., Watanabe, T., et al. (1998) Endothelium is required for 12-hydroperoxyeicosatetraenoic acid-induced vasoconstriction. *Eur. J. Pharmacol.* **341,** 57–63.

98. Kamitani, T., Little, M. H., and Ellis, E. F. (1985) Effect of leukotrienes, 12-HETE, histamine, bradykinin, and 5-hydroxytryptamine on in vivo rabbit cerebral arteriolar diameter. *J. Cereb. Blood Flow Metab.* **5,** 554–559.

99. Matsuda, H., Miyatake, K., and Dahlen, S. E. (1995) Pharmacodynamics of 15(S)-hydroperoxy-eicosatetraenoic (15-HPETE) and 15(S)-hydroxyeicosatetraenoic acid (15-HETE) in isolated arteries from guinea pig, rabbit, rat and human. *J. Pharmacol. Exp. Ther.* **273,** 1182–1189.

100. Zhu, D., Medhora, M., Campbell, W. B., Spitzbarth, N., Baker, J. E., and Jacobs, E. R. (2003) Chronic hypoxia activates lung 15-lipoxygenase, which catalyzes production of 15-HETE and enhances constriction in neonatal rabbit pulmonary arteries. *Circ. Res.* **92,** 992–1000.

101. Burhop, K. E., Selig, W. M., and Malik, A. B. (1988) Hydroxyeicosatetraenoic acids (5-HETE, and 15-HETE) induce pulmonary vasoconstriction and edema. *Circ. Res.* **62,** 687–698.

102. Uski, T. K. and Hogestatt, E. D. (1992) Effects of various cyclooxygenase and lipoxygenase metabolites on guinea-pig cerebral arteries. *Gen. Pharmacol.* **23,** 109–113.

103. Tesfamariam, B., Brown, M. L., and Cohen, R. A. (1995) 15-Hydroxyeicosatetraenoic acid and diabetic endothelial dysfunction in rabbit aorta. *J. Cardiovasc. Pharmacol.* **25,** 748–755.

104. Pomposiello, S. I., Alva, M., Wilde, D. W., and Carretero, O. A. (1998) Linoleic acid induces relaxation and hyperpolarization of the pig coronary artery. *Hypertension* **31,** 615–620.

105. Pfister, S. L., Spitzbarth, N., Nithipatikom, K., Edgemond, W. S., Falck, J. R., and Campbell, W. B. (1998) Identification of the 11,14,15- and 11,12, 15-trihydroxyeicosatrienoic acids as endothelium-derived relaxing factors of rabbit aorta. *J. Biol. Chem.* **273,** 30,879–30,887.

106. Pfister, S. L., Spitzbarth, N., Zeldin, D. C., Lafite, P., Mansuy, D., and Campbell, W. B. (2003) Rabbit aorta converts 15-HPETE to trihydroxyeicosatrienoic acids: potential role of cytochrome P450. *Arch. Biochem. Biophys.* **420(1),** 142–152.

107. Tang, X., Spitzbarth, N., Kuhn, H., Chaitidis, P., and Campbell, W. B. (2003) Interleukin-13 upregulates vasodilatory 15-lipoxygenase eicosanoids in rabbit aorta. *Arterioscler. Thromb. Vasc. Biol.* **23,** 1768–1774.

108. Gauthier, K. M., Spitzbarth, N., Edwards, E. M., and Campbell, W. B. (2004) Apamin-sensitive K+ currents mediate arachidonic acid-induced relaxations of rabbit aorta. *Hypertension* **43,** 413–419.

109. Campbell, W. B., Spitzbarth, N., Gauthier, K. M., and Pfister, S. L. (2003) 11,12,15-Trihydro-xyeicosatrienoic acid mediates ACh-induced relaxations in rabbit aorta. *Am. J. Physiol. Heart Circ. Physiol.* **285,** H2648–H2656.

110. Nadler, J., Natarajan, R., and Stern, N. (1987) Specific action of the lipoxygenase pathway in mediating angiotensin II induced aldosterone synthesis in isolated adrenal glomerulosa cells. *J. Clin. Investig.* **80,** 1763–1769.

111. Natarajan, R., Stern, N., Hseuh, W., Do, Y., and Nadler, J. (1988) Role of the lipoxygenase pathway in angiotensin II-mediated aldosterone biosynthesis in human adrenal glomerulosa cells. *J. Clin. Endocrinol. Metab.* **67,** 581–591.

112. Stern, N., Natarajan, R., Tuck, M. L., and Nadler, J. (1989) Selective inhibitory effect of the 5-lipoxygenase pathway on AII-stimulated aldosterone secretion. *Endocrinology* **125,** 3090–3095.

113. Stern, N., Golub, M., Noazwa, K., et al. (1989) Selective inhibition of angiotensin II-mediated vasoconstriction by lipoxygenase blockade. *Am. J. Physiol.* **257,** H434–H443.

114. Kisch, E. S., Jaffe, A., Knoll, E., and Stern, N. (1997) Role of the lipoxygenase pathway in angiotensin II-Induced vasoconstriction in the human placenta. *Hypertension* **29,** 796–801.

115. Natarajan, R., Gu, J. L., Rossi, J., et al. (1993) Elevated glucose and angiotensin II increase 12-lipoxygenase activity and expression in porcine aortic smooth muscle cells. *Proc. Natl Acad. Sci. USA* **90,** 4947–4951.

116. Croft, K. D., McGiff, J. C., Sanchez-Mendoza, A., and Carroll, M. A. (2000) Angiotensin II releases 20-HETE from rat renal microvessels. *Am. J. Physiol. Renal. Physiol.* **279,** F544–F551.

117. Sun, C. W., Falck, J. R., Harder, D. R., and Roman, R. J. (1999) Role of tyrosine kinase and PKC in the vasoconstrictor response to 20-HETE in renal arterioles. *Hypertension* **33,** 414–418.

118. Zou, A. P., Fleming, J. T., Falck, J. R., et al. (1996) 20-HETE is an endogenous inhibitor of the large-conductance Ca^{2+}-activated K^+ channel in renal arterioles. *Am. J. Physiol. Regul. Integr. Comp. Physiol.* **270,** R228–R237.

119. Alonso-Galicia, M., Maier, K. G., Greene, A. S., Cowley, A. W. Jr., and Roman, R. J. (2002) Role of 20-hydroxyeicosatetraenoic acid in the renal and vasoconstrictor actions of angiotensin II. *Am. J. Physiol. Regul. Integr. Comp. Physiol.* **283,** R60–R68.

120. Chen, Y., Lasaitiene, D., Gabrielsson, B. G., et al. (2004) Neonatal losartan treatment suppresses renal expression of molecules involved in cell-cell and cell-matrix interactions. *J. Am. Soc. Nephrol.* **15,** 1232–1243.

121. Scheidegger, K. J., Butler, S., and Witztum, J. L. (1997) Angiotensin II increases macrophage-mediated modification of low density lipoprotein via a lipoxygenase-dependent pathway. *J. Biol. Chem.* **272,** 21,609–21,615.

122. Alpert, E., Gruzman, A., Totary, H., Kaiser, N., Reich, R., and Sasson, S. (2002) A natural protective mechanism against hyperglycaemia in vascular endothelial and smooth-muscle cells: role of glucose and 12-hydroxyeicosatetraenoic acid. *Biochem. J.* **362(2),** 413–422.

123. Kang, S. W., Adler, S. G., Nast, C. C., et al. (2001) 12-lipoxygenase is increased in glucose-stimulated mesangial cells and in experimental diabetic nephropathy. *Kidney Int.* **59,** 1354–1362.

124. Tesfamariam, B., Brown, M. L., and Cohen, R. A. (1995) 15-Hydroxyeicosatetraenoic acid and diabetic endothelial dysfunction in rabbit aorta. *J. Cardiovasc. Pharmacol.* **25,** 748–755.

125. Spanbroek, R., Hildner, M., Kohler, A., et al. (2001) IL-4 determines eicosanoid formation in dendritic cells by down-regulation of 5-lipoxygenase and up-regulation of 15-lipoxygenase 1 expression. *Proc. Natl Acad. Sci. USA* **98(9),** 5152–5157.

126. Huang, J. T., Welch, J. S., Ricote, M., et al. (1999) Interleukin-4-dependent production of PPAR-gamma ligands in macrophages by 12/15-lipoxygenase. *Nature (London)* **400,** 378–382.

127. Yang, X. Y., Wang, L. H., Mihalic, K., et al. (2002) Interleukin (IL)-4 indirectly suppresses IL-2 production by human T lymphocytes via peroxisome proliferator-activated receptor gamma activated by macrophage-derived 12/15-lipoxygenase ligands. *J. Biol. Chem.* **277,** 3973–3978.

128. Xu, B., Bhattacharjee, A., Roy, B., et al. (2003) Interleukin-13 induction of 15-lipoxygenase gene expression requires p38 mitogen-activated protein kinase-mediated serine 727 phosphorylation of Stat1 and Stat3. *Mol. Cell. Biol.* **23,** 3918–3928.

129. Tang, X., Spitzbarth, N., Kuhn, H., Chaitidis, P., and Campbell, W. B. (2003) Interleukin-13 upregulates vasodilatory 15-lipoxygenase eicosanoids in rabbit aorta. *Arterioscler. Thromb. Vasc. Biol.* **23,** 1768–1774.

130. Schnurr, K., Borchert, A., and Kuhn, H. (1999) Inverse regulation of lipid-peroxidizing and hydroperoxyl lipid-reducing enzymes by interleukins 4 and 13. *FASEB J.* **13,** 143–154.

131. Maccarone, M., Bari, M., Battista, N., and Finazzi-Agro, A. (2002) Estrogen stimulates arachidonoylethanolamide release from human endothelial cells and platelet activation. *Blood* **100,** 4040–4048.

132. McMahon, B. and Godson, C. (2004) Lipoxins: endogenous regulators of inflammation. *Am. J. Physiol. Renal. Physiol.* **286,** F189–F201.

133. Pappayianni, A., Serhan, C. N., and Brady, H. R. (1996) Lipoxin A4 and B4 inhibit leukotriene-stimulated interactions of human neutrophils and endothelial cells. *J. Immunol.* **156,** 2264–2272.

134. Brezinski, M. E., Gimbrone, M. A. Jr., Nicolaou, K. C., and Serhan, C. N. (1989) Lipoxins stimulate prostacyclin generation by human endothelial cells. *FEBS Lett.* **45,** 167–172.

135. Maderna, P., Godson, C., Hannify, G., Murphy, M., and Brady, H. R. (2000) Influence of lipoxin A4 and other lipoxygenase–derived eicosanoids on tissue factor expression. *Am. J. Physiol.* **279,** C945–C953.

136. Brezinski, D. A., Nesto, R. W., and Serhan, C. N. (1992) Angioplasty triggers intracoronary leukotrienes and lipoxin A4. Impact of aspirin therapy. *Circulation* **86,** 56–63.

137. Leonard, M. O., Hannan, K., Burne, M. J., et al. (2002) 15-Epi-16-(para-fluorophenoxy)-lipoxin A(4)-methyl ester, a synthetic analogue of 15-epi-lipoxin A(4), is protective in experimental ischemic acute renal failure. *J. Am. Soc. Nephrol.* **13,** 1657–1662.

138. McMahon, B., Mitchell, D., Shattock, R., Martin, F., Brady, H. R., and Godson, C. (2002) Lipoxin, leukotriene, and PDGF receptors cross-talk to regulate mesangial cell proliferation. *FASEB J.* **16,** 1817–1819.

139. Fierro, I. M., Kutok, J. L., and Serhan, C. N. (2002) Novel lipid mediator regulators of endothelial cell proliferation and migration: aspirin-triggered-15R-lipoxin A(4) and lipoxin A(4). *J. Pharmacol. Exp. Ther.* **300,** 385–392.

140. Fiorucci, S., Distrutti, E., Mencarelli, A., et al. (2003) Evidence that 5-lipoxygenase and acetylated cocloooxygenase 2-derived eicosanoids regulate leukocyte-endothelial adherence in response to aspirin. *Br. J. Pharmacol.* **139,** 1351–1359.

141. Serhan, C. N. and Oliw, E. (2001) Unorthodox routes to prostanoid formation: new twists in cyclooxygenase-initiated pathways. *J. Clin. Investig.* **107,** 1481–1489.

142. Bannenberg, G., Moussignac, R. L., Gronert, K., et al. (2004) Lipoxins and novel 15-epi-lipoxin analogs display potent anti-inflammatory actions after oral administration. *Br. J. Pharmacol.* **143(1),** 43–52.

143. Serhan, C. N., Clish, C. B., Brannon, J., Colgan, S. P., Chiang, N., and Gronert, K. (2000) Novel functional sets of lipid-derived mediators with antiinflammatory actions generated from omega-3 fatty acids via cyclooxygenase 2-nonsteroidal antiinflammatory drugs and transcellular processing. *J. Exp. Med.* **192,** 1197–1204.

144. Dahlen, S. E., Raud, J., Serhan, C. N., Bjork, J., and Samuelsson, B. (1987) Biological activities of lipoxin A include lung strip contraction and dilation of arterioles in vivo. *Acta Physiol. Scand.* **130,** 643–647.

145. Feuerstein, G. and Siren, A. L. (1988) Mesenteric vascular responses to i.v. administration of lipoxin A4 and lipoxin B4 in the conscious rat. *FEBS Lett.* **232,** 51–55.

146. Xavier, N. and Brink, C. (2004) The quest for cysteinyl-lekotriene and lipoxin receptors: recent clues. *Pharmacol. Ther.* **103,** 81–94.

147. Pfister, S. L., Spit Zbarth, N., Nithipatikom, K., Falck, J. R., and Campbell, W. B. (2003) Metabolism of 12-hydroperoxyeicosatetraenoic acid to vasodilatory trioxilin C3 by rabbit aorta. *Biochim. Biophys. Acta* **1622,** 6–13.

148. Mehrabian, M., Allayee, H., Wong, J., et al. (2002) Identification of 5-lipoxygenase as a major gene contributing to atherosclerosis susceptibility in mice. *Circ. Res.* **91,** 120–126.

149. Aiello, R. J., Bourassa, P. A., Lindsey, S., Weng, W., Freeman, A., and Showell, H. J. (2002) Leukotriene B4 receptor antagonism reduces monocytic foam cells in mice. *Arterioscler. Thromb. Vasc. Biol.* **22,** 443–449.

150. Dwyer, J. H., Allayee, H., Dwyer, K. M., et al. (2004) Arachidonate 5-lipoxygenase promoter genotype, dietary arachidonic acid, and atherosclerosis. *N. Engl. J. Med.* **350,** 29–37.

151. Helgadottir, A., Manolescu, A., Thorleifsson, G., et al. (2004) The gene encoding 5-lipoxygenase activating protein confers risk of myocardial infarction and stroke. *Nat. Genet.* **36,** 233–239.

152. Rosolowsky, M., Falck, J. R., Willerson, J. T., and Campbell, W. B. (1990) Synthesis of lipoxygenase and epoxygenase products of arachidonic acid by normal and stenosed canine coronary arteries. *Circ. Res.* **66,** 608–621.

153. Shibata, N., Akagami, H., Sanma, H., and Goshima, K. (1988) Augmentation of eicosanoids in ischemic heart muscle in dogs: its role in the deterioration of the ischemic lesion. *Jpn. Circ. J.* **52,** 673–683.

154. Navab, M., Ananthramaiah, G. M., Reddy, S. T., et al. (2004) The oxidation hypothesis of atherogenesis: the role of oxidized phospholipids and HDL. *J. Lipid Res.* **45,** 993–1007.

155. Cyrus, T., Witztum, J. L., Rader, D. J., et al. (1999) Disruption of the 12/15-lipoxygenase gene diminishes atherosclerosis in apo E-deficient mice. *J. Clin. Investig.* **103,** 1597–1604.

156. George, J., Afek, A., Shaish, A., et al. (2001) 12/15-Lipoxygenase gene disruption attenuates atherogenesis in LDL receptor-deficient mice. *Circulation* **104,** 1646–1650.

157. Harats, D., Shaish, A., George, J., et al. (2000) Overexpression of 15-lipoxygenase in vascular endothelium accelerates early atherosclerosis in LDL receptor-deficient mice. *Arterioscler. Thromb. Vasc. Biol.* **20,** 2100–2105.

158. Natarajan, R., Rosdahl, J., Gonzales, N., and Bai, W. (1997) Regulation of 12-lipoxygenase by cytokines in vascular smooth muscle cells. *Hypertension* **30,** 873–879.

159. Trebus, F., Heydeck, D., Schimke, I., Gerth, C., and Kuhn, H. (2002) Transient experimental anemia in cholesterol-fed rabbits induces systemic overexpression of the reticulocyte-type 15-lipoxygenase and protects from aortic lipid deposition. *Prostaglandins Leukot. Essent. Fatty Acids* **67,** 419–428.

160. Antonipillai, I., Nadler, J. L., Robin, E. C., and Horton, R. (1987) The inhibitory role of 12- and 15-lipoxygenase products on renin release. *Hypertension* **10,** 61–66.

161. Antonipillai, I., Nadler, J., and Horton, R. (1988) Angiotensin feedback inhibition on renin is expressed via the lipoxygenase pathway. *Endocrinology* **122,** 1277–1281.

162. Antonipillai, I., Horton, R., Natarajan, R., and Nadler, J. (1989) A 12-lipoxygenase product of arachidonate metabolism is involved in angiotensin action on renin release. *Endocrinology* **125,** 2028–2034.

163. Chansel, D., Bea, M. L., and Ardaillou, R. (1989) Modulation of renin synthesis by lipoxygenase products in cultured human mesangial cells. *Mol. Cell. Endocrinol.* **62,** 263–271.

164. Katoh, T., Lakkis, F. G., Makita, N., and Badr, K. F. (1994) Co-regulated expression of glomerular 12/15-lipoxygenase and interleukin-4 mRNAs in rat nephrotoxic nephritis. *Kidney Int.* **46(2),** 341–349.

165. Stern, N., Nozawa, K., Kisch, E., et al. (1996) Tonic inhibition of renin secretion by the 12 lipoxygenase pathway: augmentation by high salt intake. *Endocrinology* **137,** 1878–1884.

166. Sasaki, M., Hori, M. T., Hino, T., Golub, M. S., and Tuck, M. L. (1997) Elevated 12-lipoxygenase activity in the spontaneously hypertensive rat. *Am. J. Hypertens.* **10(4),** 371–378.

167. Vaughan, P. F., Murphy, M. G., and Ball, S. G. (1993) Effect of inhibitors of eicosanoid metabolism on release of [3H]noradrenaline from the human neuroblastoma, SH-SY5Y. *J. Neurochem.* **60,** 1365–1371.

168. Abu-Raya, S., Bloch-Shilderman, E., Lelkes, P. I., et al. (1999) Characterization of pardaxin-induced dopamine release from pheochromocytoma cells: role of calcium and eicosanoids. *J. Pharmacol. Exp. Ther.* **288,** 399–406.

169. Sasakawa, N., Yamamoto, S., and Kato, R. (1984) Effects of inhibitors of arachidonic acid metabolism on calcium uptake and catecholamine release in cultured adrenal chromaffin cells. *Biochem. Pharmacol.* **33,** 2733–2738.

170. Zukowska-Grojec, Z., Bayorh, M. A., Kopin, I. J., and Feuerstein, G. (1982) Leukotriene D4: cardiovascular and sympathetic effects in spontaneously hypertensive rats (SHR) and Wistar–Kyoto (WKY) rats. *J. Pharmacol. Exp. Ther.* **223,** 183–189.

171. Gecse, A., Sonkondi, S., Mezei, Z., and Telegdy, G. (1987) Arachidonate cascade in mesenteric blood vessels and platelets of spontaneously hypertensive rats. *Agents Actions Suppl.* **22,** 43–48.

172. Lin, L., Balazy, M., Pagano, P. J., and Nasjletti, A. (1994) Expression of prostaglandin H2-mediated mechanism of vascular contraction in hypertensive rats. Relation to lipoxygenase and prostacyclin synthase activities. *Circ. Res.* **74,** 197–205.

173. Stern, N., Kisch, E. S., and Knoll, E. (1996) Platelet lipoxygenase in spontaneously hypertensive rats. *Hypertension* **27,** 1149–1152.

174. Stern, N., Nozawa, K., Golub, M., Eggena, P., Knoll, E., and Tuck, M. L. (1993) The lipoxygenase inhibitor phenidone is a potent hypotensive agent in the spontaneously hypertensive rat. *Am. J. Hypertens.* **6,** 52–58.

175. Takai, S., Jin, D., Kirimura, K., et al. (1999) Effects of a lipoxygenase inhibitor, panaxynol, on vascular contraction induced by angiotensin II. *Jpn. J. Pharmacol.* **80,** 89–92.

176. Mezei, Z., Kis, B., Gecse, A., Telegdy, G., Abraham, G., and Sonkodi, S. (1997) Platelet eicosanoids and the effect of captopril in blood pressure regulation. *Eur. J. Pharmacol.* **340,** 67–73.

177. Chang, W. C. and Su, G. W. (1985) Increase in 12-lipoxygenase activity in platelets of spontaneously hypertensive rats. *Biochem. Biophys. Res. Commun.* **127(2),** 642–648.

178. Munsiff, A. V., Chander, P. N., Levine, S., and Stier, C. T. Jr. (1992) The lipoxygenase inhibitor phenidone protects against proteinuria and stroke in stroke-prone spontaneously hypertensive rats. *Am. J. Hypertens.* **5,** 56–63.

179. Nozawa, K., Tuck, M. L., Golub, M., Eggena, P., Nadler, J. L., and Stern, N. (1990) Inhibition of lipoxygenase pathway reduces blood pressure in renovascular hypertensive rats. *Am. J. Physiol.* **259(6),** H1774–H1780.

180. Gowri, M. S., Reaven, G. M., and Azhar, S. (1999) Masoprocol lowers blood pressure in rats with fructose-induced hypertension. *Am. J. Hypertens.* **12,** 744–746.

181. Gowri, M. S., Azhar, R. K., Kraemer, F. B., Reaven, G. M., and Azhar, S. (2000) Masoprocol decreases rat lipolytic activity by decreasing the phosphorylation of HSL. *Am. J. Physiol. Endocrinol. Metab.* **279,** E593–E600.

182. Takizawa, H., DelliPizzi, A. M., and Nasjletti, A. (1998) Prostaglandin I2 contributes to the vasodepressor effect of baicalein in hypertensive rats. *Hypertension* **31,** 866–871.

183. Gonzalez-Nunez, D., Claria, J., Rivera, F., and Poch, E. (2001) Increased levels of 12(S)-HETE in patients with essential hypertension. *Hypertension* **37,** 334–338.

184. Arbogast, E., Schafer, W., and Zahradnik, H. P. (1996) Alterations of intrauterine eicosanoid production in pregnancy-induced hypertension: decreased production of 12-hydroxyeicosatetraenoic acid in the placenta. *Prostaglandins* **51,** 125–137.

185. Kantarci, E. and Van Dyke, T.E. (2003) Lipoxins in chronic inflammation. *Crit. Rev. Oral Biol. Med.* **4,** 4–12.

INDEX